CONTRIBUTORS

James K. Adams, M.D.
Clinical Assistant, University of Illinois at Peoria, Peoria, Illinois. Senior Resident, Department of Internal Medicine, St. Francis Medical Center, Peoria, Illinois.
Electrical Injuries

Meenakshy K. Aiyer, M.D.
Clinical Assistant, University of Illinois College of Medicine at Peoria, Peoria, Illinois. Chief Resident, Department of Internal Medicine, St. Francis Medical Center, Peoria, Illinois.
Obstetrics and Gynecology in the ICU

Mohammed Saud Anwar, M.D.
Clinical Assistant, University of Illinois College of Medicine at Peoria, Peoria, Illinois. Senior Resident, Department of Internal Medicine, St. Francis Medical Center, Peoria, Illinois.
Hypertensive Urgencies and Emergencies

Robert A. Balk, M.D.
Associate Professor of Medicine, Rush Medical College, Chicago, Illinois. Director of Pulmonary Medicine, Director of Medical Intensive Care Unit, Rush-Presbyterian-St. Luke's Medical Center, Chicago, Illinois.
Sepsis Syndrome; Essentials of the Standard Management of Septic Shock

Beverly D. Bartley, M.D.
Clinical Assistant, University of Illinois College of Medicine at Peoria, Peoria, Illinois. Chief Resident, Department of Internal Medicine, St. Francis Medical Center, Peoria, Illinois.
Hypothermia

Roderick J. Boyes, M.D.
Assistant Professor of Medicine, Wayne State University School of Medicine, Detroit, Michigan. Attending Intensivist, Oakwood Hospital, Dearborn, Michigan.
Temporary Transvenous Cardiac Pacing; Pericardiocentesis; Chest Tube Thoracostomy

Richard W. Carlson, M.D., Ph.D., F.C.C.M.
Professor of Medicine, Mayo Medical School, Rochester, Minnesota. Chairman, Department of Medicine, Maricopa Medical Center, Phoenix, Arizona.
Priorities of Initial Assessment and Management; Anaphylaxis

James E. Cisek, M.D.
Clinical Assistant Professor of Emergency Medicine, Wayne State University School of Medicine, Detroit, Michigan. Residency Director, Department of Emergency Medicine, William Beaumont Hospital, Royal Oak, Michigan.
Cocaine Intoxication; Salicylate Toxicity; Lithium Toxicity; Cardiac Glycoside Toxicity

Vivian L. Clark, M.D., F.A.C.P., F.C.C.P., F.A.C.C.
Clinical Instructor, University of Michigan Medical School, Ann Arbor, Michigan. Senior Staff Physician, Division of Cardiovascular Medicine, Henry Ford Hospital, Detroit, Michigan.
Central Venous Catheterization; Arterial Blood Pressure Monitoring; Acute Myocardial Infarction; Cardiac Dysrhythmias; Aortic Dissection; Pericardial Tamponade

David S. Cooling, M.D.
Clinical Assistant Professor of Emergency Medicine, University Medical Center, SUNY at Stony Brook, Stony Brook, New York. Attending Physician, University Medical Center at Stony Brook, Stony Brook, NY.
Theophylline Intoxication

Dennis J. Crnkovich, M.D.
Assistant Professor of Medicine, University of Illinois College of Medicine at Peoria, Peoria, Illinois. Program Director, Department of Internal Medicine, St. Francis Medical Center, Peoria, Illinois.
Preoperative Care; Hypothermia; Heat Injury and Hyperthermic Syndromes; Electrical Injuries

Cristina E. Cuevas-Korensky, M.D.
Assistant Professor of Medicine, Section of Critical Care Medicine, Wayne State University School of Medicine, Detroit, Michigan. Assistant Director, Medical Intensive Care Unit, Detroit Receiving Hospital, Detroit, Michigan.
Alcoholic Ketoacidosis; Hypoglycemia

John P. Dervan, M.D.
Associate Professor of Medicine, SUNY at Stony Brook, Stony Brook, New York. Director of Interventional Cardiology, Director of Cardiac Catheterization Laboratory, University Medical Center at Stony Brook, Stony Brook, New York.
Left Ventricular Failure; Circulatory Shock; Cardiovascular Pharmacotherapy

Herold Duroseau, M.D.
Assistant Professor of Pediatrics, SUNY at Stony Brook, Stony Brook, New York. Attending Physician, Winthrop University Hospital, Mineola, New York.
Oncologic Emergencies; Complications of Therapy of Neoplastic Disease

Peter F. Ells, M.D.
Clinical Assistant Professor of Medicine, SUNY at Stony Brook, Stony Brook, New York. Acting Chief, Division of

POCKET COMPANION TO

PRINCIPLES & PRACTICE OF MEDICAL INTENSIVE CARE

James A. Kruse, M.D.
Wayne State University School of Medicine
Detroit Receiving Hospital
Detroit, Michigan

Margaret M. Parker, M.D.
University Medical Center
State University of New York
Stony Brook, New York

Richard W. Carlson, M.D.
Mayo Medical School
Maricopa Medical Center
Phoenix, Arizona

Michael A. Geheb, M.D.
University of Alabama at Birmingham
Birmingham, Alabama

W.B. SAUNDERS COMPANY
A Division of Harcourt Brace & Company
PHILADELPHIA LONDON TORONTO
MONTREAL SYDNEY TOKYO

W.B. SAUNDERS COMPANY
A Division of Harcourt Brace & Company

The Curtis Center
Independence Square West
Philadelphia, Pennsylvania 19106

Library of Congress Cataloging-in-Publication Data

Pocket companion to Principles and practice of medical intensive care / James A. Kruse . . . [et al.].
p. cm.
Includes bibliographical references.
ISBN 0-7216-5633-1.
1. Critical care medicine—Handbooks, manuals, etc. I. Kruse, James A. II. Principles and practice of medical intensive care.
[DNLM: 1. Critical Care—handbooks. WX 39 P7413 1996]
RC86.8.P64 1996
616'.028—dc20
DNLM/DLC 96-8193

POCKET COMPANION TO PRINCIPLES AND PRACTICE OF MEDICAL INTENSIVE CARE ISBN 0-7216-5633-1

Printed in the United States of America

9 8 7 6 5 4 3 2 1

Gastroenterology, University Medical Center at Stony Brook, Stony Brook, New York.
Spontaneous Bacterial Peritonitis; Hepatic Failure and Encephalopathy

Alan B. Ettinger, M.D.
Assistant Professor of Neurology, SUNY at Stony Brook, Stony Brook, New York. Director of Adult Epileptology, University Medical Center at Stony Brook, Stony Brook, New York.
Coma; Seizures and Status Epilepticus; Neurophysiological Monitoring and Intracranial Hypertension

Jean M. Ferber, M.D.
Assistant Professor of Surgery, SUNY at Stony Brook, Stony Brook, New York. Attending Physician, University Medical Center at Stony Brook, Stony Brook, New York.
The Acute Abdomen; Diarrhea in the ICU Patient

Hussein D. Foda, M.D.
Assistant Professor of Medicine, Division of Pulmonary/Critical Care Medicine, SUNY at Stony Brook, Stony Brook, New York. Director of Medical Intensive Care Unit, Veterans Administration Medical Center, Northport, New York.
Mechanical Ventilation and Weaning; Adult Respiratory Distress Syndrome

Michael J. Freeland, M.D.
Clinical Assistant Professor of Medicine, Brown University School of Medicine, Providence, Rhode Island. Staff Intensivist, Division of Critical Care Medicine, Memorial Hospital of Rhode Island, Pawtucket, Rhode Island.
Peritoneal Dialysis; Hyponatremia and Hypernatremia; Disturbances of Calcium, Magnesium, and Phosphorous; Acid–Base Disorders; Acute Renal Failure; The Renal Transplant Patient; Diabetes Insipidus

Lonnie W. Frei, M.D.
Clinical Associate Professor of Surgery, SUNY at Stony Brook, Stony Brook, New York. Director of Surgical Intensive Care Unit, University Medical Center at Stony Brook, Stony Brook, New York.
The Acute Abdomen; Acute Pancreatitis

Jack Fuhrer, M.D.
Associate Professor of Clinical Medicine, Division of Infectious Diseases, SUNY at Stony Brook, Stony Brook, New York. Clinical Director of AIDS Center, University Medical Center at Stony Brook, Stony Brook, New York.
Candida and Other Fungal Infections; Human Immunodeficiency Virus Infection and Acquired Immune Deficiency Syndrome

Michael A. Geheb, M.D.
Professor of Medicine, Division of Pulmonary/Critical Care Medicine, Director of Medical Center and Health Systems, University of Alabama at Birmingham, Birmingham, Alabama.
Diabetic Ketoacidosis and Hyperosmolar Syndrome

Oded Gerber, M.D.
Assistant Professor of Neurology, SUNY at Stony Brook, Stony Brook, New York. Attending Physician, University Medical Center at Stony Brook, Stony Brook, New York.
Cerebrovascular Accidents; Brain Injury After Cardiac Arrest: ICU Management and Outcome, Including Brain Death

Maritza L. Groth, M.D.
Assistant Professor of Medicine, SUNY at Stony Brook, Stony Brook, New York. Director, Medical Intensive Care Unit, University Medical Center at Stony Brook, Stony Brook, New York.
Acute Respiratory Failure

Richard D. Harvey, M.D.
Clinical Assistant, University of Illinois College of Medicine at Peoria, Peoria, Illinois. Chief Resident, Department of Internal Medicine, St. Francis Medical Center, Peoria, Illinois.
Preoperative Care

Marilyn T. Haupt, M.D., F.C.C.M.
Associate Professor of Medicine, Wayne State University School of Medicine, Detroit, Michigan. Chief of Section of Critical Care Medicine, Detroit Receiving Hospital, Detroit, Michigan.
Fluid Resuscitation; Anaphylaxis

Chantal D. Henderson, M.D.
Fellow, Department of Pediatric Cardiology, Rainbow Babies and Childrens Hospital/University Hospital of Cleveland, Cleveland, Ohio.
Priorities of Initial Assessment and Management

Adam N. Hurewitz, M.D.
Associate Professor of Medicine, Division of Pulmonary/ Critical Care Medicine, SUNY at Stony Brook, Stony Brook, New York. Attending Physician, University Medical Center at Stony Brook, Stony Brook, New York.
Oxygen Therapy; Acute Asthma and Status Asthmaticus; Pulmonary Embolism; Aspiration Pneumonitis and Pneumonia; Life-Threatening Hemoptysis; Acute Smoke Inhalation; Barotrauma, Decompression Sickness, and Air Embolism

Michael T. Imperato, M.D.
Assistant Professor of Emergency Medicine, SUNY at Stony Brook, Stony Brook, New York. Attending Physician, University Medical Center at Stony Brook, Stony Brook, New York.
Sedative, Hypnotic, and Opioid Drug Overdose

Prasoon Jain, M.D.
Chief Resident, Department of Internal Medicine, University Medical Center and SUNY at Stony Brook, Stony Brook, New York.
Aspiration Pneumonitis and Pneumonia; Acute Smoke Inhalation; Barotrauma, Decompression Sickness, and Air Embolism

Slobodan Jazarevic, M.D.
Instructor of Surgery, University Medical Center and SUNY at Stony Brook, Stony Brook, New York.
Acute Mesenteric Ischemia

Victor Jimenez, M.D., M.Sc.
Assistant Professor of Medicine, Division of Infectious Diseases, SUNY at Stony Brook, Stony Brook, New York. Chief, Section of Infectious Diseases, Northport Veterans Administration Medical Center, Northport, New York.
Gram-Negative Bacterial Infections

Mark A. Kaufman, M.D.
Assistant Professor of Neurology, SUNY at Stony Brook, Stony Brook, New York. Chief of Neurology Service, Northport Veterans Administration Medical Center, Northport, New York.
Neuromuscular Diseases; Alcohol Intoxication and Withdrawal; Heat Injury and Hyperthermic Syndromes

James A. Kruse, M.D., F.C.C.M.
Associate Professor of Medicine, Division of Pulmonary/ Critical Care Medicine, Wayne State University School of Medicine, Detroit, Michigan. Director of Medical Intensive Care Unit, Medical Director of Respiratory Care and Diagnostics, Detroit Receiving Hospital, Detroit, Michigan.
Chest Radiography in the ICU; Severity of Illness Scoring in the ICU; Endotracheal Intubation in the ICU; Central Venous Catheterization; Pumonary Artery Catheterization and Hemodynamic Monitoring; Arterial Blood Pressure Monitoring; Temporary Transvenous Cardiac Pacing; Pericardiocentesis; Chest Tube Thoracostomy; Aortic Dissection; Pericardial Tamponade; Hyponatremia and Hypernatremia; Hypokalemia and Hyperkalemia; Acid–Base Disorders; Lactic Acidosis; Drug Dosing in Renal Insufficiency; Alcoholic Ketoacidosis; Diabetic Ketoacidosis and Hyperosmolar Syndrome; Antidepressant Drug Overdose; Salicylate Toxicity; Acetaminophen Poisoning; Toxic Alcohol and Glycol Poisoning

Kara H. V. Kvilekval, M.D.
Assistant Professor of Surgery, SUNY at Stony Brook, Stony Brook, New York. Attending Physician, Division of Vascular Surgery, University Medical Center at Stony Brook, Stony Brook, New York.
Acute Mesenteric Ischemia

David B. Levy, Pharm. D.
Adjunct Assistant Professor of Pharmacy Practice, Wayne State University College of Pharmacy, Detroit, Michigan. Clinical Specialist, Department of Emergency Medicine, Detroit Receiving Hospital, Detroit, Michigan.
Cocaine Intoxication; Acetaminophen Poisoning

Robert T. Mansfield, M.D.
Assistant Professor of Pediatrics, SUNY at Stony Brook, Stony Brook, New York. Attending Physician, Pediatric Intensive Care Unit, University Medical Center at Stony Brook, Stony Brook, New York.
Cardiopulmonary Resuscitation; Noninvasive Monitoring of Oxygen and Carbon Dioxide

Paul E. Marik, M.B.B.Ch., F.C.P., F.R.C.P.
Associate Professor of Medicine, University of Massachu-

setts, Worcester, Massachusetts. Director of Medical Intensive Care Unit, St. Vincent Hospital, Worcester, Massachusetts.
Chest Radiography in the ICU; Endotracheal Intubation in the ICU; Pulmonary Artery Catheterization and Hemodynamic Monitoring; Brochoscopy in the ICU

Peter R. Mariuz, M.D.
Assistant Professor of Clinical Medicine, Division of Infectious Diseases, SUNY at Stony Brook, Stony Brook, New York. Attending Physician, University Medical Center at Stony Brook, Stony Brook, New York.
Bacterial Meningitis; Urosepsis

Toshio Nagamoto, M.D.
Clinical Assistant, University of Illinois College of Medicine at Peoria, Peoria, Illinois. Senior Surgery Resident, Department of Surgery, St. Francis Medical Center, Peoria, Illinois.
Trauma

Dane J. Nichols, M.D.
Assistant Clinical Professor of Medicine, University of Illinois College of Medicine at Peoria, Peoria, Illinois. Director of Medical Intensive Care Unit, St. Francis Medical Center, Peoria, Illinois.
Priorities of Initial Assessment and Management; Hypertensive Urgencies and Emergencies; Enteral Alimentation and Nutritional Assessment; Parenteral Alimentation; Trauma; Obstetrics and Gynecology in the ICU

Margaret M. Parker, M.D., F.C.C.M.
Associate Professor of Pediatrics, SUNY at Stony Brook, Stony Brook, New York. Director of Pediatric Intensive Care Unit, University Medical Center at Stony Brook, Stony Brook, New York.
Viral Infections

Robert I. Parker, M.D.
Associate Professor of Pediatrics, SUNY at Stony Brook, Stony Brook, New York. Director of Pediatric Hematology/Oncology, University Medical Center at Stony Brook, Stony Brook, New York.
Bone Marrow Failure; Hemolysis; Coagulation Disorders; Microangiopathic Hemolytic Anemia; Blood Product Use

Brian E. Pinard, M.D.
Associate Professor of Surgery, Co-director of Surgical Residency Training Program, SUNY at Stony Brook, Stony Brook, New York. Acting Chief of Surgery, Winthrop-University Hospital, Mineola, New York.
Upper Gastrointestinal Tract Hemorrhage; Lower Gastrointestinal Tract Hemorrhage

Michael J. Ruffing, Pharm. D.
Adjunct Assistant Professor of Pharmacy Practice, Wayne State University School of Pharmacy, Detroit, Michigan. Adjunct Assistant Professor of Pharmacy, University of Michigan School of Pharmacy, Ann Arbor, Michigan. Clini-

cal Specialist, Department of Pharmacy Services, Detroit Receiving Hospital, Detroit, Michigan.
Drug Dosing in Renal Insufficiency; Antidepressant Drug Overdose

Jennifer A. Schranz, M.D., F.A.C.P., F.R.C.P.(C)
Instructor of Clinical Medicine, Division of Infectious Diseases, SUNY at Stony Brook, Stony Brook, New York. Medical Director of East End HIV/AIDS Center, University Medical Center at Stony Brook, Stony Brook, New York.
Gastrointestinal and Intra-abdominal Infections; Infections in the Immunocompromised Host

Angela Schupp, M.D.
Clinical Assistant, University of Illinois College of Medicine at Peoria, Peoria, Illinois. Senior Resident, Departments of Internal Medicine and Pediatrics, St. Francis Medical Center, Peoria, Illinois.
Heat Injury and Hyperthermic Syndromes

Magdy S. Shady, M.D.
Assistant Professor of Neurological Surgery, SUNY at Stony Brook, Stony Brook, New York. Attending Physician, University Medical Center at Stony Brook, Stony Brook, New York.
Neurophysiological Monitoring and Intracranial Hypertension

Stephen T. Smith, M.D., F.C.C.P., F.A.C.C.
Associate Director, Coronary Intensive Care Unit, Division of Cardiovascular Medicine, Henry Ford Hospital, Detroit, Michigan.
Unstable Angina Pectoris; Acute Myocardial Infarction

Roy T. Steigbigel, M.D.
Professor of Medicine and Pathology, Division of Infectious Diseases, SUNY at Stony Brook, Stony Brook, New York. Director of Comprehensive AIDS Center, Chief of Clinical Microbiology Laboratory, University Medical Center at Stony Brook, Stony Brook, New York.
Tuberculosis and Other Mycobacterial Infections; Endocarditis

David Tompkins, M.D.
Assistant Professor of Medicine, Division of Infectious Diseases, SUNY at Stony Brook, Stony Brook, New York. Attending Physician, Veterans Administration Medical Center, Northport, New York.
Gram-Positive Bacterial Sepsis; Pneumonia; Sinusitis and Other Serious Upper Respiratory Tract Infections

Margaret M. Wojnar, M.D.
Assistant Professor of Medicine and Surgery, SUNY at Stony Brook, Stony Brook, New York. Attending Physician, Surgical Intensive Care Unit, University Medical Center at Stony Brook, Stony Brook, New York.
Diarrhea in the ICU Patient

PREFACE

Critical care medicine is the final common path of general internal medicine for the acutely ill patient with organ system failure. It crosses and complements a variety of medical specialties that traditionally have been involved in part with treating patients in the ICU. As such, it represents a form of primary care, but it is restricted to those with the highest degrees of illness severity. The extent of medical knowledge required of the clinician, as well as the urgent nature of practice in the ICU, often make it necessary for reference information to be close at hand during the delivery of care in this setting.

Pocket sized so that it is easily accessible, this book is a concise and practical handbook of critical care medicine. It is designed to be useful as a bedside resource for residents, fellows, and practicing physicians, including nonintensivists caring for critically ill patients in medical ICUs. From initial assessment and resuscitation of the newly admitted patient, to differential diagnosis, to common invasive procedures and definitive therapy, the text covers the most important points of a wide variety of disorders seen in critically ill patients. In conjunction with its parent text, *Principles and Practice of Medical Intensive Care,* this book will also be useful in reviewing for examinations.

The book is organized into sections, with an emphasis on an organ systems approach. Chapters are succinctly written, often including bulleted lists and tables and figures so that the reader can find needed information quickly. For space considerations, detailed descriptions on the mechanisms of disease have been omitted here, but are available from the main textbook. Each chapter is cross-referenced to pertinent sections in the parent book, indicated directly beneath the chapter titles, thus providing easy availability to more in-depth clinical information and details of pathophysiology. While it follows a similar format, the *Pocket Companion* is not simply an extraction from the main text. In addition to being rewritten, streamlined, and focused on practical information, it has expanded sections on hematologic disorders, poisoning and drug overdose, and other topics that complement the larger text. For a full review, however, it is recommended that both books be consulted. While the main text includes an extensive bibliography, each chapter of this companion book has a short list of selected citations from the recent medical literature, as supplemental reading sources. Appended to most of these citations is a brief annotation describing an important feature of the reference.

We hope this *Pocket Companion* is a useful addition to the library of trainees and practitioners caring for acutely ill patients. Moreover, we hope it serves its purpose as a ready reference at the bedside in the ICU.

We would like to thank all of the contributors, with special thanks to Drs. Vivian Clark, Lonnie Frei, Adam Hurewitz, Robert Parker, and Roy Steibigel for their editorial assistance, and to Ms. Anna Bessette for her secretarial assistance.

JAK
MMP
RWC
MAG

CONTENTS

Resuscitation and Monitoring

CHAPTER 1

Priorities of Initial Assessment and Management

(See Chapters 10–12 and 138)

Richard W. Carlson,
Dane J. Nichols, and
Chantal D. Henderson

The first encounter with a critically ill patient can often determine the patient's survival or death. The clinician must prioritize the initial resuscitative steps to maintain life as the diagnostic evaluation is initiated and problems are identified. A step-by-step, logical approach is more likely to be successful than random, unfocused activity.

Goals for the initial evaluation include: (1) resuscitation, (2) stabilization, (3) identification of immediately life-threatening problems, (4) construction of the initial database and problem identification, and (5) use of a team effort. The immediate and ongoing priorities are assuring an **a**irway, adequate **b**reathing, and **c**ardiac function (ABCs); ensuring **v**entilation; securing **i**ntravenous access for fluid and drug infusion; and ensuring adequate **p**erfusion (VIP). These priorities are basic considerations for the management of patients with circulatory shock. These principles are important throughout the care of any unstable patient. The patient's primary physician should be involved as soon as is practical in the resuscitation and early decision making. The patient's advance directives should be respected.

After cardiopulmonary parameters have been stabilized, a more thorough history is taken and physical examination is performed. Additional laboratory and diagnostic information is obtained to complete the initial database. The sequence of maneuvers must be adjusted according to the needs of the specific patient.

This chapter reviews the principles of initial evaluation and care of critically ill patients, with special attention given to the care of the unstable medical patient. For initial management of the trauma patient, for cardiopulmonary resuscitation (CPR), and for fluid resuscitation, see the chapters on these topics in this book and also Chapters 11, 12, and 138 in the main text.

Sequential Steps of Management

The classic approach of obtaining a thorough medical history, performing a complete physical examination, and carrying out sequential diagnostic tests, followed by initiation of therapy, is not appropriate for resuscitation of the critically ill patient. Life-saving maneuvers always take precedence over other activities (therapy before diagnosis). Many life-support techniques, such as CPR, are the same or similar, regardless of the underlying clinical problem. However, as basic resuscitation efforts are carried out, the clinician must begin to introduce procedures that will not only facilitate ongoing resuscitation, but also provide diagnostic information and then must tailor the therapy to the patient's problems. Accordingly, many procedures share therapeutic and diagnostic components, and will be accomplished simultaneously.

One example of shared therapy with diagnosis is rapid fluid loading in the hypotensive patient. Fluid administration is a primary treatment of hypotension. In addition, the cardiopulmonary response to the fluid challenge provides important diagnostic information about intravascular volume and cardiac function. A variety of physical findings and hemodynamic indices may be monitored as the fluid is given, including changes in arterial pressure, neck vein distension, cardiac and pulmonary auscultatory findings, and direct measurement of cardiac filling pressures and cardiac output.

Another example of simultaneous and complementary diagnostic and therapeutic maneuvers is the administration of narcotic and benzodiazepine antagonists together with glucose and thiamine to the comatose patient. The glucose and antagonist drugs may reverse the coma as well as provide clues about its cause.

For more stable patients, the traditional approach of diagnosis followed by therapy may be used. However, for critically ill, unstable patients, life-saving facilities and personnel must be continuously and immediately available.

Cardiopulmonary Stabilization

Algorithms for the stabilization of cardiopulmonary parameters are shown in Figures 1–1 and 1–2. The resuscitation team should quickly cycle through the steps involving ventilation and gas exchange and then give their attention to cardiovascular parameters. For cardiopulmonary arrest, standard protocols for resuscitation are employed (see Chapter 2 in this book and Chapter 11 in the main text).

Ventilation and Oxygenation

An adequate airway must be assured. Blood, fluids, secretions, or malposition of the neck may compromise the air-

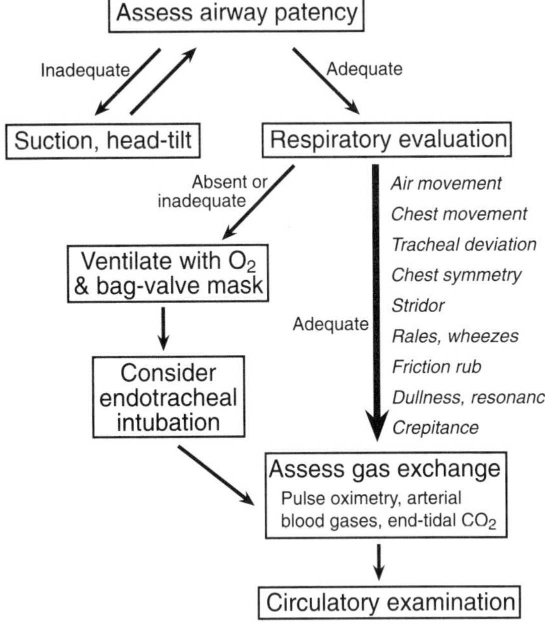

Figure 1–1. Algorithm for assessment and management of airway, oxygenation, and ventilation.

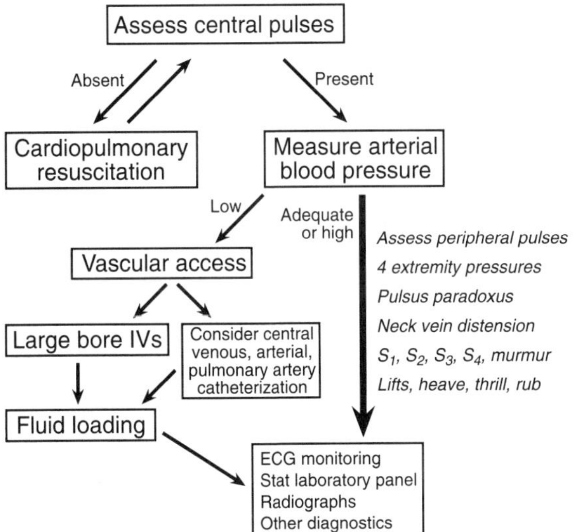

Figure 1–2. Algorithm for cardiovascular assessment and management.

way. If head or neck injury is suspected, the neck should be stabilized. If suctioning and positioning (using the head-tilt maneuver) do not ensure airway patency, endotracheal intubation should be an early consideration. Adequacy of respiratory efforts and gas exchange should be gauged. If these efforts are absent or feeble, or if gas exchange is poor, assisted ventilation with a bag-valve device is employed.

The resuscitation team should rapidly examine the nose, mouth, neck, and chest. Crucial physical findings, such as tracheal deviation, stridor, wheezes, or rales, and the quality and intensity of breath sounds of the hemithoraces are assessed. The examiner checks for the presence of crepitance, dullness, hyperresonance, or chest asymmetry. The color of the skin and mucosa and the presence of cyanosis may be helpful signs, but bedside prediction of oxygenation based on physical examination is unreliable. Quantitative information on oxygenation and ventilation by bedside or laboratory monitoring should therefore be obtained as quickly as possible (see Chapters 17, 19, and 65 in the main text and Chapter 4 in this book).

Supplemental oxygen should be administered to all patients with cardiopulmonary arrest, smoke inhalation, near-drowning and aspiration syndromes, coronary ischemic syndromes, or hypoxemia of any cause. Measures to assess and improve ventilation should also be undertaken. These measures may include provision for mechanical ventilation when arterial CO_2 tension (Pa_{CO_2}) is substantially elevated, although moderate hypercarbia may be tolerated in certain circumstances.

Cardiovascular Examination

Early examination of the cardiovascular system is crucial (Figure 1–2). Central (carotid or femoral) arterial pulses are palpated, and blood pressure is measured. Variations in pulse volume or pressure, particularly during respiratory efforts, suggest hypovolemia, pericardial disease, or airway obstruction. Peripheral pulses, capillary refill, and skin temperature and color should be assessed in all extremities to detect regional disturbances of perfusion.

Automated devices may be used to obtain repetitive measurements of blood pressure. Hypotension, hypertension, or marked variations of pressure or pulses suggest the need for arterial catheterization. If supine blood pressure is adequate and other conditions permit, the patient may be placed in an upright position to permit examination of the back and assessment of postural changes in pulse and blood pressure.

Cardiac examination should include auscultation over the base and apex and identification of lifts, heaves, thrills, gallops, and murmurs. ECG monitoring should be instituted as soon as practicable, and a chest radiograph should be obtained as well.

Venous Access

An early priority is to secure venous access. IV access serves as a lifeline for the administration of resuscitative drugs and fluids. One or two large-bore peripheral venous catheters may be sufficient, except for patients with multiple injuries or massive bleeding. Initial blood sampling for laboratory tests can be performed as the IV catheters are inserted. One or more multilumen central venous catheters may be used in place of peripheral venous access. The use of central venous catheters is necessary in patients who are likely to require vasopressor infusion. Internal jugular, femoral, or subclavian approaches may be used; the choice is related to the setting and to operator skill. In addition, a pulmonary artery catheter may subsequently be inserted at these sites. During CPR, the femoral site may be more convenient because it does not impede access to the chest and neck for resuscitative maneuvers.

Neurologic Assessment

After the patient's cardiopulmonary status has been stabilized, the team should turn to completing the diagnostic evaluation. Although the priorities will depend on the clinical problem, the neurologic status is often the next system to address.

Alterations of consciousness may be caused by a primary neurologic process, inadequate cerebral perfusion, hypoxia, hypercapnia, toxins, or significant metabolic alterations. Mental status and level of orientation must be recorded on admission. In addition, a focused, but systematic neurologic examination should be performed, including assessments of cortical function, cranial nerves, sensation, reflexes, and cerebellar responses. The Glasgow Coma Scale provides a good basis for neurologic scoring (see the chapters on severity scoring in this book and in the main text). The Glasgow score, together with additional neurologic assessments, should be tabulated as soon as possible, and may be repeated at intervals, especially when neurologic function is fluctuating.

Abdominal Examination

The abdomen is examined, with special attention given to auscultatory findings and signs of distension, tenderness, or peritoneal irritation, together with maneuvers to detect fluid, masses, pulsations, and bleeding. Pelvic and rectal examinations are performed, and any stool present is tested for blood. Naso- or orogastric intubation may be

TABLE 1–1

EXAMPLES OF BLOOD TESTS INCLUDED IN A CRITICAL CARE STAT LABORATORY PANEL

Direct assays
Arterial blood gases: pH, $Pa{O_2}$, $Pa{CO_2}$, $Sa{O_2}$*
Hemoglobin and hematocrit
Serum electrolytes, including sodium, potassium, chloride, ionized calcium, plus serum urea nitrogen (UN) and creatinine
Blood lactate concentration
Serum osmolality (freezing-point method preferred)
Serum glucose concentration
Derived results†
A-a gradient: $P_{A}O_2 - PaO_2$
a/A PO_2 ratio: $PaO_2/P_{A}O_2$
HCO_3^- concentration: calculated using the Henderson-Hasselbalch equation
Anion gap: $Na^+ - (Cl^- + HCO_3^-)$
Osmole gap: Measured osmolality − (2 × Na^+ + UN/2.8 + glucose/18 + ethanol/4.6)

*Saturation should be measured with a cooximeter, together with carboxyhemoglobin and methemoglobin (see Chapter 19 in the main text).

†$P_{A}O_2 = FIO_2 \times$ (barometric pressure − 47) − 1.2 ($PaCO_2$).

considered to relieve distension or to obtain samples for occult blood or other studies. Nasogastric intubation also may be necessary for the vomiting patient. A urinary catheter may be inserted to obtain a sample of urine for testing and to measure urine output over time.

Stat Critical Care Laboratory Panel

A basic, critical care stat panel of laboratory studies can be obtained on a small volume of arterial blood. This study provides a broad array of information on respiratory, circulatory, and metabolic parameters (Table 1–1). Blood should also be obtained for type and crossmatch and for toxicologic and other specific assays, as indicated.

Collection of Historical and Demographic Data

Traditionally, the clinical interview is the first step in evaluating a new patient. However, conventional history-taking must often be deferred, abbreviated, or modified to ensure attention to life-saving maneuvers and to focus on key historical features. Important elements of the abbreviated medical history include:

- **Demographic information,** including age, sex, name, address, next of kin, person to notify, guardian, personal physician.
- **Advance directives,** such as living wills or durable power of attorney for health care.
- **Prehospital care report,** including initial treatment required during the prehospital phase of stabilization.
- **History,** including drug allergies, current medications, previous surgery, recent hospitalization.
- **Review of systems,** abbreviated by necessity.
- **Previous medical records,** obtained from the medical records department.

This information is obtained directly if the patient is capable of communicating coherently. The comatose or confused patient or the patient whose cardiopulmonary status is unstable cannot be questioned directly. In these instances, information must be obtained from those who accompanied the patient; through telephone conversations with physicians, family, or personnel at other institutions; from medical alert tags or written material accompanying the patient; or from medical records if the patient was previously hospitalized at the same institution. The team should reassure and comfort the patient during the evaluation and also ensure that the family or friends are informed about the patient's condition.

Subsequent Assessment and Management

Vital Signs and Records. Vital signs must be sequentially determined and recorded. A rectal probe or other device may be used to monitor core temperature. For patients who are hypo- or hyperthermic, priorities of management should include measures to raise or lower body temperature (see Chapters 141 and 142 in the main text and Chapters 98 and 99 in this book). Flow sheets and automated or electronic aids to assure ongoing documentation of vital signs and related data are recommended.

Additional Procedures and Consultations. Selected diagnostic information is obtained as indicated. This information may include cultures of blood, sputum, urine, or other fluids. Lumbar puncture is indicated for patients with a high suspicion of CNS infection. Fluid from pleural, peritoneal, joint, or other anatomic sites may be aspirated, and the samples submitted for microscopic examination, cultures, and other studies. Consultants are called to participate in the evaluation and management of specific problems. The use of imaging techniques should be considered. However, until the patient has been stabilized, it may be hazardous to move the patient to the radiology, nuclear medicine, or other imaging area, or to a catheterization suite. Decisions to proceed with imaging studies or other procedures must include a risk–benefit assessment that includes the likelihood of detecting a rapidly fatal, but correctable lesion versus the risks involved in moving the patient.

Team Effort. Resuscitation and ongoing critical care management are team efforts. The critical care practitioner must work collaboratively with others, including the patient's primary physicians, nurses, therapists, and technologists. Management should be a cooperative, coordinated activity in which the optimal titrated care is considered. Often, several individuals are simultaneously needed at the bedside for resuscitation. Tasks must be assigned by the physician and nursing leaders of the team.

The senior physician should act as team leader to coordinate and integrate the overall effort. During severe crises, such as CPR and initial trauma management, the team leader should optimally direct the resuscitative effort and assign tasks to others at the bedside rather than participate actively in the resuscitation maneuvers. Vascular, airway, or other procedures performed during crisis conditions are difficult, and may be associated with considerable complications. Ideally, the most skilled operator should make the first attempt as others assist and observe the patient. If one operator is unsuccessful, basic resuscitation maneuvers should be resumed as another individual prepares to attempt the procedures. The team leader should always determine whether a procedure is needed to maintain life or to obtain essential diagnostic information. If not, in many cases, the intervention can be deferred. Inexperienced physicians frequently become too involved in one aspect of care when it would be more appropriate to focus on the global aspects of resuscitation and stabilization.

When immediate concerns, such as ensuring an adequate airway and pulse, have been addressed, the senior physician and nurse should jointly reassess and coordinate the ongoing effort. In some cases, specific individuals may be assigned to perform duties away from the bedside, such as obtaining information from the patient's family or others or acting as a liaison with the laboratory, imaging unit, or consultants. The logistics of data gathering should be coordinated. After initial stabilization, a debriefing and data summation session should be conducted.

The first examination and initial therapeutic maneuvers set the stage for the subsequent course and outcome of the critically ill patient. An orderly, team approach is essential.

Suggested Readings

Committee on Trauma, American College of Surgeons. *Advanced Trauma Life Support Program for Physicians.* Chicago, IL: American College of Surgeons, 1993.

Instructor manual for an educational course modeled after the American Heart Association's Advanced Cardiac Life Support program but directed to the initial assessment and management of the trauma patient (862 pages).

Emergency Cardiac Care Committee and Subcommittees, American Heart Association. Guidelines for cardiopulmonary resuscitation and emergency cardiac care. *JAMA* 1992;268:2199–2241.

American Heart Association standards for resuscitation and advanced cardiac life support.

Salem M, Chernow B, Burke R, et al. Bedside diagnostic blood testing. *JAMA* 1991;266:382–389.

Evaluates multichannel microchemistry analyzer usable at the bedside in the ICU.

Weigelt JA. Resuscitation and initial management. *Crit Care Clin* 1993;9:657–671.

Reviews initial survey, resuscitation, and stabilization of the trauma patient.

Weil MH. Patient evaluation, vital signs and initial care. In: Shoemaker WC, Thompson WL, eds. *Critical care state of the art,* Volume 1. Anaheim, CA: Society of Critical Care Medicine, 1980, pp 1–31.

Weil MH, Michaels S, Puri VK, et al. The stat laboratory: Facilitating blood gas and biochemical measurements for the critically ill and injured. *Am J Clin Pathol* 1981;76:34–42.

Describes the concept of critical care stat laboratory and stat panel.

Weil MH, Shubin H. The "VIP" approach to the bedside management of shock. *JAMA* 1969;207:337–340.

Classic report describing the ventilation-infusion-perfusion concept as applied to the initial resuscitation of the patient with circulatory shock.

CHAPTER 2

Cardiopulmonary Resuscitation

(See Chapter 11)

Robert T. Mansfield

This chapter focuses on the acute management of the adult patient in cardiac arrest. The goal of basic and advanced life support is to maintain perfusion to the heart and brain with oxygenated blood. The ultimate goal is to restore spontaneous circulation. Until that is achieved, the patient is supported with artificial ventilation, chest compressions, and other adjunctive measures. The sooner cardiopulmonary resuscitation (CPR) begins and defibrillation occurs, the greater the likelihood of a favorable outcome.

Airway and Breathing

Although dysrhythmias are the most common cause of cardiac arrest, providing adequate oxygenation and ventilation is vitally important. The patient in respiratory arrest should receive 100% oxygen by bag-valve mask initially and will usually require endotracheal intubation subsequently (see Chapter 7 in this book).

Circulation

Once the condition of pulselessness (or profound bradycardia) has been established, chest compressions should be initiated immediately, until a defibrillator is available. The patient must be lying supine on a firm, flat surface. The ball of the rescuer's hand is placed against the lower third of the sternum, with the other hand overlying it and the elbows straight. The chest is compressed to a depth of 1.5–2 inches, 80–100 min^{-1}, with equal time allowed for compression and relaxation. Variations on CPR have been tried, including vest CPR, intermittent abdominal compressions, and simultaneous compression–ventilation, but none have been proven to be superior to well-performed standard manual CPR.

Defibrillation

ECG monitoring must be established immediately. If ventricular fibrillation (VF) is present, defibrillation should be attempted as soon as possible to optimize the chance of a good recovery. Pulseless ventricular tachycardia (VT) is treated in the same way as VF. The objective of defibrillation is to pass an electrical current through the heart to depolarize a critical mass of myocardium, interrupting the abnormal rhythm, with the hope that the normal rhythm can resume. A shock that is too weak will not accomplish this goal; however, a shock that is too strong may induce myocardial damage or other dysrhythmias. Defibrillation should begin with 200 J. If the first shock is unsuccessful, the second shock should be 200–300 J, and the third shock no more than 360 J. These three initial shocks (if indicated) should be applied as soon as possible and in rapid succession. If this first salvo of shocks is ineffective, the patient should receive epinephrine and undergo endotracheal intubation, followed in 30–60 seconds with another attempt at defibrillation (a single shock of 360 J or, if necessary, multiple shocks). If this intervention is still unsuccessful, lidocaine, then bretylium, then additional epinephrine should be given, with each dose followed by an attempt at defibrillation (drug–shock, drug–shock . . .). Procainamide and magnesium may be included in this regimen for refractory VF. Bag-valve ventilation and chest compressions are continued as the defibrillation equipment is being readied or recharged. If VF recurs, the energy level that was previously effective should be used.

The position of the defibrillation electrodes is important. One paddle is placed just to the right of the sternum and inferior to the clavicle, and the other is applied lateral to the left nipple, in the midaxillary line. An alternative recommendation is to place one paddle anteriorly over the left precordium and the other posteriorly in the right infrascapular area. The paddle surface is covered with conducting gel and applied firmly to the skin. Factors that increase transthoracic impedance (pneumothorax, poor contact, excessive distance between electrodes) may preclude successful defibrillation.

Other cardiac dysrhythmias require synchronized cardioversion with lower energy levels (VT, 100 J; atrial flutter and paroxysmal atrial tachycardia, 50 J; atrial fibrillation, 100 J), with escalating energy levels used if necessary. Asystole will not respond to electrical conversion. If it does not delay defibrillation, a single precordial thump is acceptable in the pulseless patient with a witnessed arrest.

Transcutaneous pacing is indicated for hemodynamically unstable bradycardia, bradycardia with malignant ventricular escape beats, asystole (if it can be initiated immediately after the onset of asystole), and torsades de pointes. Transvenous pacing is preferable, but is not as easily initiated.

Drug Administration

During cardiac arrest, the priority of the rescuer is to provide basic CPR (bag-valve mask ventilation and chest compressions), defibrillation (when indicated), and endotracheal intubation. Drug administration occurs after these priorities have been addressed.

A central venous catheter is preferable for administering drugs. If the patient has no IV access, an antecubital vein should be cannulated because this approach will not interrupt resuscitative efforts (namely, chest compressions). Medications given through a peripheral vein should be followed by a 20-mL bolus of normal saline to enhance delivery to the central circulation. A central venous catheter can be inserted if circulation is not restored after the initial drug administration. If IV access is unavailable, epinephrine, atropine, and lidocaine can be given through the endotracheal tube, diluted in 10 mL normal saline or water. In general, the dose of drugs administered by endotracheal administration is double the usual IV dose.

Specific Nonantiarrhythmic Drugs

Supplemental Oxygen. One hundred percent oxygen should always be given during CPR.

Intravenous Fluids. Volume administration is not rec-...nded for routine use in the resuscitation of cardiac arrest victims who have no evidence of volume loss. Patients with acute blood loss (trauma, ruptured aneurysm, GI bleeding, etc.) or hypovolemia will require repletion with the appropriate blood products or isotonic fluids. Certain patients with myocardial dysfunction may benefit from higher filling pressures. Similarly, in patients with pulseless electrical activity, a fluid challenge may be indicated.

Epinephrine is the most important drug used routinely during cardiac resuscitation. It has potent α- and β-adrenergic properties. Its most important effects are to vasoconstrict the peripheral vasculature (with the important exception of the myocardial and cerebral vasculature), increase aortic diastolic pressure, and thereby improve myocardial and cerebral blood flow. It also has chronotropic and inotropic effects, but these occur at the expense of increasing myocardial oxygen demands. The primary indication for its use is cardiac arrest caused by VF that does not respond to initial CPR, defibrillation, and airway and ventilatory management. Another indication is asystole and pulseless electrical activity. The initial dose is 0.5–1 mg by IV injection (or 2–2.5 mg through an endotracheal tube). Higher doses of epinephrine may be beneficial, and it is acceptable to increase the dose to 3 mg, then 5 mg if needed, or to increase the dose to 0.1 mg/kg. A dose is given every 3–5 minutes during resuscitation (followed by defibrillation if VF is present). It is also used for bradycardia (after atropine is administered and while transcutaneous pacing is administered), and it can be used for its vasopressor properties for hypotension.

Atropine is a parasympatholytic agent that increases the rate of sinus node depolarization and enhances atrioventricular conduction. It is the drug of choice for symptomatic bradycardia (unless cardiac pacing is immediately available), and it is the second drug (after epinephrine) for asystole and pulseless electrical activity. For bradycardia, the dose is 0.5–1 mg IV every 5 minutes (if needed) to a total dose of 0.04 mg/kg. For asystole, 1.0 mg IV is given, and may be repeated every 3 to 5 minutes, to a total dose of 0.04 mg/kg. The endotracheal dose is 1–2 mg. A dose less than 0.5 mg may cause paradoxical bradycardia through centrally mediated mechanisms. Atropine should be used with caution in patients with myocardial ischemia.

Sodium bicarbonate is of questionable utility in the treatment of cardiac arrest. It is indicated, however, in the treatment of symptomatic hyperkalemia, in cyclic antidepressant overdose, or in the patient with a known bicarbonate-responsive acidosis. Otherwise, it may be given after a prolonged period of resuscitation. The dose is 1 mmol/kg IV, then 0.5 mmol/kg IV every 10 minutes, if indicated.

Calcium is not beneficial during CPR. Further, there is

speculation that excessive calcium intake may be detrimental because intracellular calcium accumulation seems to be the final common pathway for cellular death. However, it is indicated in the setting of hypocalcemia, hyperkalemia, hypermagnesemia, and the overdose of calcium channel blocking agents. The dose is 2 mL 10% calcium chloride solution (2–4 mg/kg).

Antiarrhythmic Drugs

Lidocaine is a class IB antiarrhythmic agent that stabilizes cell membranes and increases the threshold for VF. It is the antiarrhythmic drug of choice for the treatment of VF, VT, and ventricular ectopy. During cardiac arrest caused by VF or pulseless VT, lidocaine should be given after the second defibrillation attempt. Epinephrine is given after the first. The dose is 1.5 mg/kg IV (or by endotracheal tube) followed by defibrillation. This sequence may be repeated to a total dose of 3 mg/kg. If this treatment is successful, a continuous infusion may be initiated at 2–4 mg/min. In a patient with stable VT (i.e., good pulses, conscious, and asymptomatic), wide-complex tachycardia, or significant ventricular ectopy, an initial bolus of 1–1.5 mg/kg is followed by smaller doses (0.5–0.75 mg/kg), as needed, to a maximum cumulative dose of 3 mg/kg. Lidocaine may cause CNS toxicity (seizures, slurred speech, altered consciousness). It may be lethal if it is used to treat ventricular escape beats that result from bradycardia.

Bretylium is a class III antiarrhythmic agent. It is indicated for VF that is resistant to defibrillation, epinephrine, and lidocaine. The dose is 5 mg/kg by IV injection. Additional doses of 10 mg/kg may be given every 5 minutes if necessary, to a total dose of 30 to 35 mg/kg. In patients with VF or pulseless VT, these doses are followed by defibrillation. It may also be used for stable VT and wide-complex tachycardias (given more slowly, over 8 minutes) that are resistant to lidocaine and procainamide. If this treatment is effective, an infusion may be started at 1–2 mg/min. Bretylium may cause hypotension, nausea, and vomiting.

Procainamide is a class IA antiarrhythmic agent that may be indicated in VF or VT that is resistant to the above measures. It is the second-line drug for stable VT and wide-complex tachycardias (after lidocaine). The dose is 20–30 mg/min IV, until the dysrhythmia ceases, hypotension occurs, the QRS duration increases by 50%, or a total dose of 17 mg/kg is given. If this treatment is effective, an infusion may be given at 1–4 mg/min. Procainamide is contraindicated in patients with prolonged QT duration and in those with torsades de pointes. This agent may also cause hypotension.

Adenosine is an endogenous purine nucleotide that de-

TABLE 2–1

SUMMARY OF DYSRHYTHMIA MANAGEMENT

Situation	Appropriate Actions			
	1	2	3	4
Ventricular fibrillation, pulseless ventricular tachycardia	Defibrillation (200, 200–300, 360 J)	Endotracheal intubation	Epinephrine, defibrillation	Epinephrine, defibrillation; plus lidocaine, bretylium, procainamide, magnesium
Asystole	Confirm	Pacing, if initiated immediately	Epinephrine	Atropine
Pulseless electrical activity	Treatment of cause	Epinephrine	Atropine, if heart rate $< 60\ min^{-1}$	Volume
Wide QRS tachycardia, unknown	Cardioversion if unstable*	Lidocaine	Adenosine	Procainamide, bretylium
Wide QRS, known ventricular tachycardia	Cardioversion if unstable*	Lidocaine	Procainamide	Bretylium

Narrow QRS, paroxysmal supraventricular tachycardia	Cardioversion if unstable*	Vagal maneuver[†]	Adenosine	Verapamil
Narrow QRS, atrial fibrillation, or atrial flutter	Cardioversion if unstable*	Verapamil	Procainamide	Quinidine
Sinus bradycardia, asymptomatic[‡]	Observation if first-degree or type I second-degree block	Pacing if type II second-degree or third-degree block		
Sinus bradycardia, symptomatic[‡]	Pacing[§]	Atropine[‖]	Epinephrine	Dopamine

*Unstable as defined by the presence of signs and symptoms (see ‡) and heart rate > 150 min^{-1}.

[†]Ice should not be applied to the face of a patient with ischemia; the carotid artery should not be massaged if carotid bruits are heard.

[‡]Symptoms are chest pain, shortness of breath, and decreased level of consciousness. Signs are hypotension, pulmonary edema, shock, congestive heart failure, and acute myocardial infarction.

[§]Transvenous pacing is preferred; transcutaneous pacing is less invasive and more readily available. Transcutaneous pacing may require sedation.

[‖]Avoided in type II second-degree and third-degree heart block.

presses sinus and atrioventricular node activity. It is the drug of choice for narrow-complex tachycardia. Although it converts only reentrant-type supraventricular tachycardia, it can aid in diagnosing other dysrhythmias. Therefore, it is also indicated in wide-complex tachycardia of unknown etiology if lidocaine is ineffective. The dose is 6 mg as a rapid IV bolus, followed by 12 mg in 1 to 2 minutes, and repeated if necessary. It has a short half-life (5 seconds), and may cause transient asystole, chest pain, flushing, wheezing, and dyspnea. The effects of adenosine are potentiated by dipyridamole and carbamazepine, and attenuated by methylxanthines.

Verapamil is a calcium channel blocking agent that slows conduction and prolongs refractoriness in the atrioventricular node. It is used to convert supraventricular tachycardia when adenosine is ineffective. The dose is 2.5–5 mg IV over 2 minutes. Additional doses of 5–10 mg may be given every 15 to 30 minutes, to a total dose of 20 mg, if needed. It is contraindicated in VT and in wide-complex tachycardia with Wolff-Parkinson-White syndrome. Therefore, it should not be used in wide-complex tachydysrhythmias unless it has been confirmed that the rhythm is of supraventricular origin with aberrant conduction. Verapamil may cause hypotension, and some clinicians administer calcium before using it. Calcium channel and β-blocking agents should not be used in close temporal sequence.

Magnesium is indicated in torsades de pointes or hypomagnesemia associated with ventricular dysrhythmias. The dose is 1–2 g magnesium sulfate IV over 1–2 minutes during cardiac arrest, or over 5–60 minutes in less urgent situations.

Approach to the Patient in Cardiac Arrest

The management of a patient in cardiac arrest or impending arrest must proceed in a rapid, efficient manner. The priorities are airway, breathing, oxygenation, chest compressions, and defibrillation. Accordingly, the team leader should assign personnel responsibility for the airway, chest compressions, defibrillation, and IV access. The rescuers assess responsiveness, breathing, pulse, and cardiac rhythm to determine what interventions are required. Defibrillation (when indicated) is a priority. As the resuscitation proceeds, additional monitoring is applied, such as pulse oximetry, blood pressure, and end-tidal CO_2. If time permits, a 12-lead ECG and a chest radiograph are obtained, a physical examination is performed, and the history is reviewed. Table 2–1 summarizes the actions for the various dysrhythmias that may be encountered. Continual reassessment is important.

Suggested Readings

American Heart Association. Adult advanced cardiac life support. *JAMA* 1992;268:2199–2235.

Detailed review of advanced cardiac life support protocols and techniques.

Callaham M, Madsen CD, Barton CW, et al. A randomized clinical trial of high-dose epinephrine and norepinephrine versus standard-dose epinephrine in prehospital cardiac arrest. *JAMA* 1992;268:2667–2672.

One of several studies supporting use of high-dose epinephrine in cardiac arrest.

Cummins R, ed. *Textbook of advanced cardiac life support.* Dallas, TX: American Heart Association, 1994.

Hargarten KM, Stueven HA, Waite EM, et al. Prehospital experience with defibrillation of coarse ventricular fibrillation: A ten-year review. *Ann Emerg Med* 1990;19:157–162.

Emphasizes importance of early defibrillation.

Kern KB, Carter AB, Showen RL, et al. Twenty-four hour survival in a canine model of cardiac arrest comparing three methods of manual cardiopulmonary resuscitation. *J Am Coll Cardiol* 1986;7:859–867.

Compares three methods of chest compression and discusses the theoretical basis of cardiopulmonary resuscitation.

Zaritsky AL. Resuscitation pharmacology. In: Chernow B, ed. *The pharmacologic approach to the critically ill patient,* 3rd ed. Baltimore: Williams & Wilkins, 1994.

Provides excellent discussion of resuscitation drugs.

CHAPTER 3

Fluid Resuscitation

(See Chapter 12)

Marilyn T. Haupt

Fluid therapy is one of the most effective interventions in the treatment of critically ill patients with signs of circulatory shock. The prompt, early administration of fluids frequently reverses hypotension and oliguria, increases cardiac output, increases systemic and regional oxygen delivery, prevents or minimizes organ failure, and improves survival. Clinically available resuscitative fluids accomplish these goals with reasonable safety. Therefore, fluid therapy is recommended as initial treatment for shock associated with numerous clinical disorders. These conditions include sepsis, burns, hemorrhage, anaphylaxis, drug overdoses, pancreatitis, and many others.

Fluids available for resuscitation are frequently divided into three types: crystalloids, protein colloids, and nonprotein colloids. The hemodynamic, volume-expanding, and

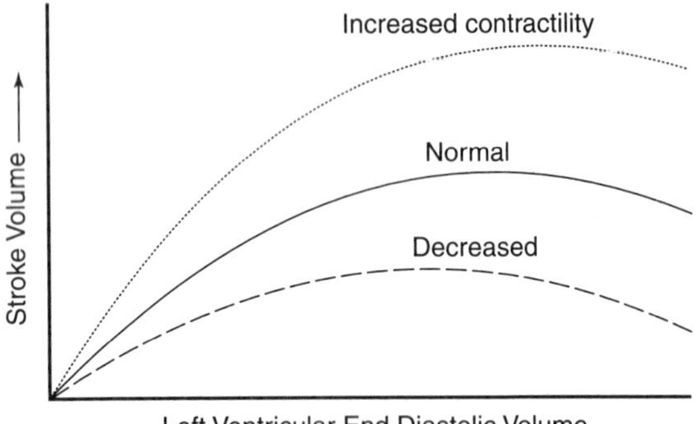

Figure 3–1. The Frank-Starling curve illustrates the relationship between left ventricular end-diastolic volume (preload) and stroke volume. Changes in contractility influence the shape and position of this curve. During fluid loading, end-diastolic volume and stroke volume are increased according to this relationship.

oxygen transport effects, as well as other clinical characteristics of these fluids, are described below.

Hemodynamic Effects of Fluid Loading

An understanding of the Frank-Starling relationship is useful because it predicts the effects of fluid loading on cardiac output, a major determinant of oxygen delivery to systemic tissues. This relationship, which has been validated in critically ill patients during volume loading (Figure 3–1), predicts that, as left ventricular end-diastolic volume increases, stroke volume and cardiac output increase until they reach plateau levels. These plateau, or maximal, levels of cardiac output vary widely in critically ill patients because of marked variations in cardiac compliance, contractility, and afterload. For example, clinical interventions, medications, and conditions that alter the shape and position of the Frank-Starling relationship include positive pressure mechanical ventilation, vasoactive and inotropic medications, myocardial ischemia, pericardial disease, and systemic inflammatory disorders, such as sepsis, pancreatitis, and aspiration pneumonitis. In most patients with sepsis, cardiac output plateaus at pulmonary artery occlusion pressures (PAOP) in the range of 12–15 mm Hg. In patients with cardiogenic shock, cardiac output typically reaches plateau levels at a PAOP of approximately 20 mm Hg. A potentially detrimental decrease in cardiac output (descending limb of the Frank-Starling curve) has been described in patients with sepsis or acute myocardial infarction as volume infusion is continued beyond maximal cardiac output levels. Although the physiologic mecha-

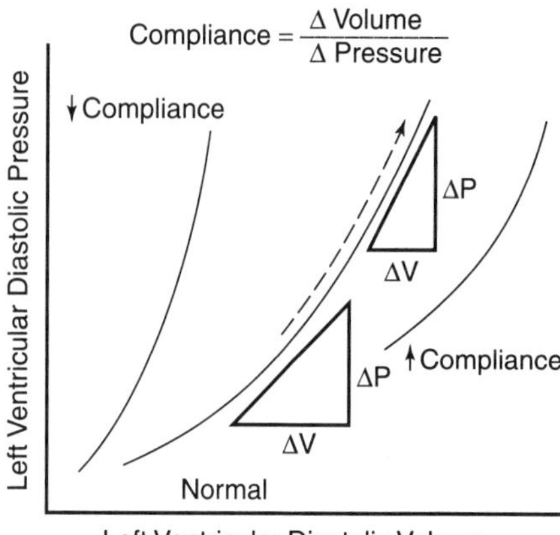

Figure 3–2. These curves describe the compliance characteristics of the left ventricle. As fluid loading continues, precipitous increases in pressure will be observed, a signal that the limits of myocardial stretch have been reached. The actual change in pressure (ΔP) for a given change in volume (ΔV) varies with chamber compliance and diastolic volume.

nisms that lead to the descending limb are not entirely understood, the clinical significance of the descending limb is clear: fluid loading beyond plateau cardiac output levels is unnecessary and may be harmful.

Fluid challenge techniques provide indirect information to the bedside clinical staff about the extent of filling of the cardiac chambers in critically ill patients. These techniques involve observing the central venous pressure (CVP) or PAOP during the rapid administration of a fluid bolus (e.g., 200 mL over 10 minutes):

- If PAOP increases by ≤ 3 mm Hg (or CVP increases by ≤ 2 mm Hg), the bolus infusion is repeated.
- If PAOP increases by > 3 but ≤ 7 mm Hg (or CVP increases by > 2 but ≤ 5 mm Hg), the infusion is held until the increase in PAOP is ≤ 3 mm Hg (or CVP increase is ≤ 2 mm Hg).
- If PAOP increases by > 7 mm Hg (or CVP increases by > 5 mm Hg), infusion is discontinued.

This technique is particularly useful for assessing patients in whom hypovolemia is suspected but uncertain. Precipitous increases in CVP (> 2 mm Hg) or PAOP (> 3 mm Hg) during the infusion period suggest that the limit of myocardial stretch has been reached. These increases correspond to the steep upslopes that are characteristic of cardiac compliance curves (Figure 3–2). When they are observed, cardiac output is likely to be maximal. At this point, additional fluids are unnecessary and may lead to increased pulmonary hydrostatic pressure and pulmonary edema. When warned by a precipitous increase in pressure, the clinician is advised to discontinue fluid administration and observe the patient for signs of clinical improvement. If a precipitous increase in CVP or PAOP is not observed, or if these pressures return to near-baseline values, the clinician may proceed cautiously with an additional fluid challenge if signs of hypoperfusion persist. Inotropic support may be required if signs of hypoperfusion have not reversed when optimal CVP or PAOP has been achieved.

Volume-Expanding Properties of Fluids

It is important to recognize that clinically available fluids for resuscitation expand the intravascular space and cardiac chambers to different extents, depending on their tonicity and oncotic properties. In general, because of their oncotic properties, colloidal fluids expand intravascular volume to a greater extent than equivalent volumes of crystalloidal fluids. In normal subjects or patients without conditions associated with increased permeability, approximately twice as much crystalloid (normal saline or Ringer's lactate) is required to achieve volume expansion equivalent to that produced by colloid (e.g., 5% albumin or 6% hydroxyethyl starch). The intra- and extravascular volume-expanding effects of some clinically available fluids are shown in Table 3–1 for conditions that are not associated with increased microvascular permeability. Clinical and laboratory studies suggest that, when microvascular permeability is increased (e.g., in sepsis, burns, and pancreatitis), three or more times as much crystalloid may be required to achieve plasma volume expansion similar to that caused by colloid.

The effect of crystalloid fluid loading on intravascular volume expansion is more transient than that of colloid loading because crystalloid moves into the interstitial space more rapidly than colloid. Accordingly, after crystalloidal fluid loading, a decline in cardiac filling pressure, cardiac output, blood pressure, and urine output may be observed after an initial improvement. These changes can be minimized in patients receiving crystalloids by giving additional fluid challenges or by increasing maintenance infusion rates.

Effects of Fluid Loading on Oxygen Transport

Because the clinically available resuscitative fluids are asanguinous, their infusion causes hemodilution. This hemodilution is dependent on the degree of intravascular vol-

TABLE 3–1

REPRESENTATIVE EFFECTS OF INFUSION OF 1 L OF VARIOUS FLUIDS ON BODY FLUID COMPARTMENTS

Fluid	Intracellular Volume (mL)	Total Extracellular Volume (mL)	Interstitial Volume (mL)	Plasma Volume (mL)
0.9% NaCl	−100	1100	825	275
5% dextrose in water	660	340	255	85
5% NaCl	−2950	3950	2960	990
5% albumin	0	1000	≥ 500	≥ 500
Whole blood	0	1000	0	1000

Reprinted with permission from Carlson RW, Rattan S, Haupt MT. Fluid resuscitation in conditions of increased permeability. *Anesth Rev* 1990; 15 (suppl 3): 14–20.

ume expansion produced by the fluid. Most asanguinous fluid challenges increase systemic oxygen delivery (the product of cardiac output and arterial oxygen content) by increasing cardiac output. However, if the hemodilution effect of the fluid challenge outweighs the increase in cardiac output, a decrease in oxygen delivery occurs. In one study of patients with septic shock, colloidal fluid loading decreased oxygen delivery in approximately one-third of patients. Although the clinical sequelae of decreases in systemic oxygen delivery from fluid loading are unclear, associated increases in blood lactate level or other signs of anaerobic metabolism may require treatment with red cells or inotropic agents.

Colloid–Crystalloid Controversy

Many studies and debates have addressed whether colloids offer advantages over crystalloids in the fluid resuscitation of patients with circulatory shock. This controversy is far from being resolved. However, most comparative studies refute an early concern that colloids might be harmful to the injured lung. When compared to crystalloids, colloidal fluid resuscitation does not appear to lead to increased interstitial edema in the lung when capillary permeability to colloidal particles is increased. Some studies suggest that there may be advantages of colloid over crystalloid fluid resuscitation in subsets of patients with increased permeability of the lung, large wound surfaces, and burns. The more sustained volume-expanding properties of colloids compared with crystalloids may be useful in hemodynamically unstable patients.

The literature suggests that some subsets of patients may not tolerate the increased interstitial edema typically observed after crystalloid resuscitation. Some studies suggest that patients with burns, adult respiratory distress syndrome, large external wound surfaces, and anaphylaxis may benefit from colloid resuscitation. However, extensive clinical experience and many controlled studies confirm that crystalloids are safe and effective, especially in patients with normal cardiopulmonary and renal function. In these patients, colloids are unnecessary and may not be justified because of their additional cost.

Characteristics of Clinically Available Fluids

Normal Saline. This crystalloidal fluid consists of 0.9% sodium chloride in water. It contains 154 mmol/L sodium and 154 mmol/L chloride, and has an osmolarity of 308 mOsm/L and a pH of approximately 5.0. It is frequently used for volume resuscitation. Large volumes of normal saline (several liters or more) may lead to hyperchloremic metabolic acidosis. This acid–base disorder, if unaccompanied by other acid–base disorders, is usually mild and has no clinical sequelae. However, preexisting metabolic acidosis exacerbated by normal saline infusion may be associated with increases in ventilation, cardiac dysrhythmias, and hyperkalemia and decreases in cardiac contractility and serum ionized calcium levels.

Ringer's Lactate Solution. This crystalloid solution is also frequently used for resuscitation. It is often favored by physicians treating surgical patients. It contains 130 mmol/L sodium, 109 mmol/L chloride, 28 mmol/L lactate, 4 mmol/L potassium, and 1.4 mmol/L calcium, and it has a pH of 6.5. The osmolarity is 273 mOsm/L, which is only slightly hypotonic to plasma. Large volumes of infused Ringer's lactate solution may lead to metabolic alkalosis when the lactate is metabolized to bicarbonate. This acid–base disorder may be associated with impaired systemic unloading of oxygen and decreased ventilatory drive. In the presence of renal or hepatic failure, conditions in which lactate excretion is impaired, elevated lactate levels may occur as a result of resuscitation with large volumes of this fluid. In addition, the calcium and potassium additives may be harmful to patients with renal failure. Blood should not be administered intravenously through tubing that contains lactated Ringer's solution because calcium can initiate coagulation and form precipitates with blood and blood products.

Other crystalloids that are clinically available include Plasma-Lyte®, Normosol®, and Isolyte®. These crystalloids are similar in composition to lactated Ringer's solution, but do not contain calcium. Thus, problems associated with mixing with blood are avoided. Hypotonic crystalloid solutions (e.g., 0.45% saline, 5% dextrose in water) are poor volume expanders (Table 3–1).

5% albumin consists of human serum albumin in a normal saline solution. It is the most frequently used protein colloid solution for fluid resuscitation. Its oncotic pressure is approximately 20 mm Hg, similar to the normal supine oncotic pressure of humans. Albumin infusions appear to be free of major toxicity. However, coagulation problems and inhibition of sodium diuresis have been described after infusion of large volumes (usually > 2 L). Coagulation problems after albumin infusions are often secondary to dilution of clotting proteins, and may be corrected with fresh-frozen plasma. Rare allergic reactions have been reported.

Hydroxyethyl starch, or hetastarch, is a synthetic nonprotein colloid. This fluid is available as a 6% solution in normal saline, and its oncotic pressure is approximately 30 mm Hg. The mechanisms for elimination of hetastarch are not entirely known, but they include excretion by the liver and kidney. Nevertheless, patients with disorders of these organs appear to tolerate this colloid well if less than 1.5 L is administered. The reticuloendothelial system eliminates large Hespan® molecules by phagocytosis. Considerable clinical experience with hetastarch suggests that it is a safe and effective volume expander, with hemodynamic effects that are similar to those of albumin. Large volumes (> 1.5 L) may be associated with impaired clotting. Rare anaphylactoid reactions have been reported. Because hetastarch complexes with plasma amylase, delaying amylase excretion, it may be associated with elevated amylase levels that do not represent pancreatitis or other intra-abdominal disorders. If the diagnosis of these conditions is uncertain in patients who have received hetastarch, serum lipase levels, which are unaffected by hetastarch, should be assessed. The major advantage of hetastarch over albumin is its lower cost. Hetastarch should be avoided in patients with severe oliguria or anuria.

Dextran solutions are available as dextran 70 (molecular weight 70,000 da) as a 6% solution in normal saline and dextran 40 (molecular weight 40,000 da) as a 10% solution. Both are hyperoncotic nonprotein colloids. Both solutions expand plasma volume to a similar extent, but the effects of dextran 40 are more transient because of the more rapid renal excretion of its smaller molecules. The dextrans are believed to be beneficial to the microcirculation, especially in the shock state, because they have antithrombogenic effects, inhibit platelet aggregation, and may prevent red cell sludging. Increased bleeding and rare anaphylactoid reactions have been observed. Dextrans are not frequently used for fluid resuscitation in critically ill patients, perhaps because of concern about bleeding complications.

Modified gelatins are synthetic protein colloids that are commercially available for fluid resuscitation outside the United States. These colloids have volume-expanding properties similar to those of 5% albumin. As is the case with all asanguinous fluids, large volumes of gelatins may lead to dilutional coagulopathy. Rarely, gelatins are associated with anaphylactoid reactions.

Pentastarch is an investigational colloid designed for use in permeability disorders. It is a macromolecular derivative of hetastarch that may have sealing properties when infused in subjects with permeability disorders. This type of colloid may have a role in the future treatment of shock.

Suggested Readings

Carlson RW, Rattan S, Haupt MT. Fluid resuscitation in conditions of increased permeability. *Anesthesiol Rev* 1990;17(suppl 3):14–24.

Haupt MT. Therapy: Effects of fluid resuscitation. In: Edward JD, Shoe-

maker WC, Vincent J-L, eds. *Oxygen transport: Principles and practice.* London: WB Saunders, 1993, pp 175–192.
Describes effects of fluid resuscitation on oxygen delivery and consumption.
Kaufman BS, ed. Fluid resuscitation of the critically ill. *Crit Care Clin* 1992;8(2):235–463.
This issue is devoted to fluid resuscitation and contains twelve articles on various aspects of fluid management.
Rackow EC, Falk JL, Fein A, et al. Fluid resuscitation in circulatory shock: A comparison of the cardiorespiratory effects of albumin, hetastarch, and saline solutions in patients with hypovolemic and septic shock. *Crit Care Med* 1983;11:839–850.
Compares the hemodynamic and pulmonary effects of colloidal and crystalloidal fluid therapy in critically ill patients.
Vincent J-L. Plugging the leaks? New insights into synthetic colloids. *Crit Care Med* 1991;19:316–318.
Brief comparative review of synthetic colloids.

CHAPTER 4

Noninvasive Monitoring of Oxygen and Carbon Dioxide

(See Chapter 17)

Robert T. Mansfield

Pulse Oximetry

Pulse oximetry allows convenient, accurate, noninvasive, continuous monitoring of arterial oxyhemoglobin (HbO_2) saturation without the need for frequent measurement of arterial blood gases. It is based on the Beer-Lambert law, which states that the concentration of a substance in a solution is proportional to the amount of light it absorbs. Hemoglobin (Hb) and HbO_2 absorb different amounts of light at different wavelengths. By comparing the relative amount of light absorbed at two different wavelengths (660 and 940 nm), the oximeter determines the relative concentrations of each, and therefore the fraction or percentage of HbO_2. The pulse oximeter senses the change in HbO_2 during pulsation and thus differentiates arterial from venous HbO_2. By design, pulse oximeters can measure only Hb and HbO_2, but not carboxyhemoglobin (HbCO) or methemoglobin, which are normally present in low concentrations. The correlation of pulse oximetry values (Spo_2) with cooximetry (Sao_2, the criterion standard) is excellent at HbO_2 saturations greater than 70%.

Because of the sigmoid shape of the oxyhemoglobin saturation curve, small changes in arterial oxygen tension (Pa_{O_2}) up to 60–70 torr cause large changes in Sa_{O_2}. Above that range, the saturation is nearly 100%. Large changes in Pa_{O_2} above this range are therefore not detectable by pulse oximetry.

Conditions Affecting Accuracy

- **Carbon monoxide** has 200 times the affinity for Hb compared with oxygen, and thus diminishes oxygen-carrying capacity. HbCO has high absorbance at 660 nm, similar to that of HbO_2, so it falsely elevates Sp_{O_2}.
- **Methemoglobin** (HbMet) is Hb with the iron moiety oxidized to the ferric state. It cannot bind oxygen. High concentrations can occur due to a congenital deficiency of reducing substances or because of exposure to certain toxins. HbMet absorbs well at both 660 and 940 nm. As the concentration of HbMet rises to 30% and higher, the pulse oximeter approaches a reading of 85%. Therefore, Sp_{O_2} overestimates Sa_{O_2} at high HbMet levels. In the presence of HbCO or HbMet, cooximetry is required to determine the true oxygen saturation.
- **Bilirubin,** even at high serum levels, does not have a significant effect on Sp_{O_2}. However, it may falsely reduce Sa_{O_2} readings.
- **Hypoperfusion,** caused by circulatory shock, vasoconstriction, cool extremities, or other factors, can preclude accurate Sp_{O_2} measurement. Warming the extremity may be helpful. Ear oximetry is more accurate and has a faster response time than digital pulse oximetry.
- **Dyes** that are occasionally used in the clinical setting, such as methylene blue and indocyanine green, can cause the pulse oximeter reading to decrease profoundly. This effect is transient.
- **External light sources** may affect the pulse oximeter. An opaque cover restores normal function.
- **Motion** hinders pulse oximeter function.

Two further caveats deserve mention. Because arterial oxygen saturation reaches a plateau when Pa_{O_2} is greater than 70 torr, the Pa_{O_2} can decrease from 500 torr to less than 100 torr with no change in Sp_{O_2}. Also, oxygen content is determined by Hb saturation and concentration, so a patient with a saturation of 100% but a Hb level of 5 mg/dL still has a low oxygen content.

Capnography

Capnography is the measurement and graphic representation of the amount of CO_2 in expired gas. Infrared spec-

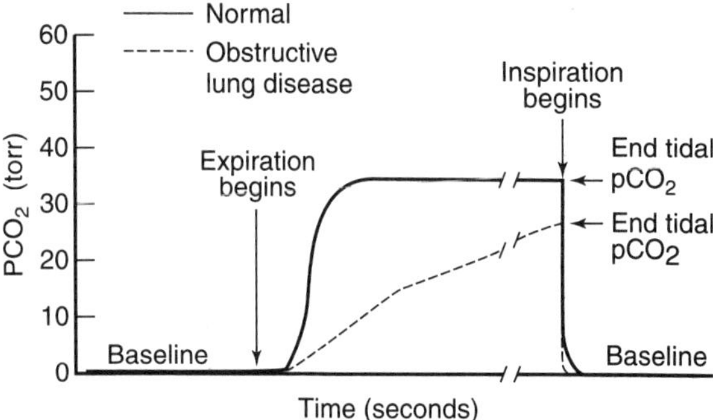

Figure 4–1. Capnogram.

troscopy is commonly used, and measurements can be made in intubated or nonintubated patients. This technology supplies useful information regarding:

- **End-tidal CO_2** (P_{ETCO_2}) as an estimate of Pa_{CO_2}.
- **Dead space volume** (V_D).
- **Respiratory rate** and pattern.
- **Cardiac output** during cardiopulmonary resuscitation (CPR).
- **Ventilator disconnection** and accidental endotracheal extubation.
- **Endotracheal tube position** verification.

P_{ETCO_2} is the tension of CO_2 in gas sampled at the end of a breath. Several physiologic variables determine the P_{ETCO_2}, including CO_2 production, pulmonary blood flow, alveolar ventilation, and dead space. Basically, alveolar gas equilibrates with the carbon dioxide tension (P_{CO_2}) of the pulmonary capillary blood, provided that ventilation and perfusion are adequate. If all alveoli are well perfused, the P_{ETCO_2} closely approximates the pulmonary capillary P_{CO_2}. If some lung units have inadequate perfusion, expired gas from these units mixes in the large airways with gas from well-perfused lung units, thus reducing P_{ETCO_2}. Therefore, a large difference between P_{ETCO_2} and Pa_{CO_2} indicates increased dead space. In normal subjects, the difference is 1 to 5 torr. The ratio of alveolar dead space to tidal volume (V_T) can be quantified as:

$$V_D/V_T = (Pa_{CO_2} - P_{ETCO_2})/Pa_{CO_2}$$

Thus, as P_{ETCO_2} approaches Pa_{CO_2}, V_D approaches zero.

A normal and an abnormal capnogram are shown in Figure 4–1. In Figure 4–1, the baseline P_{ICO_2} (inspiratory phase) is at zero, the plateau is relatively flat, and the P_{ETCO_2} approaches a normal Pa_{CO_2}. With obstructive lung disease, the upslope is slower, the plateau phase never flattens out, and the P_{ETCO_2} is well below a normal Pa_{CO_2}. Other variations are described below.

TABLE 4–1

EVENTS THAT MAY RESULT IN CHANGES IN P_{ETCO_2}*

Increased P_{ETCO_2}	Decreased P_{ETCO_2}
Increased CO_2 production	Decreased CO_2 production
Inadequate ventilation	Hyperventilation
Sudden increase in cardiac output	Sudden decrease in cardiac output
Sodium bicarbonate administration	Massive pulmonary embolism
	Air embolism
	Obstructed endotracheal tube
	Ventilator disconnection
	Extubation

*All of these changes are related to one of four variables: (1) CO_2 production, (2) alveolar ventilation, (3) pulmonary blood flow, or (4) dead space.

(Adapted from Tobin MJ. Respiratory monitoring. *JAMA* 1990; 264:244–251. Copyright 1990, American Medical Assocation.)

Respiratory rate is measured by actual movement of gases, not chest wall movement. A capnogram that shows frequent, brief dips of CO_2 that do not reach baseline may indicate weak respiratory effort requiring more ventilatory support or emergence from neuromuscular blockade. If the slope of the expiratory phase does not reach a relatively flat plateau, the patient may have obstructive airway disease, such as chronic obstructive lung disease or asthma. Failure of the P_{CO_2} to return to zero during inspiration may indicate that an expiratory valve is not closing or the flow of fresh gas is inadequate.

Several studies have demonstrated that the return of spontaneous circulation during CPR is marked by a sudden increase in the P_{ETCO_2}; failure of the P_{ETCO_2} to increase is strongly associated with a low likelihood of resuscitation. Disconnections from the ventilator, accidental extubations, obstructed endotracheal tubes, and other mechanical problems may be detected by a change on the capnogram before any other changes are noted. Correct placement of an endotracheal tube can be verified by portable or disposable semiquantitative monitors. Table 4–1 summarizes clinical events that can affect P_{ETCO_2}.

Suggested Readings

Carlon GC, Ray CJR, Miodownik S, et al. Capnography in mechanically ventilated patients. *Crit Care Med* 1988;16:550–556.

Reviews use of this technique in mechanically ventilated patients and explains how to detect inadequate ventilatory support, weaning failure, and mechanical and other problems.

Sanders AB, Kern KB, Otto, CW, et al. End-tidal carbon dioxide moni-

toring during cardiopulmonary resuscitation: A prognostic indicator for survival. *JAMA* 1989;262:1347–1351.
Prospective clinical trial demonstrating that a low end-tidal CO_2 is strongly associated with nonsurvival.

Schnapp LM, Cohen NH. Pulse oximetry: Uses and abuses. *Chest* 1990;98:1244–1250.
Focuses on practical and clinical aspects of pulse oximetry.

Tobin MJ. Respiratory monitoring. *JAMA* 1990;264:244–251.
Reviews pulse oximetry, capnography, and respiratory mechanics.

Tremper KK, Barker SJ. Pulse oximetry. *Anesthesiology* 1989;70:98–108.
Discusses historical development of the technology, the scientific basis, and its clinical applications and limitations.

CHAPTER 5

Chest Radiography in the ICU

(See Chapter 21)

Paul E. Marik and James A. Kruse

Several studies have demonstrated that obtaining routine chest radiographs daily in ICU patients often shows new, unexpected, or changing abnormalities that require changes in therapy. Daily chest radiographs should therefore be obtained in all but the most stable ICU patients.

Many problems are associated with the interpretation of chest films obtained with portable units. Magnification of the cardiac silhouette makes interpretation of the cardiothoracic ratio unreliable. Signs of pulmonary venous hypertension (upper-lobe vessel recruitment) may not be valid on a supine film. Similarly, a pneumothorax may be undetectable on the supine chest radiograph because the classic signs are frequently not present. Further, assessment of lung volumes and alveolar infiltrates may be difficult because the films often are of poor quality, are taken after a poor inspiratory effort, or are taken with the patient poorly positioned on the film plate. Even with these limitations, however, the routine ICU chest radiograph provides vital information for the management of the critically ill patient.

The chest radiograph should be studied systematically. It is helpful to devise a routine for performing this inspection. One sequence is to assess the quality of the film (i.e., degree of penetration, position of patient, depth of inspiration); then to evaluate the position of any tubes or catheters; next to examine the lung fields and pleura for abnor-

A

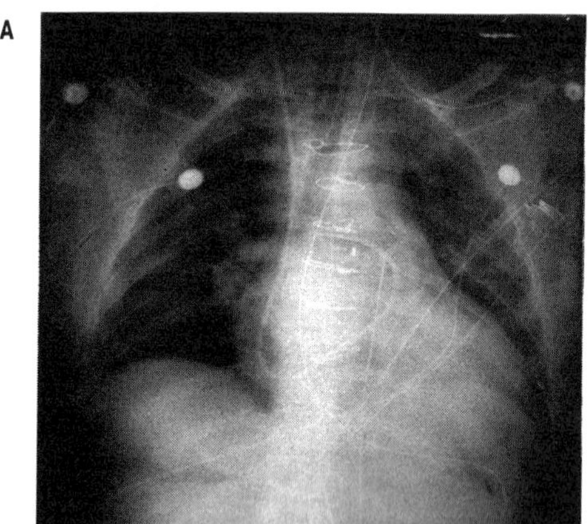

B

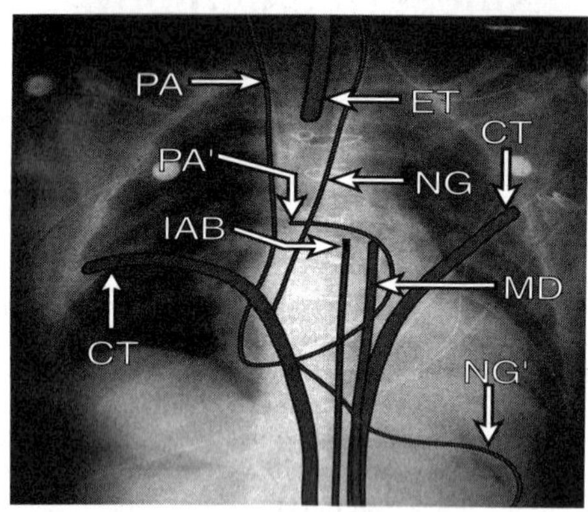

Figure 5–1. *A*. Portable frontal chest radiograph of a critically ill patient after coronary artery bypass grafting. *B*. The same film with superimposed depictions of the corresponding indwelling medical appliances. ET = endotracheal tube with tip located above carina; PA = pulmonary artery catheter coursing from the IJ to superior vena cava and right heart; PA′ = tip of pulmonary artery catheter located in proximal right main pulmonary artery; IAB = radiopaque marker at tip of an intra-aortic counterpulsation balloon catheter (position is inappropriately low in thoracic aorta; course of balloon catheter is shown below marker, but catheter itself is radiotransparent); CT = thoracostomy tubes in left and right pleural spaces, both inserted intraoperatively through anterior chest wall incisions and extending into lateral pleural spaces; MD = mediastinal drainage tube; NG = nasogastric tube coursing through esophagus; NG′ = same nasogastric tube coursing through fundus and body of stomach. (Modified from Zarshenas Z, Sparschu RA. Catheter placement and misplacement. *Crit Care Clin* 1994;10:417–436.)

malities; and finally to assess the heart, mediastinum, diaphragm, and bony and soft tissues.

Position of Indwelling Appliances (Figure 5–1)

Endotracheal Tube. If it is inserted too deeply, the tube can extend into the right mainstem bronchus, potentially causing left lung collapse or right-sided pneumothorax. If it is not inserted far enough, the cuff may impinge on the vocal cords, triggering paroxysms of coughing and placing the patient at risk for unplanned extubation. When the head is in a neutral position, the endotracheal tube should be well below the larynx, but at least 4 cm above the carina. With movement of the head from a flexed to an extended position, the tube can move by as much as 4 cm. When the carina is not visible, the tube can be assumed to be above the carina if its tip is above the level of T4.

Central Venous Catheter. The course of the catheter should follow that of the expected anatomic path. Possible aberrant courses from the subclavian vein include the ipsilateral internal jugular vein (IJ), the contralateral subclavian vein, and the azygos vein. From the IJ, the catheter occasionally courses into the distal subclavian vein. The tip of IJ and subclavian vein catheters should be located proximal to the right atrium (i.e., above the junction of the superior vena cava and right atrium). Placement in the right atrium may cause atrial perforation. Inadvertant intra-arterial placement can occur. After initial placement by the subclavian or IJ route, the chest radiograph should be examined closely for signs of pneumothorax, new pleural fluid collection (indicating possible hydro- or hemothorax), and superior mediastinal hematoma. In rare cases, a delayed pneumothorax occurs, but is not shown on the initial postprocedure radiograph.

Pulmonary Artery Catheter. The tip of the pulmonary artery catheter should be located in the proximal left or right main branch of the pulmonary artery. Pulmonary infarction or pulmonary artery rupture can occur if the tip extends too far peripherally. Generally, the tip should not extend farther than 2 cm lateral to the hilum. There should be no redundancy of the catheter within the right atrium or ventricle. Looping within these chambers is problematic because (1) it may provoke dysrhythmias; (2) it potentially represents knotting of the catheter, which can cause serious complications during removal; and (3) if the loop is in the ventricle, pressure monitored from the proximal port could represent right ventricular pressure instead of the expected right atrial pressure.

Nasogastric Tube. Both the tip and any side holes should extend into the stomach, well below the gastroesophageal junction. A tube that follows a tortuous course through the mediastinum may indicate a mass lesion, an aortic aneurysm, or another abnormality. Esophageal perforation rarely occurs when standard nasogastric tubes are used. It can occur with the use of Sengstaken-Blakemore or Minnesota tubes if the gastric balloon is inflated while in the esophagus.

Nasoenteric Feeding Tube. Ideally, the tube should extend at least into the duodenum. In all cases, the distal orifice of the feeding tube must be at least beyond the gastroesophageal junction. Serious malposition, including coiling in the pharynx or esophagus and intratracheal or intrapleural placement, should be routinely excluded. Obtunded patients and those with endotracheal tubes in place are at increased risks of tracheobroncheal placement.

Chest Thoracostomy Tube. The most proximal side hole is usually identifiable as an interruption in a radiopaque line on the tube. For tubes placed from the lateral chest wall, if this drainage hole is not medial to the inner margin of the ribs, then the chest tube insertion depth is inadequate. However, if this last side hole is medial to the inner rib margin on an anteroposterior radiograph, it does not guarantee proper insertion depth or intrapleural placement. If appropriate positioning is in doubt, a lateral radiograph or computed tomography (CT) may be necessary. The radiograph should be examined closely for evidence of persistent pneumothorax. Reexpansion pulmonary edema can occur after chest tube placement for pleural effusion, especially when large, long-standing effusions are rapidly drained.

Intra-Aortic Balloon Catheter. These devices have a radiopaque marker at the tip of the catheter. This marker should lie immediately distal to the left subclavian artery so that it does not occlude blood flow to the left arm or brain, or result in embolism to the brain. If the catheter is positioned too far inferiorly, its efficacy will be hindered, and there is risk of compromising blood flow to the renal and mesenteric arteries that branch off of the abdominal aorta. Loss of definition of the descending aorta suggests aortic perforation or dissection.

Transvenous Pacing Catheter. If used for ventricular pacing, the tip of the catheter should lie near the apex of the right ventricle. If the tip lies at or extends beyond the left margin of the cardiac silhouette, it indicates that ventricular perforation has occurred. Inadvertent placement within the coronary sinus sometimes simulates right ventricular positioning on the frontal radiograph.

Sengstaken-Blakemore Tube. It is critical that the gastric balloon is located within the stomach before and after full inflation. Therefore, the gastric balloon should be only partially inflated (50–100 mL) until its intragastric position can be confirmed radiographically. The gastric and, if necessary, esophageal balloons can then be inflated to therapeutic volumes. A nasogastric-type tube should be in place, with its tip located just above the esophageal balloon. This secondary drainage tube is unnecessary if a Minnesota tube is used.

Lung Parenchyma and Pleura

Pulmonary Infiltrates. If infiltrates are present, it should be noted whether they are interstitial or alveolar, unilateral or bilateral. Infiltrates may be caused either by water (cardiogenic or noncardiogenic pulmonary edema), blood (hematoma or intra-alveolar hemorrhage), or cellular infiltration (infection or inflammation). It may not be possible to distinguish between these causes by examination of the chest film alone. It is also sometimes difficult to distinguish infiltrates from atelectasis. Radiologic signs of pulmonary edema include a bilateral and symmetric pattern (not universally seen), vessel blurring, and perivascular cuffing. A central pattern, blurred hila, engorgement of the pulmonary vessels, Kerley B-lines, and associated cardiomegaly suggest cardiogenic pulmonary edema, but this entity often cannot be distinguished from noncardiogenic pulmonary edema. Signs associated with pneumonia include interstitial or air space disease, air bronchograms, and the silhouette sign.

Atelectasis. Radiologic signs of atelectasis include increased radio-opacity in the area of atelectasis, with silhouetting against bordering areas of the heart, mediastinum, or diaphragm. Segmental or lobar collapse can mimic pneumonia. With atelectasis, the affected area may show crowding of the pulmonary vasculature and airways. Shift of the intralobar septa or hilum toward the collapsed area, shift of the heart and mediastinum toward the affected side, and ipsilateral elevation of the hemidiaphragm may be seen. Compensatory hyperinflation can occur in unaffected areas.

Pneumothorax. The key findings are a thin, white, visceral pleural line and loss of peripheral lung markings. However, a typical apicolateral lucency may not appear on ICU supine films of patients with pneumothorax. Instead, pleural gas often collects in the anterior costophrenic sulcus because this area is the most nondependent portion of the pleural space in the supine patient. Thus, radiographic signs of pneumothorax in the supine position include a relative hyperlucency over the upper abdominal quadrants and a deep costophrenic angle (the deep sulcus sign). Redundant skin folds sometimes closely simulate the visceral pleural line of a pneumothorax. A clue to such skin folds is that they may extend beyond the thoracic cavity, whereas a pleural line cannot.

Pleural Fluid. Fluid may be caused by transudative or exudative effusion, hydrothorax from a central venous catheter that is misplaced into the pleural space, empyema, hemothorax, or chylothorax. In the supine or semiupright position, fluid tracks posteriorly, resulting in a diffuse haziness of the lung fields. The expected meniscus, commonly seen on upright posteroanterior chest radiographs, may be absent on ICU films, despite a large effusion. The presence of pleural fluid can be confirmed by lateral decubitus radiographs, ultrasonography, or CT.

Other Lung-Field Abnormalities. Other important findings include nodules, masses, cavitations, calcifications, increased pulmonary vascular markings, hyperlucency (as a result of alveolar destruction, as in emphysema, or hyperinflation, as in air trapping), fibrosis, enlarged or retracted hila, abscesses (with or without air–fluid levels), and consolidation. Air bronchograms are seen in pneumonia, pulmonary edema, pulmonary infarction, and some forms of chronic lung disease. A 3- to 5-cm, wedge-shaped, peripheral opacity abutting the pleura and extending toward the hilum (Hampton's hump) is occasionally observed in pulmonary infarction. Lung-field radiodensities that obliterate the normal roentgen silhouette of the diaphram, aortic, or cardiac border (silhouette sign) indicate that the abnormality is in physical contact with the anatomic structure. This information is useful for anteroposterior localization of water-density lesions.

Heart, Mediastinum, Diaphragm, and Bony and Soft Tissues

Cardiovascular Silhouette. Enlargement may indicate cardiomegaly or pericardial effusion. The latter sometimes causes a characteristic *water bottle* appearance of the cardiac silhouette. Separation of lenticular mural calcification from the edge of the aortic knob silhouette is a clue to the presence of aortic dissection.

Mediastinum. Widening of the mediastinum may indicate aortic dissection, lymphadenopathy, or tumor. Lateral shift of mediastinal structures, including the trachea, may be caused by simple or tension pneumothorax, atelectasis, pleural effusion, tumor, pneumonectomy, fibrosis, or other serious abnormalities.

Diaphragm. Blunting of the costophrenic angle may indicate pleural fluid. Obscuration of the medial or entire hemidiaphragm can be caused by pleural fluid, atelectasis, or infiltrate. The right hemidiaphragm is normally slightly higher than the left. More pronounced elevation or reversal of this pattern can be caused by lower-lobe collapse; pleural fluid; hepatomegaly or splenomegaly; diaphragmatic eventration, herniation, or paralysis; subphrenic abscess; or other intra-abdominal disorders.

Other Abnormal Gas Collections. Besides pneumothorax, other common manifestations of barotrauma are pneumomediastinum, subcutaneous or interstitial emphysema, and pneumatoceles. Pulmonary abscess cavities may contain gas, fluid, or both. Upper abdominal gas collections caused by gastric or colonic dilation are frequently visible on the chest radiograph. Free gas under the diaphragm suggests a perforated viscus. It can also occur after laparotomy or peritoneal catheterization.

Bony and Soft Tissues. Signs of masses or swelling may occur with a large hematoma. Unilateral mastectomy can cause disparate lung lucency. Particularly important findings are signs of traumatic or pathologic fractures and metastatic bone lesions. Air in the soft tissues can indicate subcutaneous emphysema or necrotizing soft-tissue infection.

Suggested Readings

Bekemeyer WB, Crapo RO, Calhoon S, et al. Efficacy of chest radiography in a respiratory intensive care unit: A prospective study. *Chest* 1985;88:691–696.

Concludes that routine morning chest radiographs in a patient population frequently demonstrated unexpected abnormalities or changes that prompted a change in diagnosis or treatment.

Marcy TW. Barotrauma: Detection, recognition, and management. *Chest* 1993;104:578–584.

Reviews pathogenesis and clinical manifestations of barotrauma. Ventilator management strategies to decrease its incidence are suggested (74 references).

Templeton PA, Diaconis JN. Critical care chest imaging. In: Mirvis SE, Young JWR, eds. *Imaging in trauma and critical care.* Philadelphia: Williams & Wilkins, 1992, pp 516–568.

Thorough review containing more than 90 radiographs.

Wechsler RJ, Steiner RM, Kinori I. Monitoring the monitors: The radiology of thoracic catheters, wires, and tubes. *Semin Roentgenol* 1988;23:61–84.

Extensive review of the topic (38 radiographs, 93 references).

Winer-Muram HT, Rubin SA, Miniati M, et al. Guidelines for reading and interpreting chest radiographs in patients receiving mechanical ventilation. *Chest* 1992;102(suppl):565S–570S.

Zarshenas Z, Sparschu RA. Catheter placement and misplacement. *Crit Care Clin* 1994;10:417–436.

Excellent review of the correct and incorrect radiographic positioning of vascular and other medical appliances used commonly in ICU patients (23 radiographic illustrations).

CHAPTER 6

Severity of Illness Scoring in the ICU

(See Chapters 7 and 138)

James A. Kruse

Many scoring systems have been developed for grading the severity of illness in acutely ill patients. Some systems are designed to be applied to patients with specific diseases, whereas others can be applied to critically ill patients in general. Scoring instruments have been used to objectively predict outcome in groups of patients, for risk stratification, for quality assurance studies, for evaluation of resource use, and in the context of clinical investigations. In addition to their use by physicians and researchers, these methods have been widely applied by hospital administrators, third-party payers, government agencies, and others. They are used to assess patients' severity of illness and need for therapy and to interpret institutional mortality rates. Current scoring systems range from simple instruments with only a few variables to complex proprietary systems with hundreds of variables. A few of the simpler representative systems that are in common use are described.

Glasgow Coma Scale

(see pages 79 and 1575 in the main text)

The Glasgow Coma Scale (Table 6–1) was developed in the mid-1970s as a means of grading patients with traumatic brain injury and predicting their chances of neurologic recovery. Since that time, it has been used to evaluate neurologic status in medical and surgical ICU patients without trauma. This scale is commonly used as a routine tool for neurologic assessment in the ICU setting.

Child-Turcotte Classification

(see pages 79, 1453, and 1561 in the main text)

This system is used to evaluate the severity and prognosis of a specific disease state, namely hepatic cirrhosis (see Table 95–2 in this book).

Revised Trauma Score

Several scoring systems have been adapted for grading the severity of injury in trauma patients. These instruments include the Revised Trauma Score (see Table 6–2 in this chapter), the Abbreviated Injury Scale (see Table 138–5 in the main text), and others.

Acute Physiology and Chronic Health Evaluation (APACHE) Score

The Acute Physiology and Chronic Health Evaluation (APACHE) system was first reported in 1981. It was subsequently simplified as the APACHE II system, which has become the most well known, the most extensively studied and validated, and one of the most widely applied scoring systems for general use in ICU patients. The most favorable APACHE II score is zero; the theoretically worst score is 71. Figure 6–1 shows the relationship between APACHE II scores and hospital outcome for a group of medical ICU patients at one institution. A more complex version, the APACHE III system, has recently been developed and validated. In 95% of a large group of ICU patients, the APACHE III system predicted hospital mortality rate within 3% of the actual rate.

Calculating the APACHE II Score. This instrument is usually applied to information available during the first 24 hours of a patient's admission to an ICU. A patient's APACHE II score is the sum of point values for each of the following three categories:

- The patient's acute physiology score (Table 6–3). Where more than one measurement of a given variable is available, the most abnormal measurement is used. The Glasgow Coma Scale is part of this portion of the APACHE II score.
- The patient's age points, assigned as follows: If ≤44 years, 0 points; 45–54 years, 1 point; 55–64 years, 2 points; 65–74 years, 3 points; ≥75 years, 6 points.
- The patient's chronic health evaluation points (0, 2, or 5 points).

Chronic health points (2 points for elective postoperative patients or 5 points for nonoperative or emergency postoperative patients) are added if the patient is immunocompromised or has a history of severe organ system insufficiency. The organ system insufficiency must have manifested before the current hospitalization. It consists of one or more of the following:

- **Cardiovascular:** Class IV congestive heart failure by the New York Heart Association classification system.
- **Respiratory:** Chronic obstructive, restrictive, or vascular disease resulting in severe exercise restriction.
- **Renal:** Receiving chronic dialysis.
- **Hepatic:** Cirrhosis diagnosed by biopsy or documented portal hypertension.

TABLE 6–1

THE GLASGOW COMA SCALE*

Response	Finding	Value
Eye-opening response	Spontaneous	4
	To voice	3
	To pain	2
	No response	1
Verbal response (response to voice or noxious stimulus)	Oriented	5
	Confused	4
	Inappropriate speech	3
	Incomprehensible speech	2
	No response	1
Motor response (response to command or noxious stimulus)	Obeys command	6
	Localizes pain	5
	Withdraws from pain	4
	Flexion (decorticate posturing)	3
	Extension (decerebrate posturing)	2
	No response	1

*Total score can range from 3 to 15 points.

TABLE 6–2

THE REVISED TRAUMA SCORE*

Measure	Points	Trauma Score
Glasgow Coma Scale	13–15	4
	9–12	3
	6–8	2
	4–5	1
	3	0
Systolic blood pressure (mm Hg)	> 90	4
	70–89	3
	50–69	2
	1–49	1
	0	0
Respiratory rate (min^{-1})	10–24	4
	25–35	3
	> 35	2
	1–9	1
	0	0

*Total score can range from 0 to 12 points.

TABLE 6–3

THE APACHE II SEVERITY OF DISEASE CLASSIFICATION SYSTEM

PHYSIOLOGIC VARIABLE	HIGH ABNORMAL RANGE					LOW ABNORMAL RANGE			
	+4	+3	+2	+1	0	+1	+2	+3	+4
TEMPERATURE — rectal (°C)	≥41°	39°-40.9°		38.5°-38.9°	36°-38.4°	34°-35.9°	32°-33.9°	30°-31.9°	≤29.9°
MEAN ARTERIAL PRESSURE — mm Hg	≥160	130-159	110-129		70-109		50-69		≤49
HEART RATE (ventricular response)	≥180	140-179	110-139		70-109		55-69	40-54	≤39
RESPIRATORY RATE — (non-ventilated or ventilated)	≥50	35-49		25-34	12-24	10-11	6-9		≤5
OXYGENATION: A-aDO$_2$ or PaO$_2$ (mm Hg) a. FIO$_2$ ≥ 0.5 record A-aDO$_2$	≥500	350-499	200-349		<200				
b. FIO$_2$ < 0.5 record only PaO$_2$					PO$_2$ > 70	PO$_2$ 61-70		PO$_2$ 55-60	PO$_2$ < 55
ARTERIAL pH	≥7.7	7.6-7.69		7.5-7.59	7.33-7.49		7.25-7.32	7.15-7.24	< 7.15
SERUM SODIUM (mMol/L)	≥180	160-179	155-159	150-154	130-149		120-129	111-119	≤110
SERUM POTASSIUM (mMol/L)	≥7	6-6.9		5.5-5.9	3.5-5.4	3-3.4	2.5-2.9		<2.5
SERUM CREATININE (mg/100 ml) (Double point score for acute renal failure)	≥3.5	2-3.4	1.5-1.9		0.6-1.4		< 0.6		
HEMATOCRIT (%)	≥60		50-59.9	46-49.9	30-45.9		20-29.9		<20
WHITE BLOOD COUNT (total/mm3) (in 1,000s)	≥40		20-39.9	15-19.9	3-14.9		1-2.9		<1
GLASGOW COMA SCORE (GCS): Score = 15 minus actual GCS									
A Total ACUTE PHYSIOLOGY SCORE (APS): Sum of the 12 individual variable points									
Serum HCO$_3$ (venous-mMol/L) [Not preferred, use if no ABGs]	≥52	41-51.9		32-40.9	22-31.9		18-21.9	15-17.9	< 15

[B] AGE POINTS:
Assign points to age as follows:

AGE(yrs)	Points
≤44	0
45-54	2
55-64	3
65-74	5
≥75	6

[C] CHRONIC HEALTH POINTS
If the patient has a history of severe organ system insufficiency or is immuno-compromised assign points as follows:

a. for nonoperative or emergency postoperative patients — 5 points
or
b. for elective postoperative patients — 2 points

DEFINITIONS
Organ Insufficiency or immuno-compromised state must have been evident **prior** to this hospital admission and conform to the following criteria:

LIVER: Biopsy proven cirrhosis and documented portal hypertension; episodes of past upper GI bleeding attributed to portal hypertension; or prior episodes of hepatic failure/encephalopathy/coma.

CARDIOVASCULAR: New York Heart Association Class IV.

RESPIRATORY: Chronic restrictive, obstructive, or vascular disease resulting in severe exercise restriction, i.e., unable to climb stairs or perform household duties; or documented chronic hypoxia, hypercapnia, secondary polycythemia, severe pulmonary hypertension (>40mmHg), or respirator dependency.

RENAL: Receiving chronic dialysis.

IMMUNO-COMPROMISED: The patient has received therapy that suppresses resistance to infection, e.g., immuno-suppression, chemotherapy, radiation, long term or recent high dose steroids, or has a disease that is sufficiently advanced to suppress resistance to infection, e.g., leukemia, lymphoma, AIDS.

APACHE II SCORE
Sum of [A] + [B] + [C] :

[A] APS points ________

[B] Age points ________

[C] Chronic Health points ________

Total APACHE II ________

(From Knaus WA, Draper EA, Wagner DP, et al. APACHE II: A severity of disease classification system. *Crit Care Med* 1985;13:818–829, with permission.)

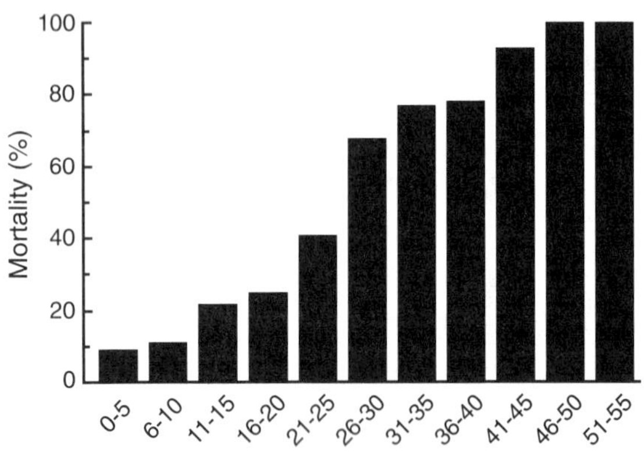

Figure 6–1. APACHE II scores versus actual hospital mortality rate for a group of consecutive medical ICU patients at one inner-city university hospital. (Kruse JA, Thill-Baharozian MC, Carlson RW. Comparison of clinical assessment with APACHE II for predicting mortality risk in patients admitted to a medical intensive care unit. *JAMA* 1988;260:1739–1742, copyright 1988, American Medical Association.)

- **Immunocompromised:** Leukemia, acquired immune deficiency syndrome (AIDS), or receiving immunosuppressive drug or radiation therapy, for example.

Therapeutic Intervention Scoring System

(see page 81 in the main text)

The Therapeutic Intervention Scoring System (TISS) was developed in the early 1970s. Unlike the other scoring systems reviewed here, TISS is based on the intensity of therapeutic support that the patient is receiving, not on physiologic variables. In the original TISS, 57 specific forms of therapy were assigned a weighted score ranging from 1 to 4 points. For example, 4 points are assigned for the use of intra-aortic balloon counterpulsation or hemodialysis. Use of a urinary catheter or supplemental oxygen by mask is assigned 1 point. The patient's final TISS score represents the total value of all points for the therapies that the patient is receiving. If treatment is not being intentionally withheld because of medical futility or other reasons, the TISS score correlates well with severity of illness and outcome.

Other Scoring Instruments

Many other scoring systems have been developed. Established and useful simple methods include the Killip (see

Table 7–1 in the main text) and New York Heart Association classification systems (see Table 7–2 in the main text) for grading the severity of congestive heart failure, Ranson's criteria (see Table 7–4 in the main text) for prediction of the severity of acute pancreatitis, and the American Society of Anesthesia Physical Status Classification (see Table 7–5 in the main text) for estimating operative risk.

Suggested Readings

Cullen DJ, Civetta JM, Briggs BA, et al. Therapeutic intervention scoring system: A method for quantitative comparison of patient care. *Crit Care Med* 1974;2:57–60.

Original full description of the TISS instrument.

Knaus WA, Draper EA, Wagner DP, et al. APACHE II: A severity of disease classification system. *Crit Care Med* 1985;13:818–829.

Original report of the APACHE II scoring instrument. Includes a mathematical method for estimating risk of death based on the APACHE II score and underlying disease state.

Knaus WA, Wagner DP, Draper EA, et al. The APACHE III prognostic system: Risk prediction of hospital mortality for critically ill hospitalized adults. *Chest* 1991;100:1619–1636.

Provides full description of the APACHE III system.

Wagner DP, Knaus WA, Draper EA. Identification of low-risk monitor admissions to medical-surgical ICUs. *Chest* 1987;92:423–428.

Examines use of the APACHE II scoring system for identifying patients at low risk of requiring ICU treatment.

Procedures

CHAPTER 7

Endotracheal Intubation in the ICU

(See Chapter 10)

Paul E. Marik and James A. Kruse

Acute respiratory failure is one of the most common reasons for admission to the medical ICU. Many critically ill patients require immediate endotracheal intubation and mechanical ventilation. The hypoxic patient is anxious, tachycardic, and often hemodynamically unstable. In addition, because of decreased functional residual capacity (e.g., as a result of pulmonary edema or pneumonia), these patients may desaturate rapidly during attempts at intubation. Further, the drugs used for sedation and anesthesia during intubation may precipitate profound hypotension or dysrhythmias. Therefore, intubating the critically ill patient requires skill and experience. Although potentially lifesaving, attempts at intubation by inexperienced clinicians may result in life-threatening complications.

Indications for Endotracheal Intubation

- **Upper-airway obstruction,** e.g., as a result of airway trauma, inhalational injury, upper-airway bleeding, or laryngeal edema.
- **Loss of airway reflexes,** necessitating airway protection, as a result of coma.
- **Increased intracranial pressure,** requiring therapeutic hyperventilation.
- **Tracheobronchial suctioning.**
- **Acute or impending respiratory failure.**
- **Apnea,** including cardiopulmonary arrest.
- **Flail chest.**

Patient Assessment

The following patient features may be associated with a difficult intubation:

- **Short neck,** with a chin-to-larynx (thyromental) distance of < 3 finger breadths.
- **Limited gape,** e.g., an interdental gap of < 2 finger breadths.

- **Protruding incisors.**
- **Limited neck extension.**
- **High, arched palate.**
- **Obesity.**

However, many patients with none of these features may be difficult to intubate. The most accepted method to assess ease of intubation involves direct visualization of the oral pharynx with the patient sitting and the tongue protruded. This type of assessment can rarely be made in an emergent situation.

Equipment Required for Intubation

All of the necessary equipment, supplies, drugs, and personnel must be present at the bedside before intubation is attempted. All items must be inspected for completeness and tested for function.

- **IV catheter.** All patients who undergo endotracheal intubation should have a free-flowing intravenous line established before the procedure is attempted.
- **Bag-valve ventilation device** to provide manual ventilation, along with an appropriately sized mask, a source of oxgen, and connecting tubing.
- **Endotracheal tubes,** including two of the anticipated size as well as a smaller and a larger tube (see below).
- **Straight laryngoscope blades,** e.g., Miller blades.
- **Curved laryngoscope blades,** e.g., MacIntosh blades.
- **Laryngoscope handle** that will accept the blades, along with working batteries and a spare lightbulb.
- **Suction source,** along with a large-bore, tonsil-tipped suction cannula and endotracheal suction catheters.
- **Magill forceps.**
- **Monitoring equipment,** ideally to include an ECG monitor and pulse oximetry apparatus.
- **Resuscitation cart** containing a defibrillator and other advanced cardiac life-support supplies and drugs.
- **Miscellaneous equipment,** including a 10-mL syringe (for cuff inflation), an oral airway, a malleable endotracheal tube stylet, local anesthetic spray, anesthethic lubricating gel, adhesive or cloth tape or other device to secure the endotracheal tube, gloves, eye protection.

Endotracheal Tube Selection

Endotracheal tubes are commonly available in internal diameter sizes ranging from 2.5 to 9.0 mm in 0.5-mm increments. Selection of the correct size tube is of the utmost importance. The resistance to airflow varies with the fourth power of the radius of the endotracheal tube. Selecting an inappropriately small tube increases the work of breathing, and may precipitate respiratory failure. Further, small tubes ($\leq$ 7.5–8.0 mm) do not permit bronchoscopic procedures to be performed through the endotracheal tube. Intubation with an inappropriately large tube may damage the larynx and vocal cords. In general, the larger the patient, the larger the endotracheal tube that should be used. Women should generally be intubated with a 7.5- or 8.0-mm tube, and men with an 8.0- or 8.5-mm tube.

IV Drugs for Intubation

Adequate sedation is crucial before orotracheal intubation is attempted. If mild IV sedation alone does not result in adequate relaxation, an induction dose can be given, alone or in conjunction with a short-acting neuromuscular blocking agent. Sedative agents may precipitate hypotension, especially in elderly patients and patients with intravascular volume depletion or underlying cardiac disease. Sedation may be achieved with incremental doses of morphine sulfate (2–5 mg), fentanyl (100 μg), midazolam (2–5 mg), or lorazepam (1 mg). The combination of an opiate and benzodiazepine may be particularly useful. Thiopental (1–2 mg/kg) can also be used, but it is a direct myocardial depressant.

Succinyl choline (1 mg/kg), atracurium (0.5 mg/kg), or vecuronium (0.1 mg/kg) may be used for neuromuscular blockade. The latter has few hemodynamic effects, and is relatively safe in patients with hyperkalemia and increased intracranial pressure. Pancuronium (0.1 mg/kg) has a longer duration of onset and also has a parasympatholytic effect that may be undesirable in the tachycardic patient. Lidocaine (1 mg/kg) IV or fentanyl (100–200 μg) given before intubation may blunt the sympathetic response to intubation. In patients who cannot be ventilated with a bag and mask, the use of paralytic agents may cause death if intubation is unsuccessful. Therefore, paralytic agents should be used only by experienced operators.

Route of Intubation

Endotracheal intubation can be accomplished by either the orotracheal or nasotracheal route. Each has advantages and disadvantages. In general, orotracheal intubation is preferred because it is rapid, is more frequently successful, and allows a larger tube to be used. However, in the conscious patient, blind nasotracheal intubation is often preferred because it affords greater patient comfort, is usually well tolerated, and does not require general anesthesia. Further, the tube is more stable and easier to secure, and mouth care is easier.

Contraindications to nasotracheal intubation include apnea, bleeding diathesis, and nasal polyps. There is a risk of intracranial placement of the endotracheal tube when the nasal route is employed in patients with basal skull fracture. Patients with suspected or confirmed cervical spine injury can be intubated by either route. If the orotracheal route is used, an assistant must provide inline cervical traction to prevent excessive extension of the neck.

Endotracheal Intubation

The initial step is to establish an airway by placing the finger of one hand under the mandible and lifting upward and backward (extending the patient's neck), or by using the index fingers of both hands to lift the mandibles from the angle of the jaw. The ability to ventilate and oxygenate the patient with a bag and mask must then be established. Care should be taken not to generate excessive pressure when ventilating by bag and mask. Airway pressure greater than 25 mm Hg is likely to overcome the resistance of the gastroesophageal sphincter, fill the patient's stomach with gas, and increase the risk of regurgitation and aspiration. When ventilation is effective, the chest rises with each squeeze of the bag. The patient should be preoxygenated in this way with 100% oxygen before intubation. If possible, arterial oxygen saturation should be monitored continuously by pulse oximetry. After a noncannulating airway is established and the patient is adequately ventilated manually, endotracheal intubation can be attempted.

Procedure of Orotracheal Intubation. The operator should stand at the head of the bed, with the height of the bed adjusted to a comfortable position. Correct positioning of the patient is an important aspect of successful intubation. The patient must be in the supine position, with the head in the *sniffing* position (i.e., with the neck flexed and the head slightly extended). This position is best achieved by placing a folded towel under the occiput. The safest approach is to assume that the patient has a full stomach and to apply pressure to the cricoid cartilage (Sellick's maneuver) to prevent aspiration of regurgitated stomach contents into the trachea.

The laryngoscope is grasped in the left hand while the patient's mouth is opened with the gloved right hand. The laryngoscope blade is inserted on the right side of the mouth and advanced to the base of the tongue, pushing the tongue to the left. If a straight blade is used, it should be extended below the epiglottis. If a curved blade is used, it is inserted into the vallecula.

With the blade in place, the operator should lift the handle of the laryngoscope forward 45 degrees from the horizontal plane to expose the vocal cords. The left wrist is kept stiff, and the arm and shoulder are used to lift the laryngoscope. It is essential to use a lifting action rather than use the patient's teeth as a fulcrum to extend the head. The endotracheal tube is then held in the right hand and inserted into the right corner of the patient's mouth. It is advanced toward the glottis and through the vocal cords, until the cuff just disappears from sight. If difficulty is encountered in advancing the tube through the cords, or when only the posterior portion of the cords is visible, it may be useful to use an introducing stylet. The plastic-coated, malleable metal stylet should be bent into the shape of a hockey stick and placed within the endotracheal tube before reinsertion. The tip of the stylet should lie close to, but not beyond, the tip of the endotracheal tube.

Orotracheal intubation is not a blind procedure; it should not be performed if the cords cannot be visualized. If the vocal cords cannot be seen with a curved blade, a straight blade may facilitate visualization. In addition, firm cricoid pressure may bring the vocal cords into view.

Procedure of Nasotracheal Intubation. The patient may be in the sitting or semirecumbant position. The nares and posterior pharynx are anesthetized with a topical anesthesic agent. A topical vasoconstrictor can also be applied intranasally. Cocaine spray or solution serves both of these functions. A 7.5- or 8.0-mm endotracheal tube can be used in most adults. Prewarming the tube in hot water softens the tube and may allow for easier intubation. The endotracheal tube should be well lubricated. It is then inserted through the nares and gently advanced until breath sounds can be heard coming from the end of the tube. At that point, the endotracheal tube is positioned just above the vocal cords. As the patient takes a breath (and the vocal cords abduct), the tube is quickly advanced through the cords and secured in position. If resistance is felt when the tube is advanced, gentle flexion (or sometimes slight extension) of the neck may facilitate correct alignment. If nasotracheal intubation is unsuccessful after two attempts, the oral route should be attempted.

Failed Intubation. As a general rule, no more than two or three attempts should be made to intubate the trachea. If these attempts are unsuccessful, airway patency should be ensured and the patient should be ventilated with 100% oxygen with a bag-valve mask until a more experienced operator is available. Further attempts at intubation may increase the risk of airway trauma and complicate subsequent attempts. Several advanced techniques are available to experienced operators. These include retrograde intubation, transtracheal ventilation, cricothyrotomy, and the use of a fiberoptic bronchoscope to facilitate intubation.

Postintubation Treatment. After successful intubation, the cuff is inflated with just enough air to prevent the loss of delivered gas from around the cuff during ventilation. The tube is then tied in position. Typically, the incisors should be at 23 cm in men and at 21 cm in women. The chest is always promptly auscultated to ensure the presence of bilateral breath sounds during positive pressure ventilation with a bag-valve mask. This observation indicates successful intubation and helps to assure that the endotracheal tube tip is above the carina. A portable chest radiograph is obtained to confirm the position of the endotracheal tube and to exclude any complications that may have occurred during the procedure. Mechanical ventilation is almost always necessary after intubation. Gas exchange should be assessed by arterial blood gas analysis.

Complications

Complications that are associated with endotracheal intubation include:

- **Upper airway trauma,** including perforation, laceration, and bleeding of the nose, mouth, oropharynx, nasopharynx, hypopharynx, larynx, or trachea.
- **Dental trauma,** including tooth avulsion.
- **Regurgitation** of stomach contents and possibly aspiration.
- **Cardiac dysrhythmias,** including cardiac arrest.
- **Esophageal intubation,** which can result in hypoxia, hypercapnia, cardiopulmonary arrest, or aspiration.
- **Mainstem bronchus intubation,** which can result in left lung atelectasis.
- **Cranial intubation,** a rare complication of nasotracheal intubation in the patient with a basal skull fracture.
- **Delayed complications,** which include laryngeal edema, sinusitis, otitis media, pneumonia, and tube blockage or kinking.
- **Late complications,** including tracheomalacia, subglottic or tracheal stenosis, tracheoesophageal fistula, and vocal cord paralysis.

In the rare instances in which an experienced operator cannot perform a successful endotracheal intubation, fiberoptic bronchoscopic intubation may be successful. In an emergency, either cricothyroidotomy or emergency tracheostomy can be performed.

Suggested Readings

Dellinger RP. Fiberoptic bronchoscopy in adult airway management. *Crit Care Med* 1990;18:882–887.
Details the procedure of endotracheal intubation using the fiberoptic bronchoscope. Briefly covers double-lumen endotracheal tube insertion and endotracheal tube changing.

Gallagher TJ. Endotracheal intubation. *Crit Care Clin* 1992;8:665–676.

Heffner JE. Timing of tracheostomy in mechanically ventilated patients. *Am Rev Respir Dis* 1993;147:768–771.
Reviews clinical studies and recommendations for timing of tracheostomy.

Concludes that most patients requiring prolonged endotracheal intubation (more than 3 weeks) should undergo tracheostomy.

Kearl RA, Hooper RG. Massive airway leaks: An analysis of the role of endotracheal tubes. *Crit Care Med* 1993;21:518–521.

In this prospective study of ICU patients, 17 patients had their endotracheal tubes removed because of the presence of massive airway leaks thought to be caused by defects in the tube. In 61% of the cases, no evidence of a mechanical defect was found after tube removal.

Sharar SR, Bishop MJ. Complications of tracheal intubation. *J Intensive Care* 1992;7:12–23.

Overview of complications associated with placement, maintenance, and removal of endotracheal tubes. Techniques to minimize these complications and their severity are suggested (85 references).

Vender JS, Shapiro BA. Essentials of artificial airway management in critical care. *Acute Care* 1987;13:97–124.

Comprehensive, illustrated review (104 references).

CHAPTER 8

Central Venous Catheterization

(See Chapter 15)

Vivian L. Clark and James A. Kruse

Indications

- IV access for patients without peripheral venous access.
- Fluid resuscitation for patients with circulatory shock, cardiopulmonary arrest, or other unstable critical illness.
- Administration of parenteral nutrition solutions.
- Access for acute hemodialysis.
- Measurement of central venous pressure.
- IV access for pulmonary artery catheterization or temporary transvenous pacing electrode placement.
- Administration of certain drugs that should not be given by peripheral IV access (e.g., vasopressors).

Contraindications

Relative contraindications include extreme obesity and severe bleeding diatheses. If a significant bleeding diathesis is present, access sites at which direct pressure cannot be applied to control bleeding should be avoided. Catheters should not be placed at the site of active local infection or in veins that are contiguous to sites of previous vascular surgical procedures, or on the same side as an arteriovenous fistula used for dialysis.

Insertion Techniques

The insertion site should be cleansed thoroughly with a suitable antiseptic, such as a povidone-iodine solution, and carefully draped. The exposed field should be kept as small as possible, although certain important proximate landmarks may remain visible. Transducers, flush solutions, IV connections, and other supplies should be ready and available before they are needed.

The preferred method for introducing central venous catheters is the Seldinger technique, in which a needle is used to insert a guidewire into the vessel and a catheter is advanced over the guidewire. In a modification of the Seldinger technique, a catheter-over-needle device, similar or identical to that commonly used for peripheral venous cannulation, is used instead of a thin-walled needle.

Femoral Catheterization

- The femoral artery is localized by palpation just below the inguinal ligament and just medial to the femoral artery.
- The site is anesthetized with 1% lidocaine without epinephrine, and a small nick in the skin is made with a #11 scalpel blade.
- The femoral artery is located, and a thin-walled 18-gauge needle, bevel up and attached to a syringe, is inserted at an approximately 45-degree angle to the skin 1 cm medial to the artery. Constant gentle suction is applied to the syringe as the needle is advanced.
- If pulsatile arterial flow is encountered, the needle should be withdrawn and pressure should be applied to the insertion site for several minutes. Subsequent attempts to enter the vein should be made slightly medial to the initial entry site.
- When venous blood is obtained and satisfactory blood return is confirmed, the syringe is disconnected. A soft-tipped, or J-tipped, guidewire is immediately advanced through the needle and into the vein several centimeters beyond the tip of the needle.
- A guidewire should not be advanced against resistance because even seemingly slight resistance may indicate subintimal or extravascular placement.
- After the guidewire has been successfully advanced into the vessel and well beyond the tip of the needle, the needle should be immediately withdrawn. The wire should then be advanced to a point slightly beyond where the tip of the catheter is to be positioned.

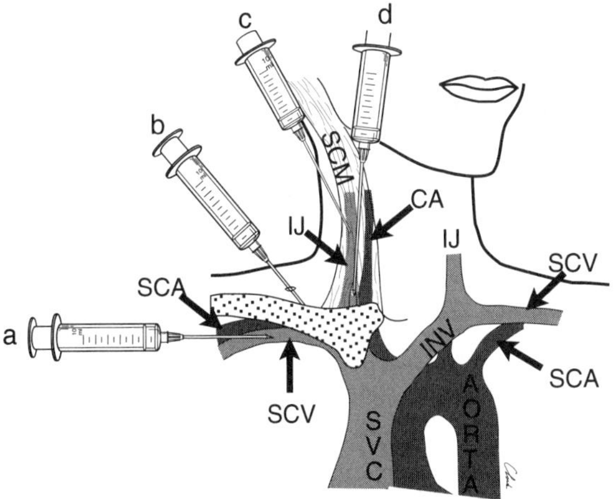

Figure 8–1. Sites of needle entry for central venous catheterization using the (a) infraclavicular subclavian approach, (b) supraclavicular subclavian approach, (c) posterior internal jugular approach, and (d) middle internal jugular approach. CA = carotid artery, IJ = internal jugular vein, INV = innominate vein, SCA = subclavian artery, SCM = sternocleidomastoid muscle, SCV = subclavian vein, SVC = superior vena cava.

- The catheter is then advanced over the wire into the vessel.
- After successful advancement of the catheter, the guidewire is removed. A syringe is immediately connected to the catheter hub. A small amount of blood is aspirated to confirm that the catheter tip is within the vessel and to remove any air from the catheter dead space before it is connected to fluid-filled intravenous tubing.

Other Central Insertion Sites. Preparation and insertion techniques are similar to the femoral technique, with the exception of the site of needle entry (Figure 8–1). For jugular or subclavian catheterization, patients should be placed in the Trendelenburg position.

- **Infraclavicular subclavian approach.** The thin-walled 18-gauge needle with attached syringe is inserted just below the middle third of the clavicle and advanced toward the suprasternal notch at a 30-degree angle from the skin. It is important to remain as close as possible to the clavicle during insertion. If the vessel is not entered, the needle should be withdrawn and redirected either slightly above or slightly below the suprasternal notch. Gentle downward traction of the ipsilateral arm may be helpful if there is difficulty locating the vessel.
- **Supraclavicular subclavian approach.** The needle is in-

serted just above the clavicle and approximately 3 cm lateral to the sternocleidomastoid muscle. It is advanced toward the contralateral nipple while constant gentle suction is maintained. The needle should be at zero degrees or a slightly negative angle to the frontal plane.

- **Posterior jugular approach.** The needle is inserted behind the sternocleidomastoid muscle, midway between the clavicle and mastoid process, and advanced toward the suprasternal notch while suction is applied with the syringe.
- **Middle jugular approach.** The needle is inserted at the apex of the triangle formed by the manubrial and clavicular heads of the sternocleidomastoid muscle and the clavicle. It is advanced toward the suprasternal notch while suction is applied with the syringe.

Peripheral Insertion Sites. Central venous catheterization can be accomplished using the basilic vein, either percutaneously or by surgical cutdown. The percutaneous basilic approach is similar to the percutaneous femoral approach, except that a tourniquet is placed on the upper extremity to increase the size of the vein before catheterization.

For an antecubital cutdown, local anesthetic is infiltrated just above the antecubital fossa, and a 2- to 3-cm transverse incision is made, extending medially from the point where the brachial artery is palpated. The subcutaneous tissue is dissected with a Kelly clamp until the vein is located. A silk tie may be used to ligate the vessel distal to the catheter insertion site. Another tie is placed loosely around the vein proximally. This tie will be used later to secure the catheter. A venotomy is made with a scalpel or eye scissors. After free blood flow is observed, a long catheter is advanced through the vein to the superior vena cava, a distance of 35–50 cm. Once the catheter tip is correctly positioned, the loose silk suture is tied around the vein to secure the catheter. The skin is closed with mattress sutures, and the catheter is anchored with a suture to the skin outside the incision.

Postcatheterization Care

- The catheter is sutured in place.
- Povidone-iodine ointment may be applied to the insertion site, and the site is covered with a sterile occlusive dressing affixed with tape.
- The IV connection tubing is secured to prevent traction on or dislodgment of the catheter.
- The location of the catheter tip is confirmed with a chest radiograph, except for short catheters inserted by the femoral approach.

- The site should be inspected daily for signs of bleeding or drainage. The dressing should be changed daily or according to institutional protocol.

Complications

Malposition occurs frequently. It can usually be identified by review of the postcatheterization chest film. In general, malpositioned catheters should be repositioned or removed to avoid additional problems.

Infectious complications include local cellulitis or abscess, septic phlebitis, bacteremia, and sepsis. The incidence of infection ranges from 0% to more than 25%, and it increases with the duration of catheterization. The insertion site should be inspected during each dressing change for signs of erythema, induration, purulent drainage, or undue tenderness. If there is evidence of infection at the catheter site, or if the patient has unexplained fever, the catheter should be removed and the tip cultured.

Pneumothorax occurs primarily after subclavian catheterization, with an incidence ranging from 0–6%. It occurs less frequently with internal jugular catheterization. A small pneumothorax may require no intervention; however, chest tube thoracostomy is often necessary, particularly in critically ill patients and those receiving positive pressure ventilation.

Inadvertent arterial puncture accounts for many of the complications associated with internal jugular catheterization. It is less common during catheterization at other sites. Arterial puncture is rarely associated with significant bleeding, even in patients with coagulopathy.

Other complications include venous thrombosis, which can result in superior vena cava syndrome or pulmonary embolism, air embolism, perforation of the right atrium or superior vena cava, brachial plexus injuries, and shearing of the catheter, with embolization of fragments to the right heart or pulmonary vessels.

Suggested Readings

CVC Working Group, Office of Training and Assistance, Food and Drug Administration. *Central venous catheter complications.* Capitol Heights, MD: National Audio-Visual Center, 1994.

Three-part videotape series covering central venous catheter complications and including a review of surgical landmarks and underlying anatomy, insertion techniques, radiologic implications, and use of peripherally inserted central venous catheters.

Kruse JA, Shah NJ. Central venous catheter-related infection. *Nutr Clin Pract* 1993;8:163–170.

Detailed review of infectious complications related to central venous catheterization, including methods of detection and prevention.

McGee WT, Ackerman BL, Rouben LR, et al. Accurate placement of central venous catheters: A prospective, randomized, multicenter trial. *Crit Care Med* 1993;21:1118–1123.

Shows that, to achieve correct positioning, central venous catheters placed by the internal jugular and subclavian route should not be routinely inserted to a depth of greater than 20 cm. The intravascular electrogram method of estimating appropriate insertion depth is explained.

Richet H, Hubert B, Nitemberg G, et al. Prospective multicenter study of vascular catheter related complications and risk factors for positive central catheter cultures in intensive care unit patients. *J Clin Microbiol* 1990;28:2520–2525.

Finds that duration of catheterization, use of semipermeable transparent dressings, and internal jugular insertion site are associated with positive cultures of central venous catheters.

Sznajder JI, Zveibil FR, Bitterman H, et al. Central vein catherization: Failure and complication rates by three percutaneous approaches. *Arch Intern Med* 1986;146:259–261.

Finds similar success and complication rates when comparing internal jugular, infraclavicular subclavian, and supraclavicular subclavian methods, with the exception of pneumothorax, which occur less frequently with the internal jugular approach.

CHAPTER 9

Pulmonary Artery Catheterization and Hemodynamic Monitoring

(See Chapters 15 and 95)

Paul E. Marik and James A. Kruse

Since its introduction in the early 1970s, millions of patients have undergone pulmonary artery (PA) catheterization. The original balloon-tipped, flow-directed catheters made possible the bedside measurement of PA pressures. Newer catheters have a variety of features that can provide additional physiologic measurements, such as:

- **Cardiovascular pressures,** including PA pressure, pulmonary artery occlusive pressure (PAOP), right atrial (RA) pressure, and right ventricular (RV) pressure.
- **Cardiac output,** measured by the thermodilution principle. Cold water of known temperature is injected through a right atrial port. As it flows past a thermistor near the tip of the catheter, a bedside computer calculates cardiac output from the area under the temperature–time curve.
- **RV ejection fraction,** also obtained by thermodilution using PA catheters equipped with a rapid-response thermistor. This modification further allows for determinations of RV end-systolic and end-diastolic volumes.

- **Mixed venous oxygen saturation,** ($S\bar{v}O_2$), assessed by drawing a blood specimen from the distal port of the catheter and analyzing the sample with a laboratory oximeter. $S\bar{v}O_2$ can also be monitored continuously with specialized catheters. A fiberoptic bundle transmits light to the tip of the catheter. Light reflected from blood within the PA is conducted through a second fiberoptic bundle back to a bedside instrument that uses the principle of reflectance spectrophotometry to measure $S\bar{v}O_2$.
- **Temporary transvenous pacing** can be performed through specialized PA catheters that have an RV port. A compatible pacing electrode is advanced through the catheter and into the right ventricle.

With the exception of temporary transvenous pacing, PA catheterization is a diagnostic rather than a therapeutic intervention. Therefore, in itself, it does not improve patient outcome. However, in certain clinical settings, interventions that optimize the physiologic variables obtained from PA catheterization may improve patient outcome. Complications associated with the procedure, or incorrect determination or interpretation of the variables obtained, may increase morbidity and mortality rates. In each patient a risk–benefit ratio must be carefully evaluated before the procedure is undertaken.

Indications for Pulmonary Artery Catheterization

Invasive hemodynamic monitoring with a PA catheter may be useful in the following circumstances:

- **Circulatory shock,** to assist with the differential diagnosis and facilitate optimization of cardiac output and other hemodynamic and oxygen-transport variables.
- **Acute myocardial infarction,** to identify and assist with the management of associated hemodynamic derangements (e.g., RV myocardial infarction or acute left ventricular failure) and mechanical complications (e.g., ventricular septal defect or papillary muscle rupture).
- **Severe heart failure,** to characterize hemodynamic derangements, optimize hemodynamic function, and assess response to therapy.
- **Respiratory distress,** to evaluate for pulmonary hypertension, differentiate cardiogenic pulmonary edema from adult respiratory distress syndrome, and assist with titration of therapy.
- **Acute oliguria,** to evaluate and optimize intravascular volume and systemic perfusion.
- **Perioperative management,** to monitor patients undergoing open-heart surgery and high-risk patients under-

going noncardiac surgery, e.g., abdominal aortic aneurysm repair.
- **Pericardial tamponade,** to confirm or exclude the diagnosis.

The information obtained from PA catheterization can guide titration of therapeutic interventions such as fluid loading; vasopressor, vasodilator, or inotropic drug infusions; ultrafiltration; positive end-expiratory pressure; and intra-aortic balloon counterpulsation.

Method of Insertion

- The patient is prepared and draped. The operator dons cap, mask, eye protection, sterile gown and gloves. Aseptic technique is used.
- The infusion and pressure monitoring lumina of the catheter are connected and flushed. All air bubbles are removed, the transducers are leveled and calibrated, and the monitoring equipment is checked to ensure proper operation. The balloon is tested for integrity and symmetric inflation. The balloon of a standard adult PA catheter should be tested with 1.5 mL air.
- The tip of the catheter is gently shaken to confirm that an undamped pressure wave can be obtained on the monitor screen.
- The jugular or subclavian vein is cannulated with an introducer sheath. The femoral vein may also be used; however, it is often more difficult to correctly position the catheter by this route. Directing the catheter into the pulmonary artery is easiest with either the left subclavian or right internal jugular approach.
- The catheter is inserted through the introducer sheath and advanced 20 cm. A central venous pressure waveform should be visible on the monitor. The balloon is fully inflated, and the catheter is advanced until an RV waveform is identified (Figure 9–1). The RV pressures are recorded.
- The catheter is advanced until a PA waveform is identified and a PAOP (wedge) tracing is obtained. The balloon is deflated to confirm that an undamped PA waveform returns. It is then slowly reinflated to reconfirm the ability to obtain a PAOP tracing. If less than 1.5 mL of air inflation results in conversion to a PAOP tracing, the catheter tip is too distal and should be partially withdrawn (after balloon deflation).
- If the catheter does not advance into the pulmonary artery, the balloon is deflated, the catheter is withdrawn back into the right atrium, the balloon is fully inflated, and the catheter is advanced again.
- After the introducer is sutured in place and the site is dressed, a chest radiograph is obtained with a portable

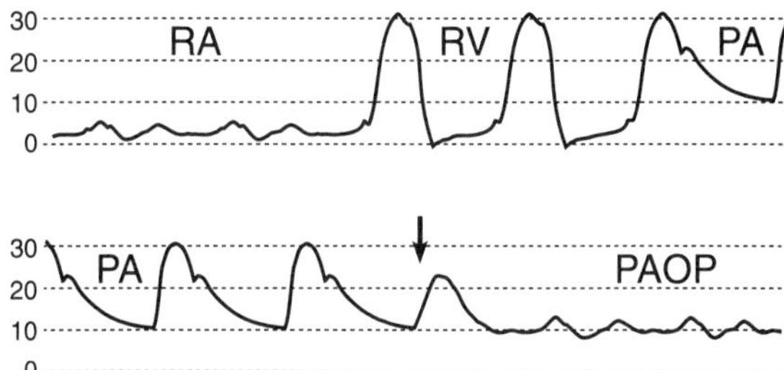

Figure 9–1. Pressure waveform sweep obtained as the PA catheter is advanced through the right heart. Upper tracing shows transition from the right atrium (RA) to the right ventricle (RV), to the pulmonary artery (PA). Arrow in lower tracing indicates balloon inflation, showing the transition from PA pressure to the PAOP waveform.

unit to exclude complications and confirm the position of the catheter.

In difficult cases, fluoroscopy, if available, may be helpful in correctly positioning the catheter. However, this procedure is rarely necessary.

Caveats During Insertion

- The balloon should not be inflated if there is undue resistance or while a PAOP tracing is visible.
- The catheter should not be advanced or withdrawn if there is undue resistance.
- The catheter should not be withdrawn with the balloon inflated.
- The balloon should not remain inflated longer than is necessary to obtain a measurement of PAOP (usually < 30 seconds).
- The monitor should be watched as the catheter is advanced. The configuration of the pressure waveform is what guides the operator.
- As the catheter is advanced, the ECG monitor should be watched for possible ventricular dysrhythmias. The balloon should be quickly deflated and the catheter tip withdrawn to the right atrium if ventricular tachycardia develops.

Hemodynamic and Oxygen Transport Variables

Table 9–1 shows the common abbreviations and the normal ranges for measured and derived hemodynamic and oxygen transport values. It also lists the formulas used to

Text continued on page 68

TABLE 9–1

HEMODYNAMIC, OXYGEN TRANSPORT, AND RELATED PHYSIOLOGIC VARIABLES, THEIR NORMAL RANGES, AND FORMULAS FOR DERIVED VARIABLES

Variable	Formula	Normal Range
Right atrial pressure (central venous pressure [CVP])	Determined by pressure transduction	1–6 mm Hg
Pulmonary artery systolic (PA_S) and diastolic (PA_D) pressure	Determined by pressure transduction	PA_S: 15–30 mm Hg PA_D: 4–12 mm Hg
Mean pulmonary artery pressure (PA_M)*	$\frac{PA_S - (2 \times PA_D)}{3}$	10–18 mm Hg
Pulmonary artery occlusive pressure (PAOP)	Determined by pressure transduction	4–12 mm Hg
Mean arterial pressure (MAP)*	$\frac{BP_S - (2 \times BP_D)}{3}$	85–100 mm Hg
Cardiac output (CO)	Determined by thermodilution	4.5–6.0 L • min^{-1}
Body surface area (BSA)	$0.007184 \times W^{0.425} \times H^{0.725}$	1.4–2.1 m^2

Cardiac index (CI)	$\frac{CO}{BSA}$	2.6–4.0 L • min^{-1} • m^{-2}
Stroke volume (SV)	$\frac{CO \times 1000}{\text{Heart rate}}$	60–90 mL
Stroke index (SI)	$\frac{SV}{BSA}$	35–50 mL • m^{-2}
Right ventricular stroke work index (RVSWI)	$0.0136 \times SI \times (PA_M - CVP)$	4–8 g • m • m^{-2}
Right ventricular ejection fraction (RVEF)	Determined by thermodilution	0.45–0.65
Right ventricular end-diastolic volume index (RVEDVI)	$\frac{SI}{RVEF}$	60–100 mL • m^{-2}
Right ventricular end-systolic volume index	$RVEDVI \times (1 - RVEF)$	30–60 mL • m^{-2}
Left ventricular stroke work index (LVSWI)	$0.0136 \times SI \times (MAP - PAOP)$	40–60 g • m • m^{-2}

Table continued on following page

TABLE 9–1 *Continued*

HEMODYNAMIC, OXYGEN TRANSPORT, AND RELATED PHYSIOLOGIC VARIABLES, THEIR NORMAL RANGES, AND FORMULAS FOR DERIVED VARIABLES

Variable	Formula	Normal Range
Systemic vascular resistance (SVR)	$\frac{(MAP - CVP) \times 80}{CO}$	900–1400 dynes • s • cm^{-5}
Systemic vascular resistance index (SVRI)	SVR × BSA	1600–2400 dynes • s • m^2 • cm^{-5}
Pulmonary vascular resistance (PVR)	$\frac{(PA_M - PAOP) \times 80}{CO}$	100–250 dynes • s • cm^{-5}
Pulmonary vascular resistance index (PVRI)	PVR × BSA	200–400 dynes • s • m^2 • cm^{-5}
Arterial O_2 content (CaO_2)	$(Hb \times 1.39 \times SaO_2) + (0.0031 \times PaO_2)$	18–20 mL/dL
Mixed venous O_2 content ($C\bar{v}O_2$)	$(Hb \times 1.39 \times S\bar{v}O_2) + (0.0031 \times P\bar{v}O_2)$	14–16 mL/dL
Alveolar oxygen tension (PAO_2)	$FIO_2 \times (P_{bar} - P_{H_2O}) - \left(\frac{PaCO_2}{RQ}\right)$	Depends on FIO_2, $PaCO_2$, and P_{bar}

Pulmonary capillary O_2 content ($Cc\text{O}_2$)	$(Hb \times 1.39) + (0.0031 \times P\text{AO}_2)$	Depends on $P\text{AO}_2$
Venous admixture ($\dot{Q}s/\dot{Q}t$)	$\frac{Cc\text{O}_2 - Ca\text{O}_2}{Cc\text{O}_2 - C\bar{v}\text{O}_2} \times 100$	$< 5\%$
Arterial–venous O_2 difference ($a\bar{v}D\text{O}_2$)	$Ca\text{O}_2 - C\bar{v}\text{O}_2$	3.6–5.0 mL/dL
Oxygen extraction	$\frac{a\bar{v}D\text{O}_2}{Ca\text{O}_2} \times 100$	20%–30%
Oxygen delivery index ($\dot{D}\text{O}_2I$)	$CI \times Ca\text{O}_2 \times 10$	550–600 mL • min^{-1}
Oxygen consumption index ($\dot{V}\text{O}_2I$)	$CI \times a\bar{v}D\text{O}_2 \times 10$	110–160 mL • min^{-1} • m^{-2}

*Calculated mean vascular pressures are only estimates. It is more accurate to obtain mean vascular pressures with pressure transduction and electronic averaging.

BP_S = systolic systemic blood pressure (mm Hg); BP_D = diastolic systemic blood pressure (mm Hg); W = body weight (kg); H = body height (cm); $F\text{IO}_2$ = fraction of inspired oxygen; P_{bar} = barometric pressure (torr); $P\text{H}_2\text{O}$ = partial pressure of water vapor at body temperature (torr); RQ = respiratory quotient (normally approximately 0.8); $Sa\text{O}_2$ = fractional arterial oxyhemoglobin saturation; Hb = blood hemoglobin concentration (g/dL); $Pa\text{O}_2$ = partial pressure of oxygen in arterial blood (torr); $S\bar{v}\text{O}_2$ = fractional mixed venous oxyhemoglobin saturation; $P\bar{v}\text{O}_2$ = partial pressure of oxygen in mixed venous blood (torr).

calculate the derived variables. The following section highlights some important facts about the most basic of these measurements obtained with the PA catheter. Optimal interpretation of these variables requires an in-depth understanding of the physiology represented by each variable as well as the ability to recognize common clinical patterns in these variables, known as hemodynamic profiles (Table 9–2).

Cardiac output is the amount of blood pumped by the heart each minute. It is a quantitation of cardiac function and systemic perfusion. The determinants of cardiac output are heart rate, preload, afterload, and intrinsic contractility. It is more meaningful to normalize this measurement to body size by converting it to cardiac index. Thermodilution measurements of cardiac output may be inaccurate in the presence of right-sided valvular insufficiency or intracardiac shunts.

Stroke volume is the volume ejected by the ventricles with each heartbeat. Stroke volume represents an adjustment of the cardiac output value for the heart rate, thus providing a measurement of cardiac function that reflects the combined effects of preload, afterload, and contractility. Like cardiac output, stroke volume should be indexed to body surface area.

Central venous pressure is the pressure within the great veins that lie in close proximity to the right atrium. For practical purposes, it is tantamount to right atrial pressure. It provides an estimate of RV preload and relative intravascular volume.

PAOP is the pressure obtained from the distal tip of the PA catheter when the balloon is inflated within the PA. It provides an estimate of left ventricular preload and relative intravascular volume. If measured correctly, PAOP should be less than the mean PA pressure. If there is more than slight variation in the PAOP waveform because of the effects of respiration, special techniques are necessary to determine PAOP accurately (see pages 1085–1086 in the main text). PAOP will not accurately reflect left ventricular preload in the presence of mitral stenosis.

PA diastolic pressure is slightly higher (approximately 1–4 mm Hg) than PAOP. A greater discrepancy indicates the presence of pulmonary hypertension. If PA diastolic pressure closely parallels PAOP in a given patient, it may be used in place of PAOP, obviating the need for periodic balloon inflation. If measured correctly, PA diastolic pressure should not be less than PAOP.

Mixed venous oxygen saturation is a reflection of overall systemic oxygen use. A decrease in $S\bar{v}O_2$ (normal is approximately 66%–74%) can be caused by arterial hypoxemia, a decrease in cardiac output, a decrease in hemoglobin concentration, or an increase in oxygen consumption. Conversely, a relative increase in $S\bar{v}O_2$ may reflect an improvement in cardiac output, arterial oxygenation, anemia, or a decrease in oxygen utilization.

Ventricular stroke work index can be calculated for the left or right ventricle. It quantifies the physical work performed by the left or right heart. The left ventricular stroke work index is a useful bedside indicator of overall pump performance. Serial values can be plotted against PAOP to obtain a clinical Starling curve, which is useful in evaluating ventricular function.

RV ejection fraction is a measure of overall RV function. It may be impaired in pulmonary embolism, RV myocardial infarction, severe acute or chronic lung disease, and states of global myocardial dysfunction. In conjunction with stroke index, it can be used to calculate RV end-diastolic volume, a direct measure of RV preload.

Systemic vascular resistance is a quantification of the degree of overall vasoconstriction or vasodilation of the systemic vascular tree. It also provides an estimate of left ventricular afterload.

Pulmonary vascular resistance is analogous to systemic vascular resistance, except that it relates to the pulmonary circulation. It is elevated in a wide variety of critical illnesses, particularly those associated with acute lung injury, many forms of chronic lung disease, pulmonary hypertension, and hypoxemia of any etiology. It is preferable to index systemic and pulmonary vascular resistance values to body surface area.

Oxygen delivery index is the volume of oxygen delivered to the systemic circulation each minute, indexed to body surface area. Its value depends on cardiac output, arterial oxygenation, and hemoglobin concentration. Normalization of inadequate oxygen delivery is a rational goal in the treatment of circulatory shock. There is emerging, but conflicting information that augmenting oxygen delivery to supranormal levels may decrease morbidity and mortality rates in certain critically ill patients. This hypothesis is the subject of continuing clinical research.

Oxygen consumption index is the volume of oxygen consumed by the body each minute, indexed to body surface area. It can be determined with expired gas analysis or derived with the Fick equation from cardiac output and arterial and mixed venous blood oxygen content. Oxygen consumption is normally determined by systemic oxygen demand. However, in circulatory shock, its value is limited by and varies directly with oxygen delivery.

Oxygen extraction is the ratio of oxygen consumption to oxygen delivery, or the overall fraction or percentage of oxygen extracted by the systemic tissues. It increases in most conditions associated with systemic hypoperfusion. It is often decreased in severe sepsis, severe hepatic disease, and several uncommon clinical conditions (e.g., arteriovenous fistula, thiamine deficiency, and Paget's disease).

TABLE 9–2

TYPICAL PROFILES OF VARIABLES OBTAINED FROM PA CATHETERIZATION IN VARIOUS FORMS OF CRITICAL ILLNESS

Illness	CI	MAP	CVP	P_{RV_D}	P_{PA_D}	PAOP	SVRI	PVRI	$S\bar{v}O_2$
Cardiogenic shock	↓	↓	↑	↑	↑	↑	↑	N–↑	↓
Severe left ventricular failure	↓	↓–N	N	N	↑	↑	↑	N–↑	↓
Acute ventricular septal defect	↓	↓	↑	↑	↑	↑	↑	N–↑	↓
Right ventricular myocardial infarction	↓	↓	↑	↑	↓–N	↓–N	↑	N	↓
Cardiac tamponade	↓	↓	↑ ≈	↑ ≈	↑ ≈	↑	↑	N–↑	↓
Critical mitral stenosis	↓	↓–N	N–↑	N–↑	↑	↑	↑	N–↑	↓
Massive pulmonary embolism	↓	↓	↑	↑	↑	↓–N	↑	↑	↓
End-stage cor pulmonale	↓	↓–N	↑	↑	↑	N	↑	↑	↓
Septic shock	↑	↓	↓–↑	↓–↑	↓–↑	↓–↑	↓	↑	↑
Hemorrhagic shock	↓	↓	↓	↓	↓	↓	↑	N–↑	↓
End-stage hepatic disease	↑	↓	↓–↑	↓–↑	↓–↑	↓–↑	↓	N–↑	↑

CI = cardiac index; MAP = mean arterial pressure; CVP = central venous pressure; P_{RV_D} = RV diastolic pressure; P_{PA_D} = PA diastolic pressure; PAOP = PA occlusive pressure; SVRI = systemic vascular resistance index; PVRI = pulmonary vascular resistance index; $S\bar{v}O_2$ = mixed venous oxyhemoglobin saturation; ↓ = decreased; ↑ = increased; N = normal; ≈ = equalization of adjacent pressures.

Venous admixture is the fraction or percentage of blood flow through the pulmonary circulation that bypasses fully or partially ventilated alveoli. It is increased in many forms of acute lung disease, notably pulmonary edema. If significantly elevated, the result is hypoxemia that is relatively refractory to therapy with supplemental oxygen. It is also called intrapulmonary shunt.

Complications Associated with PA Catheterization

PA catheterization can result in minor or life-threatening complications, including:

- **Access-related complications** that occur during central venous cannulation, such as pneumothorax, bleeding, and air embolism.
- **Cardiac dysrhythmias,** e.g., ventricular tachycardia, or condunction disturbances, e.g., complete heart block.
- **Catheter-related infection,** either localized or systemic sepsis.
- **Thrombosis** around the outside of the in-dwelling portion of the catheter, with potential for venous obstruction or pulmonary embolism.
- **Pulmonary infarction** caused by spontaneous distal migration of the catheter tip, prolonged inflation of the balloon, or thromboembolism.
- **Endocarditis** or traumatic damage to the endocardium or to the tricuspid or pulmonary valve.
- **Balloon rupture** as a result of excessive balloon inflation volume, repeated inflations, or the use of expired catheters.
- **Catheter knotting** within the heart or great veins. Risk increases with excessive manipulation, with excessive insertion distance, and in patients with dilated right heart chambers.
- **Pulmonary artery rupture,** with the potential for pulmonary hemorrhage, massive hemoptysis, and death.
- **Thrombocytopenia** as a result of the use of heparin-bonded catheters.

Suggested Readings

Bressack MA, Raffin TA. Importance of venous return, venous resistance, and mean circulatory pressure in the physiology and management of shock. *Chest* 1987;92:906–912.

Reviews physiology of venous return, its role as a determinant of cardiac output, and its clinical relevance.

Daily EK, Schroeder JS. *Techniques in bedside hemodynamic monitoring,* 4th ed. St. Louis: CV Mosby, 1989.

Ermakov S, Hoyt JW. Pulmonary artery catheterization. *Crit Care Clin* 1992;8:773–806.

Contains useful information on indications, contraindications, insertion tech-

niques, acquisition of hemodynamic information, clinical utility, and complications (115 references).

Hayes MA, Timmins AC, Yau EHS, et al. Elevation of systemic oxygen delivery in the treatment of critically ill patients. *N Engl J Med* 1994;330:1717–1722.

Randomized trial examining the effect of augmenting cardiac index and oxygen delivery using dobutamine in fluid-resuscitated patients. The treatment group had a significantly higher mortality rate than the control patients.

Mimoz O, Rauss A, Rekik N, et al. Pulmonary artery catheterization in critically ill patients: A prospective analysis of outcome changes associated with catheter-prompted changes in therapy. *Crit Care Med* 1994;22:573–579.

Shows that pulmonary artery catheterization in certain patients frequently identifies unexpected hemodynamic findings and is associated with improved outcome, independent of other variables affecting prognosis.

Sprung CL, Elser B, Schein RMH, et al. Risk of right bundle-branch block and complete heart block during pulmonary artery catheterization. *Crit Care Med* 1989;17:1–3.

In this prospective study involving 279 evaluable pulmonary artery catheterizations, 3% were associated with the development of a new right bundle branch block. Recommends that external and transvenous pacemakers be available on standby for patients with preexisting left bundle branch block who undergo pulmonary artery catheterization.

Tuchschmidt J, Fried J, Astiz M, et al. Elevation of cardiac output and oxygen delivery improves outcome in septic shock. *Chest* 1992; 102:216–220.

Randomized trial showing that increasing cardiac index to supranormal levels significantly improves chance of survival in patients with septic shock.

CHAPTER 10

Arterial Blood Pressure Monitoring

(See Chapters 15 and 20)

James A. Kruse and Vivian L. Clark

Indications and Contraindications

Catheterization of a systemic artery is indicated for continuous arterial blood pressure monitoring and for frequent arterial blood sampling. The former indication is commonly required for optimal management of critically ill patients with hypotension or severe hypertension or those who are otherwise unstable. The latter indication is usually reserved for patients who require serial arterial blood gas analysis.

Relative contraindications include marked bleeding diatheses and severe peripheral vascular disease. Arterial puncture should be avoided in vessels with bruits or locally diminished pulsation. It should not be performed at sites of previous vascular surgery, through synthetic graft material, or in the vicinity of previous arterial thromboembolism.

Site Selection

The most common access sites are the radial, femoral, brachial, and axillary arteries. The radial artery is frequently employed because of the low risk of serious vascular complications and because the site offers optimal patient comfort. For patients with circulatory shock, the femoral artery may be more easily cannulated and may yield more accurate measurements.

Before the site is selected, the adequacy of the peripheral circulation should be evaluated by examining the distal pulses and looking for other signs of arterial insufficiency. Before radial artery catheterization is performed, an Allen test should be performed to ensure adequate collateral circulation to the hand by way of the ulnar artery (see page 236 in the main text).

Catheterization Technique

A variety of catheter types is available for arterial cannulation, including catheter-over-needle and catheter-plus-guidewire devices. Radial artery catheterization with the Seldinger method is described:

- The hand and forearm are supinated and immobilized. A small folded towel is placed under the wrist to maintain extension. The site is cleansed with povidoneiodine.
- By palpation, the radial artery just proximal to the wrist crease is located. A small amount of local anesthetic (lidocaine) is instilled at the site.
- The needle is inserted parallel to the vessel at an approximately 30- to 45-degree angle. It is advanced slowly until blood return is obtained. A syringe should not be attached to the needle during arterial cannulation because it is unnecessary and may interfere with immediate recognition of arterial puncture.
- If the vessel is not entered, the needle is withdrawn. The entry site or angle of insertion is changed slightly, and insertion is attempted again. To prevent laceration of the vessel, the direction of needle insertion should never be changed until the needle is completely or nearly completely withdrawn.
- When pulsatile blood return is obtained, the guidewire is advanced well beyond the tip of the needle, and the needle is withdrawn. Guidewire placement should not be attempted unless pulsatile blood is flowing from the

needle hub, and the guidewire should not be advanced against resistance. The guidewire is advanced sufficiently so that the tip of the wire lies farther upstream than the planned position of the catheter tip.

- After successful guidewire insertion, a small nick is made in the skin with a #11 scalpel blade, and the catheter is advanced over the wire. Pausing occasionally to check the guidewire for undue resistance assures that the catheter and wire are not kinking within the subcutaneous space.
- The catheter hub is connected to the previously readied, fluid-filled monitoring tubing, pressure transducer, and flush device. The catheter is flushed briefly, and the operator confirms that a typical arterial pressure waveform is visible on the monitor.

A catheter-over-needle device may be used for radial, but not femoral, artery cannulation instead of the needle-and-guidewire method. Placement is similar to that of a peripheral venous catheter. After pulsatile blood return is observed, the catheter is advanced over the needle and into the vessel, and the needle is then removed. Blood return from the catheter should be confirmed before it is connected to the transducer and flush device.

Postcatheterization Care

The catheter must be connected to the pressure transducer and continuous-flush device with low-compliance tubing. The height of the air–fluid interface of the zeroing stopcock on the transducer is adjusted to the level of the midchest. The electronic system is calibrated according to the manufacturer's instructions. The site is dressed and maintained as for central venous catheters. The involved extremity is gently immobilized to prevent flexion at the insertion site, which can result in spuriously low pressure readings. The extremity and pulses distal to the insertion site should be checked regularly. If there is evidence of arterial insufficiency (e.g., diminished or absent pulses, coolness, or mottling of the skin), the catheter should be removed to avert more serious complications.

Evaluating Dynamic Response

When using fluid-filled catheter–transducer systems to measure arterial pressures, the operator should assess the resonant frequency and dynamic response of the system. A poor dynamic response will result in inaccurate pressure measurements. Although there are more sophisticated methods of evaluating dynamic response, the simplest is the fast-flush technique. This procedure is quickly and easily performed at the bedside with the pressurized flush

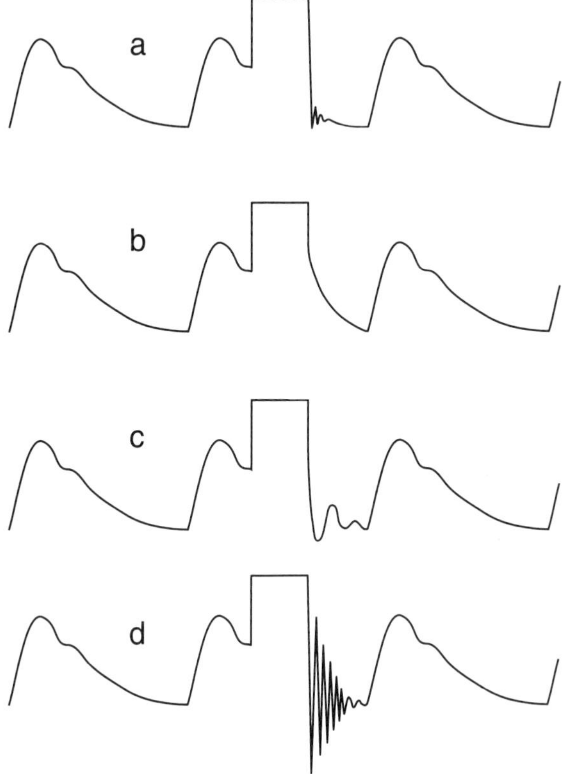

Figure 10–1. Stylized pressure versus time waveforms illustrating the results of the fast-flush test for evaluating dynamic response of arterial pressure monitoring systems. *A*. Optimal dynamic response. *B*. Overdamped system. *C*. Unacceptably low-resonant frequency. *D*. Hyperresonant, underdamped system.

mechanism that is part of standard continuous irrigation devices commonly used to maintain the patency of arterial catheters.

The catheter is flushed for approximately 1 second, and the operator observes the waveform on the monitor as the flush is abruptly discontinued. A square waveform will be visible on the monitor during the flush, followed by a brief period of damped oscillation (Figure 10–1). Lack of any oscillation indicates overdamping; excessive oscillation (ringing) indicates underdamping or a suboptimal resonant frequency. An overdamped waveform produces artifactually low systolic pressure readings; an underdamped waveform yields a spuriously elevated systolic pressure measurement.

An underdamped, hyperresonant system can be caused by:

- Use of small-bore catheters.
- Excessive numbers of stopcocks or connections.
- Inappropriately long or short connecting tubing.
- Certain patient characteristics (e.g., severe tachycardia, increased inotropic state, or noncompliant vasculature).

Overdamping can be caused by:

- Air bubbles in the transducer or connecting tubing.
- Kinking of the catheter or connecting tubing.
- Use of an excessive number of stopcocks.
- Use of high-compliance tubing (such as regular IV tubing) instead of low-compliance tubing.
- Blood clots within the catheter or tubing.
- Excessively long connecting tubing.

Accurate systolic pressure measurement is dependent on an adequate dynamic response. Diastolic pressure accuracy is less dependent, and mean arterial pressure is practically immune from these effects.

Complications

- **Infection** risk is similar to but less than that for venous catheters. It increases with the duration of catheterization. To minimize infectious complications, catheters should be removed as soon as the clinical situation warrants. If infection is suspected, the catheter tip should be cultured.
- **Bleeding** complications are more common in patients with coagulopathy or in those receiving anticoagulants, particularly thrombolytic agents. If possible, anticoagulants should be stopped or reversed before insertion or removal of arterial catheters.
- **Ischemia** may occur as a result of thrombosis or embolization, vascular spasm, dissection, or rarely, cholesterol emboli. Significant sequelae are uncommon, although surgical thrombectomy may be necessary. In rare instances, loss of digits or of the limb may occur. The risk of ischemic complications is augmented by use of the brachial approach, long-term catheterization, increasing catheter diameter, concomitant use of vasopressor agents, and the presence of atherosclerosis, hypertension, hypotension, or low-flow states. A pulse deficit or any manifestation of limb ischemia mandates prompt removal of the catheter. Removal alone often results in restoration of the pulse and alleviation of ischemia without need for further intervention. Persistent clinical evidence of ischemia is generally an indication for exploration and thrombectomy.

- **Other potential complications** include pseudoaneurysm and arteriovenous fistula formation. These conditions are most often noted after catheter removal and may not become apparent for several days after removal. Pain at the insertion site is common, and a pulsatile mass and bruit may be present. Doppler ultrasound imaging or digital subtraction angiography can be used to confirm the diagnosis. Surgical repair may be required.

Suggested Readings

Clark VL, Kruse JA. Arterial catheterization. *Crit Care Clin* 1992; 8:687–697.

Reviews arterial catheterization including indications, insertion techniques, and complications.

Gardner RM. Hemodynamic monitoring: From catheter to display. *Acute Care* 1986;12:3–33.

Detailed review of technical yet practical aspects of transducer-based pressure monitoring.

Leroy O, Billiau V, Beuscart C, et al. Nosocomial infections associated with long-term radial artery catheterization. *Intensive Care Med* 1989;15:241–246.

Although other investigations have shown a low but finite incidence of catheter-related infection using the radial artery, there were no cases of infection in this study involving 164 catheters maintained in place for an average of 6.5 days.

Mathers LH Jr. Anatomical considerations in obtaining arterial access. *J Intensive Care Med* 1990;5:110–119.

Reviews anatomical landmarks, selection criteria, and risks involved in arterial catheterization of the radial, ulnar, brachial, axillary, femoral, posterior tibial, dorsalis pedis, and superficial temporal arteries (96 references).

Pauca AL, Wallenhaupt SL, Kon ND, et al. Does radial artery pressure accurately reflect aortic pressure? *Chest* 1992;102:1193–1198.

In this study of 51 patients, measurements of systolic blood pressure from radial artery catheters correlated poorly with systolic pressures measured in the ascending aorta. Radial artery mean and diastolic pressure were within 3 mm Hg of corresponding aortic pressures in approximately 90% of patients.

CHAPTER 11

Temporary Transvenous Cardiac Pacing

(See Chapter 15)

James A. Kruse and Roderick J. Boyes

Temporary cardiac pacing is commonly performed with either transcutaneous or transvenous electrical pacing.

The former is accomplished with externally applied electrodes. It is simple to use, but is sometimes limited by its reliability and by patient discomfort. Transcutaneous pacing is often used in emergency circumstances before a transvenous pacing electrode is inserted. This chapter describes the indications, techniques, and complications of temporary transvenous cardiac pacing.

Indications

- Symptomatic bradycardia unresponsive to pharmacologic drugs.
- Symptomatic high-degree or complete heart block.
- Acute myocardial infarction with new bundle branch block (see Tables 90–16 and 94–2 in the main text and Table 29–3 in this book).
- Overdrive pacing for control of certain tachyarrhythmias.
- High-degree heart block in patients going to surgery.

Equipment

Insertion of a temporary pacemaker is facilitated by ensuring that all needed supplies and equipment are available before the procedure is performed. These include:

- Supplies necessary for obtaining central venous access (antiseptic, local anesthetic, syringes, needles, guidewire, etc.).
- Masks, hats, eye protection, sterile gowns, gloves, and drapes.
- Introducer sheath (introducer size must be selected to conform to the pacing catheter diameter to prevent air embolism or blood loss through the sheath).
- Transvenous ventricular pacing electrode.
- Pacemaker generator and batteries, in working condition.
- ECG machine or suitable portable monitor.
- Alligator clip connecting wire.

Transvenous pacing catheters range from 4 to 7 Fr in diameter. Bipolar catheters are the most frequently used. Some are equipped with a balloon at the tip to facilitate floatation into the right ventricle.

Procedure

An introducer sheath is first inserted with the Seldinger technique (see Chapter 8 in this book). The right internal jugular vein and left subclavian vein are the preferred access sites. The femoral veins may be used when fluoroscopy is available or when other sites are not accessible. Rigid adherence to aseptic technique is mandatory throughout the procedure. If the pacing catheter is flow directed (i.e., balloon tipped), the balloon should be checked before insertion to ensure that it is intact. Two insertion techniques are described, the blind method and the ECG-guided method. With either technique, the pacing catheter is first advanced through the introducer sheath (with the balloon deflated) to just beyond the end of the sheath. At that point, the balloon is fully inflated.

With the blind technique, the pacing electrodes are connected to the pulse generator and the pacing catheter is advanced into the right ventricle with the balloon inflated. Correct placement is usually approximately 25 or 30 cm from the right internal jugular or left subclavian access site, respectively. The balloon is then deflated. The pacemaker is turned on, and its rate control is adjusted to a level greater than the patient's intrinsic heart rate. Narrow pacemaker spikes should be evident on the ECG monitor. The catheter is advanced a few more centimeters while the ECG is observed for capture. Capture is recognized by the finding of wide-complex, ventricular-type beats, with a left bundle branch block pattern occurring consistently after each pacemaker spike. If capture is successful and the pacing and sensing thresholds are adequate (see below), the catheter is assumed to be appropriately positioned. If pacing is not achieved or is suboptimal, repositioning is required. This method of placement is useful during initial placement in emergency situations.

In most cases, the ECG-guided method is recommended over blind insertion. With the ECG-guided technique, the limb leads of a 12-lead ECG machine are preconnected to the patient's extremities before the procedure is begun. With attention given to maintaining the sterility of the rest of the catheter, the distal electrode connection of the pacing catheter is attached to the V_1 precordial lead of the ECG machine with an alligator clip connecting wire. After the catheter is introduced to just beyond the end of the sheath, the balloon is inflated and the catheter advanced under continuous internal ECG monitoring. If the atria are contracting, large inverted P waves are observed as the electrode enters the right atrium (Figure 11–1b). As the electrode is advanced into the right ventricle, a large ventricular complex is seen (Figure 11–1e). The balloon is then deflated, and the catheter is further advanced until it contacts the endocardium. This contact is heralded by an injury pattern on the intracavitary electrogram (Figure 11–1f). The external connectors of the pacing electrodes are attached to the pulse generator, and pacing is attempted.

A third method is placement under fluoroscopic guidance. This method allows visual positioning of the catheter, but it cannot be performed at the bedside at most cen-

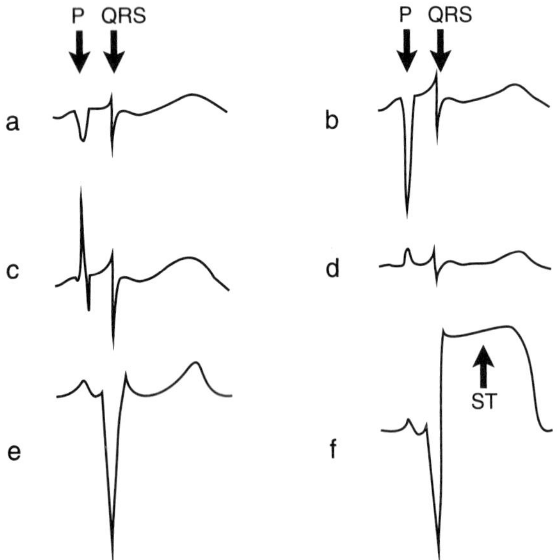

Figure 11–1. Intracavitary electrograms obtained from a transvenous pacing electrode as it is advanced into (a) the superior vena cava, (b) the high right atrium, (c) the mid-right atrium, (d) the inferior vena cava, and (e) the right ventricle. Note the relative height of P waves when the electrode is within the right atrium and also that the P wave deflection changes from predominantly negative to predominantly positive as the electrode passes through the atrium. Contact with the right ventricular endocardium (f) results in an injury pattern (ST elevation).

ters. Regardless of the method of placement, a chest radiograph should be obtained to assess the position of the pacing electrode and to exclude complications (see page 269 in the main text).

Pulse Generator Controls

Typical controls available on a minimally configured, non-AV sequential, demand-mode, external pulse generator include:

- **On/off control.** Turns the pulse generator on and off. Most pacemakers employ a safety lock device to prevent accidentally switching the generator off.
- **Rate control.** Sets the pacing frequency. Typically, this dial is calibrated for rates between 30 and 180 min^{-1}.
- **Output control.** Sets the electrical current (amperage) delivered during pulse generation. Typically, the out-

put control is calibrated from 0.1 to 20 mA. It is normally set to a level just above the minimum current necessary to achieve reliable pacing (see below).

- **Sensitivity control.** Sets the voltage threshold at which the patient's R wave suppresses pulse generation. The control typically ranges from 1 to more than 20 mV, and it is used to optimize the pulse inhibition threshold during demand pacing. The lower the voltage threshold setting, the higher the sensitivity for detecting intrinsic QRS complexes.

For treatment of bradyarrhythmias, the rate control is usually set to a level greater than the patient's intrinsic heart rate. For patients who currently have an adequate intrinsic rate, this control can be set to a backup rate of 50 to 60 min^{-1}. Optimal settings for the output and sensitivity controls are arrived at by determining the pacing and sensing thresholds.

Determining Pacing Threshold

To measure the pacing, or stimulation, threshold, the rate is set to a level at least 10 min^{-1} higher than the patient's intrinsic rate, the output is set to approximately 5 mA, the sensitivity set at 1.5–3 mV, and the pulse generator is turned on. A light-emitting diode (usually labeled *pace*) on the generator control panel blinks in synchrony with each fired pulse. Pacing spikes should be evident on the surface ECG, and consistently followed by ventricular capture beats. The output level is gradually reduced until capture no longer occurs and the heart reverts to its intrinsic rate. At this point, pacing spikes may be seen on the monitor, but they are not followed by captured complexes. The threshold current level at which capture is first lost is the pacing threshold. This level is reconfirmed by increasing the output slightly to show that capture is regained. The optimal pacing threshold is less than 2 mA. As a safety margin, the output control is set to a level greater than the patient's stimulation threshold. For example, if the threshold is 1.5 mA, the output control may be set to 5 mA. The electrode catheter should be repositioned if the stimulation threshold exceeds approximately 5 mA.

Determining Sensing Threshold

When the sensitivity control is set to the highest voltage value (often labeled *async* on the generator dial), the generator operates in the asynchronous mode. In this mode, pulse generation occurs regardless of the patient's intrinsic rhythm or rate. This setting is not generally used because it can precipitate ventricular tachycardia if the pulse fires at the right moment immediately after an intrinsic

TABLE 11–1

TEMPORARY TRANSVENOUS PACEMAKER TROUBLESHOOTING

Problem	Likely Cause	Intervention
Failure to capture	Catheter malposition	Reposition catheter
	Battery expended	Change battery
	Low current output	Increase current output
	Disconnected or loose wire	Check connections
Failure to sense	Catheter malposition	Reposition catheter
	Low sensitivity setting	Increase sensitivity level
	Electrical interference	Eliminate source of interference
Oversensing	High sensitivity setting	Decrease sensitivity
	Electrical interference	Eliminate source of interference

(Adapted from Jafri SM, Kruse JA. Temporary transvenous cardiac pacing. *Crit Care Clin* 1992;8:713–725.)

beat. When the sensitivity control is set to any other position, the generator is said to be in demand mode, i.e., the generator fires only when there are no intrinsic beats, or when the intrinsic beat has an R wave voltage less than the sensitivity voltage setting. When the pacemaker detects an R wave that exceeds the sensitivity setting, a light-emitting diode (usually labeled *sense*) on the generator control panel blinks on, and pulse generation is inhibited. The sensing threshold is the highest voltage setting at which the pacemaker detects the patient's intrinsic ventricular beats. If the sensitivity control is set to a higher voltage, sensing ability is lost, the pulse generator is not inhibited by the patient's intrinsic ventricular beats, and the pacemaker is in effect operating asynchronously. In practice, the sensitivity control is set to a voltage much lower than the sensing threshold. False sensing (oversensing) may occur if the sensitivity control is set too low. In this situation, interfering electrical discharges from T waves, somatic myopotentials, or other artifacts are interpreted as R waves, and they erroneously inhibit pulse generation. The sensitivity control should be adjusted to determine whether oversensing occurs. This adjustment is made by increasing the sensitivity (decreasing the voltage threshold setting) until false sensing is noted. If false sensing occurs, the sensitivity control is optimally set to a level midway between the sensing threshold and the oversensing threshold.

Complications

- Complications associated with central venous access (e.g., bleeding, pneumothorax, air embolism, thrombosis).
- Dysrhythmias precipitated by contact of the electrode tip with the endocardium.
- Perforation of the right atrium or right ventricle, with possible pericardial tamponade or ventricular septal defect.
- Diaphragmatic or skeletal muscle (chest wall) pacing.
- Infection, including insertion-site infection, bacteremia, endocarditis, or sepsis.
- Pacemaker failure (e.g., battery or electronic failure, displacement or disconnection of electrode).
- Other causes of capture failure, sensing failure, or oversensing (see Table 11–1).

Suggested Readings

Fitzpatrick A, Sutton R. A guide to temporary pacing. *Br Med J* 1992;304:365–369.

Practical review of the procedure.

Jafri SM, Kruse JA. Temporary transvenous cardiac pacing. *Crit Care Clin* 1992;8:713–725.

Detailed review of indications, equipment, techniques, complications, and troubleshooting of temporary transvenous pacemakers.

Madsen JK, Meibom J, Videbak R, et al. Transcutaneous pacing: Experience with the Zoll noninvasive temporary pacemaker. *Am Heart J* 1988;116:7–10.

Describes a case series of patients undergoing temporary pacing using an external, noninvasive, transcutaneous pacemaker. Pacing was achieved in 33 of 35 patients. All patients had contractions of thoracic and shoulder muscles, and the majority of conscious patients reported feeling some discomfort during electrical discharges.

CHAPTER 12

Pericardiocentesis

(See Chapters 15, 92, and 95)

Roderick J. Boyes and James A. Kruse

Indications and Contraindications

Pericardiocentesis is used as a diagnostic procedure to obtain pericardial fluid for analysis or as a therapeutic procedure to treat cardiac tamponade. The differential diagnosis of pericardial effusion is broad (see Table 14–6 in the main text). Common causes of pericardial effusion and tamponade are malignancy, infection, and trauma. Because it provides a higher diagnostic yield, open pericardiotomy with biopsy should be considered when the diagnosis is unknown and if time permits. Relative contraindications to pericardiocentesis include thrombocytopenia, coagulopathy, an uncooperative patient, operator inexperience, and lack of proper monitoring and resuscitation equipment. There are no absolute contraindications for using pericardiocentesis to treat cardiac tamponade.

Procedure

Except in emergencies, pericardiocentesis should be performed in a monitored setting with full resuscitation equipment immediately available. The presence of pericardial effusion should be confirmed with an imaging technique such as echocardiography or computed tomography. If echocardiographic guidance is to be used during the procedure, arrangements are made for having an echocardiograph available. For electrocardiographic guidance, two ECG machines may be employed, one for continuous surface ECG monitoring and one for monitoring the pericardiocentesis needle position. Alternatively, a single ECG monitor capable of displaying two simultaneous ECG channels can be used. The ECG electrodes are connected to the patient's limbs. Supplemental oxygen, resuscitation equipment and drugs, and all supplies needed for the procedure must be available before the procedure is begun. The patient is positioned in a 30- to 45-degree upright position to facilitate accumulation of pericardial fluid on the diaphragmatic surface. The stomach is decompressed with a nasogastric tube, and the patient may be given a sedative or narcotic. If not already available, reliable IV access is established. The subxiphoid area is thoroughly prepared with a suitable antiseptic (e.g., povidone-iodine), and a sterile field is created with sterile drapes. The operator wears hat, mask, eye protection, sterile gloves and gown.

Although several trajectories have been described and used successfully, the left subxiphoid approach with left shoulder trajectory is commonly used. It is described in the following sequence:

- A site 1–2 cm below the xiphoid process, 1–2 cm toward the left arm, and 1–2 cm below the left costal margin is located by palpation.
- A 22-gauge needle is used to inject local anesthetic (1% lidocaine without epinephrine) at the intended insertion site and along the intended tract.
- An 18-gauge, thin-walled spinal or similar needle and a 20-mL syringe are used to aspirate fluid from the pericardial space. Before the needle is introduced, the proximal portion of the metal needle shaft is first connected to the V lead of the guiding ECG machine channel with a sterile alligator clip connecting wire (see Figure 12–1 in this chapter and Figure 14–9 in the main text).
- The needle enters the skin at the described surface location and is directed toward the left shoulder at a 45-degree angle to the body. As the needle is advanced, the subsurface electrogram is monitored for the appearance of a characteristic high-amplitude epicardial injury pattern that signifies needle contact with the epicardium. The needle must be at least partially withdrawn if this contact occurs.
- In most patients, pericardial fluid should be aspirated when the needle is inserted to a depth of 2 to 8 cm.

If fluid is not obtained, a second attempt may be performed using the same trajectory, but at a 60-degree angle, or instead, aiming toward the right shoulder while the subsurface ECG is monitored. Once the needle enters the pericardial space, fluid is aspirated into the syringe. A J-tipped guidewire may be inserted through the needle, and a plastic catheter may be placed in the pericardium prior to

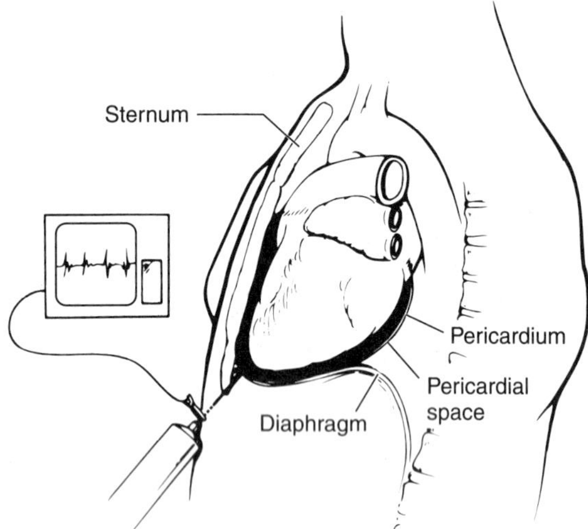

Figure 12–1. Equipment and position of the needle during a subxiphoid approach to pericardiocentesis. (Adapted from Kirkland LL, Taylor RW. Pericardiocentesis. *Crit Care Clin* 1992;8:699–712.)

drainage. Aspirated fluid is sent for the desired diagnostic laboratory studies. These may include complete cell count and differential; hematocrit; glucose and protein concentrations; pH; cytologic examination; Gram, fungal, and acid-fast stains; and microbiologic cultures. If grossly hemorrhagic fluid is aspirated, an aliquot should be observed to determine whether it spontaneously clots. Clotting indicates that circulating blood was obtained, rather than true hemopericardium. A postprocedure chest radiograph is required to exclude complications, such as pneumothorax.

Complications

(see Table 14–7 in the main text)

Inadvertent perforation of the pleura, lung, liver, diaphragm, bowel, cardiac chambers, coronary arteries, or other vessels can occur, resulting in hemorrhage, myocardial infarction, pneumothorax, infection, or other complications. Induced hemopericardium can also occur. Complications are reduced with the use of electrocardiographic or echocardiographic guidance. Blind pericardiocentesis entails considerable risk and should be used only during a crisis.

Suggested Readings

Ameli S, Shah PK. Cardiac tamponade: Pathophysiology, diagnosis, and management. *Cardiol Clin* 1991;9:665–674.

Reviews cardiac tamponade, including the electrocardiographic, echocardiographic, Doppler flow, and hemodynamic findings (50 references).
Kirkland LL, Taylor RW. Pericardiocentesis. *Crit Care Clin* 1992; 8:699–712.
Reviews the etiologies and pathophysiology of cardiac tamponade, use of various diagnostic imaging modalities, and indications, contraindications, and complications of pericardiocentesis and surgical pericardial drainage.
Markiewicz W, Borovik R, Ecker S. Cardiac tamponade in medical patients: Treatment and prognosis in the echocardiographic era. *Am Heart J* 1986;111:1138–1142.
Report of 36 patients with cardiac tamponade treated with various interventions. Pericardiocentesis was used initially in 34 patients and successfully relieved the tamponade in 30. Delay in diagnosis was frequent, and was a factor in three deaths.
Park SC, Pahl E, Ettedgui JA, et al. Experience with a newly developed pericardiocentesis set. *Am J Cardiol* 1990;66:1529–1531.
Detailed description of percutaneous placement of pericardial catheters using the Seldinger technique.

CHAPTER 13

Chest Tube Thoracostomy

(See Chapter 14)

Roderick J. Boyes and
James A. Kruse

Indications and Contraindications

(see Table 14–2 in the main text)

Urgent or emergent closed chest tube thoracostomy is a common procedure in the ICU for the treatment of pneumothorax and drainage of pleural fluid collections. Specific indications include:

- **Hemothorax** as a result of spontaneous bleeding (e.g., from an aneurysm or arteriovenous malformation), iatrogenic injury during a procedure (e.g., thoracentesis or central venous catheterization), or trauma.
- **Pneumothorax,** either spontaneous (e.g., from a ruptured emphysematous bleb or asthma), iatrogenic (e.g., resulting from an invasive procedure or positive pressure ventilation), surgical (e.g., after thoracotomy), or traumatic (e.g., from a stab or gunshot wound) (also see pages 868–871 in the main text).
- **Empyema** and certain parapneumonic effusions.
- **Miscellaneous indications,** e.g., chylothorax or pleurodesis.

Relative contraindications include coagulopathy, thombocytopenia, and pleural malignancy or adhesions at the intended site of insertion. In patients with tension pneumothorax, the potential benefit of emergency chest tube placement outweighs the added risk associated with these conditions.

Preparation

The chest radiograph documenting the indication for the procedure should be reviewed by the operator (see Chapter 21 in the main text). All necessary supplies and equipment should be available before the procedure is begun. Needles, syringes, povidone-iodine, local anesthetic, a Kelly or similar clamp, scalpel, gauze sponges, and adhesive tape should be at hand. Many hospitals have premade equipment trays for thoracostomy tube placement. The size of the chest tube selected depends on the viscosity of the fluid to be drained. A 32 to 42 Fr tube should be used to drain viscous fluid from a hemothorax or empyema. Smaller tubes (e.g., 20 to 30 Fr) can be used for removing air or serous fluid. A commercially available integral thoracostomy drainage system is usually employed (see below). It should be set up in advance of the procedure.

Before the procedure is started, it is explained to the patient to reduce anxiety and increase cooperation. All patients should have IV access. If appropriate, supplemental oxygen and a sedative or narcotic may be administered. The operator should wear a surgical mask, hat, eye protection, sterile gown and gloves.

If a patient has a suspected tension pneumothorax, an immediately life-threatening condition, a 14- to 18-gauge IV catheter-over-needle device should be placed quickly. It is inserted into the pleural space at the second intercostal space on the side of the pneumothorax as a temporizing procedure to release the tension. A standard chest tube can then be inserted as described below.

Procedure

(see pages 164–166 in the main text)

The two most common sites are the second intercostal space at the midclavicular line, and either the fourth, fifth, or sixth intercostal space at the midaxillary line. The former site is most frequently used for treating pneumothorax, and the latter is used for removing either air, pleural effusions, or blood from the pleural cavity. The procedure for the lateral approach, with entry into the pleura at the fifth intercostal space, is described below. Evidence of previous thoracic surgery, obtained from either the history, physical examination, or chest radiograph, should prompt reconsideration of the intended entry site to avoid encountering adhesions.

- The sixth intercostal space is located by counting down from the second rib (identified as adjacent to the sternal angle of Louis). The skin incision is made at the sixth intercostal space at the midaxillary line, one intercostal space inferior to the intended site of pleural entry.
- The patient is placed in a 30-degree upright position with the ipsilateral arm above the head. A wide area of the lateral chest wall is thoroughly prepared with povidone-iodine, and sterile drapes are positioned around the intended insertion site to create a sterile field.
- With a 22-gauge needle, the skin is infiltrated with 1% lidocaine with epinephrine at the site of the intended incision.
- Additional anesthetic is injected into the underlying soft tissue and intercostal muscles at the intended incision site and also below the immediately superior (in this case, fifth) intercostal space. Finally, the parietal pleura is anesthetized immediately above the sixth rib. Before each injection, the syringe is aspirated to ensure that a blood vessel has not been entered. During deep instillation of anesthesia, air or pleural fluid may be aspirated unintentionally, or intentionally to confirm that the pleura has been anesthetized.
- A 2- to 4-cm skin incision is made in the sixth intercostal space parallel to the ribs, and hemostasis is obtained. Blunt dissection is performed with a Kelly or similar clamp to create a subcutaneous tract into the sixth intercostal space, over the superior margin of the sixth rib, and into the fifth intercostal space (Figure 13–1A). Because a neurovascular bundle is located on the inferior aspect of each rib, the dissection should be made closely over the superior aspect of the sixth rib to avoid these structures.
- The wound is enlarged sufficiently to allow insertion of a finger to palpate the tract, rib margin, and parietal pleura (Figure 13–1B).
- Once the parietal pleura has been reached, the clamp is grasped firmly in the closed position. The tip is pressed against the pleura to puncture the tough membrane in a controlled manner. A pop may be heard or felt as the membrane is pierced. Often, the sound of air entering or leaving the wound is heard, or escaping pleural fluid is noted.
- After the pleural space has been entered with the clamp, the orifice is gently enlarged by repeatedly spreading the jaws of the clamp while they are within the orifice. The operator's finger is then inserted into the wound and the pleural defect to ensure that the pleural cavity has been entered and that no adhesions are present.
- A clamp is used to grasp the chest tube and introduce

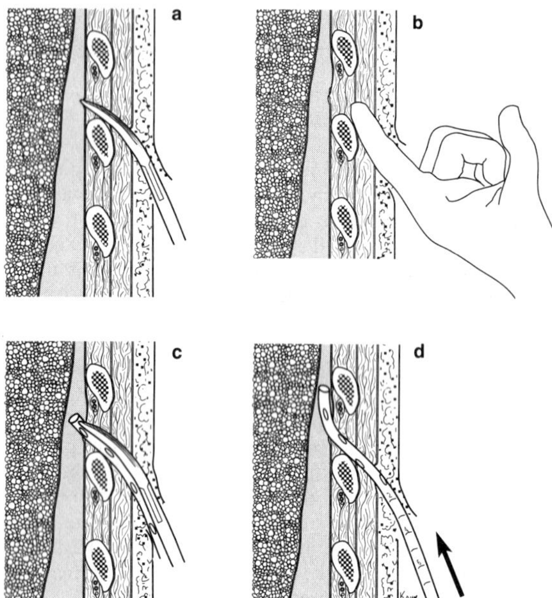

Figure 13–1. *A.* After a skin incision is made with a scalpel, a surgical clamp is used for blunt dissection through the subcutaneous tissue, muscle, and pleura. The dissection begins one interspace below the intended point of entry into the pleural space. *B.* Digital exploration of the tract is performed to ensure that it reaches the pleural space and to ensure that the lung parenchyma is not fixed to the pleura. *C.* The thoracostomy tube is introduced into the pleural space with the surgical clamp. *D.* The clamp is removed, and the tube is advanced into the chest until the last side hole is within the pleural space (further than shown here). Graduated markings on the chest tube indicate the distance from the last drainage hole. (Adapted from Boyes RJ, Kruse JA. Selected nonvascular procedures. In: Carlson RW, Geheb MA, eds. *Principles and practice of medical intensive care.* Philadelphia: WB Saunders, 1993, pp 160–176.)

it into the wound tract, over the superior margin of the rib, and into the pleural space (Figure 13–1C).

- The clamp is removed, and the tube is advanced (Figure 13–1D). The last drainage hole on the chest tube must lie well inside the pleural cavity. If this side hole is outside the body or in the subcutaneous tissue, subcutaneous emphysema, an open pneumothorax, or leakage of pleural fluid can occur.
- The tube is attached to the drainage device. Two heavy (size 2–0) silk sutures are placed on either side of the

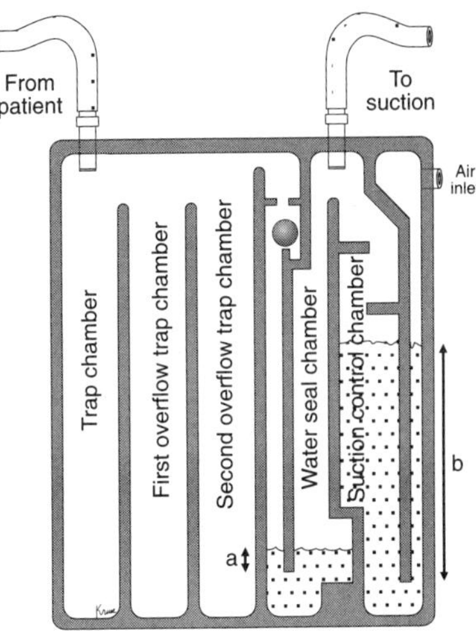

Figure 13–2. Cross-section of a modern integral thoracostomy tube drainage system. The height of the water level (a) determines the pressure that must be overcome for gas to escape from the pleural space. The hydrostatic height in the suction control chamber (b) determines the maximum suction that can be applied to the drainage system and thoracostomy tube. (Adapted from Boyes RJ, Kruse JA. Selected nonvascular procedures. In: Carlson RW, Geheb MA, eds. *Principles and practice of medical intensive care.* Philadelphia: WB Saunders, 1993, pp 160–176.)

chest tube and tied to the skin, leaving two long ends of suture. These ends are then wrapped repeatedly around the tube and tied to secure it in position.

A sterile occlusive dressing is applied to the site. Each tubing connection is tightened and secured with tape to guard against accidental disconnection or leakage. Suction may be applied to the drainage device as appropriate. A chest radiograph is ordered, and the operator documents the procedure in the medical record. The chest radiograph is examined to ensure acceptable intrathoracic positioning of the chest tube, to verify that there is no pneumothorax, and to exclude other complications.

Drainage Devices

(see pages 166–167 in the main text)

The chest tube may be connected to a simple one-bottle water seal, a Heimlich valve, or a multiple-bottle drainage system (see Figures 14–3 through 14–6 and accompanying text in the main book). However, a commercial one-piece drainage system is most frequently used (see Figure 13–2). This device consists of several successive chambers, each with a specific purpose:

- **Trap chamber,** commonly consisting of several successive chambers that collect evacuated pleural fluid. Graduations on the chamber allow the volume of evacuated fluid to be quantified.
- **Water seal chamber,** which allows gas to exit the pleural space through the chest tube and into the atmosphere, but prevents atmospheric air from entering the chest tube and pleural space. The water seal acts, in effect, as a one-way valve.
- **Suction control chamber,** used if suction is to be applied to the system to hasten the evacuation of pleural air or fluid. This chamber prevents the applied suction from exceeding a predetermined level of negative pressure. This maximum degree of vacuum is regulated by the vertical height of water added to the suction control chamber. For example, if this chamber is filled to a vertical height of 25 cm, the system vacuum will not exceed -25 cm H_2O, regardless of the degree of applied suction.

If suction is used, it should be sufficient to cause bubbling in the suction control chamber. Bubbles usually appear in the water seal chamber immediately after initial chest tube placement. This bubbling signifies that air is being evacuated from the pleural cavity. Prolonged bubbling from the water seal chamber indicates either a bronchopleural fistula or a leak somewhere in the system between the chest tube insertion site and the water seal chamber. Loose tubing connections are a frequent cause. A chest tube drainage side hole that is outside the pleural space can also result in bubbling in the water seal chamber. Briefly clamping the chest tube will show whether the water seal chamber bubbling is caused by gas entering proximal or distal to the clamp.

Complications

The overall incidence of complications is approximately 1%. These include bleeding; lung laceration; empyema and other infections; reexpansion pulmonary edema; lung entrapment; injury to the diaphragm, phrenic nerve, liver, spleen, heart, or esophagus; Horner's syndrome; abdominal or subcutaneous placement; and death. Unilateral reexpansion pulmonary edema is particularly likely to occur after drainage of large effusions (> 1000 mL) and after relief of a tension or long-standing pneumothorax. Close postprocedure monitoring of vital signs and respiratory status is mandatory, as is obtaining a chest radiograph to detect possible complications.

Chest Tube Removal

When the chest tube is no longer indicated, it is removed by releasing the securing sutures and quickly withdrawing the tube while the patient expires or performs a Valsalva maneuver. However, if the patient is intubated and receiving positive pressure ventilation, the tube is removed during inspiration. Withdrawal is coordinated with respiration to ensure that intrathoracic (and hence intrapleural) pressure is greater than atmospheric pressure at the moment the tube is removed. This coordination will minimize the possibility of atmospheric air entering the pleural space through the wound, inducing a pneumothorax during the removal process.

Suggested Readings

Miller KS, Sahn SA. Chest tubes: Indications, technique, management and complications. *Chest* 1987;91:258–264.

Pavlin DJ, Raghu G, Rogers TR, et al. Reexpansion hypotension: A complication of rapid evacuation of prolonged pneumothorax. *Chest* 1986;89:70–74.

Describes three patients who had unilateral pulmonary edema, hypotension, and oliguria after rapid evacuation of persistent pneumothorax. The pneumothorax had been present for 1 week or more in each case. Preexisting volume depletion, rapid pooling of fluid within the thorax, and postevacuation myocardial depression are cited as possible mechanisms.

Schoenenberger RA, Haefeli WE, Weiss P, et al. Evaluation of conventional chest tube therapy for iatrogenic pneumothorax. *Chest* 1993;104:1770–1772.

Retrospective analysis of 47 patients undergoing chest tube placement for iatrogenic pneumothorax in a medical ICU setting. Gas egress ceased within 72 hours in all patients without underlying pulmonary disorders. Of those with underlying lung disease, 71% and 92% were healed within 3 and 10 days, respectively.

Shapira OM, Aldea GS, Kupferschmid J, et al. Delayed perforation of the esophagus by a closed thoracostomy tube. *Chest* 1993; 104:1897–1898.

Case report of a patient who had esophageal perforation from a chest tube. Notes that early recognition and repositioning of the tube is key to preventing this rare, but serious, complication.

CHAPTER 14

Bronchoscopy in the ICU

(See Chapter 16)

Paul E. Marik

Flexible fiberoptic bronchoscopy has largely replaced rigid bronchoscopy as the procedure of choice for most endoscopic evaluations of the airway. Flexible bronchoscopy is easily performed, is generally associated with few complications, and allows greater visualization of the tracheobronchial tree compared with rigid bronchoscopy. Indications for fiberoptic bronchoscopy in the ICU include:

- **Atelectasis** that has not improved despite aggressive chest physiotherapy. There are no data to suggest that bronchoscopy is more efficacious than chest physiotherapy for treating atelectasis.
- **Diffuse parenchymal disease in the human immunodeficiency virus (HIV)-positive patient.** Bronchoscopy with bronchoalveolar lavage is the initial diagnostic procedure of choice in HIV-positive patients with diffuse alveolar infiltrates.
- **Diagnosis of ventilator-associated pneumonia.** Bronchoscopy with protected specimen brushings or bronchoalveolar lavage, together with quantitative culture, can be used for the diagnosis of ventilator-associated pneumonia.
- **Acute inhalational injury.** In patients exposed to smoke inhalation, fiberoptic laryngoscopy and bronchoscopy are used to identify the anatomic level and severity of injury.
- **Diagnosis of traumatic airway fracture.** Bronchoscopy can be used to assess for airway fracture in patients with atelectasis, pneumomediastinum, or pneumothorax after blunt chest trauma.
- **Endotracheal intubation.** In difficult or failed intubation, a flexible bronchoscope may be used as an obturator for endotracheal intubation. Fiberoptic bronchoscopy is particularly useful for checking the position of double-lumen endobronchial tubes. A bronchoscope can also be used to facilitate changing an endotracheal tube.
- **Hemoptysis.** Massive airway hemorrhage necessitates the use of rigid bronchoscopy and consideration of thoracic surgery. However, flexible bronchoscopy can be useful for localizing and evaluating nonmassive hemoptysis. Fiberoptic bronchoscopy can also facilitate the placement of double-lumen endobronchial tubes and Fogarty catheters for control of airway bleeding.
- **Foreign bodies.** Forceps are available for use with flexible bronchoscopes. They can be used to remove foreign bodies from the airways. Rigid bronchoscopy is indicated for the removal of large foreign bodies that may be difficult to remove with a flexible bronchoscope.

Except for HIV-positive patients, fiberoptic bronchoscopy has limited diagnostic value in the evaluation of immunocompromised patients with respiratory failure and diffuse pulmonary infiltrates. Open-lung biopsy has a higher diagnostic yield and, in some critically ill patients, a lower complication rate than bronchoscopic transbronchial biopsy.

Contraindications

- **Refractory hypoxemia.** Arterial oxygen tension (PaO_2) typically decreases by approximately 20 torr during the procedure.
- **Poorly controlled asthma** or severe bronchospasm.
- **Hemodynamic instability** or acute coronary ischemic syndromes.
- **Thrombocytopenia** (relative contraindication).
- **Positive pressure ventilation** with high airway pressures and high levels of positive end-expiratory pressure increases the risk of complications.

Performance of Bronchoscopy

- **Sedation and anesthesia.** It is important to ensure that the patient is calm, yet cooperative during the procedure. Nonintubated patients should be lightly sedated using, e.g., a short-acting benzodiazepine. Intubated, mechanically ventilated patients should be well sedated because coughing during the procedure increases airway pressure, interferes with ventilation, and hampers the procedure. Local anesthesia is used to limit the irritation caused by the bronchoscope. As the endotracheal tube (or tracheostomy tube) bypasses the upper airways, topical anesthesia of the upper airway is not required in intubated patients. Local anesthetic agents should not be used when protected specimen brushings are performed.
- **Oxygenation.** Pulse oximetry monitoring is essential throughout the procedure and for several hours thereafter. Should the patient desaturate during the procedure, the bronchoscope should be removed immediately. Intubated, mechanically ventilated patients should be preoxygenated with 100% oxygen. The fraction of inspired oxygen (FIO_2) should remain at 1.0 during the procedure. After the procedure, the FIO_2 should be maintained at a higher than baseline level for some hours because ventilation–perfusion mismatching increases after bronchoscopy.
- **Insertion of the bronchoscope.** In the nonintubated patient, the two standard approaches to the lower airways are transnasal and transoral. Patients generally tolerate the transnasal approach better. In the intubated patient, the bronchoscope is passed through the endotracheal tube with an adapter that allows for simultaneous mechanical ventilation through one port and passage of the bronchoscope through the other. An 8-mm (in

some cases, 7.5-mm) or larger endotracheal tube is required to both ventilate the patient and allow for the passage of the bronchoscope. A pediatric bronchoscope may be used in patients intubated with a smaller endotracheal tube, or the patient can be reintubated with a larger tube.

Complications

Flexible fiberoptic bronchoscopy is generally a safe procedure. The complication rate increases significantly when transbronchial biopsy is performed. Complications include:

- Those associated with the use of sedative and anesthetic agents.
- Hypoxemia or hypercapnia.
- Bleeding, especially in patients with thrombocytopenia, hepatic disease, or uremia.
- Pneumothorax (increased risk with transbronchial biopsy and use of positive pressure ventilation).
- Vasovagal reactions, such as bradycardia or hypotension.
- Fever, bacteremia, or pneumonia.
- Aspiration of gastric contents or upper-airway secretions.
- Bronchospasm and, in nonintubated patients, laryngospasm.
- Cardiac dysrhythmias.
- Acute coronary ischemia or myocardial infarction.

Suggested Readings

Dellinger RP, Bandi V. Fiberoptic bronchoscopy in the intensive care unit. *Crit Care Clin* 1992;8:755–772.

Contains excellent illustrations and descriptions explaining the techniques of endotracheal intubation and changing endotracheal tubes using the fiberoptic bronchoscope.

Hertz MI, Woodward ME, Gross CR, et al. Safety of bronchoalveolar lavage in the critically ill, mechanically ventilated patient. *Crit Care Med* 1991;19:1526–1532.

Retrospective study of 81 patients undergoing bronchoalveolar lavage. No procedures were prematurely terminated. Two patients had hypotension, and one had bronchospasm after the procedure. Concludes that bronchoalveolar lavage is well tolerated in this patient population.

Kitamura S, ed. *Color atlas of clinical applications of fiberoptic bronchoscopy*, 2nd ed. St. Louis: Mosby-Year Book, 1990.

Meduri GU. Ventilator-associated pneumonia in patients with respiratory failure: A diagnostic approach. *Chest* 1990;97:1208–1219.

Summary of various methods, including a variety of bronchoscopic methods, for diagnosing pneumonia in patients receiving mechanical ventilation (65 references).

Meduri GU, Chastre J. The standardization of bronchoscopic techniques for ventilator-associated pneumonia. *Chest* 1992; 102(suppl):557S–564S.

Specific recommendations are given, including identification of high-risk pa-

tients, management considerations during the peribronchoscopy period, sampling techniques, and specimen analysis.

Montravers P, Gauzit R, Dombret MC, et al. Cardiopulmonary effects of bronchoalveolar lavage in critically ill patients. *Chest* 1993; 104:1541–1547.

In this prospective study, hemodynamic and gas-exchange variables were sequentially recorded in patients undergoing bronchoalveolar lavage. Marked decreases in Pa_{O_2} occurred during the procedure. Two hours after the procedure, 40% of patients had Pa_{O_2} values that were 20% lower than prelavage values.

CHAPTER 15

Peritoneal Dialysis

(See Chapter 109)

Michael J. Freeland

Several dialysis modalities are available, including traditional hemodialysis and peritoneal dialysis (intermittent forms of dialysis) as well as the increasingly popular continuous forms of renal replacement therapy, continuous arteriovenous hemofiltration, and continuous arteriovenous hemodialysis. Each has advantages and disadvantages relative to the others. In addition, technical limitations and the medical or surgical condition of the patient may make some of these techniques impossible or subject the patient to increased risk of complications from a particular mode (see Table 109–3 in the main text). The knowledge, skill, and experience of the physician and nursing staff should also be a major consideration in selecting any form of dialytic therapy. Peritoneal dialysis (PD) is the most widely available form of acute dialysis. It can be performed with a minimal amount of simple equipment and does not require highly skilled dialysis nursing. The survival of patients is similar when intermittent PD is compared with intermittent hemodialysis in the treatment of acute renal failure.

Principles of Peritoneal Dialysis

Simply stated, PD is performed by instilling 1–3 L of a dextrose-containing salt solution (dialysate) into the peritoneal cavity. Solute clearance is achieved by diffusion of solute from the peritoneal microcirculation into the dialysate. Ultrafiltration is achieved by the establishment of an osmotic gradient with hypertonic dextrose, which favors the net flux of water into the peritoneal cavity.

Manipulation of the dialysate dextrose concentration and intraperitoneal dwell time allows the operator to control the amount of solute and ultrafiltrate removed with each exchange. Patients with acute renal failure are often uremic, fluid overloaded, acidemic, and hypercatabolic. These patients require a PD prescription that achieves rapid solute removal and ultrafiltration. This process is best accomplished by frequent exchanges (e.g., hourly exchanges with dwell times of 30 minutes).

Indications and Contraindications

PD is useful when vascular access cannot be readily established or when anticoagulation is absolutely contraindicated. The relatively slow removal of solute and ultrafiltrate is also advantageous in patients who are prone to disequilibrium syndrome or who are hemodynamically unstable. Patients who need rapid removal of fluid, correction of severe electrolyte and acid–base derangements, or removal of certain toxins are better served by hemodialysis.

The only absolute contraindication to PD is severe loss of peritoneal surface because of adhesions or recurrent peritonitis. Unfortunately, the condition of the peritoneum may not be known before PD is attempted. Problems become obvious only after difficulty is encountered on catheter insertion or during the dialytic course (e.g., poor catheter flow or ineffective dialysis). Relative contraindications include:

- Recent abdominal surgery or trauma.
- Large space-occupying mass in the abdomen.
- Peritonitis (especially unusual forms, e.g., tuberculous, fungal).
- Extreme obesity.
- Presence of ostomy (e.g., colostomy, ileostomy, nephrostomy).
- Pleuroperitoneal communication.
- Compromised respiratory status.
- Abdominal wall hernia.

Equipment and Supplies for Peritoneal Dialysis

The basic equipment required for PD includes a peritoneal catheter, dialysate, and tubing to connect the dialysate container to the catheter and the catheter to a drainage bag.

Commercially available dialysate (e.g., Dianeal®, Dialyte®) is typically available in bags containing 1.5–2.5 L. Its

TABLE 15–1

COMPOSITION OF A TYPICAL PERITONEAL DIALYSATE*

Component	Concentration
Sodium	132 mmol/L
Potassium	0 mmol/L
Chloride	95–102 mmol/L
Lactate	35–40 mmol/L
Calcium	1.25–1.75 mmol/L
Magnesium	0.25–0.75 mmol/L
Dextrose†	1.5% (347 mOsm/L)
	2.5% (398 mOsm/L)
	4.25% (486 mOsm/L)

*Actual prescription varies with individual patient requirements.
†Concentration refers to glucose plus electrolytes.

composition is such that plasma electrolytes are maintained within the physiologic range (Table 15–1). The most frequently manipulated component, other than the dextrose concentration, is the potassium content. When the patient is normo- or hypokalemic, 2 to 4 mmol/L of potassium chloride should be added. Calcium-free dialysate is available for use in the hypercalcemic patient. Insulin can be added to the dialysate for hyperglycemic patients. Heparin is often added (200–500 units/L) to prevent obstruction of the catheter from blood that may be present in the effluent immediately after catheter insertion or from fibrin clots that may form. For patients receiving aminoglycosides, these may be added to the dialysate in the same concentration as desired for steady-state blood levels.

Although automated cyclers are available, acute PD is usually performed manually with a long Y transfer tubing set with one limb of the Y leading to the dialysate bag for inflow and the other limb leading to a sterile drainage bag. With the manual technique, a new dialysate bag is attached to the inflow limb after each exchange (through a hollow spike punched through a sterile capped port on the dialysate bag). Clamps on the arms of the Y allow routing of fresh dialysate into the peritoneal cavity and emptying of spent dialysate into the drainage bag. The dialysate should be warmed to 37°C immediately before use. Special ovens are available for this purpose but, alternatively, a heating pad or warming blanket can be used. Use of a microwave oven or water-immersion bath should be avoided.

Peritoneal Access

For acute PD, a straight or slightly curved, semirigid plastic catheter with multiple side holes or a soft Tenckhoff catheter is usually inserted at the bedside. The semirigid catheters are easily inserted. However, because they enter the peritoneal cavity directly (rather than being tunneled subcutaneously), they do not have cuffs to protect against bacterial infection. They can be used safely for up to 72 hours. The soft Tenckhoff catheter requires surgical placement. Because they are tunneled and have an internal and external cuff, they can be left in place for a prolonged period, however.

Procedure. Insertion of semirigid catheters is guided by either a metal stylet (trocar) or a flexible wire over which the catheter slides. Preparation for insertion by either method begins with examination of the abdomen for surgical scars, enlarged abdominal organs, distended bowel loops, masses, or aneurysms. The stomach and bladder should be emptied or decompressed, with a nasogastric tube and bladder catheter, if necessary. A site that will avoid abdominal wall vessels should be selected. Scars or areas of previous catheter insertion should be avoided by at least 2 to 3 cm. Usual puncture sites include the midline, approximately 3 cm below the umbilicus, and the area lateral to the border of the rectus muscle, on a line between the umbilicus and the anterior superior iliac spine. On the right side, the lateral site will thus lie slightly superior and medial to McBurney's point. The left lateral site may be safer because it avoids the cecum.

Wearing proper attire and using standard aseptic technique, the operator prepares and drapes the area around the puncture site in routine fashion. Local anesthesia should be achieved with 1% lidocaine. The skin is injected using a 25-gauge needle, and deeper tissue (including the peritoneal membrane) with a 21-gauge needle. A 3- to 5-mm incision is then made through the skin and superficial subcutaneous tissue with a #11 scalpel blade. Subsequent steps vary depending on the type of catheter being inserted.

Stylet Method (for Stylocath® or Trocath®)

- After the patient has been asked to tense the abdominal wall, a 16-gauge, 2-inch plastic catheter-over-needle device is inserted into the abdomen through the skin incision. After the inner needle is removed, 1 to 2 L of prewarmed, heparinized dialysate containing 1.5% dextrose is infused into the peritoneal cavity while the patient is observed for respiratory embarrassment. The dialysate should flow freely by gravity, and should not cause significant discomfort. The short catheter is then removed.
- With the abdominal wall again tensed, the stylet-catheter is inserted through the same site with a firm twisting motion. The direction should be 20 degrees off of the perpendicular, toward the sacrum. The operator controls the depth of penetration by grasping the stylet-catheter 6 to 8 cm from the end with the thumb and index finger.

- While the catheter is held in place, the stylet is withdrawn 2 to 3 cm. Some prefer to remove the stylet completely to check for escape of peritoneal fluid and then reinsert the stylet, stopping short of full insertion. If a curved catheter is used, it should be rotated until the tip (indicated by markings on the catheter) is directed toward the pelvic gutter. With the stylet angled to a plane as close as possible to that of the abdominal wall, the catheter is then advanced over the stylet, without advancing the stylet itself, until it meets firm resistance or until the suture points descend to the skin surface. Some catheters are secured with a clip attached after the catheter is properly positioned. The stylet is then removed.
- The Y transfer tubing set is then connected to the catheter, and the peritoneum is immediately drained. If no flow occurs, or if drainage is sluggish, the catheter should be withdrawn a short distance or rotated slightly and better flow established before the catheter is sutured into position with 2–0 silk sutures and dressed with sterile gauze.

Guidewire Method (described for Cook® catheter)

- For insertion of wire-guided catheters, it is not necessary to prefill the abdomen, although some choose to do so.
- With the abdominal wall tensed, the introducer needle is advanced through the skin incision into the peritoneal cavity. The flexible end of the guidewire is then passed through the hub of the introducer needle and advanced 10 to 15 cm toward the pelvic gutter. The needle is then withdrawn over the wire.
- After the silicone retention disk has been positioned on the catheter, the catheter is passed over the wire. With the catheter held near the tip, it is pushed through the abdominal wall with a firm twisting motion. It is then advanced as far as possible into the peritoneal cavity before the guidewire is withdrawn.
- After adequate flow has been established, the retention disk should be positioned at the skin surface, cinched to the catheter (with the pull tie located on the neck of the disk), and secured to the skin.

Many physicians routinely send a sample of the first (and last) effluent for cell count, culture, and sensitivity. Several rapid 1-L exchanges should be performed immediately after catheter insertion.

Assessment and Monitoring of the Peritoneal Dialysis Patient

The fluid and electrolyte status of the patient should guide selection of the appropriate dextrose and potassium concentration in the dialysate. The patient should be weighed before and after dialysis as well as daily during the dialytic course, with the peritoneum drained. Appropriate laboratory parameters (e.g., serum electrolytes, glucose, urea nitrogen, and creatinine) should be reassessed at least daily, and the dialysis prescription modified accordingly. The tip of the removed catheter may be sent for microbiologic culture and susceptibility testing.

Every patient should have a PD flow sheet at the bedside documenting the following:

- Date and time of each exchange (inflow, dwell, drain).
- Drugs added per liter of dialysate.
- Volume of fluid instilled and recovered (per exchange and cumulative).
- Pre-, postdialysis, and intradialytic weights (peritoneum drained).
- Color and consistency of effluent.
- Unusual clinical events.

Complications of Peritoneal Dialysis

The complications of PD are listed in Table 15–2. Most are preventable by proper catheter insertion, strict adherence to aseptic technique, and careful assessment and monitoring of the patient. One of the more frustrating problems encountered during PD is catheter malfunction. Malposition of the catheter or obstruction of the catheter or its side holes can result in poor flow and incomplete drainage. Obstruction may occur as a consequence of blood or fibrin clots or surrounding omentum. Incomplete drainage may be caused by pooling of dialysate and ultrafiltrate in loculated compartments.

Efforts to prevent or correct these problems include heparinizing the dialysate, inspecting the catheter and tubing for kinks, turning the patient to either side, raising or lowering the head of the bed, squeezing the compliant portion of the inflow tube, irrigating the catheter or extension tubing, and administering oral lactulose or nonphosphate enemas to stimulate bowel motility. If these measures do not improve function, the PD catheter may need to be replaced at a new site.

Sample Peritoneal Dialysis Prescription

(actual parameters are adjusted for each patient)

- PD for 36 hours (up to 72 hours).
- Strict bedrest.
- Immediately after PD catheter insertion, perform three rapid (zero dwell) I-L exchanges with 1.5% Dianeal®.
- After the rapid exchanges, increase the exchange volume to 2 L, alternating 1.5% with 4.25% Dianeal®, and

TABLE 15-2

POTENTIAL COMPLICATIONS ASSOCIATED WITH PERITONEAL DIALYSIS

Catheter insertion	Bowel, bladder, or blood vessel perforation
Technical	Pericatheter leaks (leakage, subcutaneous dissection of dialysate), outflow obstruction (clots, extrinsic), catheter malposition, fluid loculation
Infectious	Peritonitis, wound- and catheter-related infection
Noninfectious peritonitis	Possibly caused by peritoneal air or plasticizers
Cardiovascular	Hypovolemia, volume overload, dysrhythmias
Respiratory	Pleural effusion, atelectasis, pneumonia, respiratory embarrassment
Abdominal wall	Abdominal wall hernias, scrotal or labial swelling
Metabolic	Hypernatremia and other electrolyte disturbances, hyperglycemia, hypoglycemia, metabolic alkalosis or acidosis, protein loss

using 10-minute inflow, 30-minute dwell, and 20-minute drain.

- Add 2 mmol potassium chloride to each liter of Dianeal®.
- Add 250 units heparin to each liter of Dianeal®.
- Maintain PD flow sheet at the bedside.
- Take vital signs every 4 hours (or as indicated).
- Measure intake and output every 4 hours (intravenous, enteral, urine).
- Weigh the patient predialysis, daily (with peritoneum drained), and postdialysis.
- Send a sample of the first and last effluent for cell count, culture, and susceptibility.
- Send blood for electrolytes, urea nitrogen, creatinine, glucose, calcium, magnesium, phosphorus, and complete blood count every morning.
- Call the physician for catheter malfunction, cloudy or bloody effluent, excessive pericatheter leak, severe abdominal pain, sudden increase in urine output, hematuria, watery diarrhea, cumulative patient positive dialy-

sate balance >1500 mL, or change in vital signs (parameters specified).

Suggested Readings

Daugirdas JT, Ing TS, eds. *Handbook of dialysis.* Boston: Little, Brown and Co, 1988.

Concise, extremely readable, pocket-sized book that deals with all aspects of dialysis therapy: hemodialysis, continuous forms of renal replacement therapy, and peritoneal dialysis.

Dickson DM, Hillman KM. Continuous renal replacement in the critically ill. *Anaesth Intensive Care* 1990;18:76–101.

Mandal AK, Hebert LA, eds. Renal disease. *Med Clin North Am* 1990;74(4):859–1083.

Contains several articles related to dialysis techniques, including one on the physiology of the peritoneum and its implications for peritoneal dialysis and one on the principal uses and complications of hemodialysis.

Respiratory Disorders

CHAPTER 16

Acute Respiratory Failure

(See Chapters 67–71)

Maritza L. Groth

Respiratory failure is the inability of the lungs to provide oxygen or to remove carbon dioxide. It is often defined clinically on the basis of arterial blood gas findings, as an arterial oxygen tension (PaO_2) less than 60 torr or an arterial carbon dioxide tension ($PaCO_2$) greater than 45 torr. Blood gas tensions are a function of alveolar ventilation and the adequacy of gas exchange between alveoli and pulmonary capillary blood. $PaCO_2$ is also directly related to CO_2 production (a function of metabolic rate). At sea level, normal blood gas values are PaO_2 between 90 and 100 torr and $PaCO_2$ between 35 and 45 torr. Arterial pH is normally between 7.35 and 7.45. The value for PaO_2 decreases gradually with aging, whereas that for $PaCO_2$ generally remains stable in the absence of serious disease.

From the simplified alveolar gas equation, the alveolar–arterial oxygen tension gradient ($A\text{-}aDO_2$) may be calculated as:

$$A\text{-}aDO_2 = [(P_{bar} - 47) \times FIO_2) - (PaCO_2/R)] - PaO_2,$$

where P_{bar} is the prevailing barometric pressure, FIO_2 is the fraction of inspired oxygen, and R is the respiratory quotient (which, if unavailable, can be assumed to be 0.8). It reflects the overall degree to which the lungs are able to oxygenate mixed venous blood. The normal $A\text{-}aDO_2$ is 5–10 torr while breathing room air, but increases to approximately 50 torr when breathing pure oxygen. An increased $A\text{-}aDO_2$ indicates the presence of an impairment in gas exchange. Hypoxemia associated with a normal $A\text{-}aDO_2$ indicates that the cause of the hypoxemia is hypoventilation.

Hypoxemic Respiratory Failure

In acute hypoxemic respiratory failure, PaO_2 is less than 60 torr, $A\text{-}aDO_2$ is increased, there is respiratory alkalosis, and the patient is usually in respiratory distress, with dyspnea and tachypnea. Excluding hypoxemia caused by high altitude or subnormal FIO_2, nonhypercapnic hypoxemia is the result of one of four mechanisms:

- **Ventilation–perfusion mismatch** is the most frequently encountered cause of hypoxemia. Common etiologies include chronic obstructive lung disease (COPD) and pneumonia. The response to oxygen supplementation in hypoxemia caused by this mechanism is usually good.

- **Right-to-left shunting** occurs because of intrapulmonary shunting (e.g., from pulmonary edema) or because of the presence of an intracardiac shunt (e.g., a ventricular septal defect). Unlike ventilation–perfusion mismatch, the response to oxygen supplementation is usually poor.
- **Diffusion impairment** at the level of the alveolar–capillary interface can occur with certain forms of lung disease, such as interstitial fibrosis and sarcoidosis, and may cause hypoxemia during exercise. It rarely causes clinically significant degrees of hypoxemia at rest. The response to supplemental oxygen is good.
- **Low cardiac output.** Severely reduced systemic perfusion leads to low mixed venous oxygen content ($Cv{O_2}$) because of increased systemic oxygen extraction. In the presence of any degree of intrapulmonary shunting, reduced $Cv{O_2}$ will result in decreased arterial blood oxygenation.

Management. As a general therapeutic guideline, in the absence of hypercapnia, supplemental oxygen can be given by any means sufficient to increase the $Pa{O_2}$ to more than 60 torr or the arterial oxygen percent saturation ($Sa{O_2}$) to more than 90%. Several methods are available for administering supplemental oxygen (see Chapter 17 in this book). Hypoxemia caused by right-to-left shunting is frequently refractory. In some cases, even using an $FI{O_2}$ of 1.00 may be insufficient to increase the level of arterial oxygenation to an acceptable level. The use of continuous positive airway positive (CPAP) or positive end-expiratory pressure (PEEP) is often effective in these cases. CPAP may be given by mask in selected patients who can ventilate adequately, but cannot be oxygenated with other methods of delivering supplemental oxygen. However, endotracheal intubation and mechanical ventilation with PEEP are required for most patients with high levels of shunting (see Chapter 18 in this book). The above treatment is supportive. Therapy directed at the underlying cause, e.g., antibiotics for pneumonia, diuretics for pulmonary edema, is essential (see chapters on the specific pulmonary disorders in this book and the main text).

Hypercapnic Respiratory Failure

In acute hypercapnic respiratory failure, $Pa{CO_2}$ is greater than 45 torr and there is associated respiratory acidosis. The patient may be in respiratory distress, or may have a depressed sensorium. $Pa{CO_2}$ is a direct reflection of the adequacy of alveolar ventilation relative to carbon dioxide production. Thus, factors that increase $Pa{CO_2}$ and therefore can lead to hypercapnic respiratory failure include:

- **Decreased respiratory rate** as a result of, e.g., sedative drugs, catastrophic CNS disease or injury, or obesity hypoventilation syndrome.
- **Increased physiologic dead space** in which there is excessive ventilation relative to pulmonary perfusion. Examples include pulmonary embolism and emphysema. This condition can be compensated for at the expense of increased work of breathing.
- **Decreased tidal volume** may be caused by factors that decrease pulmonary compliance (e.g., pulmonary fibrosis, atelectasis, or consolidation), factors that decrease chest wall compliance (e.g., thoracic cage deformities), or factors that decrease respiratory muscle strength (e.g., neuromuscular disorders). It can also be caused by the same factors that can decrease the respiratory rate. By increasing the ratio of dead space to tidal volume, a decrease in tidal volume has an effect that is tantamount to increasing dead space.
- **Increased CO_2 production** because of increased metabolism secondary to, e.g., sepsis, active muscle contractions, thyrotoxicosis, or excessive carbohydrate feeding. This situation is easily compensated for in patients without underlying lung disease.

A variety of neuromuscular disorders can lead to respiratory failure, including:

- **Spinal cord disorders,** e.g., spinal cord injury, amyotrophic lateral sclerosis, multiple sclerosis, polymyelitis, encephalomyelitis.
- **Disorders of peripheral nerves,** e.g., Guillain-Barré syndrome, phrenic nerve dysfunction.
- **Disorders of the neuromuscular junction,** e.g., myasthenia gravis, Eaton–Lambert syndrome, use of neuromuscular blocking agents, organophosphates poisoning, botulism.
- **Disorders of the muscles,** e.g., myopathies, polymyositis, muscular dystrophy, respiratory muscle fatigue.
- **Metabolic causes,** e.g., myxedema, hypophosphatemia, hypokalemia.

Respiratory failure from a neuromuscular cause usually occurs as a decrease in tidal volume associated with an increase in respiratory rate. $Paco_2$ levels begin to increase when muscle strength is less than approximately 30% of normal. This situation usually occurs when the vital capacity is less than 10–15 mL/kg and the maximal negative inspiratory force generated is less than −20 cm H_2O.

Some patients with severe COPD retain carbon dioxide on a chronic basis, even with optimal treatment. Through compensatory mechanisms, these patients survive with chronic respiratory insufficiency, despite sometimes high levels of chronic hypercapnia. An acute exacerbation, such as worsening bronchospasm, superimposed infection, or progression of underlying disease, can lead to further hypercapnia and precipitate respiratory failure.

Hypercapnic respiratory failure can also occur as a consequence of hypoxemic respiratory failure caused by respiratory muscle fatigue or exhaustion. Respiratory muscle fatigue is a reversible state caused by extreme effort that exceeds the strength and endurance of the respiratory muscles. Clinically, it occurs as paradoxical breathing (inward movement of the abdomen during inspiration) or respiratory alternans (alternately using the diaphragm and the intercostal and accessory muscles to effect inspiration). These clinical signs may be seen during weaning from mechanical ventilation if the patient is not ready to have positive pressure ventilation discontinued.

Management. Unless the degree of hypoventilation is extreme, the response to oxygen supplementation is good. However, treatment is aimed at improving ventilation. Most cases that cannot be rapidly reversed by treatment of the underlying condition require mechanical ventilation (see Chapter 18 in this book).

For exacerbations of chronic carbon dioxide retention, mechanical ventilation can sometimes be avoided by using low-flow oxygen (typically, 0.5–1.0 L/min oxygen by nasal cannula, or 24% oxygen by venturi mask) while providing intensive bronchodilator and other therapy (see Table 71–1 in the main text). The level of supplemental oxygen must be titrated according to serial arterial blood gas results and the patient's sensorium. The goal is to provide adequate oxygenation without significantly exacerbating hypercapnia. Sa_{O_2} values somewhat less than 90% may be acceptable in patients with chronic hypoxemia and hypercapnia. Although patients with advanced COPD sometimes become chronically dependent on mechanical ventilation once initiated, it should not be withheld if it is needed.

Patients with neuromuscular disorders who are at risk for respiratory failure should be monitored closely with serial bedside spirometry measurements. Management of neuromuscular respiratory failure requires mechanical ventilatory assistance. An occasional patient may tolerate ventilation by noninvasive means, but eventually, almost all require endotracheal intubation or tracheostomy.

Suggested Readings

Aldrich TK. Respiratory muscle fatigue. *Clin Chest Med* 1988;9:225–236.
Reviews pathophysiologic mechanisms, clinical implications, and types of respiratory muscle fatigue, emphasizing function of diaphragm.

Bergofsky EH. Respiratory failure in disorders of the thoracic cage. *Am Rev Respir Dis* 1979;119:643–669.
Thorough analysis of pathogenic mechanisms involved in development of re-

spiratory failure in chest wall disorders, including increased work of breathing, ventilation–perfusion inequality, impairment in cough, and acquired defects of respiratory center.

Greene KE, Peters JI. Pathophysiology of acute respiratory failure. *Clin Chest Med* 1994;1:1–12.
Overview of normal physiology of pulmonary gas exchange and pathophysiologic mechanisms responsible for respiratory failure.

Kelly B, Luce J. The diagnosis and management of neuromuscular diseases causing respiratory failure. *Chest* 1991;99:1485–1494.
Approach to diagnosis and management of neuromuscular diseases causing hypercapneic respiratory failure, emphasizing neuroanatomic basis for respiratory muscle weakness.

Mancebo J, Benito S. Pulmonary mechanics in acute respiratory failure. *Intensive Care World* 1993;10:64–67.
Reviews measurement and interpretation of compliance, specific compliance, resistance, and functional residual capacity in patients with respiratory failure.

Swinburne AJ, Fedullo AJ, Bixby K, et al. Respiratory failure in the elderly: Analysis of outcome after treatment with mechanical ventilation. *Arch Intern Med* 1993;153:1657–1662.
Retrospective study comparing 282 patients 80 years and older with 1578 patients younger than 80 years, all of whom were treated with mechanical ventilation. Concludes that, for the majority of elderly patients, the short-term survival rate is nearly as good as in younger patients.

CHAPTER 17

Oxygen Therapy

(See Chapters 65, 86, and 87)

Adam N. Hurewitz

Indices of Oxygenation

Several measured and derived indices are used in the ICU setting for assessing oxygenation. These include:
Arterial oxygen tension (Pa_{O_2}), the partial pressure of oxygen in arterial blood.

- **Normal range** is 90–100 torr while breathing ambient air.
- **Significance:** Proportional to the amount of oxygen dissolved in plasma.
- **Practical value:** Values below the normal range indicate impairment of pulmonary gas exchange. Pa_{O_2} values greater than 60 torr correlate with oxygen saturations greater than 90%, are on the flat portion of the oxyhemoglobin dissociation curve, and indicate an adequate level of arterial blood oxygenation.

Arterial oxyhemoglobin saturation (Sa_{O_2}), the fraction or percentage of hemoglobin sites bound with oxygen.

- **Normal value** ≥ 97% while breathing ambient air.
- **Significance:** Proportional to the amount of oxygen carried by hemoglobin, but not the amount dissolved in plasma. The therapeutic goal of oxygen therapy is to maintain $Sa_{O_2} \geq 90\%$. Sa_{O_2} can be monitored invasively by arterial blood sampling and analysis, or noninvasively with pulse oximetry.

Arterial oxygen content (Ca_{O_2}), the volume of oxygen gas contained in 100 mL of arterial blood.

- **Calculation:** $Ca_{O_2} = 1.39 \times \text{Hemoglobin} \times Sa_{O_2}$, where hemoglobin is expressed as grams per deciliter and Sa_{O_2} is expressed as a decimal fraction.
- **Normal value** is approximately 20 mL/dL.
- **Significance:** Indicates the amount of molecular oxygen carried in arterial blood. This value is used to calculate other derived oxygen transport variables.

Mixed venous oxygen tension and saturation, the oxygen tension ($P\bar{v}_{O_2}$) and oxyhemoglobin saturation ($S\bar{v}_{O_2}$) of mixed venous blood. A pulmonary artery catheter is required to obtain these measurements.

- **Normal value** for $P\bar{v}_{O_2}$ is approximately 40 torr; $S\bar{v}_{O_2}$ is approximately 70%.
- **Significance:** An estimate of the average tissue oxygen tension. Values of $P\bar{v}_{O_2} < 30$ torr or $S\bar{v}_{O_2} < 60\%$ may indicate tissue hypoxia.

Systemic oxygen delivery (DO_2), the amount of oxygen transported to the tissues each minute.

- **Calculation:** $D_{O_2} = 10 \times Ca_{O_2} \times \text{Cardiac output}$, where cardiac output is expressed as liters per minute.
- **Normal value** is approximately 1000 mL/min.
- **Significance:** A single value that shows the combined contributions of pulmonary function, cardiac function, and hemoglobin concentration to providing oxygen to the systemic tissues.

Indications for Oxygen Supplementation

The primary purpose of supplemental oxygen administration is to correct an impairment of oxygen delivery. The most common reason for using oxygen therapy is reduced arterial oxygen tension, usually because of abnormal pulmonary gas exchange. The goal of treatment is to increase Pa_{O_2} and Sa_{O_2}, thereby increasing Ca_{O_2} and ensuring adequate oxygen delivery. If the mechanism of hypoxemia is ventilation–perfusion mismatch, even low levels of supplemental oxygen are usually effective at improving arterial blood oxygenation. Conversely, when the mechanism is predominantly intrapulmonary shunting, even high levels of supplemental oxygen may not have a major effect on increasing arterial Pa_{O_2}. However, hypoxemia caused by intrapulmonary shunting usually responds to treatment with positive end-expiratory pressure (PEEP).

Anemia also results in reduced Ca_{O_2}, but Pa_{O_2} and Sa_{O_2} may remain normal. The usual goal of treatment is to increase the hemoglobin level with red blood cell transfusions, thereby raising Ca_{O_2}. Just increasing Pa_{O_2} with supplemental oxygen will have a negligible effect on Ca_{O_2} if Sa_{O_2} is already greater than 90%. An F_{IO_2} of 1.0 has been used in cases of severe anemia when transfusions cannot be used, but in general, this intervention still has a minor effect on Ca_{O_2}.

In carbon monoxide poisoning, the toxic gas displaces oxygen from hemoglobin. One goal of treatment is to increase Pa_{O_2} to allow competitive displacement of carbon monoxide by oxygen. Administering 100% oxygen decreases the carboxyhemoglobin level more rapidly than the use of lower levels of F_{IO_2} (see Chapter 24 in this book).

Supplemental oxygen has also been used to hasten the resolution of pneumothorax by accelerating pleural gas reabsorption (see the discussion on reabsorption atelectasis below).

Devices

A variety of devices are available for delivering supplemental oxygen to nonintubated patients. The decision as to which to use hinges chiefly on the severity of the hypoxemia, the required accuracy of controlling the F_{IO_2}, the need for humidification, and patient tolerance.

- **Nasal cannula:** This device provides a comfortable means of supplying low levels of supplemental oxygen. It allows the patient to easily talk, eat, and cough. Oxygen flow rates of 0.5–15 L/min can be delivered; however, flows > 6 L/min are poorly tolerated, do not substantially increase F_{IO_2}, and therefore are not used. This method provides limited humidification and can be drying to the upper airway, particularly at higher flow rates. The actual F_{IO_2} varies not only with the oxygen flow rate but also with the patient's minute volume, inspiratory flow rate, inspiratory-to-expiratory ratio, and upper airway dead space. For example, a high inspiratory flow rate or high minute volume results in a lower than expected F_{IO_2}.
- **Simple face mask:** This method can be used to provide somewhat higher flow rates (up to 10 L/min) than can

be comfortably used with nasal cannulas. As with nasal cannulas, the F_{IO_2} cannot be precisely predicted or controlled. As with all mask devices, it interferes with eating and expectoration. Flow rates of at least 5 L/min are required to prevent rebreathing exhaled carbon dioxide.

- **Venturi face mask:** Unlike the above methods, this device uses the Bernoulli principle to provide a stable level of F_{IO_2}, even as the patient's respiratory pattern changes. It is particularly useful for patients with chronic hypercapnia that may worsen if excessive oxygen is administered. The F_{IO_2} can be specified at preset, stepwise levels, typically between 0.24 and 0.50. The delivery system may not provide sufficient gas flow to maintain the specified F_{IO_2} in patients with a high minute ventilation or high inspiratory flow rates, especially at higher F_{IO_2} levels.
- **Aerosol face mask:** This method uses a nebulizer to provide an aerosolized water mist that decreases the drying effect of high-flow gas delivery. It provides for added patient comfort, and is particularly useful immediately after endotracheal intubation. It can be combined with a venturi device so that F_{IO_2} can be specifically regulated.
- **Reservoir face mask:** Also known as a partial rebreather mask, this device has a reservoir bag that collects the delivered gas mixture, making it available even when the patient's inspiratory flow rate exceeds that of the oxygen source. F_{IO_2} levels as high as 0.60 may be achievable as long as the oxygen flow is sufficiently high to prevent the bag from deflating during inspiration.
- **Nonrebreather face mask:** This device uses a reservoir bag and one or more one-way valves to allow exhaled gas to exit from the mask while minimizing the amount of ambient air entrainment during inspiration. Because the mask is not perfectly gas-tight, achievable F_{IO_2} levels are only approximately 0.80.
- **Gas-tight face mask:** This type of face mask is used with a bag-valve device for resuscitation, or used for ventilating patients under anesthesia who are not endotracheally intubated. It is also used for administering continuous positive airway pressure to nonintubated patients. The cuffed mask must be tightly secured to the patient's head with elastic straps to form a gas-tight seal covering the mouth and nose. A high-flow source of oxygen is necessary. It is the only type of noncannulating airway that can achieve an F_{IO_2} of 1.0. However, it is uncomfortable for the patient, and poses a risk of aspiration.

Nasal cannulas and simple face masks can be connected to humidifiers that add water to the inhaled gas mixture. The simplest devices work by bubbling the gas through a water reservoir. If not heated, the amount of moisture added by this method is minimal. Nebulizers, on the other hand, generate an aerosol of water, delivering significantly more moisture than humidifiers, particularly when the nebulizer is heated. There is a risk of nosocomial infection if these devices become contaminated by bacterial growth.

Complications of Oxygen Therapy

Administration of oxygen at concentrations higher than ambient levels can be considered a form of pharmacotherapy. As such, this intervention has the potential for adverse effects, including:

Hypercapnia. As discussed above, administration of supplemental oxygen to patients with chronic obstructive airway disease and chronic carbon dioxide retention can result in worsening of hypercapnia because of central hypoventilation and alterations in ventilation–perfusion ratios.

Reabsorption Atelectasis. Use of 100% oxygen results in depletion of alveolar nitrogen. In alveoli that are poorly ventilated, ongoing capillary oxygen uptake decreases the total gas pressure. If the degree of ventilation to these alveoli is insufficient to match this oxygen uptake, total alveolar gas pressure decreases and leads to microatelectasis. The result is an increase in intrapulmonary shunting and worsening of oxygenation.

Oxygen Toxicity. Prolonged breathing of high levels of inspired oxygen results in pulmonary toxicity. The mechanism is probably related to the production of oxygen-derived free radicals within the lung. The clinical consequences of oxygen toxicity are reduced lung volume, atelectasis, impaired mucociliary clearance, increased alveolar permeability, and adult respiratory distress syndrome. F_{IO_2} levels greater than 0.50 to 0.60 continued for several days probably have some degree of toxic effect in humans. F_{IO_2} levels at or below this range are not associated with toxicity. A variety of experimental agents have been proposed for treatment or prophylaxis, including superoxide dismutase, glutathione peroxidase, and vitamin E, but none are currently used clinically. Patients who require potentially toxic F_{IO_2} levels are treated with PEEP to improve oxygenation and allow the use of lower inspired oxygen concentrations while achieving an adequate Sa_{O_2}.

Suggested Readings

Bazuaye EA, Stone TN, Corris PA, et al. Variability of inspired oxygen concentration with nasal cannulas. *Thorax* 1992;47:609–611.
Illustrates potential variability of F_{IO_2} *when a nasal cannula is used at a given oxygen flow rate.*

Branson RD. The nuts and bolts of increasing arterial oxygenation: Devices and techniques. *Respir Care* 1993;38:672–686.
Describes various systems and devices for oxygen delivery (92 references).
Chechani V, Scott G, Burnham B, et al. Modification of an aerosol mask to provide high concentrations of oxygen in the inspired air: Comparison to a nonrebreathing mask. *Chest* 1991;100:1582–1585.
Describes simple modifications to standard aerosol mask to achieve higher FIO_2.
Hudes ET, Marans HJ, Hirano GM, et al. Recovery room oxygenation: A comparison of nasal catheters and 40 percent oxygen masks. *Can J Anaesth* 1989;36:20–24.
Lodato RF. Oxygen toxicity. *Crit Care Clin* 1990;6:749–765.
Reviews physiologic and pathologic effects of therapeutic oxygen use, including good discussion of possible mechanisms (59 references).
McPherson SP. *Respiratory therapy equipment,* 4th ed. St. Louis: CV Mosby, 1990.
Deals mostly with details of mechanical ventilators, but also has excellent chapters covering various types of masks, gas regulators and controlling devices, humidifiers and nebulizers, artificial airways and resuscitator devices, and other useful information.

CHAPTER 18

Mechanical Ventilation and Weaning

(See Chapter 84)

Hussein D. Foda

Indications for Mechanical Ventilation

Many disease processes can lead to respiratory failure requiring mechanical ventilation (see Chapter 16 in this book). General indications for initiating mechanical ventilation are ventilatory failure and oxygenation failure. Ventilatory failure can be caused by a reduction in respiratory drive (e.g., in sedative drug overdose), mechanical defects of the chest wall (e.g., flail chest injury), or respiratory muscle fatigue (e.g., end-stage chronic obstructive lung disease). If sufficiently severe, ventilatory failure results in hypercapnia and respiratory acidosis. Oxygenation failure can be caused by a reduction in functional residual capacity (e.g., with interstitial lung disease), ventilation–perfusion mismatch (e.g., status asthmaticus or pulmonary embolus), or intrapulmonary shunting (e.g., pneumonia or pulmonary edema). If sufficiently severe, supplemental oxygen administration alone will be insufficient to correct hypoxemia, and positive pressure ventilation becomes necessary.

Another general indication is circulatory shock that cannot be rapidly reversed. Mechanical ventilation should be instituted early, even if the arterial blood gas values are relatively normal, because of the high likelihood of imminent respiratory failure in patients with severe cardiovascular instability.

Specific physiologic criteria for initiating mechanical ventilation include:

- **Respiratory rate** > 35 min^{-1}.
- **Negative inspiratory force** < −20 mm Hg.
- **Vital capacity** < 10 mL/kg.
- **Minute ventilation** < 3 or > 20 L/min.
- **Arterial oxygen tension** ($Pa{O_2}$; on high-flow supplemental oxygen) < 55 torr.
- **Arterial carbon dioxide tension** ($Pa{CO_2}$) acutely increased in association with arterial blood pH < 7.20.

Types of Mechanical Ventilation

Negative pressure ventilation is rarely used today. In this mode, negative pressure is created around the patient's chest, causing gas to flow into the lung. Exhalation is passive. Negative pressure ventilators include the cumbersome iron lung; the more portable cuirass, or body shell; and the bodysuit. Indications are essentially limited to neuromuscular diseases with minimal or no associated lung disease. Drawbacks are that the airway is unprotected (no endotracheal tube is used) and that pooling of blood can occur in the splanchnic vasculature, leading to *tank shock.*

Positive pressure ventilation can be implemented with either pressure-cycled or volume-cycled mechanical ventilators. In a pressure-cycled ventilator, gas is delivered until the airway pressure reaches a preset value, when inspiration stops. It is used mainly in the pediatric ICU. An advantage is that it may minimize the risk of barotrauma. A drawback is that any change in airway resistance (e.g., as a result of bronchospasm) or lung compliance (e.g., as a result of pulmonary edema) may lead to decreased delivered tidal volume, and result in hypoventilation.

Volume-cycled ventilators are the most common type used in the adult ICU. Gas is delivered by positive pressure until a preset volume is achieved. Changes in airway resistance and compliance do not affect the volume delivered. Therefore, minute ventilation is unaffected. However, there is a risk of barotrauma because of the resulting increased airway pressures. In addition, venous return may be impaired, leading to reduced cardiac output and systemic hypoperfusion.

Modes of Positive Pressure Ventilation

Controlled ventilation (CMV) is a mode in which tidal volume and rate are set by the operator. Breaths are thus delivered under positive pressure at preset intervals and tidal volumes. The patient cannot trigger any machine breaths or take any spontaneous breaths, and thus cannot alter minute ventilation to adjust for changes in $Pa{CO_2}$ or acid–base status. This mode is used only in heavily sedated or anesthetized patients.

Assist-control ventilation (A/C) provides a preset tidal volume and a preset minimum (backup) rate controlled by the operator. The patient may initiate and receive extra breaths if desired. All breaths are delivered under positive pressure until the preset tidal volume is reached. The patient can increase minute ventilation with minimal effort and can adapt minute ventilation to acid–base status. This method is the most commonly used initial mode of mechanical ventilation.

Intermittent mandatory ventilation (IMV) delivers a preset number of positive pressure breaths per minute at a preset tidal volume. Additional breaths may be taken by the patient, but without any mechanical support. This mode is commonly used during weaning. By adjusting the rate setting, partial ventilatory support can be provided in the sense that a certain fraction of breaths each minute will be fully machine supported, and the remainder will be fully generated by the patient. Modern ventilators provide a synchronization feature (synchronous IMV) so that a positive pressure breath is not delivered during a spontaneous breath.

Pressure support ventilation (PSV) permits partial ventilator support during each breath. The patient initiates every breath and is assisted by a preset amount of positive pressure as long as the inspiratory effort continues. The patient thus determines inspiratory time and respiratory rate. The tidal volume is determined by a combination of the duration of the patient's inspiratory effort (determined in large part by respiratory muscle strength) and the level of pressure support selected. This mode is useful in weaning, but is not usually used as an initial setting. It can also be combined with the IMV mode.

Initial Settings

When a patient initially receives mechanical ventilation, reasonable initial settings are:

- **Mode:** assist-control.
- **Tidal volume:** 8–14 mL/kg ideal body weight.
- **Rate:** 12 min^{-1}.
- **Fraction of inspired oxygen** ($F{IO_2}$): 1.00.
- **Flow rate:** 40 L/min, or to achieve an inspiratory–expiratory ratio close to 1:3.
- **Triggering sensitivity:** −2 cm H_2O.

Lower-range tidal volumes are suggested in patients with chronic obstructive or restrictive lung disease. There is growing evidence that high tidal volumes may exacerbate the lung injury of adult respiratory distress syndrome. The ventilator-delivered flow rate or inspiratory–expiratory ratio may need to be adjusted in patients with bronchospasm because intrinsic positive end-expiratory pressure (auto-PEEP) may occur as a result of air trapping. Lower tidal volumes and higher flow rates may alleviate this problem. Triggering sensitivity sets the level of negative pressure that the patient must generate to initiate a positive pressure breath.

The adequacy of oxygenation and ventilation is assessed by measuring PaO_2 and $PaCO_2$ 15 minutes or so after mechanical ventilation is initiated. In general, the respiratory rate is adjusted to affect the $PaCO_2$; FIO_2 is adjusted to maintain adequate oxygenation. FIO_2 is initially set to 1.00 to avoid the possibility of subjecting the patient to hypoxemia. In most cases, FIO_2 can be decreased after the operator verifies that PaO_2 is more than adequate.

Patients ventilated in the A/C or IMV mode set their own $PaCO_2$ by setting their own respiratory rate, assuming that the operator-selected rate is less than that desired by the patient. If the operator-selected rate is set too high, the patient will be forced to breathe at the high rate, and respiratory alkalosis will develop. Thus, the selected rate should not be so high that this problem develops. In some disease processes, the patient will trigger the ventilator at a higher respiratory rate than is necessary for maintaining normal $PaCO_2$. This situation, or psychogenic hyperventilation caused by anxiety, may lead to significant respiratory alkalosis. Reducing the rate setting in the A/C mode will not correct this problem. Switching the mode from A/C to synchronized intermittent mandatory ventilation, adding dead space to the ventilator circuit, or decreasing the tidal volume is usually ineffective. If necessary, sedation can be used to correct this condition.

Positive End-Expiratory Pressure

Positive end-expiratory pressure (PEEP) is effected by impeding the expiratory phase of respiration such that a constant positive pressure is created in the airways at end-expiration. It is used to correct hypoxemia that is refractory to supplemental oxygen. Optimum PEEP has been defined in several ways. These include, in order of general acceptance:

- The minimal level of PEEP that allows FIO_2 to be decreased to a nontoxic level (i.e., < 0.60).
- The level associated with maximal systemic oxygen delivery.

- The level associated with maximal pulmonary compliance.
- The level associated with minimal intrapulmonary shunting.

By increasing intrathoracic pressure throughout the respiratory cycle, PEEP can decrease venous return and hence cardiac output. Even if arterial blood oxygen content is improved, a PEEP-induced reduction of cardiac output may result in decreased oxygen delivery to the tissue. This result is the basis for defining optimum PEEP as that associated with maximal oxygen delivery. When the level of PEEP is greater than 10 to 12 cm H_2O, pulmonary artery catheterization is often used to monitor the effects on hemodynamics and to allow assessment of oxygen delivery.

Complications of Mechanical Ventilation

Barotrauma. Patients mechanically ventilated with positive pressure are at risk for barotrauma, including pneumothorax, bronchopleural fistula, and pneumomediastinum. If possible, peak airway pressures should be maintained at less than 50 cm H_2O. Peak pressures greater than 60 cm H_2O place the patient at a high risk for barotrauma.

Volutrauma. Alveolar overdistension exacerbates acute lung injury. It may be desirable to use lower tidal volumes (e.g., 8–10 mL/kg) in patients with adult respiratory distress syndrome. To prevent atelectasis, low levels of PEEP or intermittent sighs may be added when tidal volumes are reduced.

Hemodynamic Effects. The effects of PEEP on venous return and cardiac output have been alluded to above. Hypotension can also occur, especially in patients who are hypovolemic or when there is intrinsic PEEP in addition to extrinsic PEEP. Fluid loading will often reverse PEEP-induced hypotension and restore cardiac output.

Auto-PEEP. In conditions associated with increased resistance to exhalation, the tidal volume may not be exhaled completely before the next breath is delivered. This problem leads to breath stacking and increased airway pressure, known as intrinsic PEEP, or auto-PEEP. Auto-PEEP is detected and quantified by measuring the ventilator circuit pressure while briefly occluding the exhalation port of the ventilator at end-expiration. Auto-PEEP can impair alveolar ventilation, leading to a rise in Pa_{CO_2}, and decrease cardiac output by the same mechanism as extrinsically applied PEEP. The patient's ability to trigger the ventilator may also be impaired because the patient must generate additional negative pressure to overcome the level of auto-PEEP and reach the preset triggering level.

Decreasing the tidal volume and increasing the inspiratory flow rate may be helpful in reducing air trapping. Adding external PEEP at levels below the level of auto-PEEP may facilitate patient triggering of the ventilator.

Other Consequences. Patients receiving positive pressure ventilation are prone to fluid retention. Positive pressure mechanical ventilation may increase intracranial pressure.

Alternatives to Conventional Volume-Cycled Ventilation

High-frequency ventilation is mechanical ventilation with rates in excess of approximately 60 min^{-1}. There are three modes, defined by the respiratory rate employed:

- **High-frequency positive pressure ventilation,** in which respiratory rates from 60–100 min^{-1} are used.
- **High-frequency jet ventilation,** in which respiratory rates of 100–600 min^{-1} (approximately) are used.
- **High-frequency oscillation,** using rates of up to 3000 min^{-1}.

High-frequency ventilation typically results in lower peak pressures than conventional positive pressure ventilation. On this basis, these methods have been advocated for use in patients with bronchopleural fistula to decrease the loss of volume through the fistula and facilitate its healing. Their use in other disease states, such as adult respiratory distress syndrome or chronic obstructive lung disease, has not been proven to be clearly beneficial.

Pressure-controlled inverse ratio ventilation has been attempted in patients with diffuse lung disease and refractory hypoxemia. Patients must be well sedated or paralyzed; the inspiratory–expiratory ratio is then increased to 2:1 or as much as 4:1. This increase results in a lower peak airway pressure, but an increase in mean airway pressure, with a consequent increased risk of barotrauma. Complications include pneumothorax and hypotension. This modality is still considered experimental.

Permissive hypercapnia has been most frequently employed in patients with severe status asthmaticus. After heavy sedation, with or without therapeutic paralysis, the respiratory rate is set to a low level, e.g., 4 to 6 min^{-1}. The slow rate allows a longer time for exhalation, preventing auto-PEEP and barotrauma and allowing for better distribution of ventilation. $Pa{CO_2}$ is intentionally allowed to increase; if pH decreases to less than 7.2, an infusion of sodium bicarbonate may be started. The use of permissive hypercapnia is also being investigated in other disease states, such as adult respiratory distress syndrome.

Weaning from Mechanical Ventilation

When the condition that necessitated mechanical ventilation has improved or resolved, the patient should be evaluated for weaning from the ventilator.

Weaning criteria are used to assess the ability of the patient to oxygenate and ventilate without the mechanical ventilator. The patient may be assumed to be able to adequately oxygenate if PaO_2 greater than 60 torr can be maintained with FIO_2 less than 0.50. A variety of criteria are in common use for assessing a patient's ability to adequately ventilate without mechanical ventilation. These include:

- Spontaneous respiratory rate $< 20\ min^{-1}$.
- Inspiratory pressure (with maximal effort) < -20 cm H_2O.
- Spontaneous tidal volume > 250 mL (or > 5 mL/kg).
- Vital capacity > 10 mL/kg.
- Minute ventilation < 10 L/min.
- Maximum voluntary ventilation at least twice the resting minute ventilation.

Many patients can be successfully removed from mechanical ventilation if they meet most of these criteria.

Methods of weaning. When the patient is ready for weaning, several methods may be used. A few rules must be followed for all methods. The patient should be awake, alert, and (ideally) able to understand what is happening. Weaning is preferably performed during the day, and the patient is allowed to rest at night with full ventilatory support. It is important to avoid inducing respiratory muscle exhaustion because recovery may take 24 hours or longer.

- **T-piece weaning.** Supplemental oxygen is given through a T-piece (Brigg's adaptor), and the patient is closely monitored for 5–10 minutes. Arterial blood gas is obtained, and mechanical ventilation is resumed. If the patient is comfortable and PaO_2 and $PaCO_2$ are adequate, increasing periods on the T-piece are tried, with rest periods of at least 1 hour in between.
- **IMV weaning.** The IMV rate is reduced by 1 or 2 min^{-1}, and the patient is observed for 2–3 hours. If tolerated, the rate is reduced further, with another period of observation. When the patient tolerates a rate of 3–4 min^{-1}, a T-piece is substituted for the ventilator. If it is tolerated for 1–2 hours, the patient is extubated. Patients should not use a T-piece for prolonged periods.
- **PSV weaning.** Inspiratory pressure support is added until the tidal volume is 300–400 mL and the patient is comfortable. The level of pressure support is periodically decreased by 2–3 cm H_2O until the patient is weaned to a pressure support of ≤ 5 cm H_2O.

This method is often used in combination with IMV, with pressure support assisting the patient-generated breaths. After the patient is weaned from the IMV, the pressure support is progressively decreased.

Extubation. Additional criteria must be satisfied before a patient can be extubated. The chief principle is that the patient must be able to maintain a clear and patent airway. The sensorium should be normal or near-normal, an adequate cough and gag reflex should be present, and sputum production should not be excessive. Extubation is accomplished by the following steps:

- Ensuring that the patient is awake and alert, with an empty stomach.
- Ensuring that the mouth and endotracheal tube are suctioned thoroughly just before extubation.
- Removing the air from the endotracheal tube cuff.
- Removing the endotracheal tube at the peak of a deep inspiration.
- Encouraging the patient to cough and take deep breaths.

An aerosol oxygen mask should be set up and ready before extubation is performed. The physician should be prepared for the possibility that the patient may require emergency reintubation. Reintubation may be necessary because the patient was not ready for full weaning or because of the development of stridor caused by laryngeal edema. If stridor is present but not severe enough to require immediate reintubation, inhaled racemic epinephrine and IV corticosteroids may be administered.

Suggested Readings

Banner MJ, Kirby RR, Blanch PB, et al. Decreasing imposed work of the breathing apparatus to zero using pressure-support ventilation. *Crit Care Med* 1993;21:1333–1338.

Imposed work of the breathing apparatus was calculated at incremental levels of pressure support until the work decreased to zero. Imposed work was zero at mean pressure support levels of approximately 14 cm H_2O. The authors recommend that patients with respiratory failure and compromised pulmonary mechanics receive at least a minimal level of pressure support while breathing spontaneously to decrease the work of breathing.

Hickling KG, Henderson SJ, Jackson R. Low mortality associated with low volume pressure limited ventilation with permissive hypercapnia in severe adult respiratory distress syndrome. *Intensive Care Med* 1990;16:372–377.

Report of one group's experience with limiting peak inspiratory pressure by decreasing tidal volume and allowing hypercapnia in 50 patients with severe adult respiratory distress syndrome. Hospital mortality rate was 16%, with an APACHE II-predicted mortality rate of 40% ($P < 0.001$).

MacIntyre NR. Respiratory function during pressure support ventilation. *Chest* 1986;89:677–683.

Thorough description of pressure support ventilation.

Marini JJ, Rodriguez RM, Lamb V. The inspiratory workload of patient-initiated mechanical ventilation. *Am Rev Respir Dis* 1986;134:902–909.
Discusses work of breathing in synchronized intermittent mandatory ventilation and assist-control modes of ventilation.
Parker JC, Hernandez LA, Peevy KJ. Mechanisms of ventilator-induced lung injury. *Crit Care Med* 1993;21:131–143.
Describes physiologic mechanisms of ventilation-induced lung injury. Predisposing factors for lung injury are high peak inspiratory volumes and pressures, high mean airway pressure, surfactant insufficiency or inactivation, and pre-existing lung disease.
Pepe PE, Marini JJ. Occult positive end-expiratory pressure in mechanically ventilated patients with airflow obstruction: The auto-PEEP effect. *Am Rev Respir Dis* 1982;126:166–170.
Article that first described the phenomenon of auto-PEEP and coined that term.
Tobin MJ. Mechanical ventilation. *N Engl J Med* 1994;330:1056–1061.
Concise review of mechanical ventilation, covering common and alternative modes, settings, adjunctive therapy, avoidance of complications, and weaning.

CHAPTER 19

Adult Respiratory Distress Syndrome

(See Chapter 73)

Hussein D. Foda

Adult respiratory distress syndrome (ARDS) is a form of acute lung injury that results in pulmonary edema caused by increased permeability of the pulmonary capillary endothelium. The lung injury typically progresses to respiratory failure within 6 to 48 hours. It manifests clinically as refractory hypoxemia (e.g., arterial oxygen tension [PaO_2] < 50 torr with fraction of inspired oxygen [FIO_2] > 0.5), radiographic evidence of diffuse pulmonary infiltrates, and a severe decrease in lung compliance.

Clinically, it may be difficult to differentiate this form of pulmonary edema from the hydrostatic pulmonary edema that occurs with left-sided heart failure. However, unless there is concomitant heart failure, the pulmonary artery occlusion pressure (PAOP) in ARDS is generally less than 18 mm Hg.

More than 50 causes of ARDS have been identified.

TABLE 19–1

COMMON ETIOLOGIES OF ADULT RESPIRATORY DISTRESS SYNDROME

Sepsis
Circulatory shock
Multiple trauma
Pulmonary contusion
Drug overdose
Aspiration of blood
Massive transfusions
Venous air embolism
Near-drowning
Pneumonia
Aspiration of gastric contents
Multiple organ system failure
Neurogenic pulmonary edema
Extensive burns
Diffuse alveolar hemorrhage
Leukoagglutinin transfusion reaction
Relief of upper-airway obstruction
Reaction to radiocontrast media

Some of the more common clinical states that may lead to the development of ARDS are shown in Table 19–1.

Physiologic Disturbances Occurring in ARDS

- **Hypoxemia** is caused by intrapulmonary shunting. It responds poorly to supplemental oxygen, but usually responds well to positive end-expiratory pressure (PEEP).
- **Increased dead space,** requiring high levels of minute ventilation to maintain normal arterial carbon dioxide tension ($PaCO_2$).
- **Decreased pulmonary compliance,** indicating stiff lung parenchyma as a result of pulmonary edema. In its simplest form, static compliance can be calculated as:

$$\frac{\text{Tidal volume}}{\text{Plateau pressure} - \text{PEEP}}.$$

  Plateau pressure is the airway pressure during a 0.3- to 0.5-second end-inspiratory pause. The ventilator must be set to provide this pressure. Normal compliance is approximately 100 mL/cm H_2O, but in ARDS, the compliance is often as low as 10 mL/cm H_2O. Static compliance may be followed daily in ARDS as an indicator for determining improvement.
- **Increased airway resistance** can occur, and it produces expiratory air trapping (auto-PEEP). Increased resistance and decreased compliance both increase the work of breathing.

- **Pulmonary hypertension** is usually present in ARDS. It can range from mild to severe, in some cases causing right-sided heart failure.

Treatment

There is no specific treatment for ARDS that has proven efficacy. Therefore, therapy is directed toward sustaining life with the fewest possible complications until the underlying cause resolves and the inflammatory process subsides. Pharmacologic doses of corticosteroids have not been shown to be of benefit in preventing ARDS in patients who are at risk or in improving the outcome in patients with established ARDS. Central points of clinical management are described below:

- **Treatment of the underlying cause.** Examples include resuscitation from circulatory shock, stabilization of long bone fractures, and antibiotic treatment for sepsis.
- **Supplemental oxygen** is given to maintain arterial oxyhemoglobin saturation ($Sa{O_2}$) $\geq$ 0.90. Because of the high level of intrapulmonary shunting that typically occurs in ARDS, high levels of $F{IO_2}$ may be required. In severe cases, even these high levels may be insufficient to alleviate hypoxemia.
- **Mechanical ventilation** is indicated in essentially all patients with established ARDS. It becomes necessary when the patient cannot be adequately oxygenated with supplemental oxygen administered by face mask, when acute hypercapnia or respiratory acidosis develops, or when respiratory failure is imminent.
- **Positive end-expiratory pressure** is used to improve oxygenation ($Sa{O_2} \geq 0.90$) and to allow $F{IO_2}$ to be reduced (to < 0.6 if possible) to avoid oxygen toxicity. PEEP recruits atelectatic and partially fluid-filled alveoli, increases lung functional residual capacity, decreases intrapulmonary shunting, and improves pulmonary compliance. Adverse effects of PEEP include barotrauma and decreased venous return. The latter can result in decreased cardiac output and hypotension. Even if PEEP improves oxygenation, the reduction of cardiac output may lead to decreased oxygen delivery to the tissue. In some cases, fluid loading or inotropic agents may be necessary to overcome the adverse hemodynamic effects of PEEP and improve oxygen delivery. This requirement is the basis for one common method of defining optimal PEEP, namely, the level of PEEP that is associated with the highest systemic oxygen delivery.
- **Reduction of PAOP.** PAOP provides an estimate of pulmonary capillary hydrostatic pressure. In the face of permeability pulmonary edema, reducing PAOP, re-

gardless of the starting level, should result in decreased fluid flux from the pulmonary capillaries to the lung interstitium and alveoli. Many clinicians advocate reducing PAOP by diuresis or, if necessary, ultrafiltration in an attempt to decrease the degree of pulmonary edema. Although this approach intuitively appears beneficial, no convincing clinical studies exist to show that it affects the outcome of ARDS.

ARDS commonly occurs in the setting of multiple organ system failure (MOSF), usually in conjunction with sepsis. The increased vascular permeability that frequently occurs in MOSF can lead to hypovolemia, which can result in decreased cardiac output and oxygen delivery. In severe cases, treatment aimed at reducing pulmonary capillary pressure may precipitate or exacerbate hemodynamic instability. On the other hand, fluid loading can augment venous return, ameliorate hemodynamic embarrassment, allow the use of high levels of PEEP, and augment oxygen delivery. However, it may worsen the degree of pulmonary edema. In treating ARDS and MOSF, the clinician must balance the goal of correcting the hypovolemia and decreasing pulmonary capillary pressure to reduce pulmonary edema with the task of ensuring adequate systemic oxygen delivery. Inotropic agents may be helpful. Invasive hemodynamic monitoring is frequently employed, although the interpretation of PAOP may be difficult in patients receiving high levels of PEEP (see Chapter 95 in the main text).

Experimental Forms of Therapy

A variety of experimental pharmacologic modalities are under investigation. These include aerosol delivery of artificial surfactants and liposome-encapsulated antioxidants. Controlled hypothermia has been used to decrease systemic oxygen demand when hypoxemia cannot be corrected despite the use of mechanical ventilation and PEEP. Several newer modes of mechanical ventilation, such as inverse-ratio ventilation, airway pressure release ventilation, high-frequency ventilation, and permissive hypercapnia, have been used to treat ARDS. Unconventional modes of gas exchange that have been used include extracorporeal membrane oxygenation, extracorporeal carbon dioxide removal, and more recently, the use of an IV oxygenator. Although widely studied, these methods are of unproven benefit.

Suggested Readings

Bone RC, Fisher CJ Jr, Clemmer TP, et al. A controlled clinical trial of high-dose methylprednisolone therapy in the treatment of severe sepsis and septic shock. *N Engl J Med* 1987;317:653–658.

This large-scale clinical investigation concludes that corticosteroids are not beneficial in the treatment of severe sepsis and septic shock.

High KM, Snider MT, Richard R, et al. Clinical trials of an intravenous oxygenator in patients with adult respiratory distress syndrome. *Anesthesiology* 1992;77:856–863.

Report on the use of an experimental oxygenation device (IVOX) inserted into the vena cava, providing oxygen to the blood by diffusion from gas-filled hollow fibers.

Marini JJ. Monitoring during mechanical ventilation. *Clin Chest Med* 1988;9:73–100.

Reviews aspects of monitoring the cardiopulmonary system in mechanically ventilated patients.

Murray JF, Matthay MA, Luce JM, et al. An expanded definition of the adult respiratory distress syndrome. *Am Rev Respir Dis* 1988; 138:720–723.

Elaborates on criteria used to define adult respiratory distress syndrome.

Said SI, Foda HD. State of the art: Pharmacologic modulation of lung injury. *Am Rev Respir Dis* 1989;139:1553–1564.

Provides good review of some potential treatments for adult respiratory distress syndrome.

Shanholtz C, Brower R. Should inverse ratio ventilation be used in adult respiratory distress syndrome? *Am J Respir Crit Care Med* 1994; 149:1354–1358.

Concludes that this mode of mechanical ventilation remains of unproven value in the management of adult respiratory distress syndrome.

Yu M, Tomasa G. A double-blind, prospective, randomized trial of ketoconazole, a thromboxane synthetase inhibitor, in the prophylaxis of the adult respiratory distress syndrome. *Crit Care Med* 1993; 21:1635–1642.

ICU patients with sepsis received either ketoconazole or placebo. Ketoconazole group had a significantly lower frequency of adult respiratory distress syndrome (15% vs. 64%) and a lower mortality rate (15% vs. 30%).

CHAPTER 20

Acute Asthma and Status Asthmaticus

(See Chapter 72)

Adam N. Hurewitz

Status asthmaticus is an exacerbation of asthma that is severe, persistent, and refractory to conventional therapy. Although asthma is usually not a life-threatening disease, it accounts for the deaths of 4500 Americans each year, and the mortality rate is increasing. In those with status asthmaticus, however, the risk of death is as high as 10%.

Recognizing those patients who are at particular risk and providing careful monitoring and aggressive intervention are important aspects of the management of severe asthma.

Pathogenesis and Pathophysiology

- **Precipitating factors** include allergens (e.g., animal dander, pollens, and housedust mites), inhaled irritants (e.g., cigarette smoke, paints, and perfumes), infections (particularly viral), neural stimuli (e.g., cold air, emotions, and exercise), and intrinsic factors that are poorly defined.
- **Immunologic response** may be extrinsic (i.e., allergic) or intrinsic. Early (30–60 minutes) and late (8–12 hours) responses can occur. The late reaction results from the release of inflammatory mediators, and can occur in the absence of an early response. It increases reactivity to triggering factors for as long as several weeks.
- **Airway obstruction** may be caused by bronchospasm, mucosal edema, and mucus plugging. All of these conditions may lead to hyperinflation, increased airway resistance, air trapping, hyperinflation, reduced compliance, and hypercapnia.
- **Impaired gas exchange** may be caused by ventilation–perfusion mismatch, increased dead space, abnormal lung and chest wall mechanics, increased airway resistance, reduced compliance, increased work of breathing, and respiratory muscle fatigue.

Clinical Presentation

Rapid assessment of the severity of disease is essential. Patients whose disease is refractory to standard therapy (i.e., with status asthmaticus) or who have high-risk factors should be admitted to the ICU. Symptoms include:

- **Dyspnea** at rest, labored speech, orthopnea.
- **Diffuse wheezing,** both inspiratory and expiratory, with a prolonged expiration phase.
- **Cough,** with viscid sputum, described as pseudopurulent because of the presence of many eosinophils.

A number of findings are potentially indicative of life-threatening asthma (Table 20–1). The absence of wheezing on auscultation (quiet chest) indicates either relatively mild asthma, a diagnosis other than asthma, or such severe airway obstruction that airflow is insufficient to permit hearing wheezing. A severely dyspneic patient with a quiet chest is therefore regarded as having life-threatening disease. Likewise, normal or elevated arterial carbon dioxide tension ($Pa{CO_2}$) indicates either mild airway disease,

TABLE 20–1

FINDINGS POTENTIALLY INDICATIVE OF A LIFE-THREATENING ACUTE ASTHMA EPISODE

History of status asthmaticus
History of endotracheal intubation and mechanical ventilation for asthma
Absence of wheezing coupled with severe dyspnea
Increasing or elevated $Paco_2$
Marked hypoxemia
Impaired level of consciousness
Use of accessory muscles of respiration
Pulsus paradoxus > 20 mm Hg
Cyanosis
Difficulty speaking
Inability to lie flat

$Paco_2$ = arterial carbon dioxide tension.

chronic obstructive airway disease, or acute, severe asthma with a combination of marked airway obstruction and respiratory muscle fatigue. In this setting, mild asthma is suggested by minimal dyspnea; chronic hypercapnia is indicated by signs of renal compensation (minimal acidemia, elevated plasma bicarbonate level). Respiratory muscle fatigue is most likely in a patient with sustained bronchospasm, the use of accessory respiratory muscles, and paradoxical movement of the rib cage and chest wall during inspiration.

Differential Diagnosis

Many diseases can cause wheezing and mimic asthma. Examples include:

- **Acute bronchiolitis** caused by infectious or chemical causes.
- **Chronic obstructive airway disease,** including emphysema and chronic bronchitis.
- **Congestive heart failure** and pulmonary edema, in which wheezing is a frequent auscultatory finding and is commonly called cardiac asthma.
- **Upper airway obstruction,** which produces symptoms and signs much like those of acute asthma. However, the examination shows inspiratory obstruction (stridor) with little or no expiratory wheezing. Causes include epiglottitis, foreign body aspiration, vocal cord dysfunction syndrome, and tumor.
- **Pulmonary embolism,** which is sometimes associated with wheezing. It may be difficult to diagnose because bronchospasm can lead to false-positive perfusion scan results.
- **Tracheal or endobronchial tumor** or extrinsic compres-

sion of the airways as a result of mediastinal or hilar adenopathy or tumor.

- **Tracheomalacia** or tracheal stenosis, e.g., associated with previous prolonged endotracheal intubation.
- **Miscellaneous causes,** including eosinophilic pneumonia, carcinoid syndrome, endobronchial sarcoidosis, superior vena cava syndrome, systemic mastocytosis, and systemic vasculitis.

Laboratory Findings

The diagnosis of bronchial asthma hinges on a history of episodic dyspnea and wheezing, corroborated by pulmonary function test results that reflect reduced expiratory flow. Other tests are primarily useful in assessing the severity of disease or excluding associated medical disorders. The following tests are helpful in the diagnosis during an acute episode:

- **Sputum** appears grossly mucoid and viscid, with eosinophils, Charcot-Leyden crystals, and Curschmann spirals seen on microscopic examination.
- **Pulmonary function test** results show a forced expiratory volume in 1 second (FEV_1) to forced vital capacity (FVC) that is reduced ($FEV_1/FVC < 70\%$ is abnormal; $< 40\%$ indicates severe disease). Functional residual capacity, residual volume, and total lung capacity are increased ($> 120\%$). Diffusion capacity is normal or supranormal. It is not possible to obtain these formal pulmonary function tests in patients with moderate or severe acute asthma. However, peak expiratory flow rate can be obtained in most cases. Peak flow rates < 100 L/min indicate severe airway obstruction.
- **Chest radiography** is of limited diagnostic value in asthma. Findings may include hyperinflation, with flat diaphragms, reduced vascular markings, linear atelectasis, and occasionally lobar atelectasis. Radiography is useful to confirm a clinical suspicion of pneumonia, pulmonary edema, or other disorders. It also facilitates detection of pneumothorax or pneumomediastinum, which may complicate acute asthma.
- **Arterial blood gases** may show hypoxemia, hypocapnia, or hypercapnia. Respiratory acidosis (caused by hypercapnia) and metabolic acidosis (caused by lactic acidosis) may also occur in status asthmaticus. Classically, a sequential pattern of gas exchange abnormalities occurs as an acute asthma episode increases in severity (see Table 20–2).

Treatment

Bronchodilators and corticosteroids are the mainstays of treatment for acute and severe asthma.

TABLE 20–2

THE CLASSIC, SEQUENTIAL PATTERN OF GAS EXCHANGE ABNORMALITIES OCCURRING AS AN ACUTE ASTHMA EPISODE PROGRESSES FROM MILD BRONCHOSPASM TO RESPIRATORY FAILURE

Stage	$Paco_2$	Pao_2
0	Normal	Normal
1	↓	Normal
2	↓	↓
3	Normal	↓
4	↑	↓

$Paco_2$ = arterial carbon dioxide tension; Pao_2 = arterial oxygen tension.

Standard Pharmacologic Agents

- **Inhaled β_2-adrenergic agonists** are potent bronchodilators. They are the first line of therapy. Administration by nebulizer is the preferred route. This approach is as effective as parenteral treatment, having an onset of action within 1–2 minutes, with fewer cardiac and systemic side effects than parenteral administration. If necessary, continuous nebulization or repetitive aerosol dosing (e.g., every 20–30 minutes for the first 60–90 minutes) can be used. Representative agents and their dosing for status asthmaticus include:

  - **Metaproterenol** 15 mg (0.3 mL of a 5% solution) in 2.5 mL saline every 1–2 hours.
  - **Albuterol** 2.5 mg (0.5 mL of a 0.5% solution) in 2.5mL saline every 1–2 hours.
  - **Isoproterenol** 2.5 mg (0.5 mL of a 0.5% solution) in 2 mL saline as often as every 20 minutes.

  Isoproterenol may induce marked tachycardia or dysrhythmias, and is avoided in the elderly and in patients with heart disease.
- **IV aminophylline** has a role in treating refractory bronchospasm. Its drawbacks are that it has limited bronchodilator benefit when added to a β-agonist regimen, it has a high toxic-to-therapeutic ratio, and it requires monitoring of serum levels (generally, to maintain 10–15 μg/mL). The loading dose is 4–6 mg/kg IV. The maintenance IV infusion rate is 0.5 mg/kg/hr (0.25 mg/kg/hr in patients with cardiac failure, with hepatic disease, or receiving interacting drugs), titrated according to serum drug levels.
- **Corticosteroids** are effective, but have a delayed onset of action. Optimal dosing is controversial. Typical doses are 60–125 mg methylprednisolone, or 300 mg hydro-

cortisone, given IV every 6 hours for at least the first 24–48 hours. There is a more rapid improvement in expiratory flow rate with high doses, but this advantage dissipates after the initial 48 hours.

Nonstandard Pharmacologic Agents

- **Inhaled anticholinergic agents** (ipratropium bromide, 6 puffs every 4 hours 500 μg as an aerosol solution every 6–8 hours) may have a limited role in the treatment of acute severe asthma. The onset of action is relatively slow.
- **Calcium channel blocking agents** have modest bronchodilator properties.
- **Magnesium sulfate.** There is limited evidence that administration of this compound may ameliorate bronchospasm.
- ***N*-acetylcysteine** is a mucolytic agent delivered by inhalation. Although mucous inspissation and plugging can occur in severe asthma, this drug is best avoided in most cases because it may provoke or worsen bronchospasm.
- **General anesthetic agents,** such as halothane, isoflurane, enflurane, and ketamine, have bronchodilator properties and have been given in rare instances in which ventilation is inadequate and airway pressures are severely elevated.

Mechanical Ventilation. Approximately 10% of patients with status asthmaticus progress to respiratory failure and require endotracheal intubation and mechanical ventilation. Indications include:

- **Hypercapnia** or a $Paco_2$ that is increasing despite therapy in a patient who is not improving.
- **Hypoxemia** that is refractory to supplemental oxygen given by face mask.
- **Signs of fatigue,** such as poor cough, inability to cooperate with therapy, and increasing $Paco_2$.
- **Altered mental status,** which may indicate hypercapnia, profound fatigue, or impending respiratory arrest.

Mechanical ventilation does not relieve increased airway resistance. However, it results in high airway pressures that predispose to barotrauma. In addition, positive pressure ventilation impairs venous return and cardiac filling, which can lead to decreased cardiac output or hypotension. One of the challenges of using mechanical ventilation in the patient with status asthmaticus is ensuring adequate minute ventilation and correcting hypoxemia while avoiding high inflation pressures.

A variety of maneuvers can be used to mitigate excessive airway pressure during mechanical ventilation, including:

- **Bronchodilator therapy,** which reduces airway pressures by lowering airway resistance.

- **Sedation,** which avoids respiratory efforts that are out of synchrony with the mechanical ventilator. Benzodiazepine agents are often successful at achieving the desired level of sedation.
- **Therapeutic paralysis** with nondepolarizing neuromuscular blocking agents. The patient must be fully sedated before using these agents. There is a risk of prolonged motor paralysis in asthmatic patients treated with both corticosteroids and certain neuromuscular blocking agents.
- **Positive pressure ventilation adjustment.** Positive end-expiratory pressure (PEEP) should not be used. Achieving a slower respiratory rate, using lower tidal volumes, and using lower inspiratory flow rates will all lower inspiratory pressure, but may also decrease alveolar ventilation. Decreasing inspiratory flow rate also has the disadvantge of increasing the likelihood of creating intrinsic-PEEP.
- **Permissive hypercapnia** is a mode of mechanical ventilation wherein the patient is sedated and the delivered minute ventilation is intentionally decreased to allow $Paco_2$ to remain greater than 44 mm Hg. If there is an unacceptable decrease in pH, an infusion of sodium bicarbonate may be used. By allowing more complete exhalation, airway pressures are reduced and oxygenation may improve.

Suggested Readings

Braman SS, Kaemmerlen JT. Intensive care of status asthmaticus: A 10 year experience. *JAMA* 1990;264:366–368.

Ten-year experience with 80 episodes of status asthmaticus, reporting no mortality with in-hospital management.

Dompeling E, van Schayck CP, van Grunsven PM, et al. Slowing the deterioration of asthma and chronic obstructive pulmonary disease observed during bronchodilator therapy by adding inhaled corticosteroids. *Ann Intern Med* 1993;118:770–778.

Prospective study of 56 patients followed for 2 years with bronchodilator therapy and then for 2 years with the addition of inhaled steroids. FEV_1 decreased less during inhaled steroid therapy than during the previous 2 years, especially in asthmatic patients.

Haskell RJ, Wong BM, Hansen JE. A double blind randomized clinical trial of methylprednisolone in status asthmaticus. *Arch Intern Med* 1983;143:1324–1327.

Study of the benefit of high doses of intravenous corticosteroids in treatment of severe asthma.

Huang D, O'Brien RG, Harman E, et al. Does aminophylline benefit adults admitted to the hospital for an acute exacerbation of asthma? *Ann Intern Med* 1993;119:1155–1160.

This randomized, placebo-controlled study examined 21 patients hospitalized with acute asthma. Patients who received aminophylline required fewer nebulization treatments and had greater improvement in FEV_1 at 3 and 48 hours.

Menitove SM, Goldring RM. Combined ventilator and bicarbonate strategy in the management of status asthmaticus. *Am J Med* 1983;74:898–901.

Early investigation showing value of permissive hypercapnia in reducing air-

way pressure and risk of barotrauma in patients with status asthmaticus and severe respiratory failure.

National Asthma Education Program. *Guidelines for the diagnosis and management of asthma.* Bethesda, MD: National Institutes of Health, 1991 (DHMS publication no. NIH 91-3042).

Clear and concise report on current guidelines for asthma from NIH consensus recommendations.

Zimmerman JL, Dellinger RP, Shah AN, et al. Endotracheal intubation and mechanical ventilation in severe asthma. *Crit Care Med* 1993;21:1727–1730.

Retrospective review of 57 adults who required mechanical ventilation for asthma during 69 hospital admissions. Complications were common, but the mortality rate was low (6%).

CHAPTER 21

Pulmonary Embolism

(See Chapter 75)

Adam N. Hurewitz

Approximately 630,000 cases of pulmonary embolism occur each year in the United States. The diagnosis may go unrecognized as much as 70% of the time. The mortality rate is approximately 30% if untreated, but improves to 8% if treated with anticoagulation. There is a 10% incidence of sudden death.

Approximately 85% of pulmonary emboli arise from thrombi formed in the deep veins of the legs (deep vein thrombosis [DVT]). Recent European autopsy studies suggest that approximately 10% arise from the large central thoracic veins (in some cases because of central venous catheterization), and at least 5% originate from the pelvic veins and right atrium.

Deep Vein Thrombosis

Hypercoagulability, endothelial trauma, and venous stasis comprise Virchow's triad of pathophysiologic factors predisposing to venous thromboses. Important clinical risk factors for pulmonary embolism include:

- History of pulmonary embolism or DVT.
- Immobilization or stasis (e.g., prolonged bed rest, obesity, pregnancy, long bone fracture).
- Hypercoagulability state (e.g., malignancy; deficiency of antithrombin III, protein S, or protein C).

- Recent surgery or trauma.

Abnormal physical findings are present in only half of patients with DVT. These findings include asymmetric enlargement of the thigh or calf (measured at a fixed distance from the knee or ankle), increased warmth and tenderness of the leg, a palpable venous cord, and resistance to dorsiflexion of the foot (Homan's sign). However, half of patients with signs suggestive of DVT have another cause for these findings (e.g., ruptured popliteal cyst or muscle trauma).

Because symptoms and physical findings are of little help in confirming a diagnosis of DVT, imaging or flow studies are mandatory. These studies are discussed in the evaluation of pulmonary embolism below. The standard treatment for DVT is anticoagulation with heparin. Because heparin treatment is managed the same as for pulmonary embolism, it is also discussed here.

DVT can be largely prevented in hospitalized patients by routinely administering low-dose heparin (5000 units subcutaneously every 12 hours) to bedridden patients. When heparin is contraindicated, intermittent pneumatic compression devices can be applied to the lower extremities.

Pulmonary Embolism

Clinical Presentation. Patients with pulmonary embolism may have either sudden onset of dyspnea and hypoxemia or acute hypotension. The classic triad of dyspnea, pleuritic chest pain, and hemoptysis is seen in fewer than 15% of patients. A chronic presentation, with progressive dyspnea, can also occur, and may be the result of multiple small emboli and pulmonary hypertension.

Many diseases mimic pulmonary embolism. Common examples include bronchial asthma, cardiac ischemia with congestive failure, and aspiration of oropharyngeal or gastric contents. Thus, the initial evaluation of patients with sudden onset of dyspnea is more helpful in excluding other diseases than in making a diagnosis of pulmonary embolism. Initial assessment should focus on:

- **History,** which frequently includes sudden onset of dyspnea or onset while getting out of bed or defecating, chest pain, and recent risk factors for DVT.
- **Examination,** which often shows tachycardia and tachypnea; however, findings on auscultation of the chest are often normal.
- **Arterial blood gas** results, which show hypoxemia and an abnormal alveolar–arterial oxygen gradient. In addition, hypocapnia and respiratory alkalosis are common findings. Normal oxygen and carbon dioxide tensions

are rare in pulmonary embolism, although this situation can occur.

- **ECG reading** generally shows sinus tachycardia, and frequently shows right bundle branch block, an S wave in lead I, a Q wave in lead III, or right axis deviation.
- **Chest radiograph** is commonly either normal or shows nonspecific findings, such as minor atelectasis, a small pleural effusion, or an elevated hemidiaphragm. Occasionally, there is a more specific finding, such as a prominent central pulmonary artery and a zone of focal hypoperfusion (Westermark's sign), or a pleural-based, wedge-shaped lesion (Hampton's hump). The primary value of the chest radiograph is to exclude other diagnoses, such as pneumothorax, pulmonary edema, or pneumonia.

Presentation of pulmonary embolism with acute hypotension is generally associated with either a large, central clot (saddle embolus) or with massive embolism in a patient with limited cardiovascular reserve. Death within the first hour is common, limiting the possibilities for medical intervention.

Another presentation of pulmonary embolism is chronic pulmonary hypertension and cor pulmonale. These patients have progressive dyspnea over a period of months or years, with a more recent exaggeration of symptoms, associated with signs of acute right heart failure and perhaps hypotension. Some of these patients may have had multiple small pulmonary emboli over a long period.

More recently, the concept of chronic central clot syndrome has been described. In this situation, there is a large or central vessel clot that occurred during a remote embolism, perhaps years earlier, and did not resolve. The clinical presentation is the result of chronic pulmonary hypertension and heart failure.

Diagnostic Tests. When pulmonary embolism is considered a serious possibility, a logical diagnostic path, such as that shown in Figure 21–1, should be followed. Similar weight is placed on confirming a diagnosis of either DVT or pulmonary embolism because the treatment for both is anticoagulation.

Perfusion Lung Scan. Assessment of the probability of pulmonary embolism by lung perfusion scanning is typically graded into four categories:

- **Normal,** i.e., no perfusion defects.
- **Low probability,** i.e., either nonsegmental perfusion defects, a single segmental unmatched perfusion defect, or multiple segmental perfusion defects matched by ventilation defects.
- **High probability,** i.e., either two large (≥ 75% of a segment) unmatched perfusion defects, two moderate (25–75% of a segment) unmatched defects plus one

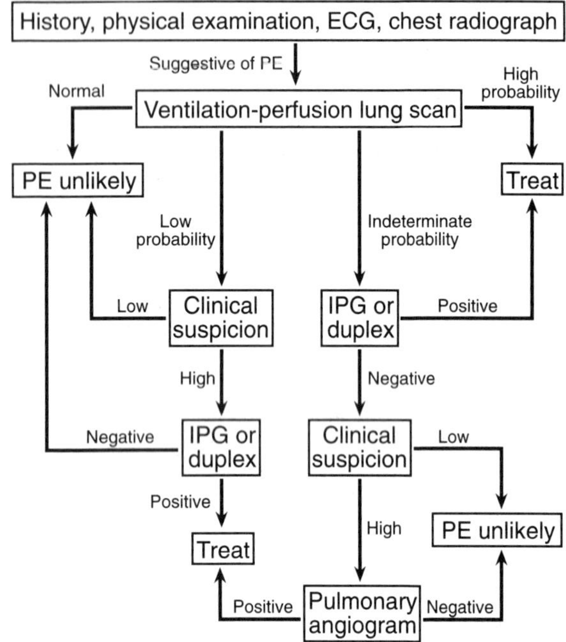

Figure 21–1. Suggested diagnostic approach to suspected pulmonary embolism. IPG = impedance plethysmography; duplex = duplex Doppler ultrasound testing; PE = pulmonary embolism.

large unmatched defect, or four moderate unmatched perfusion defects.

- **Indeterminate probability,** i.e., all results other than normal, low, or high probability.

Patients with low-probability scans and low clinical suspicion for pulmonary embolism need no further testing. All other patients with abnormal, but not high-probability scans, plus moderate to high clinical suspicion, warrant further diagnostic testing.

Noninvasive Leg Vein Studies. Two widely available noninvasive techniques for detecting DVT of the legs are impedance plethysmography (IPG) and duplex Doppler ultrasonography. The sensitivity and specificity of these techniques are excellent in patients with suspected pulmonary emboli, but are not good for routine screening in asymptomatic patients (e.g., preoperative evaluation). IPG is a bedside procedure that is well tolerated and free of significant risks, but it measures locally reduced venous flow, not the presence or absence of clot. Therefore, false-positive findings are seen in right heart failure, obesity, and low-flow states. Duplex studies also can be performed at the bedside, and their accuracy depends on the technical skill of the user. The Doppler component, like IPG, reflects alterations in venous flow, and therefore can lead to false-positive results. The ultrasound component is aimed at detecting clot in large veins, and is believed to be less prone to false-positive results.

Radiocontrast Venography. The diagnosis of DVT of the lower extremities can be accurately made with this procedure. However, venography is expensive, can cause phlebitis, is dependent on the skill of the radiologist, and carries risks associated with the use of radiocontrast material. Therefore, noninvasive leg vein studies are more commonly used. Once a decision to use contrast radiography has been made, many clinicians prefer to obtain a pulmonary angiogram.

Pulmonary Angiography. The criterion standard test for the diagnosis of pulmonary embolism is pulmonary angiography. However, the procedure is invasive, cannot be performed at the bedside, and carries a small risk of morbidity (< 1%) and mortality (< 0.01%). Bleeding can occur from the venous access site, and ventricular dysrhythmias can occur during passage of the catheter through the heart. Other possible adverse effects include radiocontrast-induced renal failure and allergic reactions. Patients with a history of allergic reactions from contrast are at higher risk of the former, whereas those with underlying renal dysfunction have an increased risk of the latter complication. There is also a remote risk of cardiopulmonary arrest during the dye injection. This complication is seen mainly in patients with severe pulmonary hypertension.

Treatment

Heparin. Guidelines for heparin therapy for DVT or pulmonary embolism are as follows:

- Administration of 5000–7500 units heparin (not more than 100 units/kg) by IV injection.
- Initiation of continuous IV infusion of heparin at 1250 units/hr.
- Measurement of partial thromboplastin time (PTT) every 6 hours.
- If PTT is < 45 seconds, administration of an additional 5000 units by IV injection and increase of the infusion rate by 100 units/hr.
- If PTT is 45–50 seconds, increase of the infusion rate by 100 units/hr.
- If PTT is 50–70 seconds, maintenance of the same infusion rate.
- If PTT is 70–80 seconds, reduction of the infusion rate by 50 units/hr.

- If PTT is 80–100 seconds reduction of the infusion rate by 100 units/hr.
- If PTT is > 100 seconds, the infusion is discontinued for 30 minutes, then reinitiated at 150 units/hr less than the previous rate.

Inadequate anticoagulation is a common problem in the first 24 to 48 hours, and is the most common cause of recurrent embolization. Common mistakes leading to inadequate anticoagulation are failure to give a bolus injection of heparin initially or when PTT is < 45 seconds and use of an inadequate initial infusion rate. The risk of bleeding is more closely related to underlying mucosal lesions than to excessive prolongation of PTT.

Warfarin can be initiated as early as 24 hours after heparin administration; however, the frequent need to reverse anticoagulation in the critically ill patient favors withholding warfarin until the patient is no longer critically ill. In the stable patient, warfarin 5 to 10 mg PO is given once daily until the prothrombin time is 1.5 times the control time. The newer standard for warfarin anticoagulation is the international normalized index (INR), which reflects the prothrombin time corrected for local variability in reagents. An INR of 3 is desirable.

Thrombolytic therapy is commonly reserved for patients with pulmonary embolism associated with either systemic hypotension, pulmonary hypertension, or extensive emboli, in whom additional clots might prove fatal. Extensive emboli are evidenced by perfusion scan images suggesting that more than 40% of the pulmonary vasculature is occluded. Contraindications for thrombolytic therapy for pulmonary embolism are more common in the critically ill patient. Absolute contraindications include:

- Recent trauma (e.g., 1–2 weeks).
- Recent surgery (e.g., 1–2 weeks).
- Recent neurosurgery or retinal surgery (3–6 months).
- Recent cerebral infarction or intracranial hemorrhage.
- Acute pericarditis.

Relative contraindications include severe uncontrolled hypertension, invasive hemodynamic monitoring, pregnancy, liver disease, and advanced age.

Streptokinase is administered as 250,000 units by IV infusion over 30 minutes, then 100,000 units/hr for the next 24 hours. Urokinase or tissue plasminogen activator may be used in lieu of streptokinase. Heparin is reinitiated at 1250 units/hr (without a bolus) after thrombolytic therapy is discontinued.

Vena Caval Interruption. When patients cannot tolerate anticoagulation because of bleeding complications, vena caval interruption is necessary unless the source of venous thrombosis is believed to be an upper extremity or central thoracic vein or the right side of the heart. Other indications are recurrent thromboembolism despite adequate anticoagulation and the presence of moderate or severe pulmonary hypertension when recurrent embolism is thought to be life threatening.

Embolectomy. Surgical or catheter extraction of pulmonary embolus in the central pulmonary artery or its main branches is associated with a high mortality rate, approaching 30% in stable patients. In the treatment of massive, acute pulmonary embolism, this technique is rarely successful. However, in patients with persistent central clot syndrome and progressive cor pulmonale, embolectomy can have good results, including improvement in pulmonary artery pressures, even after many years of pulmonary hypertension as a result of the chronic thrombosis.

Suggested Readings

Cruikshank MK, Levine MN, Hirsh J, et al. A standard heparin nomogram for the management of heparin therapy. *Arch Intern Med* 1991;151:333–337.

Provides recommendations for instituting IV heparin therapy and obtaining therapeutic anticoagulation within 24 hours.

Grant BJ. Noninvasive tests for acute venous thromboembolism: Clinical commentary. *Am J Respir Crit Care Med* 1994;149:1044–1047.

Good review of data indicating strengths and weaknesses of current noninvasive tests for both venous thrombi and pulmonary embolism.

Hull RD, Hirsh J, Carter CJ. et al. Diagnostic value of ventilation-perfusion lung scanning in patients with suspected pulmonary embolism. *Chest* 1985;88:819–828.

PIOPED Investigators. Value of the ventilation/perfusion scan in acute pulmonary embolism: Results of the prospective investigation of pulmonary embolism diagnosis (PIOPED). *JAMA* 1990;263:2753–2759.

Analysis of sensitivity and specificity of lung scans in 931 patients participating in a multicenter study. Emphasizes value of a clinical estimate of a positive diagnosis in interpreting lung scan data.

Sreeram N, Cheriex EC, Smeets JLRM, et al. Value of the 12-lead electrocardiogram at hospital admission in the diagnosis of pulmonary embolism. *Am J Cardiol* 1994;73:298–303.

In this study of 49 patients with pulmonary embolism, 73% had an S wave in leads I and aVL, 69% had complete or incomplete right bundle branch block, 49% had a Q wave in leads III and aVF, 33% had right-axis deviation, 33% had T wave inversions in leads III and aVF, and 26% had completely normal ECG findings on admission.

Stein PD, Hull RD, Saltzman HA, Pineo G. Strategy for diagnosis of patients with suspected acute pulmonary embolism. *Chest* 1993; 103:1553–1559.

From the PIOPED study, a useful schema for the evaluation of patients using noninvasive techniques to help minimize the need for angiography.

CHAPTER 22

Aspiration Pneumonitis and Pneumonia

(See Chapter 77)

Prasoon Jain and
Adam N. Hurewitz

Aspiration of gastric or oropharyngeal contents into the tracheobronchial tree occurs more often than is clinically recognized. Clinical presentations vary from asymptomatic aspiration to fulminant respiratory failure and death. Aspiration of highly acidic gastric contents leads to acute chemical pneumonitis, called Mendelson's syndrome. Aspiration of a solid foreign body may lead to life-threatening upper airway obstruction (cafe coronary syndrome). Aspiration of food particles into the airways causes a foreign body reaction, with mononuclear cell inflammation, fibrosis, and bronchostenosis, leading to postobstructive pneumonia and bronchiectasis. Aspiration pneumonia secondary to aspiration of oropharyngeal or gastric contents can have an indolent presentation, or may be recurrent.

Predisposing Conditions

- **Altered sensorium,** e.g., caused by anesthesia, coma, seizures, ethanol intoxication, sedative drugs, or drug overdose.
- **Impaired swallowing,** e.g., caused by neurologic disorders (e.g., stroke), anatomic disorders (e.g., tracheoesophageal fistula), or esophageal disorders (e.g., achalasia).
- **Impaired laryngeal function,** e.g., caused by laryngeal nerve palsy, or the presence of an endotracheal, tracheostomy, or nasoenteric tube.

Aspiration Pneumonitis

The extent of lung damage depends on the pH, volume, and osmolality of the aspirated material. In severe cases, the patient may have adult respiratory distress syndrome (ARDS) and respiratory failure. Mortality rates of 30–60% have been reported in patients with aspiration pneumonitis, despite aggressive management.

Clinical Features of aspiration pneumonitis include:

- **Symptoms** include cough, wheezing, cyanosis, fever, and diffuse rales, all of which may develop within minutes to hours of aspiration.
- **Arterial blood gas** results show hypoxemia, with a widened alveolar–arterial oxygen gradient and hypocapnia.
- **Chest radiography** may show localized or diffuse infiltrates. Aspiration occurring in the supine position often leads to the development of infiltrates in the posterior segment of the upper lobe and the superior segment of the right lower lobe.
- **Bronchoscopy** is indicated when foreign body aspiration is suspected and also in some patients with lobar collapse.

Treatment is supportive. Supplemental oxygen and tracheal suction should be instituted immediately. For refractory hypoxemia, apnea, or the development of ARDS or respiratory failure, endotracheal intubation and mechanical ventilation are necessary. Tracheal lavage with alkaline solutions should not be used. Corticosteroids have no role in the management of aspiration pneumonitis. Their use is associated with a higher risk of secondary infection.

Bacterial infection complicates chemical pneumonitis after gastric aspiration in as many as 50% of patients. In most cases, the initial injury is a sterile inflammation. Use of antibiotics at this stage does not alter mortality rate or risk of subsequent bacterial infection. Appearance of an enlarging infiltrate after initial stabilization, increasing fever, purulent sputum, leukocytosis, and positive results of blood or appropriately collected sputum culture indicate the onset of infection and the need for antibiotic tre... ment. However, it is often difficult to distinguish ch... aspiration pneumonitis from pneumonia, part... critically ill patients.

Aspiration Pneu...

Patients with an altered level ... ess, an abnormal glottic closure mecha... dental hygiene are at increased risk fo... nonia. Aspiration is often recurrent a...

Clinical Featu... symptoms is longer than 1 week ... of patients. The clinical cours... the development of cavitary o... which can lead to the form... gh, sputum production, fever, ... smelling, purulent sputum pro- ... possibility of lung abscess.

- **Chest radiography** may show lung infiltrate, cavity, or evidence of empyema.
- **Blood culture** findings are not usually positive.
- **Expectorated sputum** sample may be contaminated with oropharyngeal contents and therefore nondiagnostic. Samples obtained after endotracheal intubation or by protected specimen bronchoscopy are more reliable.

Microbiology. Anaerobic organisms account for most pleuropulmonary infections secondary to aspiration in nonhospitalized patients. Mixed infection with aerobic gram-negative organisms, such as *Pseudomonas aeruginosa, Escherichia coli, Klebsiella* species, or *Proteus* species, in addition to anaerobic organisms, occurs when aspiration takes place in hospitalized, critically ill, and debilitated patients. This mixed infection is caused by the high incidence of oropharyngeal colonization with gram-negative organisms in these patients. *Staphylococcus aureus* is isolated in some cases.

Treatment. Antibiotics are the mainstay of therapy. Penicillin G or clindamycin is standard treatment for community-acquired aspiration pneumonia. Clindamycin may have a lower rate of therapeutic failure. Aspiration pneumonia that develops in hospitalized patients requires additional coverage effective against gram-negative bacteria (see Chapter 73 in this book). Supplemental oxygen is given to correct hypoxemia. Mechanical ventilation may be necessary in severe cases. Bronchodilators, chest physiotherapy, and postural drainage are useful adjunctive measures. Fiberoptic bronchoscopy should be performed when a foreign body or tumor causing bronchial obstruction is suspected. Lung abscess may be able to be drained ...cutaneously under computed tomographic guidance. In ...e cases, lobectomy has been used when a lung abscess ... not resolve despite appropriate medical treatment ...

Ap... to Patients with Suspected Aspiration

Many patie... ...er from aspiration pneumonitis
or pneumoni... ... further episodes of aspiration.
A careful histo... ...xamination can provide valuable informat... ...ld be observed for drooling, coughing, a... ... attempted swallowing.
The presence of ... ...xes does not confer
absolute protection a... ...everal other methods of evaluation ar...

- **Blue dye test:** Aspi... ...nts may be
detected by the addi... ...ans blue

or methylene blue) to the enteral nutrition formula and visual examination of tracheal aspirate for blue coloration.

- **Glucose oxidase test strip method:** Detection of glucose ($\geq$ 20 mg/dL) in bloodless tracheal aspirate with glucose oxidase test strips has been reported to be more sensitive than dye testing in detecting clinically significant aspiration.
- **Fiberoptic laryngoscopy:** Direct visualization of the larynx can detect unilateral or bilateral vocal cord paralysis and upper airway inflammatory or neoplastic diseases predisposing to aspiration. Pooling of food or secretions in the pyriform sinus and valleculae may be observed.
- **Scintigraphy studies:** Imaging is performed after ingestion of radiolabeled (^{99m}Tc sulfur colloid) food bolus. Pharyngeal transit time, number of swallows needed to clear the pharynx, and aspiration of bolus into the lungs can be detected.
- **Modified barium swallow videofluoroscopy:** Dynamic evaluation of the oropharyngeal and esophageal phase of swallowing is most commonly performed by this technique. It involves swallowing of barium solution of varying consistency. Any delay, pooling of barium, or aspiration is readily apparent. Initially, a small amount of barium solution is swallowed to avoid potentially dangerous aspiration.

Preventive Measures

Posture. The risk of aspiration is lower in intubated patients when they receive tube feedings in the semirecumbent rather than the supine position.

Antacids and H_2-Receptor Antagonists. Despite their extensive use, the efficacy of antacids and H_2-blocking agents in preventing chemical pneumonitis is controversial.

Enteral Feeding. In patients with suspected or proven aspiration, oral intake should be suspended. Aspiration rates may be similar in patients fed by nasogastric and nasojejunal feeding tubes. Surgical or endoscopic percutaneous gastrostomy does not eliminate the risk of aspiration in most patients. Although an unequivocal advantage has not been found, jejunostomy tube feeding may be the safest approach to enteral feeding. Continuous feeding is preferable to bolus feeding. When the gastric route of feeding is used, gastric residuals should be checked periodically.

Tracheostomy. Some authorities recommend tracheostomy for additional protection against aspiration. However, the usefulness of this practice is unclear because as many as 70% of patients continue to aspirate despite having had a tracheostomy.

Suggested Readings

DePippo KL, Holas MA, Reding MJ. Validation of the 3-oz water swallow test for aspiration following stroke. *Arch Neurol* 1992;49:1259–1261.
Simple bedside water swallowing test identified 80% of patients who aspirated during a subsequent videofluoroscopic swallow study.

DeVita MA, Spierer-Rundback L. Swallowing disorders in patients with prolonged orotracheal intubation or tracheostomy tubes. *Crit Care Med* 1990;18:1328–1330.
Despite presence of a gag reflex, various abnormalities were found during a modified barium swallow with videofluoroscopy in patients after prolonged orotracheal intubation.

Jarnagin WR, Duh QY, Mulvihill SJ, et al. The efficacy and limitations of percutaneous endoscopic gastrostomy. *Arch Surg* 1992;127:261–264.
Nearly one-third of patients with a history of aspiration continue to aspirate after percutaneous endoscopic gastrostomy.

Potts RG, Zaroukian MH, Guerrero PA, et al. Comparison of blue dye visualization and glucose oxidase strip methods for detecting pulmonary aspiration of enteral feedings in intubated adults. *Chest* 1993; 103:117–121.
Concludes that the glucose oxidase test strip method is more sensitive and may detect aspiration earlier than the traditional blue dye visualization technique.

Torres A, Serra-Batlles J, Ros E, et al. Pulmonary aspiration of gastric contents in patients receiving mechanical ventilation: The effect of body position. *Ann Intern Med* 1992;116:540–543.
Using ^{99m}Tc sulfur colloid–labeled gastric contents, a considerably higher incidence of aspiration was detected in the recumbent than in the supine position.

Weltz CR, Morris JB, Mullen JL. Surgical jejunostomy in aspiration risk patients. *Ann Surg* 1991;215:140–145.
In this study, jejunostomy placement eliminated the preexisting risk of aspiration in most patients.

CHAPTER 23

Life-Threatening Hemoptysis

(See Chapter 78)

Adam N. Hurewitz

A cough productive of gross blood is a frightening event for both physician and patient. Massive hemoptysis is variously defined as between 300 and 600 mL of blood expectorated within a 24-hour period. It is a true medical emergency. The mortality rate is influenced by the rate of bleeding, the underlying medical condition and, to a lesser extent, the total volume of blood lost. Hemoptysis of 600 mL in 4 hours has an associated mortality rate of

70%. When the same amount of blood is expectorated in 4 to 16 hours, the mortality rate decreases to 45%, and over 16 to 48 hours, the mortality rate is 5%. The primary cause of death is aspiration of blood and asphyxia, not exsanguination.

Etiologies of massive hemoptysis include:

- **Infection,** e.g., tuberculosis, bronchiectasis, lung abscess, or mycetoma.
- **Neoplasm,** e.g., endobronchial cancer.
- **Cardiovascular,** e.g., mitral stenosis, pulmonary infarction, pulmonary arteriovenous fistula or malformation.
- **Trauma,** e.g., airway fracture, pulmonary laceration, pulmonary contusion, or foreign body aspiration.
- **Alveolar hemorrhage** as a result of systemic diseases, e.g., Goodpasture's syndrome, Wegener's granulomatosis, or pulmonary hemosiderosis.
- **Iatrogenic,** e.g., pulmonary artery rupture during right heart catheterization, nonsurgical lung biopsy (fiberoptic or transthoracic needle biopsy), or thoracentesis.

Laboratory Evaluations

- **Sputum** is bright red and foamy. The pH is alkaline. Alveolar macrophages may be seen on microscopic examination. Gram, acid-fast, and fungal stains and cultures are performed.
- **Hemoglobin and hematocrit** levels are evaluated, but the severity of hemoptysis is not always reflected by their reduction.
- **Bleeding diathesis** is excluded by assaying prothrombin time, partial thromboplastin time, and platelet count. If they are abnormal, the diathesis is treated by blood product transfusion.
- **Arterial blood gas** analysis may show hypoxemia, which can result from the underlying lung condition or from aspiration of blood.
- **Chest radiograph** in some cases suggests the etiology, but localization of the site of bleeding by this method is not reliable.
- **Urinalysis** showing red blood cells and red cell casts suggests an underlying immunologic disease.
- **Specific blood markers,** such as anti-basement membrane or antinuclear antibodies, are tested if diffuse alveolar hemorrhage is suspected.

General Management

In many cases, these steps are a prelude to bringing the patient to the operating room for partial lung resection. If a patient cannot tolerate resection, these measures may help to minimize the risk of death. Consultation with a pulmonologist or thoracic surgeon is necessary. It is useful to collect all expectorated secretions in individually labeled cups for each 8-hour shift and to store the cups in the patient's room so that the entire health care team can directly observe the amount, appearance, and rate of hemoptysis. Emergency treatment is centered on the following principles:

Maintaining a Patent Airway. Endotracheal intubation is unnecessary if the patient is conscious and has an effective cough. Oral, rather than nasal, intubation is preferred if the patient is fatigued, unconscious, or has an impaired cough. An orotracheal tube can be advanced more distally into a mainstem bronchus if needed to emergently isolate a bleeding bronchus.

Stabilizing the Circulation. Adequate venous access is established, and hypovolemia is corrected, if present. Four units of packed red blood cells are typed and screened.

Localizing the Bleeding Site. The patient's perception of which lung is bleeding is unreliable. The following methods can be used to determine the origin of bleeding.

- **Radiographic findings:** Unilateral lung abnormality (e.g., neoplasm or abscess) strongly suggests the side from which bleeding originates. Alveolar (blood) infiltrates may be similarly helpful if unilateral. Frequently, however, blood is aspirated throughout both lungs.
- **Fiberoptic bronchoscopy** does not allow adequate visualization if there is active, massive bleeding because the suction channel of the flexible bronchoscope is too small to allow removal of massive volumes of blood.
- **Rigid bronchoscopy** has a larger capacity for suctioning, and therefore provides better airway maintenance and visualization when there is active and massive bleeding.
- **Arteriography** is 90% successful if there is a bronchial artery source.

Curtailing the Spread of Blood in the Airways. The thoracic surgeon is contacted immediately because of the occasional need for surgery to stop the bleeding. Partial lung resection may be necessary; however, in many instances of massive hemoptysis, procedures other than lung resection may suffice. Bedside interventions include:

- **Bedrest,** with the patient positioned with the bleeding lung dependent.
- **Correction of bleeding diatheses,** i.e., coagulopathy or platelet deficiency.
- **Cough suppressant** use is controversial. Codeine 30 mg PO or IM every 4 to 6 hours as needed may be considered if persistent coughing is believed to increase the risk of hemoptysis.
- **Treatment of the underlying etiology,** e.g., administration of antibiotics for infection.

- **IV vasopressin** given at 0.2 to 0.3 units/min has been used, but is of uncertain value.

Special interventions include:

- **Iced saline or epinephrine** (1:20,000) may be instilled bronchoscopically at the bleeding site.
- **Balloon catheter occlusion** may be performed bronchoscopically to allow isolation of the bleeding site bronchus.
- **Mainstem intubation** with the endotracheal tube can be performed, if bleeding is from the left lung, by advancing the tube into the right mainstem bronchus and ventilating the right lung.
- **Vascular embolization** of an involved bronchial artery can be performed angiographically. This procedure is immediately successful in nearly 90% of cases, although 20% of patients bleed again. Spinal artery embolization and paralysis is a serious potential complication.

Management of Specific Causes

Tuberculosis is still the most common cause of massive hemoptysis. This condition can occur as a result of erosion into a pulmonary artery (Rasmussen's aneurysm) at an old cavity or at the site of active infection. The mortality rate is high, and surgical resection is usually necessary.

Bronchiectasis can be caused by previous infection, cystic fibrosis, or immune deficiency. Hemoptysis is common, but usually not massive. In patients with bronchiectasis, bronchitis, or lung infection, systemic antibiotics should be administered. With diffuse disease, embolization is preferable to surgical resection.

Lung cancer accounts for up to half of all cases of hemoptysis, but massive hemoptysis is not common. If the patient is an operative candidate for cure, surgical resection is indicated. If not, radiation and laser therapy are both effective.

Arteriovenous malformations can occur as multiple lung nodules and hypoxemia from arteriovenous shunting across the lung. Radiography may show a feeding vessel that is confirmed by arteriography. Embolization is preferable to surgical resection when multiple lesions are present.

Mitral stenosis causes hemoptysis when pulmonary capillary pressure becomes significantly elevated. Bleeding is usually mild, but is rarely massive. Emergency valve replacement is indicated.

Pulmonary mycetomas can bleed massively. Although there are reports of improvement with intracavitary and systemic amphotericin, surgical resection is usually necessary.

Systemic diseases with alveolar hemorrhage are more likely to cause mild to moderate hemoptysis rather than massive bleeding. Systemic immunosuppressive therapy can be effective, but the onset of action may be days to weeks. In these patients, attempts to medically stabilize the bleeding should be pursued.

Suggested Readings

Athayde J, Shore ET. Invasive pulmonary aspergillosis presenting as massive hemoptysis in a nonimmunocompromised host. *Chest* 1993;103:960–961.

Case report of an elderly, nonimmunocompromised patient who had massive hemoptysis as a result of invasive pulmonary aspergillosis.

Conlan AA. Massive hemoptysis: Diagnostic and therapeutic implications. *Surg Annu* 1985;17:337–354.

Haponik EF, Chin R. Hemoptysis: Clinicians' perspectives. *Chest* 1990;97:469–475.

Survey of clinicians experienced in caring for patients with hemoptysis describing their approaches to diagnosis and management.

Lederle FA, Nichol KL, Parenti CM. Bronchoscopy to evaluate hemoptysis in older men with nonsuspicious chest roentgenograms. *Chest* 1989;95:1043–1047.

Of 106 older men with hemoptysis undergoing bronchoscopy, 6 were found to have cancer. Four were surgically resectable. Emphasizes that a nonsuspicious radiograph in a patient with hemoptysis does not exclude the possibility of cancer, which may be resectable.

Thompson AB, Teschler H, Rennard SI. Pathogenesis, evaluation and therapy for massive hemoptysis. *Clin Chest Med* 1992;13:69–82.

Uflacker R, Kaemmerer A, Picon PD, et al. Bronchial artery embolization in the management of hemoptysis: Technical aspects and long term results. *Radiology* 1985;157:637–644.

Case series of patients undergoing therapeutic bronchial artery embolization. Of 64 cases, immediate control of hemoptysis was achieved in 49.

CHAPTER 24

Acute Smoke Inhalation

(See Chapter 79)

Prasoon Jain and
Adam N. Hurewitz

Toxic inhalation injury occurs most commonly in the setting of residential fires in the United States. It accounts for the majority of deaths from these fires. Carbon monoxide (CO) is the most dangerous gas produced in fires; a relatively brief exposure may lead to tissue hypoxia. Other toxic gases that may be present in fires are hydrogen cyanide and hydrogen chloride, both of which are produced from the burning of polyvinylchloride. In addition to toxic gas exposure, direct thermal injury to the airways may lead to laryngeal edema, upper airway obstruction, and severe bronchospasm.

Complications of Smoke Inhalation

- **CNS:** cerebral edema, seizures, coma.
- **Cardiac:** acute myocardial infarction, congestive heart failure, cardiac dysrhythmias.
- **Pulmonary:** laryngeal edema, tracheobronchitis, bronchospasm, noncardiogenic pulmonary edema, pulmonary infections.
- **Miscellaneous:** lactic acidosis, myonecrosis, acute renal failure, diabetes insipidus, disseminated intravascular coagulation.

Clinical Evaluation

In mild cases, symptoms may be limited to eye irritation, nonproductive cough, nausea, vomiting, and mild respiratory distress. Mental status should be carefully assessed. Although hypoxemia is the major cause of altered mental status in these patients, alcohol intoxication, head trauma, and drug abuse should also be considered. The presence of acute respiratory distress, significant tachycardia, cyanosis, hypotension, or altered mental status indicates significant tissue hypoxia and severe inhalation injury. The presence of facial burns, intense erythema of the oropharynx, singed nasal hair, and soot in the airways indicates thermal injury to the airways. Fiberoptic laryngoscopy is indicated for evaluation of the upper and lower airways in patients with thermal airway injury. The presence of mucosal erythema, ulceration, hemorrhage, edema, and carbonaceous material in the airways indicates thermal and chemical injury. In endotracheally intubated patients, bronchoscopy may not be necessary unless there is lobar collapse or suspicion of a foreign body. Clinical manifestations of airway compromise, such as the development of stridor and bronchospasm, may be delayed for as long as 24 hours. Thus, these patients should be closely monitored during this period.

Laboratory Tests

- **Arterial oxygen tension (Pa_{O_2})** is low if there is significant airway injury. In CO poisoning, Pa_{O_2} may be normal if there is no significant airway injury, or it may be supranormal if the patient is receiving supplemental oxygen. In spite of a normal or supranormal Pa_{O_2}, the patient may be hypoxemic.
- **Measured arterial oxygen percent saturation (Sa_{O_2})**, obtained by multiple-wavelength spectrophotometric oximetry of arterial blood, decreases in proportion to the

carboxyhemoglobin (COHb) level, even if Pa_{O_2} is normal or supranormal. Thus, patients with high COHb levels who are receiving supplemental oxygen can have a supranormal Pa_{O_2}, but a low Sa_{O_2}. Because oxyhemoglobin saturation is quantitatively more important than oxygen tension in determining arterial blood oxygen content, hypoxemia can occur despite high Pa_{O_2}.

- **Calculated Sa_{O_2}** derived mathematically from Pa_{O_2}, as is done by some automated blood gas analyzers that do not employ spectrophotometric oximetry, is falsely normal if Pa_{O_2} is normal or elevated. Hence, direct oximetry and measurement of carboxyhemoglobin levels is essential in all cases of smoke inhalation or suspected CO poisoning to detect hypoxemia.
- **Pulse oximetry** values are falsely elevated in the presence of COHb because these instruments cannot distinguish between COHb and oxyhemoglobin.
- **COHb level** is elevated, at least initially, in CO poisoning. In nonsmokers, the COHb level is normally less than 2%, whereas in smokers, it may be as high as 5–10%. Signs and symptoms of CO poisoning roughly correlate with the COHb level, with symptoms progressing from headaches at COHb levels of 20–30% to respiratory failure, coma, and convulsions at levels of 50–60%. COHb levels $> 60\%$ are generally fatal.
- **Blood lactate** level will be elevated if there is lactic acidosis caused by tissue hypoxia as a result of severe hypoxemia or CO poisoning. If lactic acidosis is present, arterial blood gas analysis will show evidence of metabolic acidosis, i.e., low pH and low bicarbonate concentration. Cyanide poisoning is a consideration in patients with smoke inhalation and lactic acidosis, but normal COHb levels.
- **ECG** may show sinus tachycardia, cardiac dysrhythmias, or signs of myocardial ischemia.
- **Chest radiograph** may be normal, despite significant airway thermal injury. Radiographic findings usually lag several hours behind clinical findings. Pulmonary edema, focal or general infiltrates, and atelectasis develop in some cases.
- **Xenon lung scanning** may be used to detect lung injury. Lung imaging is performed after IV administration of xenon gas. Inhalation injury is indicated by delayed clearance, trapping of radioactivity, and inequality of clearance from different lung segments.
- **Sputum gram stain** and culture should be performed when pulmonary infection is suspected.

Treatment

Endotracheal intubation and mechanical ventilation may be required in patients with altered sensorium, laryngeal edema, laryngospasm, significant thermal airway injury, adult respiratory distress syndrome, or respiratory failure.

Oxygen therapy with 100% oxygen given with a tight-fitting nonrebreathing reservoir mask is a priority in managing CO poisoning. The half-life of COHb is significantly shortened (to approximately 1 hour) if the fraction of inspired oxygen (FIO_2) is increased to 1.0. Serial COHb levels should be followed and 100% oxygen continued at least until COHb saturation is less than 5%. Pregnant women may benefit from prolonged oxygen therapy.

Hyperbaric therapy (HBO) is an effective treatment for carbon monoxide poisoning. Retrospective studies suggest improved neurologic outcome in patients receiving HBO. However, its utility is limited because it is not available in most centers. Whenever available, HBO should be used if the COHb level is more than 40% in asymptomatic patients and in any patient with cardiac or neurologic symptoms, regardless of the COHb level. If such patients are being managed in centers without this capability, transportation to a center with HBO is recommended if no improvement is noted with 100% oxygen administration within 4 hours. In many cases, the risk of transporting the patient to an HBO-equipped center may be higher than the potential benefit. Therefore, the decision to transport a patient to such a facility must be individualized. Normobaric oxygen therapy is as effective as HBO for treating CO poisoning in patients without initial impairment of consciousness.

Bronchodilators, specifically inhaled β_2-adrenergic agonists, should be used in patients with wheezing and in those with a history of chronic obstructive pulmonary disease or asthma. Racemic epinephrine aerosol inhalation may be effective in cases of upper airway obstruction.

Corticosteroids are contraindicated in patients with inhalation injury and surface burns because their use is associated with higher mortality rates and infectious complications. In patients without thermal surface burns, corticosteroids (e.g., methylprednisone 2 mg/kg/day) may be used for 24 to 48 hours to treat upper airway obstruction or severe bronchospasm.

Antibiotics and aggressive pulmonary toilet should be instituted in patients with evidence of pneumonia.

Suggested Readings

Ilano AL, Raffin TA. Management of carbon monoxide poisoning. *Chest* 1990;97:165–169.

Moylan JA, Chan CK. Inhalation injury: An increasing problem. *Ann Surg* 1978;188:34–37.

In this study, 33% of seriously burned patients had bronchoscopic evidence of inhalation injury. Steroid use in this subset of patients was associated with lower survival rates because of a higher incidence of infectious complications.

Norkool DM, Kirkpatrick JN. Treatment of acute carbon monoxide poisoning with hyperbaric oxygen: A review of 115 cases. *Ann Emerg Med* 1985;14:1168–1171.
Retrospective study of carbon monoxide poisoning, suggesting improved patient outcome with use of hyperbaric oxygen.
Raphael J-C, Elkharrat D, Jars-Guincestre M-C, et al. Trial of normobaric and hyperbaric oxygen for acute carbon monoxide intoxication. *Lancet* 1989;2:414–419.
Prospective, randomized study showing no benefit of hyperbaric oxygen over normobaric oxygen therapy in patients with carbon monoxide poisoning without initial loss of consciousness.

CHAPTER 25

Barotrauma, Decompression Sickness, and Air Embolism

(See Chapter 82)

Prasoon Jain and Adam N. Hurewitz

As scuba diving has become increasingly popular in the United States, the number of diving injuries and cases of decompression sickness (DCS) have increased. In addition, iatrogenic causes of air embolism are increasingly being recognized, although the incidence is unknown.

At underwater depth, ambient pressure and tissue uptake of nitrogen increase, especially in tissues with high lipid content. With rapid ascent, nitrogen is rapidly released from tissues, leading to the formation of intravascular gas bubbles that cause mechanical obstruction to blood flow. Air bubbles originating in veins may enter the arterial circulation through a patent foramen ovale or pulmonary arteriovenous fistula. Air embolism to the coronary or cerebral circulation may have devastating consequences.

Pulmonary Barotrauma

Rapid ascent from underwater depth may lead to marked distension of the lungs because of overexpansion of compressed air as the ambient pressure decreases. The result is similar to the barotrauma that can occur during positive pressure ventilation, i.e., alveolar rupture with possible pneumothorax, pneumomediastinum, or pneumopericardium. Physical examination may show subcutaneous emphysema and an auscultatory crackling sound over the precordium during systole (Hamman's sign). Ventilation with 100% oxygen is recommended to hasten nitrogen elimination. Immediate chest decompression is required when tension pneumothorax develops (see Chapter 13 in this book).

Ear Barotrauma

Tympanic membrane hemorrhage and rupture may occur during underwater diving if the middle ear pressure does not match the external ear pressure as a result of eustachian tube blockage. Divers report ear pain, sensation of ear blockage, hearing loss, tinnitus, and vertigo. Occasionally, rupture of the round window occurs when a diver performs a Valsalva maneuver in an effort to equalize middle ear pressure. Treatment of ear barotrauma includes suspension of diving activities, oral decongestants, analgesics, and otologic evaluation.

Sinus Barotrauma

Sinus barotrauma may occur during descent and ascent when pressure inside the skull sinuses does not equalize with ambient pressure as a result of sinus ostia blockage. As a consequence, mucosal edema and inflammation occurs, causing headache, sinus pain, and epistaxis. Occasionally, sinus rupture and pneumocephalus may develop. Prophylactic antibiotics are recommended in such cases.

Decompression Sickness

Formation of gas bubbles in the intravascular space during rapid ascent from underwater depth leads to variable clinical symptoms. Nearly three-fourths of patients have symptoms within 1 hour of decompression. In a few patients, symptoms may not develop for 24 to 48 hours after diving. Symptoms may be precipitated by air travel in nonpressurized aircraft. Predisposing factors associated with increased risk of DCS include dehydration, poor physical conditioning, obesity, advanced age, and multiple dives by unacclimatized individuals.

Clinical manifestations of DCS include:

- **Constitutional,** e.g., fatigue or malaise.
- **Cutaneous,** e.g., pruritus, localized erythema, scarlatiniform rash, mottled cyanosis, or peau d'orange.
- **Musculoskeletal,** e.g., pain in the joints, such as the shoulder or elbow. This symptom is referred to by divers as *the bends.*

- **Neurologic,** e.g., spinal cord dysfunction, cerebral dysfunction, or peripheral neuropathy.
- **Vestibular,** e.g., tinnitus, vertigo, hearing loss, nausea, vomiting, or ataxia.
- **Pulmonary,** e.g., dyspnea or cough.

Management of Decompression Sickness. Oxygen should be initiated immediately by nonrebreathing reservoir mask. Improvement in symptoms is noted in most cases because of a decrease in the size of nitrogen-containing bubbles. This intervention is, however, a temporizing measure, and relapse of symptoms may occur after initial improvement. Hyperbaric oxygen therapy (HBO) is the cornerstone of management of DCS. Overall, a success rate of as high as 90% has been reported with recompression treatment in a hyperbaric oxygen chamber. Although delay in the institution of therapy adversely affects outcome, therapeutic success has been reported in patients treated days after the initial injury. Adequate hydration is ensured. Use of corticosteroids in the management of DCS is controversial.

Air Embolism

Arterial and venous gas embolism can occur from a variety of etiologies, including:

- **Ambient depressurization,** such as rapid decompression from underwater depth, rapid decompression within a hyperbaric chamber, and loss of cabin pressure in an aircraft.
- **Gynecologic etiologies,** such as insufflation of air into the vagina, childbirth, and air-cooled laser surgery of the uterine cavity.
- **Surgical procedures,** such as open-heart procedures, brain surgery, and hepatic transplantation.
- **Vascular access–related etiologies,** including air entrainment through cannulae during arteriography, hemodialysis, and central venous catheter placement.

Manifestations include:

- **Pulmonary:** pulmonary embolism, pulmonary hypertension, acute cor pulmonale.
- **Cardiovascular:** obstructive circulatory shock, cardiac arrest, myocardial infarction, dysrhythmias.
- **Cerebrovascular:** loss of consciousness, seizures, aphasia, motor or sensory deficits, confusion, blindness, cranial nerve dysfunction, increased intracranial pressure.
- **Renal:** hematuria, proteinuria, renal failure.
- **Miscellaneous:** GI bleeding, uterine bleeding, cyanotic marbling of skin.

Funduscopic examination may show air bubbles in the retina. Occasionally, a sharply defined area of tongue pallor caused by air (Liebermeister's sign) is observed on physical examination. Signs of pulmonary hypertension and right heart failure may be apparent. Occasionally, a continuous (*millwheel*) murmur is heard over the precordium throughout the cardiac cycle.

Management. Patients with suspected air embolism should be immediately given 100% oxygen to reduce bubble size and promote diffusion of nitrogen out of the air bubbles. Patients may be transiently placed head-down in the left lateral decubitus position (Durant position), which keeps air bubbles away from the coronary ostia and right ventricular outflow tract. Maintaining patients in this position for prolonged periods may be harmful because it can lead to cerebral edema. Evacuation of air through a right heart catheter may be attempted, especially when the catheter is already in place. Adequate hydration should be maintained.

HBO is an effective form of therapy for air embolism. It decreases the size of internal air bubbles, improves oxygenation of ischemic tissues and, with early institution, results in improved prognosis. Relapse of symptoms occurs occasionally after initial improvement. These patients need recompression treatment. In many instances, aeromedical evacuation is required to transport the patient expeditiously to a center with HBO facilities. Decreased ambient pressure at high altitudes may cause expansion of internal gas bubbles, leading to worsening of clinical status. Therefore, such patients should be transported in pressurized aircraft. The lowest safe altitude should be maintained during helicopter transport.

Some centers routinely use steroids to treat patients with suspected cerebral arterial embolism. However, no controlled trials have demonstrated the efficacy of this treatment.

Suggested Readings

Dick AP, Massey EW. Neurologic presentation of decompression sickness and air embolism in sport divers. *Neurology* 1985;35:667–671.

Retrospective study describing the neurologic profile of 70 patients with decompression sickness and 39 patients with air embolism.

Graf-Deuel E, Knoblauch A. Simultaneous bilateral spontaneous pneumothorax. *Chest* 1994;105:1142–1146.

Series of 12 patients is described, each of whom sustained simultaneous bilateral spontaneous pneumothorax. This group represented 4% of the spontaneous pneumothoraces at the authors' institution over two decades.

Green RD, Leitch DR. Twenty years of treating decompression sickness. *Aviat Space Environ Med* 1987;58:362–366.

Describes treatment protocols and results of recompression treatment.

Jerrard DA. Diving medicine. *Emerg Med Clin North Am* 1992;10:329–338.

Concise review of various diving-related injuries.

Leitch DR, Green RD. Pulmonary barotrauma in divers and the treatment of cerebral arterial gas embolism. *Aviat Space Environ Med* 1986;57:931–938.

Prompt institution of hyperbaric oxygen and steroids was associated with favorable outcome in patients with arterial gas embolism.

Orebaugh SL. Venous air embolism: Clinical and experimental considerations. *Crit Care Med* 1992;20:1169–1177.

Detailed review of venous air embolism. Various therapeutic options are discussed.

Cardiovascular Disorders

CHAPTER 26

Left Ventricular Failure

(See Chapter 91)

John P. Dervan

Left-sided heart failure is a common problem among critically ill patients. It is useful to classify left ventricular (LV) failure on the basis of its underlying mechanism, systolic versus diastolic dysfunction.

Systolic Dysfunction

Etiology. The term systolic dysfunction refers to impairment in myocardial contractility, with a reduction in effective stroke volume. Patients with systolic dysfunction have impaired LV ejection fractions. Potential causes of LV systolic dysfunction include:

- **Myocardial ischemia** or infarction, usually secondary to obstructive coronary artery disease.
- **Mechanical complications** of acute myocardial infarction, i.e., mitral insufficiency secondary to papillary muscle rupture or dysfunction, ventricular septal rupture, and ventricular free-wall rupture.
- **Dilated cardiomyopathy,** which may be idiopathic, familial, postpartum, or related to drug exposure (e.g., ethanol or doxorubicin [Adriamycin®]).
- **Valvular heart disease,** either congenital or acquired (e.g., related to endocarditis or rheumatic heart disease).
- **Long-standing hypertension,** particularly when it has been poorly controlled.
- **Volume-overload states,** such as pregnancy or renal failure.
- **High-output states,** including thyrotoxicosis, severe anemia, beriberi, Paget's disease, and arteriovenous fistula.
- **Miscellaneous** conditions, including sepsis and myocarditis.

LV failure may manifest as pulmonary edema or cardiogenic shock, or it may be a chronic condition that has insidious onset and is exacerbated by changes in myocardial oxygen supply or demand.

Diagnosis

- **History and physical examination** can provide important clues about the presence and etiology of LV failure. Clinical manifestations are generally secondary to pulmonary congestion or low cardiac output (Table 26–1). An S_3 gallop may be present. Other findings may point to the underlying etiology, e.g., history of doxorubicin use or a heart murmur of mitral or aortic insufficiency.

- **Electrocardiography** may show evidence of ischemia, prior infarction, conduction disturbances, or chamber enlargement. Rhythm disturbances, such as ventricular ectopy or atrial fibrillation, are often present.
- **Chest radiography** is useful in assessing cardiac size and confirming the presence of pulmonary congestion and pleural effusions. Radiographic evidence of cardiomegaly is common in advanced systolic dysfunction.
- **Echocardiography** can be performed at the bedside to confirm the presence and estimate the severity of systolic dysfunction. LV ejection fraction is decreased, and the left atrial and LV chambers are often dilated. Echocardiography may also provide information about the cause of LV failure, such as valve dysfunction or regional wall motion abnormalities.
- **Pulmonary artery catheterization** allows measurement of right-sided and pulmonary artery occlusive pressure and cardiac output, and permits calculation of derived hemodynamic variables, such as systemic vascular resistance. These data provide a quantitative assessment of LV function and are helpful both diagnostically and in guiding therapy.

Treatment. An effort should be made to determine the underlying cause of LV systolic function because it can have important implications for treatment and prognosis. Precipitating factors should be identified and treated. These include dysrhythmias, anemia, ischemia, hypertension, fluid overload, and the use of drugs that have negative inotropic properties. Arterial blood gases are performed to assess oxygenation and gas exchange, and supplemental oxygen is given as necessary. Endotracheal intubation and mechanical ventilation may be necessary in cases of severe LV failure, if respiratory failure is present or threatened (pH < 7.25, arterial carbon dioxide tension [Pa_{CO_2}] > 50 torr, arterial oxygen tension [Pa_{O_2}] < 50 torr) and cannot be immediately reversed with pharmacologic management. Drugs useful in managing systolic dysfunction include:

- **Diuretics,** which are used to reduce preload and relieve pulmonary congestion. In the acute situation, this goal is accomplished with a loop diuretic, such as furosemide or bumetanide, given IV. Urine output monitoring and daily weighing aid in determining the effectiveness of diuresis.
- **Nitroglycerin,** which may be given IV, PO, or transder-

TABLE 26–1

SIGNS AND SYMPTOMS OF LEFT VENTRICULAR FAILURE

Symptoms	Signs
Shortness of breath	Tachycardia
Fatigue	Tachypnea
Cough	Pulmonary rales
Orthopnea	Gallop rhythm
Paroxysmal nocturnal dyspnea	Apical impulse shifted leftward
Anorexia	Oliguria

mally to further reduce preload as well as relieve ischemia.

- **Vasodilators,** such as sodium nitroprusside, hydralazine, angiotensin-converting enzyme (ACE) inhibitors, or high-dose IV nitroglycerin, which are used to reduce LV afterload. Long-term treatment with ACE inhibitors has been shown to improve the long-term prognosis in patients with systolic dysfunction.
- **Inotropic agents,** such as dobutamine, dopamine, or amrinone, which are used to increase cardiac contractility. Because dopamine increases myocardial oxygen demand and may increase pulmonary capillary occlusive pressure, its use should be reserved for patients who are hypotensive.
- **Morphine sulfate,** which acts as both a venodilator and an anxiolytic. It is particularly useful in treating acute cardiogenic pulmonary edema. Important side effects are respiratory depression and hypotension.
- **Heparin** (5000 units subcutaneously every 12 hours), which is given for prophylaxis against venous thrombosis. Full-dose IV heparin therapy is considered in the setting of LV dysfunction secondary to acute myocardial ischemia and in patients with documented LV thrombus.

Insertion of an intra-aortic balloon pump should be considered in patients who do not respond to the above measures or who have ongoing ischemia. Intra-aortic balloon counterpulsation reduces LV afterload and improves coronary perfusion. It may allow diagnostic cardiac catheterization and other definitive interventions to be undertaken with improved safety. Intra-aortic balloon insertion is contraindicated in patients with aortic insufficiency or aortic dissection.

Diastolic Dysfunction

Etiology. Diastolic dysfunction is characterized by impaired LV compliance, often with well-preserved or even hyperdynamic systolic function. Common causes of diastolic LV dysfunction include:

- **Ischemia,** either acute or chronic. Patients who have diastolic dysfunction as a result of ischemia frequently also have a component of systolic dysfunction.
- **Left ventricular hypertrophy,** e.g., secondary to longstanding, poorly controlled hypertension or as a result of aortic stenosis.
- **Hypertrophic cardiomyopathy,** i.e., idiopathic hypertrophic subaortic stenosis.
- **Restrictive or infiltrative cardiomyopathies,** e.g., as a result of amyloidosis, sarcoidosis, or hemochromatosis.
- **Constrictive pericarditis,** e.g., caused by neoplasm, tuberculosis, radiation therapy, or connective tissue disease.

Diagnosis. It is important to recognize diastolic dysfunction as the underlying cause of LV failure because its management can differ significantly from that of systolic dysfunction. In some cases, however, the diagnosis must be inferred based on the lack of evidence of LV systolic dysfunction. Both forms of LV dysfunction coexist in some patients.

- **History and physical examination.** The signs and symptoms of LV failure are similar to those seen with systolic dysfunction (see Table 26–1). An S_4 gallop suggests reduced LV compliance. Other symptoms and physical findings (e.g., hypertension) may provide clues about the underlying cause.
- **Electrocardiography** may show evidence of LV hypertrophy. ECG signs of ischemia or previous infarction may be present. Reduced QRS voltage may suggest amyloid heart disease.
- **Chest radiography** may, as with systolic dysfunction, show signs of pulmonary vascular congestion or pleural effusions.
- **Echocardiography** is helpful in distinguishing between systolic and diastolic LV dysfunction. With the latter, hypertrophy and normal or even increased LV ejection fraction may be seen. Chamber size is often normal unless there is concomitant systolic dysfunction.
- **Pulmonary artery catheterization** may show distinctive hemodynamic patterns in constriction (i.e., equalization of diastolic pressures), but it generally is not helpful in differentiating systolic from diastolic dysfunction. However, it does allow quantitative hemodynamic assessment, and it is useful for titrating therapy.

Treatment. Pulmonary congestion should be treated with a loop diuretic; however, overzealous diuresis can be deleterious because these patients have impaired ventricular filling. Similarly, nitrates and vasodilators must be used with care to avoid excessive preload and afterload reduction. Digitalis and other inotropic drugs may actually be detrimental in these patients because they further reduce LV compliance. Underlying ischemia or hypertension should be treated with β-adrenergic receptor antagonists or verapamil. These agents tend to decrease LV contractility, but improve compliance. It is important to maintain a sinus rhythm and avoid tachycardia if possible. These patients tolerate atrial fibrillation and tachycardia poorly, and either can result in hypotension or an increase in congestive symptoms.

Suggested Readings

Braunwald E. ACE inhibitors: A cornerstone of the treatment of heart failure. *N Engl J Med* 1991;325:351–353.
Discusses addition of angiotensin-converting enzyme inhibitors to the management of heart failure.

Cohn JN. Current therapy of the failing heart. *Circulation* 1988; 78:1099–1107.
Useful review of overall management strategies for cardiac failure.

Dudwania PC, ed. Congestive heart failure. *Cardiol Clin* 1994;12:1–168.
Issue is devoted to heart failure, including several monographs on pharmacologic therapy.

Katz AM. The myocardium in congestive heart failure. *Am J Cardiol* 1989;63:12A–6.
Concise discussion of cellular mechanisms involved in the pathophysiology of the failing heart.

Lorell BH. Significance of diastolic dysfunction of the heart. *Ann Rev Med* 1991;42:411–436.
Useful expanded discussion on the management of diastolic dysfunction.

Sabia P, Abbott RD, Afrookteh A, et al. Importance of two-dimensional echocardiographic assessment of left ventricular systolic function in patients presenting to the emergency room with cardiac related symptoms. *Circulation* 1991;84:1615–1624.
Retrospective study on prognostic and diagnostic information obtained by early echocardiography.

CHAPTER 27
Circulatory Shock

(See Chapter 89)

John P. Dervan

Circulatory shock is a clinical state characterized by inadequate systemic tissue perfusion. Its clinical manifestations include the following:

- **Hypotension,** often defined as a systolic pressure of < 90 mm Hg, is usually present. In the early stages of shock, some patients may not be hypotensive.
- **Oliguria** is defined as a urinary output of < 20 mL/hr. However, this criterion may not be useful in patients with established renal failure or those who have polyuria secondary to osmotic or drug-induced diuresis.
- **Altered mental status** is an important, although nonspecific finding. It usually occurs as confusion, agitation, or a reduced level of consciousness. Focal neurologic findings suggest a primary neurologic injury or illness.
- **Skin temperature** is generally reduced, with cool, clammy extremities. In patients with septic shock, skin temperature may be normal or increased.
- **Hyperlactatemia** is the result of anaerobic metabolism. It is defined as a blood lactate level of ≥ 2.5 mmol/L.

General Assessment

- **Physical examination** should include assessment of vital signs, mental status, and skin temperature. Other findings are often nonspecific, but can provide important clues to the underlying cause of shock. Examples include fever, pulmonary congestion, pulse deficits, and pulsus paradoxus.
- **Laboratory studies** should include complete blood count, routine serum chemistries, urinalysis, arterial blood gas studies, and lactate concentration. If sepsis is considered a possible cause of the shock state, samples of blood and other body fluids should be obtained for culture. Other specific laboratory tests are obtained as clinically indicated.
- **Electrocardiography** identifies cardiac ischemia, infarction, and rhythm disturbances, which may be the precipitating cause of, or a consequence of, shock.
- **Chest radiography** should be performed to detect pulmonary vascular congestion, cardiomegaly, pleural effusions, pneumothorax, or infiltrates. Additional imaging studies may be warranted to determine the etiology of shock (e.g., ventilation–perfusion scan, computed tomography, echocardiography).
- **Hemodynamic monitoring** with arterial and pulmonary artery catheterization should be employed for accurate, continuous monitoring of systemic blood pressure, cardiac output and filling pressures, and other hemodynamic and gas-exchange variables (Table 27–1).

Clinical Shock Syndromes

Circulatory shock is generally divided into four categories based on hemodynamic characteristics.

Cardiogenic shock is usually secondary to severe impairment of left ventricular function. It usually occurs in the setting of massive myocardial infarction, with or without associated mechanical complications. Cardiogenic shock may also be seen in end-stage cardiomyopathy, acute myocarditis, and severe, acute valvular heart disease. Hemodynamically, it is characterized by low cardiac output, elevated pulmonary artery occlusive pressure (PAOP), and increased systemic vascular resistance (SVR).

Hypovolemic shock most often occurs in patients with blood loss, such as from traumatic or GI hemorrhage. It is also seen in severe dehydration (e.g., secondary to diabetic ketoacidosis or infectious diarrhea). Its hemodynamic characteristics include low cardiac output, low PAOP, and increased SVR.

Distributive shock is seen most commonly in severe sepsis. It is characterized in its early stages by increased cardiac output, low or normal PAOP, and significantly reduced SVR. Other causes include anaphylaxis, spinal cord injury, and effects of drugs and anesthetic agents.

Obstructive shock is caused by mechanical factors that significantly impede blood flow through the central circulation. Causes include pulmonary embolism, pericardial tamponade, aortic dissection, and prosthetic heart valve thrombosis. Obstructive shock is characterized by elevation in right atrial pressure, low cardiac output, and increased SVR.

Treatment

General principles. Identifying the underlying cause is crucial to the management of patients in circulatory shock. However, a number of general therapeutic measures are applicable to all patients.

- **Resuscitation** to ensure adequate airway, ventilation, and perfusion. Mean arterial blood pressure is maintained > 60 mm Hg to provide adequate end-organ perfusion. This goal may be accomplished through fluid resuscitation with blood, colloid, or crystalloid solutions, or with the use of inotropic or vasoactive agents, as indicated (see Table 27–2 and Chapter 34 in this book).
- **Intravenous access** must be maintained with one or more large-bore cannulae for infusion of fluids and drugs. Central venous catheterization is usually desirable.
- **Arterial catheterization** allows continuous monitoring of blood pressure, direct determination of mean arterial pressure, and frequent determination of arterial blood gases and other blood parameters.
- **Pulmonary artery catheterization** should be considered in all patients to assist in confirming the diagnosis and

TABLE 27–1

USE OF PULMONARY ARTERY CATHETERIZATION IN THE DIAGNOSIS AND CLASSIFICATION OF CIRCULATORY SHOCK

Type of Shock	Pulmonary Artery Occlusion Pressure	Cardiac Output	Comments
Cardiogenic			
Myocardial dysfunction	↑↑	↓↓	Usually occurs with evidence of extensive myocardial infarction, severe cardiomyopathy, or myocarditis
Acute ventricular septal defect	↑ or Nl	↓↓	Left-to-right shunt with oxygen saturation step-up in right ventricle
Acute mitral regurgitation	↑↑	↓↓	V waves in pulmonary artery occlusion pressure tracing
Right ventricle infarction	↓ or Nl	↓↓	Elevated right atrial and right ventricular end-diastolic pressures

Extracardiac Obstructive			
Pericardial tamponade	↑↑	↓ or ↓↓	Mean right atrial, right ventricular end-diastolic, and pulmonary artery occlusion pressures are all within 5 mm Hg of one another
Pulmonary embolism (massive)	↓ or Nl	↓↓	Right-sided heart pressures may be elevated
Oligemic			
Hypovolemia	↓↓	↓↓	Right atrial pressure is low
Distributive			
Septic shock	↓ or Nl	↑↑ or Nl (rarely ↓)	High mixed venous oxygen saturation and low systemic vascular resistance
Anaphylactic shock	↓ or Nl	↑ or Nl	—

↑↑ = moderate to severe increase; ↓↓ = moderate to severe decrease; ↑ = mild to moderate increase; ↓ = mild to moderate decrease; Nl = normal.

(Modified from Parrillo JE. Septic shock: Clinical manifestations, pathogenesis, hemodynamics, and management in a critical care unit. In: Parrillo JE, Ayres SA, eds. *Major issues in critical care.* Baltimore: Williams & Wilkins, 1984, p 111.)

TABLE 27–2

CATECHOLAMINE DRUGS USED IN TREATING CIRCULATORY SHOCK

Catecholamine	Dose μg/kg/min (μg/min)	Inotropic Effect (β_1)	Vasoconstriction (α_1)	Vasodilation (β_2)	Dopaminergic Effect	Indication (MAP < 60, mm Hg, PAOP > 12 mm Hg, plus:)
Dopamine	1–10	++	+	++	+++	↑ or normal CO
	10–20	+++	+++	+	0	Single pressor used
Norepinephrine	(2–10)	+++	++++	0	0	Dopamine failure
Phenylephrine	(20–200)	0	++++	0	0	Dysrhythmias, IHSS
Epinephrine	(1–8)	++++	++++	++	0	↓ CO, norepinephrine failure
Dobutamine	1–10	++++	+	++	0	↓ CO, may need to combine with norepinephrine therapy

+ = mild increase; ++ = moderate increase; +++ = large increase; ++++ = very large increase; 0 = no significant change; MAP = mean arterial blood pressure; PAOP = pulmonary artery occlusion pressure; CO = cardiac output; IHSS = idiopathic hypertrophic subaortic stenosis.

(Modified from Natanson C, Hoffman WD. Septic shock and other forms of distributive shock. In: Parrillo JE, ed. *Current therapy in critical care medicine,* 2nd ed. Philadelphia: BC Decker, 1991, p 62, by permission of Mosby–Year Book, Inc.)

determining the adequacy of volume replacement and other therapy.

- **Arterial blood gas** studies are necessary to ensure adequate oxygenation and ventilation and to evaluate the presence and severity of acidosis. Measurements of arterial blood lactate levels are also useful in assessing the degree of shock and the response to therapy.
- **Foley catheterization** allows accurate hourly measurement of urinary output. This information is useful for assessing systemic perfusion and guiding fluid loading.

Hypovolemic shock is treated with volume replacement, using blood, colloid, or crystalloid solutions. The type of fluid used depends on the underlying cause of the hypovolemia. Hemodynamic monitoring can be used to evaluate the adequacy of volume replacement. In the absence of underlying cardiopulmonary disease, central venous monitoring may be used instead of pulmonary artery catheterization. In addition, treatment efforts should be directed at correcting the underlying problem.

Cardiogenic shock is usually treated with preload reduction through diuresis and inotropic support. Dobutamine is the inotropic agent of choice. However, if there is severe hypotension, dopamine should be used because dobutamine may further reduce blood pressure. Intra-aortic balloon counterpulsation may help by improving coronary perfusion and reducing afterload. However, the use of this device is only a temporizing measure and, alone, will not improve long-term survival, although it may serve as a bridge to more definitive therapy, such as coronary revascularization, valve replacement, or cardiac transplant.

Septic shock is the most common form of distributive shock. Appropriate antibiotic use is the cornerstone of therapy. Selection is initially based on clinical presentation and the likely offending organisms, and later tailored to the results of cultures and susceptibility tests. Any focus of infection should be directly addressed. Possibilities include drainage of an abscess and removal of an indwelling vascular catheter suspected of being a nidus. Adequate fluid resuscitation is also crucial. Most patients with septic shock are hypovolemic and respond to fluid loading. Because sepsis is often associated with depressed cardiac function, an inotropic agent, such as dobutamine, may be of value in improving perfusion. For patients who remain hypotensive despite adequate volume loading and inotropic support, the use of a vasopressor agent, such as dopamine, will be necessary.

Obstructive shock includes a variety of causes. Therefore, treatment depends on the specific etiology. Unless there is a contraindication, pulmonary embolism associated with shock may be treated with thrombolytic therapy followed by heparinization (see Chapter 21 in this book).

In pericardial tamponade, removal of fluid by either pericardiocentesis or surgical pericardial window placement is the definitive treatment (see Chapters 12 and 33 in this book). Fluid resuscitation is useful in stabilizing patients with obstructive shock before more definitive therapy is administered.

Suggested Readings

Califf RM, Bengtson JR. Cardiogenic shock. *N Engl J Med* 1994; 330:1724–1730.
Reviews pathophysiology and management.

Kruse JA. The cellular basis of conventional and experimental pharmacotherapies for circulatory shock. *Anaesth Pharmacol Rev* 1994; 2:115–127.

Leor J, Goldbourt U, Reicher-Reiss H, et al. Cardiogenic shock complicating acute myocardial infarction in patients without heart failure on admission: Incidence, risk factors, and outcome. *Am J Med* 1993;94:265–272.
From analysis of 5839 patients with acute myocardial infarction, the authors found that a significant proportion of those who had cardiogenic shock were free of heart failure on admission.

Lollgen H, Drexler H. Use of inotropes in the critical care setting. *Crit Care Med* 1990;18:S56–S60.
Comparative discussion of inotropes in the management of the critically ill patient.

Packman MI, Rackow EC. Optimum left heart filling pressure during fluid resuscitation of patients with hypovolemic and septic shock. *Crit Care Med* 1983;11:165–169.
The average optimal pulmonary artery occlusive pressure in patients with hypovolemic and septic shock was 12 mm Hg in this study.

Parrillo JE, Parker MM, Natanson C, et al. Septic shock in humans: Advances in the understanding of pathogenesis, cardiovascular dysfunction and therapy. *Ann Intern Med* 1990;113:227–242.
Detailed discussion of pathophysiologic mechanisms and treatment.

Rackow ES, Astiz ME, eds. Circulatory shock. *Crit Care Clin* 1993; 9:183–399.
Issue is devoted to circulatory shock. It includes monographs on fluid resuscitation and septic, hemorrhagic, and cardiogenic shock.

CHAPTER 28

Unstable Angina Pectoris

(See Chapter 90)

Stephen T. Smith

Unstable angina pectoris (UA) is a changing pattern of symptoms indicating the development of an acute ischemic syndrome. It may be secondary to coronary arterial endothelial disruption or plaque rupture, with subsequent intramural and intraluminal thrombus formation caused by activation of clotting factors, platelet aggregation, and enhanced vascular tone. Synonyms of UA include acute coronary insufficiency, preinfarction angina, crescendo angina, accelerating angina, and intermediate coronary syndrome. Typical presentations include the following:

- New-onset angina at low levels of exertion.
- Rest, or nocturnal, angina.
- Increase in the frequency, severity, duration, or ease of provocation of previously stable angina.
- Postinfarction angina (within 30 days of acute myocardial infarction) and angina after revascularization with thrombolysis, coronary artery bypass grafting, or percutaneous transluminal coronary angioplasty (PTCA).

Clinical Features

History. The discomfort of UA is similar to that of stable angina pectoris, with variations in severity, frequency, timing, precipitating factors, duration, and the occurrence of new associated symptoms. Episodes of UA may last 30 minutes or more. The longer the episode, the more likely it is that an acute myocardial infarction (AMI) has occurred.

Physical examination findings are nonspecific; however, transient findings with symptomatic episodes may include:

- S_3 or S_4 gallop rhythm.
- Systolic murmur of mitral insufficiency because of papillary muscle dysfunction.
- Palpable cardiac apical dyskinesis.
- Hypertension or, less commonly, hypotension.

ECG findings are variable, and often transient. The most frequent abnormality is ST segment depression of 1 mm or greater that is horizontal, downsloping, or sagging. ST segment elevation may be seen transiently with transmural or epicardial ischemia in any lead except aVR, and is often seen with vasospasm or intermittent coronary occlusion. ST elevation is more likely to occur with left mainstem stenosis, high-grade proximal coronary stenosis, or triple-vessel disease. T wave changes include symmetric T wave inversion, T wave peaking, or changes in the T wave vector. New, persistent Q waves represent myocardial infarction, not UA. Other findings in UA may include U wave inversion, changes in R wave amplitude, QT prolongation, ventricular ectopy, and transient conduction disturbances, such as bundle branch blocks. Holter monitoring and telemetry may show the above findings, with and without symptoms, and may provide prognostic information about silent ischemia, helping to guide therapy or indicating the need for further intervention.

Stress Testing and Imaging Studies

- **Stress testing,** with or without adjunctive imaging, may be performed, after medical stabilization, for risk stratification. A negative finding on a treadmill test for ischemia confers a favorable prognosis. Tests showing ischemia at low workloads, exercise-induced hemodynamic disturbances, or severe dysrhythmias with ischemia may indicate the need for invasive studies.
- **Nuclear imaging** with ^{201}Tl or ^{99m}Tc sestaMIBI can be used to show reversible defects during spontaneous symptoms, and may confirm the diagnosis in equivocal cases.
- **Echocardiography** during symptoms may show focal reversible wall motion abnormalities, ventricular dilatation, or acute, transient mitral insufficiency, and thus may aid in the diagnosis.
- **Transesophageal echocardiography** can be used to exclude aortic dissection, and may demonstrate proximal coronary artery stenosis.
- **Cardiac catheterization** and coronary angiography are rarely needed for diagnosis, but should be performed in patients who do not respond to medical therapy and, therefore, may benefit from early revascularization.

Treatment

General Treatment. Low-risk patients with no history of ischemia, minimal or no ECG changes, prompt symptom relief, and no evidence of myocardial infarction can be admitted to a medical ward with telemetry. Higher-risk patients (i.e., those with ongoing symptoms, recent AMI or revascularization, high likelihood of new AMI, or other complicating factors) should be admitted to an intensive or coronary care unit. Initial management includes:

- Bed rest.
- Supplemental oxygen.
- Continuous ECG monitoring.
- IV access.
- Evaluation for precipitating factors for UA (e.g., anemia or hypertension).
- Serial ECG evaluations and cardiac enzyme assays.
- Frequent determination of vital signs and clinical evaluation (e.g., every 4 hours).

Pharmacologic Therapy

- **Aspirin** (80–325 mg, not enteric coated) should be chewed or swallowed, unless contraindicated. Aspirin appears to protect against AMI, late death, and probably early death in unstable angina. Ticlopidine is an alternative antiplatelet agent for patients who are allergic to aspirin, although its efficacy in unstable angina has not been proven.

- **Heparin** (5000 units by IV injection, followed by an infusion of 1000–1500 units/hr to maintain the partial thromboplastin time (PTT) at 1.5 to 2.5 times the control value, for 3 to 5 days), like aspirin, reduced the likelihood of death and reinfarction in several large trials. Newer, more specific antithrombin agents, such as hirudin, are under evaluation.
- **Nitrates** should be given by the PO, sublingual, or transdermal route. The IV route may also be used, and is preferable in patients with refractory symptoms. Infusion should begin at 5–10 μg/min, increasing every 5 minutes, and titrated to symptom relief or to a 15% reduction in mean arterial blood pressure, or to a maximum dose of 200–300 μg/min. Pharmacologic tolerance may develop after 24 hours. Adverse reactions include hypotension, headache, minor rhythm disturbances, methemoglobinemia, and heparin resistance. High-dose infusions of nitroglycerin may reduce the effectiveness of heparin by as much as 50%, perhaps by antithrombin III depletion, but this problem is usually overcome by increasing the heparin infusion rate.
- **β-Adrenergic receptor antagonists** (e.g., metoprolol 5 mg IV over 2 minutes, repeated every 5 minutes, for a total loading dose of 15 mg, followed in 1 hour by 25–50 mg PO every 12 hours) reduce myocardial oxygen consumption by decreasing heart rate, blood pressure, and myocardial contractility. Other IV formulations include esmolol, propranolol, and atenolol. Esmolol, with its half-life of 9 minutes, offers the advantages of a rapidly titratable, quickly eliminated IV drug. Endpoints include relief of symptoms and heart rate $\leq 50 \text{ min}^{-1}$. Contraindications to β-adrenergic antagonist therapy include symptomatic congestive heart failure, severe bronchospasm, bradydysrhythmias, and conduction disturbances.
- **Calcium channel antagonists** may be useful in treating symptoms in some patients, although they do not appear to reduce the mortality rate or risk of infarction. Nifedipine (a dihydropyridine) appears to increase mortality rate unless it is given with adjunctive β-adrenergic antagonist therapy. Other calcium channel antagonists may be best used as adjuncts to β-receptor antagonists or when contraindications to their use exist.
- **Thrombolytic agents** do not appear to be useful in the treatment of UA, and are not recommended.
- **Morphine sulfate** (e.g., 2–5 mg by IV injection) may be administered to patients whose pain is unrelieved by sublingual nitroglycerin and other anti-ischemic therapy.

Nonpharmacologic Treatment. Intra-aortic balloon counterpulsation may be used to stabilize medically refractory patients by increasing proximal aortic diastolic coronary perfusion pressure and by reducing afterload. Intra-aortic balloon counterpulsation alone has not been shown to improve survival rates, and should not be considered an endpoint in therapy. Contraindications include aortic aneurysm or dissection, aortic valvular insufficiency, severe dysrhythmias, and peripheral vascular disease. Complications include arterial insufficiency, which can result in limb loss; aortic dissection or perforation; bleeding; and infection.

Cardiac Catheterization and Revascularization. Early diagnostic catheterization may be associated with higher complication rates. It is generally deferred until patients are stabilized with medical therapy. The most common indication for urgent catheterization is continued ischemia despite medical management. Angiographically, most patients have eccentric lesions, with a high incidence of intraluminal thrombus. Intra-aortic balloon counterpulsation is often instituted at the time of urgent catheterization.

After medical stabilization, diagnostic catheterization may be indicated for patients with recurrent symptoms, treadmill test results showing ischemia at low workloads, or intolerance to medical therapy.

Urgent coronary angioplasty in patients with UA is associated with lower success rates, higher complication rates, and higher mortality rates than in those with stable angina pectoris. Nevertheless, it may be required in medically refractory cases.

In patients with left main coronary disease or three-vessel coronary disease, coronary artery bypass graft surgery may improve survival, relieve symptoms, and reduce the incidence of future hospitalizations. However, urgent bypass surgery is associated with higher mortality and complication rates compared with elective operations. Unfortunately, there are no large, randomized, prospective studies comparing medical therapy, balloon angioplasty, and bypass surgery in patients with unstable angina pectoris.

Prognosis

The in-hospital mortality rate is 2% to 5%, and approaches 15% at 1 year. Myocardial infarction occurs in as many as 20% of patients. A poorer short-term prognosis is seen in patients with advanced age, triple-vessel coronary artery disease, complex coronary anatomy, ongoing ischemic symptoms, intracoronary thrombi, ischemia at low workloads, and evidence of silent ischemia.

Suggested Readings

Agency for Health Care Policy and Research and the National Heart, Lung, and Blood Institute. *Unstable angina: Diagnosis and management.*

Clinical Practice Guideline No. 10. Washington, DC: U.S. Department of Health and Human Services, 1994.
Authoritative guidelines derived from systematic analysis of scientific literature and opinions of an expert panel. Copies are available from AHCPR Publications Clearinghouse; P.O. Box 8547; Silver Spring, MD 20907 (AHCPR publication no. 94-0602; 154 pages).

Betriu A, Heras M, Cohen M, Fuster V. Unstable angina: Outcome according to clinical presentation. *J Am Coll Cardiol* 1992;19:1659–1663.
Reviews clinical presentation of unstable angina and its importance.

Prisant ML, Von Dohlen T, Rogers W, et al. Pharmacotherapy of unstable angina. *J Clin Pharmacol* 1992;32:390–399.
Reviews current therapy for unstable angina pectoris.

Theroux P, Lidon RM. Unstable angina: Pathogenesis, diagnosis and treatment. *Curr Probl Cardiol* 1993;18:157–231.
In-depth review of unstable angina.

Theroux P, Waters D, Qiu S, et al. Aspirin versus heparin to prevent myocardial infarction during the acute phase of unstable angina. *Circulation* 1993;88:2045–2048.
Useful discussion of beneficial effects of aspirin and heparin in unstable angina.

The TIMI IIIB Investigators. Effects of tissue plasminogen activator and a comparison of early invasive and conservative strategies in unstable angina and non-Q wave myocardial infarction. *Circulation* 1994; 89:1545–1556.
Analysis of the TIMI III data, showing lack of efficacy for front-loaded recombinant tissue-type plasminogen and equivalence of invasive and conservative strategies in these ischemic syndromes.

CHAPTER 29

Acute Myocardial Infarction

(See Chapter 90)

Stephen T. Smith and Vivian L. Clark

Acute myocardial infarction (AMI) is a clinical syndrome that begins with coronary ischemia and culminates in myocardial cellular damage and, ultimately, necrosis, over minutes to hours. AMI usually results from acute coronary thrombosis in the setting of underlying coronary artery disease, but can also occur as a result of coronary embolization, spasm (either spontaneous or secondary to vasospastic drugs, such as cocaine), aortic dissection, vasculitides, congenital anomalies, or trauma.

Clinical Presentation

Symptoms

- **Pain** is the cardinal symptom of AMI. It is severe, prolonged (i.e., >30 minutes), and substernal in location.

It frequently radiates to the shoulders, arms, neck, or back. However, as many as 25% of infarctions are unrecognized because there is no pain or because symptoms are atypical. Painless AMI is particularly likely to occur in patients with diabetes mellitus or those who have undergone cardiac transplantation.

- **Associated symptoms** are frequently present, and include diaphoresis, shortness of breath, nausea, and vomiting. The latter two are particularly common in inferior wall AMI.
- **Prodromal symptoms,** usually crescendo chest pain, may precede AMI by hours or days.
- **Differential diagnosis** includes aortic dissection, pulmonary embolism, pericarditis, pneumonia, pneumothorax, and GI and musculoskeletal disorders.

Physical Examination. There are no specific physical findings in AMI. Patients often appear anxious, pale, and distressed, and usually indicate their chest as the source of discomfort.

- **Cardiovascular findings** may include bradycardia (especially with inferior wall AMI) or tachycardia. The rhythm may be irregular because ventricular ectopy is common. The precordium may show an abnormal apical impulse (dyskinesis) or an S_3 or S_4 gallop. Murmurs are uncommon, but can occur when there is associated mitral or tricuspid valve dysfunction or ventricular septal defect. Pericardial rubs are present in fewer than 25% of patients with AMI, but may persist for days. Distended jugular veins are indicative of right-sided heart failure, which may be caused by right ventricular infarction.
- **Pulmonary findings** may include tachypnea or orthopnea. The lungs may be clear or may show dependent rales as a result of pulmonary vascular congestion.
- **Other physical findings** may include fever, diaphoresis, and stigmata associated with underlying risk factors, e.g., digital tobacco staining, fundoscopic changes of hypertension or diabetes mellitus, or xanthomata of hyperlipidemia.

Diagnostic Testing

Electrocardiography. ST segment elevation of 1 mm or greater in two or more contiguous leads is strongly indicative of acute injury. Development of Q waves is variable but, when present, usually manifests within 24 hours after acute ST elevation. AMI may occur without the development of classic ST elevation and Q waves; comparison with earlier ECG readings may be helpful. Left bundle branch block may obscure the classic findings of AMI. A new left bundle branch block accompanied by prolonged chest discomfort may indicate the need for thrombolytic therapy.

Reciprocal changes (i.e., ST segment depression away from the zone of infarction) may represent reflective electrical changes or separate ischemic zones. ST elevation in V_1 or in the right precordial leads (e.g., V_3R and V_4R) suggests the possibility of right ventricular infarction. ST depression along with increased R wave amplitude in V_1 and V_2 may indicate posterior AMI.

Enzyme Analysis. Serum creatine phosphokinase (CK) level increases within 8 hours of myocardial damage, peaks within 24 hours, and usually returns to baseline over the next several days. CK typically increases twofold or more in AMI. The degree of elevation correlates roughly with the size of the infarction. To be diagnostic, the MB isoenzyme of CK is expected to increase to at least 4% of the total CK value in AMI. Serum lactate dehydrogenase (LDH) enzyme levels peak at 24 to 48 hours, and may help to confirm AMI, particularly in patients who do not seek treatment immediately. A ratio of LDH_1 to LDH_2 isoenzymes of greater than one is consistent with AMI.

Imaging Studies

- **Chest radiography** results may be entirely normal or may show signs of congestive heart failure, including cardiomegaly, pulmonary vascular congestion, Kerley B lines, or pleural effusion. It can also help to exclude other causes of chest pain, such as aortic dissection, pneumonia, or pneumothorax.
- **Echocardiography** is the most useful noninvasive imaging technique for detecting acute myocardial infarction. Its advantages include the ability to: (1) exclude other potential causes of chest pain (e.g., aortic dissection, pericarditis); (2) provide an assessment of ventricular performance, regional wall motion, and the location and size of the infarction; (3) detect mechanical complications, such as papillary muscle dysfunction and ventricular septal defect; and (4) detect intracardiac thrombus.
- **Radionuclide imaging,** using infarction-avid agents, such as ^{99m}Tc pyrophosphate or radiolabeled antimyosin antibody, can be used to confirm infarction if the ECG reading is equivocal. Perfusion imaging using ^{201}Tl or ^{99m}Tc sestaMIBI may show defects consistent with AMI.
- **Cardiac catheterization** and coronary angiography can document myocardial infarction by the presence of a characteristic occlusion of a coronary artery, coronary stenosis, or intracoronary thrombus, coupled with a focal wall motion abnormality seen by ventriculography. Usually, catheterization is not required for the diagno-

sis, and is reserved for patients who are likely to require urgent revascularization.

Treatment

General Measures

- The patient is admitted to the coronary care unit with continuous ECG monitoring.
- The patient is kept at bed rest (stable patients can use a bedside commode).
- Oxygen is administered by nasal cannula or mask, and oxygenation is assessed by pulse oximetry or blood gas analysis.
- IV access is established.
- Analgesics are administered for control of ischemic pain (e.g., IV morphine sulfate in 2-mg increments every 2–5 minutes to a total dose of approximately 10 mg).
- Low- to intermediate-dose anxiolytics (usually benzodiazepines) are useful for sedation.

Thrombolytic therapy is the most important pharmacotherapy for AMI. Many trials for AMI have been performed, and most have shown improved survival rates in patients receiving thrombolysis. The characteristics of the available thrombolytics are shown in Table 29–1. Indications include:

- Chest pain consistent with AMI, lasting > 30 minutes and unrelieved by nitrates.
- ST segment elevation (> 1 mm) in two or more contiguous leads, new bundle branch block, or posterior AMI (anterior ST segment depression and increased R wave amplitude in V_1 and V_2).
- No absolute contraindications to thrombolysis.

Regardless of the thrombolytic agent used, the survival benefit correlates with the rapidity of initiating treatment. Recombinant tissue-type plasminogen (rtPA) may have a small advantage in young patients with large anterior AMI who seek treatment within 4 hours. Clinicians should focus on the prompt recognition of AMI and prompt initiation of thrombolytic therapy.

Contraindications to thrombolytic therapy include factors that increase the risk of bleeding (e.g., major trauma, major neurologic surgery within 2 months, history of cerebrovascular accident, active internal bleeding, predisposition to hemorrhage, diabetic hemorrhagic retinopathy, prolonged or traumatic cardiopulmonary resuscitation (CPR), or severe uncontrolled hypertension). An allergic reaction to a thrombolytic within the previous 6 months is also a contraindication for that particular agent.

Relative contraindications include major surgery or

TABLE 29–1

CHARACTERISTICS AND DOSAGE OF THROMBOLYTIC AGENTS

Agent	Streptokinase	Urokinase*	APSAC	rtPA
Dose	1.5 million units over 60 minutes	3.0 million units over 60 minutes	30 mg over 5 minutes	15-mg bolus; 0.75 mg/kg over 30 minutes; 0.5 mg/kg over 60 minutes
Allergic potential	Yes	Minimal	Yes	Minimal
Repeat dose allowed	≤ 5 days, ≥ 6 months	Any time	≤ 5 days; ≥ 6 months	Any time
Approximate cost	$300	>$3000	$1800	$2400
Adjunctive heparin recommended	No	Yes	No	Yes

*Urokinase is approved only for intracoronary use.
APSAC = anisoylated plasminogen–streptokinase activator complex; rtPA = recombinant tissue plasminogen activator.

trauma within the previous 10 days, pregnancy, a high likelihood of intracardiac thrombus, acute pericarditis or endocarditis, or any condition in which bleeding is likely or would be difficult to manage. When relative contraindications exist, potential benefits of the therapy must be weighed against the risks.

Other Pharmacologic Therapy

- **Aspirin,** 160 mg initially followed by a 325-mg oral dose daily, improves survival, especially in combination with thrombolysis.
- **β-adrenergic receptor antagonists** without intrinsic sympathomimetic activity are advised early in AMI based on data suggesting a survival benefit, reduction of infarct size, and reduction of recurrent ischemia and infarction. In the absence of contraindications (e.g., heart failure, bronchospasm, high-degree heart block, PR interval > 0.24 seconds, severe hypotension, or severe bradycardia), β-blocking drugs should be administered as described in Table 29–2. Although it has no documented survival benefit, esmolol, with a half-life of 9 minutes, may be of value in cases in which complications are likely and prompt reversibility is desired.
- **Nitroglycerin** is of benefit in reducing infarct size, infarct expansion, and infarct-related complications; however, it has not been shown to improve survival. Nitrates have a role in controlling ischemic pain and ameliorating heart failure and recurrent ischemia, but they must be used cautiously in right ventricular infarction. These agents may be administered IV, starting at 5–10 μg/min and increased by 5–10 μg/min increments every 5 minutes until chest pain resolves, a dose of 200–300 μg/min is reached, or mean arterial pressure is < 80–90 mm Hg.
- **Calcium channel blocking agents** are useful in the treatment of myocardial ischemia, but their place in the treatment of AMI is questionable. One study using diltiazem suggested a benefit in non-Q wave AMI without heart failure; however, most data suggest that these drugs have a minimal role in the treatment of AMI, and some studies suggest that their use may be harmful in this setting.
- **Heparin** is frequently employed after thrombolytic therapy with rtPA. Major trials studying the potential of heparin alone to reduce mortality rate or prevent reinfarction have not been completed. Heparin is of benefit in patients with large anterior infarctions who are at increased risk of embolic events and in those with recurrent ischemia.

Primary Percutaneous Transluminal Coronary Angioplasty. Early cardiac catheterization and primary angio-

TABLE 29–2

CHARACTERISTICS OF β-ADRENERGIC BLOCKING AGENTS USED IN THE TREATMENT OF ACUTE MYOCARDIAL INFARCTION

Agent	Dose	β_1-Selective	Solubility	Half-Life
Metoprolol	5 mg IV every 1 hour for 3 doses, then 50–100 mg PO every 12 hours	+	Hydrophilic	3 hours
Atenolol	5–10 mg IV, then 100 mg PO every 24 hours	+	Hydrophilic	6–9 hours
Propranolol	20–80 mg PO every 8 hours	−	Lipophilic	1–6 hours
Timolol	0.4–1 mg IV, then 15–45 mg PO every 8 hours	−	Hydrophilic	4–5 hours
Esmolol	0.5 mg/kg IV loading dose, then 50–300 μg/kg/min IV	+	Hydrophilic	9 minutes

plasty of the infarct-related vessel should be considered when there is an absolute contraindication to thrombolytic therapy in patients presenting within 4 to 6 hours of symptom onset or in patients with suspected failure of thrombolytic therapy. In each clinical situation, the risks of early angiography and angioplasty must be weighed against the benefits. Primary percutaneous transluminal coronary angioplasty is an expensive therapy with limited availability (20% of United States hospitals have catheterization laboratories). It has not been proven superior to thrombolytic therapy.

Risk Stratification in Acute Myocardial Infarction

Early risk stratification in AMI is based on clinical examination, hemodynamic measurements, or the occurrence of complications. The degree of pulmonary congestion correlates with increasing mortality. One study showed that patients with a low cardiac index (< 2.2 L/min/m^2) and high pulmonary artery occlusion pressure (PAOP; > 18 mm Hg) had the highest mortality rate. Other factors indicating a poorer prognosis include large infarctions, anterior infarctions, previous AMI, diabetes mellitus, hypertension, ejection fraction less than 40%, female sex, advanced age, and evidence of residual ischemia, either spontaneous or provoked at low workloads on a predischarge exercise test. Patients with indicators of poor prognosis may benefit from early catheterization and revascularization.

Complications of Acute Myocardial Infarction

Heart Failure. Hemodynamic complications range from mild pulmonary congestion to frank cardiogenic shock. The latter is associated with mortality rates approaching 80%. In patients with cardiogenic shock, a search for correctable mechanical causes, such as mitral insufficiency, ventricular septal defect, or ventricular rupture, should be undertaken. In the absence of another remediable cause, reperfusion by angioplasty of the infarct-related artery may improve survival.

Mechanical intervention, such as the intra-aortic balloon pump or ventricular assist devices may be helpful, but are probably best used as a bridge to more definitive therapy, i.e., revascularization or repair of a mechanical defect. These devices alone do not appear to reduce the mortality rate.

See Chapters 26 and 27 in this book for a discussion of

further aspects of treatment of heart failure and cardiogenic shock.

Mechanical Complications. Ventricular free-wall rupture, which is usually a fatal complication, accounts for approximately 10% of deaths in patients with AMI. Its peak incidence is at 1 to 4 days, but can occur as long as 3 weeks after the event. Predisposing factors include anterior infarction, advanced age, female sex, first infarction, preexisting hypertension, and possibly late thrombolytic therapy. Rupture permits blood to enter the pericardial space, leading to tamponade, electromechanical dissociation, and death. Occasionally, a pseudoaneurysm forms, possibly as a result of localized pericardial adhesions, with a more protracted clinical course and the potential for surgical intervention.

Papillary muscle rupture or dysfunction and ventricular septal defect (VSD) also commonly occur within 1 to 4 days after AMI. The former can lead to mitral insufficiency, and the latter, to acute volume overload. Both of these complications occur clinically as worsening heart failure, pulmonary edema, or cardiogenic shock, associated with a new systolic murmur. The diagnosis in either case can be made by Doppler echocardiography. In addition, VSD can be identified by an increase in oxygen saturation at the level of the right ventricle. Treatment includes afterload reduction and inotropic support with pharmacotherapy or intra-aortic balloon counterpulsation and urgent surgical repair of the mechanical lesion, accompanied by revascularization where indicated.

Right ventricular infarction (RVMI) is usually seen in the setting of inferior wall infarction. Clinical findings suggesting RVMI include elevated jugular venous pressure and systemic hypotension, especially when unaccompanied by signs of pulmonary vascular congestion. ECG findings include evidence of inferior wall AMI accompanied by ST elevation in the right precordial leads V_3R and V_4R, or in lead V_1. Hemodynamic characteristics include elevated right atrial pressure (particularly when accompanied by a prominent y descent and a low PAOP), elevated right ventricular end-diastolic pressure with a dip-and-plateau pattern, and low cardiac index. Volume loading often reverses shock in RVMI, although inotropic support may also be required, particularly in patients with significant associated left ventricular involvement.

Intraventricular thrombus is detectable by echocardiography in 20 to 40% of patients, and in approximately 5% it leads to a clinically apparent embolic event. Patients with thrombus are especially at risk for embolism during the first 3 to 6 months after AMI. Anticoagulation with heparin and warfarin is used when there is a documented intracardiac thrombus, when an embolic event has occurred, or in cases of large anterior infarction, ventricular aneurysm, or pseudoaneurysm.

Pericardial syndromes after AMI include pericardial effusion, early pericarditis, and late pericarditis (Dressler's syndrome). Myocardial infarction is a common cause of a small, self-limited pericardial effusions that usually require no specific treatment, unless hemorrhagic pericarditis or myocardial rupture is suspected. Pericarditis can occur within 1 day, as in the common, early form, or as late as 10 weeks, as in the less common Dressler's syndrome. Most episodes respond promptly to nonsteroidal anti-inflammatory agents, preferably aspirin. Anticoagulation should be avoided in patients with pericarditis, unless deemed essential.

Dysrhythmias and conduction disturbances are common in AMI. They may arise because of ischemic injury to the conducting system, abnormal vagal responsiveness, or electrical instability of the injured myocardium.

- **Sinus tachycardia** occurs in as many as 25% of patients, and may significantly increase myocardial oxygen demands. Treatment includes correction of precipitating factors, such as hypoxemia, pain, left ventricular dysfunction, and increased catecholamine state. β-receptor antagonists may be useful in reducing heart rate and oxygen demands.
- **Atrial fibrillation** with symptomatic, rapid ventricular response is seen in approximately 15% of patients. Digoxin, calcium channel blockers (intravenous diltiazem or verapamil), and β-receptor antagonists may be used to control heart rate. Spontaneous conversion to sinus rhythm usually occurs. Electrical cardioversion should be considered in symptomatic patients.
- **Accelerated junctional rhythm,** which is generally benign and self-limited, requires no specific therapy.
- **Ventricular dysrhythmias** are most common in the early stages of AMI. They have a variety of forms and frequencies, including simple and complex ventricular ectopy, accelerated idioventricular rhythms, ventricular tachycardia, and ventricular fibrillation. Ventricular ectopy is common in AMI and is more likely to occur in the setting of extensive left ventricular dysfunction. Symptomatic or frequent ventricular ectopy may be treated with lidocaine; however, prophylactic treatment with this agent does not appear to reduce the mortality rate. It is therefore not recommended because of its inherent risks. Ventricular tachycardia is seen in 10 to 40% of patients with AMI, and may herald ventricular fibrillation. Treatment of sustained ventricular tachycardia and ventricular fibrillation includes immediate cardioversion, IV lidocaine for 24 hours, and correction of any precipitating factors (e.g., hypoxemia, electrolyte

TABLE 29–3

MANAGEMENT OF ATRIOVENTRICULAR CONDUCTION DISTURBANCES ASSOCIATED WITH ACUTE MYOCARDIAL INFARCTION

Type of Heart Block	Clinical Setting	Treatment
First-degree AV block	Any AMI	Observe
Type I second-degree AV block	Any AMI	Observe
Type II second-degree AV block	Stable inferior AMI	Observe
	Unstable inferior AMI	Pacemaker
	Anterior AMI	Pacemaker
Third-degree AV block	Stable inferior AMI	Atropine; consider pacemaker
	Anterior AMI	Pacemaker
Right or left bundle branch block	Any AMI	Observe; consider pacemaker
Left anterior or posterior hemiblock	Any AMI	Observe

AMI = acute myocardial infarction; AV = atrioventricular.

disturbances, digitalis toxicity). Antiarrhythmic drugs are discussed in Chapter 34 in this book.

- **Heart block** may be related to ischemia of the conduction system or to abnormal vagal responses seen in some patients with AMI (especially inferior wall infarction). Bundle branch block in the setting of anterior myocardial infarction implies major conduction system damage and carries a poor prognosis. Guidelines for temporary pacemaker insertion are shown in Table 29–3.

Recurrent ischemia that occurs as postinfarction angina, new ECG changes, or reinfarction, is seen in 10 to 20% of patients within the first 10 days after AMI. It is more common after successful thrombolytic therapy. Because of its unfavorable prognosis, recurrent ischemia is an indication for cardiac catheterization and revascularization. It may be treated initially with anticoagulation, repeat thrombolysis (in the case of reinfarction), and anti-ischemic agents, as appropriate.

Suggested Readings

Chatterjee K. Pathogenesis of low output in right ventricular myocardial infarction. *Chest* 1992;102:590S–595S.

The major mechanism is a decrease in left ventricular filling volume. This decrease is caused by right ventricular dilation within a constrained pericardial sac, decreased right ventricular stroke volume, and increased right ventricular afterload as a result of increased pulmonary capillary pressure and increased right ventricular wall stress.

Gruppo Italiano per lo Studio della Streptochinasi nell' Infarto Miocardio (GISSI). Effectiveness of intravenous thrombolytic treatment in acute myocardial infarction. *Lancet* 1986;1:397–402.

One of the original large-scale thrombolytic trials.

Gunnar RM, Passamani ER, Bourdillon PD, et al. Guidelines for the early management of patients with acute myocardial infarction: A report of the American College of Cardiology/American Heart Association Task Force on Assessment of Diagnostic and Therapeutic Cardiovascular Procedures (subcommittee to develop guidelines on the early management of patients with acute myocardial infarction). *J Am Coll Cardiol* 1990;16:249–292.

In-depth position paper that outlines several issues in the management of acute myocardial infarction, including pharmacologic therapy, the use of pacemakers, and the role of revascularization with percutaneous transluminal coronary angioplasty or bypass surgery.

The GUSTO Investigators. An international randomized trial comparing four thrombolytic strategies for acute myocardial infarction. *N Engl J Med* 1993;329:673–682.

Recent trial comparing thrombolytic agents in 40,000 patients.

ISIS-2 (Second International Study of Infarct Survival) Collaborative Group. Randomised trial of intravenous streptokinase, oral aspirin, both or neither among 17,187 cases of suspected acute myocardial infarction: ISIS-2. *Lancet* 1988;2:349–360.

Landmark study that showed the independent and additional benefit of adjunctive aspirin with thrombolytic therapy.

Lee L, Bates ER, Pitt B, et al. Percutaneous transluminal coronary angio-

plasty improves survival in acute myocardial infarction complicated by cardiogenic shock. *Circulation* 1988;78:1345–1351.
One of several small studies that suggest that angioplasty of the infarct-related artery may substantially improve survival in cardiogenic shock caused by myocardial infarction.

CHAPTER 30

Cardiac Dysrhythmias

(See Chapter 94)

Vivian L. Clark

Cardiac dysrhythmias are frequently encountered in critically ill patients. Prompt recognition and appropriate management of dysrhythmias is important because some of these disorders can have a substantial effect on a patient's clinical course.

Supraventricular Dysrhythmias

Sinus tachycardia is the most common rhythm disturbance encountered in the ICU. It does not occur as a primary dysrhythmia, but is a compensatory response to a physiologic or pathologic condition such as pain, exertion, agitation, hypoxemia, fever, anemia, hypovolemia, excess thyroid hormone, or heart failure. It can also occur as a response to certain drugs, e.g., vasodilators and β-adrenergic agonists. When sinus tachycardia is present, it is important to look for and treat the underlying cause because efforts to simply slow the rate are rarely appropriate.

Premature atrial contractions (PACs) are also common, and they may precede or precipitate other atrial dysrhythmias. These are generally narrow-complex beats that occur early and are preceded by a P wave that may differ morphologically from the patient's normal P waves. PACs are not followed by a compensatory pause, and rarely require treatment.

Atrial fibrillation is a rapid, irregularly irregular rhythm caused by chaotic atrial activity, with variable conduction of impulses to the ventricles. The characteristics of atrial fibrillation (Figure 30–1) include:

- Irregular baseline without discernible P waves.
- Narrow QRS complexes, although aberrant conduction may occur, particularly if the ventricular rate is fast.
- Ventricular rate that is dependent on atrioventricular

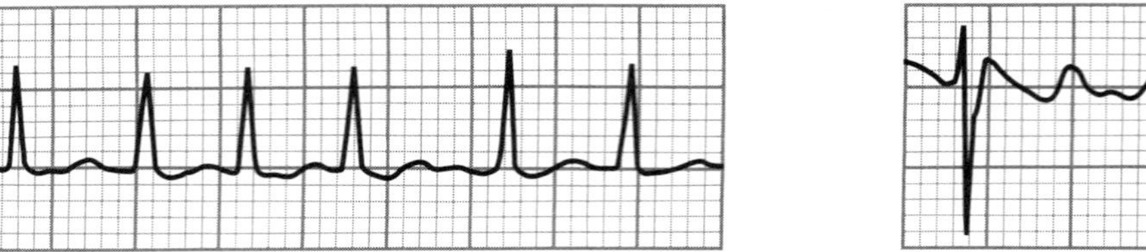

Figure 30–1. Atrial fibrillation with ventricular rate of approximately 200 min^{-1}. Irregular RR intervals are seen, and P waves are absent.

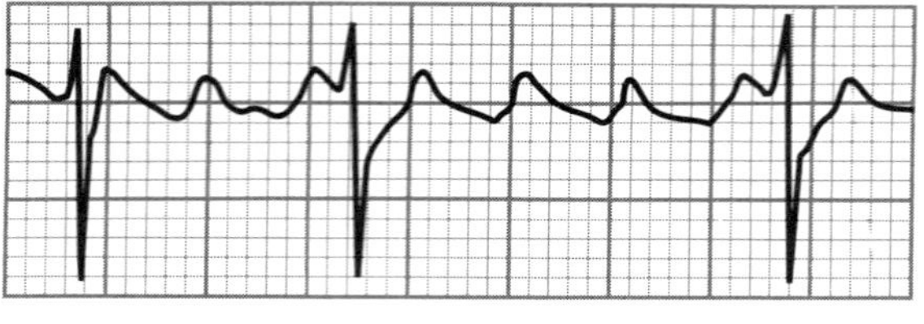

Figure 30–2. Atrial flutter with variable atrioventricular conduction. Flutter waves are regular. Rate is 300 min^{-1}.

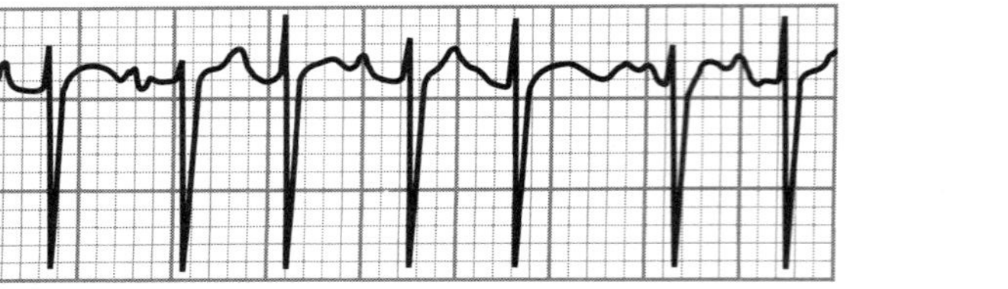

Figure 30–3. Multifocal atrial tachycardia at a rate of approximately 230 min^{-1}. P wave morphology and PR intervals are variable.

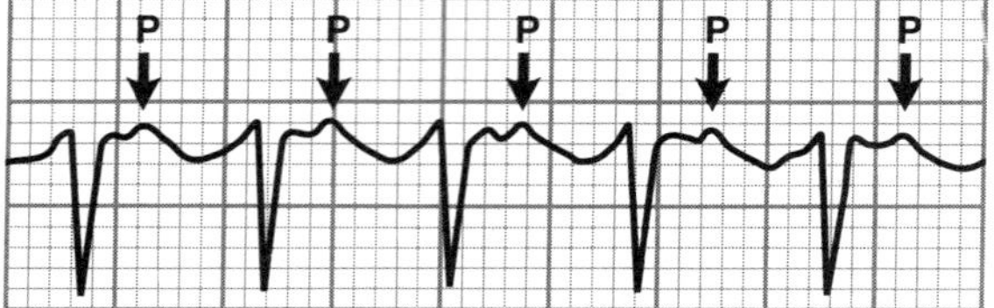

Figure 30–4. Supraventricular tachycardia with a ventricular rate of 170 min^{-1}. Retrograde P waves are superimposed on T waves (arrows).

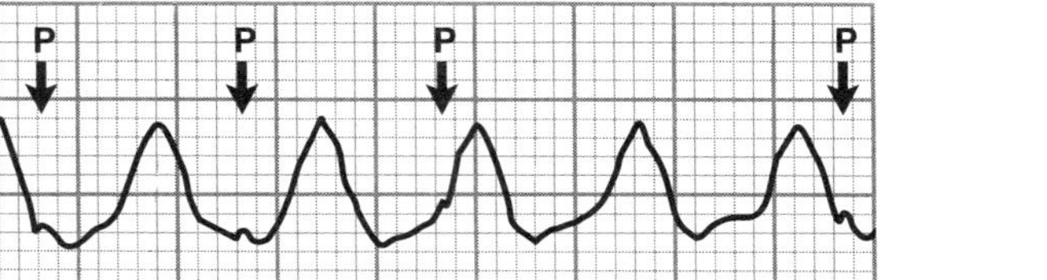

Figure 30–5. Ventricular tachycardia at a rate of 190 min^{-1}. The dissociated P waves are sometimes visible (arrows).

Figure 30–6. Torsades de pointes at a rate of approximately 300 min^{-1}. The QRS morphology is continually varying, and there is a sine wave pattern to the waveform envelope.

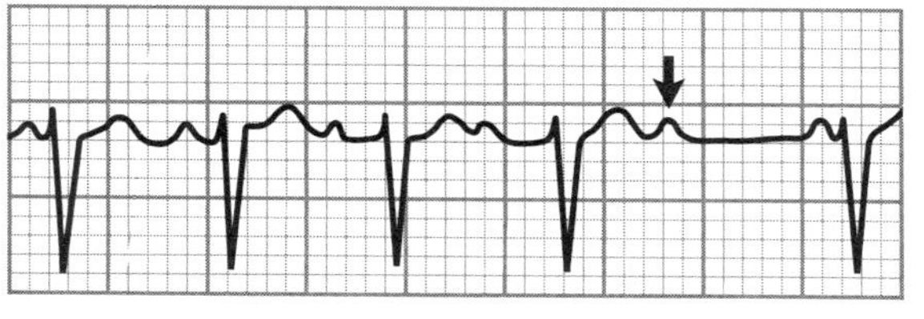

Figure 30–7. Wenckebach atrioventricular block, with gradual prolongation of the PR interval culminating in a nonconducted P wave (arrow).

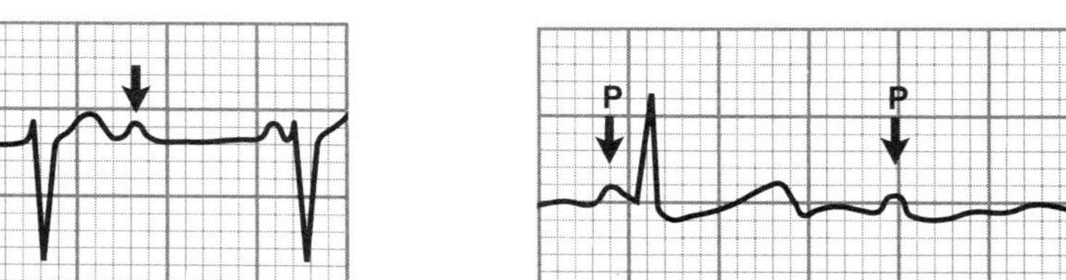

Figure 30–8. Third-degree atrioventricular block with junctional escape rhythm at a rate of 55 min^{-1}. P waves are dissociated (arrows).

(AV) nodal conduction, sympathetic and parasympathetic tone, and the duration of the atrial fibrillation. Generally, in untreated patients, the rate exceeds 120 min^{-1}.

Precipitating factors include hypertension, coronary artery disease, and valvular heart disease, particularly when there is associated left atrial enlargement. It can occur postoperatively, particularly after thoracic and cardiac procedures, and with pulmonary embolism.

The treatment of atrial fibrillation is generally aimed at controlling the ventricular rate, but it depends on the patient's clinical status. If marked hemodynamic instability is present, electrical cardioversion should be performed. Digoxin is usually effective in controlling ventricular rate, but it does not have rapid onset of effect. IV adenosine and verapamil are rapidly effective in controlling ventricular rate, but have relatively short half-lives, although these drugs may be useful in conjunction with digoxin. IV diltiazem can be given as a continuous infusion. β-adrenergic blocking agents, such as propranolol and esmolol, are also useful for controlling ventricular rate, particularly in atrial fibrillation in the setting of ischemia.

Atrial flutter (Figure 30–2) is related to atrial fibrillation and is characterized by:

- Regular atrial activity at rates between 250 and 400 min^{-1}, with a sawtooth pattern most often evident in the inferior leads or in lead V_1.
- Conduction to the ventricle, which usually occurs at a ratio of 2:1 or 3:1 in untreated patients.

This rhythm is associated with valvular heart disease, pericardial disease, and thyrotoxicosis. Treatment is similar to that for atrial fibrillation. In addition, flutter can sometimes be converted by rapid atrial pacing. Treatment sometimes results in conversion to atrial fibrillation.

Multifocal atrial tachycardia (MAT; Figure 30–3) is frequently encountered in patients with severe pulmonary disease. It may be a precursor of respiratory failure. MAT is characterized by:

- Irregular rhythm, with P waves of at least three different morphologies, and with 1:1 ventricular conduction.
- Variable rate, although it may be as high as 200 min^{-1} and can be difficult to control.

The initial management goal is to identify and treat the underlying cause. Mechanical ventilation may be beneficial in patients with impending respiratory failure. Digoxin is of little benefit in controlling the rate, and the response to calcium channel blocking agents has also been disappointing. Cardioselective β-blocking drugs, such as metoprolol, may be effective, but must be used cautiously in the setting of bronchospasm. Recent studies have suggested that high-dose magnesium may be of benefit.

Paroxysmal supraventricular tachycardia (PSVT; Figure 30–4) is common and often occurs in patients with underlying heart disease. It is frequently seen in patients with bypass tracts (e.g., Wolff-Parkinson-White syndrome). PSVT is characterized by:

- Rapid regular rhythm.
- A QRS complex that is usually narrow, but may be wide, particularly if there is a bypass tract.
- P waves that may not be visible, or may occur after the QRS complex.
- Abrupt onset and termination.

PSVT can often be successfully terminated by vagal maneuvers, such as the Valsalva maneuver, carotid massage, or facial immersion in cold water. When the QRS complex is wide, a bypass tract should be suspected, and treatment should be selected accordingly, with drugs that slow conduction through the bypass tract (see Chapter 34 in this book).

Ventricular Dysrhythmias

Premature ventricular contractions (PVCs) are the most common ventricular dysrhythmia encountered clinically. They are characterized by:

- Wide QRS beats that occur early and are followed by a compensatory pause.
- No associated P waves.
- QRS morphology and axis that differ from those of the normal QRS complex.

The presence of PVCs does not imply underlying cardiovascular disease, although they can be a marker of ischemia. Other precipitating factors include high catecholamine states, acid–base disturbances, drugs (e.g., digoxin, antiarrhythmic agents, cyclic antidepressants), and hypothermia.

Asymptomatic PVCs generally do not require treatment. If a precipitating cause is identified, it should be treated. In the setting of ischemia, frequent ventricular ectopy may be treated with lidocaine. Life-threatening ventricular dysrhythmias may or may not be heralded by PVCs.

Ventricular tachycardia (VT) is generally defined as more than three consecutive PVCs (Figure 30–5). It is considered sustained when it continues for more than 30 seconds. The morphologic characteristics of VT are the same as those of PVCs. The rate may vary from less than 100 to more than 250 min^{-1}. Ventricular tachycardia is often, but not always, associated with symptoms and hemodynamic compromise. The absence of significant symptoms does not exclude VT.

In some cases, it is difficult to determine whether a wide QRS dysrhythmia is ventricular or supraventricular in origin. Characteristics used to differentiate between the two types of dysrhythmia are listed in Table 30–1. An intra-atrial electrogram recorded from a transvenous pacing wire will usually allow differentiation between the two if they cannot be distinguished by the surface ECG reading. The presence of AV dissociation suggests that the rhythm is of ventricular origin. Drugs used in the treatment of ventricular dysrhythmias are outlined in Chapter 34 in this book. Prompt electrical cardioversion should be administered for VT associated with hemodynamic instability.

A distinct type of polymorphic ventricular tachycardia, commonly referred to as torsades de pointes, is characterized by periodic reversal in the axis of the QRS complex that gives the waveform envelope a characteristic sine-wave appearance (Figure 30–6). This dysrhythmia is most often seen in the setting of prolongation of the QT interval. Its recognition is critical because the management is different from that of ordinary VT. Causes of torsades de pointes include antiarrhythmic drugs, particularly class I agents (quinidine, procainamide, and disopyramide); hypokalemia; severe bradycardia; congenital prolongation of the QT interval; and other drugs, such as certain psychotropic agents. Although prolonged QT interval is frequently seen with ischemia and CNS events, torsades de pointes rarely occurs in these settings. Treatment of the underlying cause is important in the management of this dysrhythmia. Overdrive pacing or increasing the heart rate with drugs such as isoproterenol will often prevent its recurrence. Phenytoin has been used, but its efficacy is uncertain. Magnesium replacement may be of value. In patients with congenital long QT syndromes, β-adrenergic receptor blocking drugs are often effective in preventing recurrent episodes.

Ventricular fibrillation is characterized by chaotic electrical activity, with absence of recognizable complexes. Untreated, death usually ensues, although occasionally this dysrhythmia spontaneously reverts. Ventricular fibrillation may be preceded by PVCs, ventricular tachycardia or, less commonly, by a supraventricular dysrhythmia, but it can also occur de novo. Ventricular fibrillation occurs most often in the setting of myocardial ischemia or infarction, although any critically ill patient is at some risk. A significant electrolyte or acid–base imbalance, drug toxicity, or hypothermia can be a precipitating factor. Prompt electrical defibrillation is the treatment of choice. If the arrest is witnessed, a precordial thump may convert ventricular fibrillation to an organized rhythm. On conversion, it is

TABLE 30–1

CHARACTERISTICS USEFUL IN DETERMINING THE ORIGIN OF WIDE QRS TACHYDYSRHYTHMIAS

Characteristic	Ventricular	Supraventricular
Rate	Rarely helpful	Rarely helpful
Axis	Marked axis shift	Axis similar to normal QRS
QRS duration	$\geq$ 0.16 seconds	$<$ 0.14 seconds
QRS morphology	Atypical right (uni- or biphasic) or left bundle branch block configuration	Typical right bundle branch block configuration
Atrioventricular dissociation	Usually present	Usually absent
QRS concordance	Often present	Often absent
Underlying heart disease	Usually present	Often absent

imperative to search for and treat any underlying factors that may have precipitated the episode.

Bradycardia and Atrioventricular Block

Bradycardia is encountered frequently in the ICU setting. Sinus bradycardia (rate $< 50\ \text{min}^{-1}$) may occur with sinus node disease, drugs (particularly β-blocking drugs), CNS catastrophes, or hypothermia. It occurs normally in trained athletes. Sinus bradycardia should not be treated in the absence of symptoms. Symptomatic sinus bradycardia may respond to atropine or β-adrenergic drugs, such as isoproterenol. Temporary or permanent cardiac pacing is sometimes required.

Atrioventricular junctional rhythm is another type of bradycardia occasionally encountered in critically ill patients. This rhythm occurs as an escape mechanism during AV block or during periods of sinus node dysfunction. It can occur normally in response to increased vagal tone. AV junctional rhythm has the following characteristics:

- Regular narrow QRS rhythm at rates of 35–60 min^{-1}.
- P waves that are absent or that occur just before, buried within, or after the QRS complex or, in the setting of complete AV block, are dissociated from the QRS.

AV junctional rhythms are frequently asymptomatic and generally respond to the same measures used to treat sinus bradycardia.

Atrioventricular nodal block. There are three degrees of AV nodal block, signifying different stages of AV nodal dysfunction. First-degree AV block is defined as a PR interval of greater than 0.20 sec. It does not require treatment, although in its presence, drugs that suppress AV conduction should be used cautiously.

Second-degree AV nodal block is of two types. Mobitz type I, also known as Wenckebach AV block (Figure 30–7), is characterized by gradual prolongation of the PR intervals, along with gradual reduction in the RR intervals, ultimately culminating in a nonconducted P wave. Wenckebach AV block usually occurs with 3:2 or 4:3 conduction. It may be intermittent, and 2:1 conduction can occur. Mobitz type II second-degree AV block is characterized by nonconducted P waves in the absence of changes in the PR interval. This type of block is often associated with some prolongation in QRS. Its presence implies disease lower in the conducting system than Mobitz type I block, and it carries a more ominous prognosis. When second-degree AV block occurs with 2:1 conduction, it may not be possible to distinguish between the two types, although gradual prolongation of the PR interval seen on other parts of the rhythm strip suggest Mobitz type I block.

Second-degree AV block generally does not require urgent teratment unless it is accompanied by significant symptoms. Because Mobitz type II block may progress to higher-degree AV block, pacing might be required.

Third-degree, or complete, AV block (Figure 30–8) has the following characteristics:

- AV dissociation, i.e., no relationship between atrial and ventricular activity.
- A junctional (rate 35–60 min^{-1}) or ventricular (wide QRS complex with rate $\leq$ 40 min^{-1}) escape mechanism.
- An atrial rate that exceeds the ventricular rate, thus distinguishing complete AV block from escape rhythms caused by sinus pauses or sinus arrest.

Third-degree AV block occurs as a result of degeneration or ischemia in the AV nodal conducting tissue. Less commonly, it results from pressure on or infiltration into the AV node as a result of endocarditis with abscess formation, sinus of an Valsalva aneurysm, or infiltrative myocardial disease. As with other types of AV block, complete AV block may not require urgent treatment. When ischemia is the cause, block is often transient, and it resolves over a period ranging from less than 24 hours to more than 2 weeks. Only occasionally does complete AV block respond to atropine. Therefore, temporary or permanent cardiac pacing may be required (see Chapter 11 in this book).

Treatment of Dysrhythmias

In treating cardiac dysrhythmias, several general principles should be noted:

- The degree of hemodynamic compromise caused by the rhythm disturbance should dictate the type of therapy selected. Patients who are in severe distress may require electrical cardioversion or defibrillation. On the other hand, an asymptomatic patient may require no treatment.
- If the origin (i.e., supraventricular or ventricular) of a wide QRS tachycardia cannot be determined with certainty, it should be assumed to be of ventricular origin, and treated accordingly.
- Dysrhythmias may be precipitated or exacerbated by a number of factors, including ischemia, electrolyte or acid–base disturbances, sepsis, circulatory shock, and pulmonary embolism. It is important to identify and treat any underlying precipitating factors.

Drugs commonly used to treat dysrhythmias are discussed in Chapter 34 in this book.

Suggested Readings

Akhtar M. Clinical spectrum of ventricular tachycardia. *Circulation* 1990;82:1561–1573.
Excellent review of ventricular tachycardia.

Akhtar M, Shenasa M, Jazayeri M, et al. Wide QRS complex tachycardia: Reappraisal of a common problem. *Ann Intern Med* 1988; 109:905–912.
Of 150 consecutive cases of wide-complex tachycardia, 122 had ventricular tachycardia, 21 had supraventricular mechanism, and 7 had accessory pathway conduction.

Jackman WM, Friday KJ, Anderson JL, et al. The long QT syndromes: A critical review, new clinical observations and a unifying hypothesis. *Prog Cardiovasc Dis* 1988;31:115–172.
Comprehensive review of the long QT syndrome.

Kastor JA. Multifocal atrial tachycardia. *N Engl J Med* 1990; 322:1713–1717.
Excellent review of MAT.

Roden DM. Torsades de pointes. *Clin Cardiol* 1993;16:683–686.
Reviews clinical findings and mechanisms underlying this form of ventricular tachycardia.

Wang K, Hodges M. The premature ventricular complex as a diagnostic aid. *Ann Intern Med* 1992;117:766–770.
Explaining how analysis of premature ventricular complexes can provide clues to physical or electrocardiographic diagnosis, such as allowing visualization of P waves or flutter waves and distinguishing an S_3 from an S_4 gallop.

CHAPTER 31

Hypertensive Urgencies and Emergencies

(See Chapter 114)

Mohammed Saud Anwar and Dane J. Nichols

Hypertensive crises include a group of clinical syndromes in which rapid blood pressure reduction is necessary to prevent serious, permanent, or fatal complications. These syndromes may be categorized into hypertensive urgencies and emergencies according to their severity and the recommended rate at which blood pressure reduction should be achieved. Hypertensive emergencies are characterized by progressing end-organ damage. Susceptibility to pressure injury is dependent not only on the degree of elevation of blood pressure, but also on the rate of increase. Table 31–1 summarizes the clinical features, complications, and goals of treatment for hypertensive emergencies and urgencies.

Clinical Assessment

History. A complete medical history is obtained, with a focus on eliciting symptoms suggesting end-organ damage and identifying underlying conditions or factors that may have precipitated the hypertensive crisis. Important points include the patient's age; sex; race; history of CNS or cardiovascular symptoms; history of previously diagnosed hypertension, chronic renal disease, or pregnancy; and current drug use.

Physical and Laboratory Findings. The physical examination is directed at identifying evidence of end-organ damage, and thus should focus on ocular, neurologic, cardiovascular, and renal manifestations. Funduscopic changes, alterations in mental status, and focal neurologic deficits suggest CNS involvement. Cardiovascular dysfunction may occur as acute heart failure or pulmonary edema, ischemic ECG changes, or findings suggesting aortic dissection. These findings may include blood pressure disparity in the extremities, physical signs of aortic insufficiency, and widened mediastinum detected by chest radiography (see Chapter 32 in this text). Rising serum levels of urea nitrogen and creatinine in the presence of anemia suggest renal-induced hypertension. Urinalysis may provide evidence of renal parenchymal disease. In patients with neurologic abnormalities, computed tomographic imaging of the brain is frequently necessary to exclude intracranial hemorrhage or infarction.

Treatment

The rapidity and extent of blood pressure reduction is dictated by the precipitating event, the organ system involved, and the severity and chronicity of the hypertension. Several general principles guide the treatment of hypertensive crisis. During reduction in mean arterial pressure (MAP) of as much as 25%, vascular autoregulation within the brain preserves cerebral blood flow (CBF). On the other hand, more severe reductions may compromise CBF and lead to cerebral ischemia. To avoid this complication, a general initial goal of acute antihypertensive treatment is to limit the reduction of MAP to 20 to 25%, or to a diastolic pressure of 100 to 110 mm Hg. Close monitoring is required, particularly serial neurologic examinations, preferably with an objective assessment tool such as the Glasgow Coma Scale (see Chapter 6 in this book). Deterioration in neurologic condition should prompt consideration for reducing or discontinuing antihypertensive therapy.

Text continued on page 204

TABLE 31–1

DIAGNOSTIC FEATURES AND THERAPEUTIC APPROACH TO HYPERTENSIVE URGENCIES AND HYPERTENSIVE EMERGENCIES

	Hypertensive Urgency	Hypertensive Emergency
Diagnostic Features		
Diastolic blood pressure*	Typically > 120 mm Hg	Typically > 130 mm Hg
Retinopathy (Keith-Wegener funduscopic changes)	Grade I or II	Grade III or IV
Coexisting end-organ damage, clinical settings, and complications	No end-organ damage	Cerebrovascular complications
		Hypertensive encephalopathy
		Cerebral ischemia or stroke
		Intracranial hemorrhage
	Uncontrolled preoperative hypertension	Cardiovascular complications
	Postoperative hypertension	Aortic dissection
	Accelerated hypertension	Coronary insufficiency
	Malignant hypertension	Left ventricular failure

		Acute renal failure Eclampsia Adrenergic crises Tyramine and monoamine oxidase inhibitor drug interaction Accelerated and malignant hypertension
Therapeutic Approach	Control blood pressure within 24 hours May not need invasive blood pressure monitoring ICU admission may not be required Oral antihypertensive agents preferred	Control blood pressure within minutes to hours Invasive blood pressure monitoring needed ICU admission required Parenteral antihypertensive agents preferred

*Both hypertensive urgency and emergency can be associated with diastolic blood pressure less than 120 mm Hg if baseline blood pressure is low and the rate of rise is rapid.

TABLE 31–2

SPECIFIC TREATMENT STRATEGIES FOR CLINICAL CONDITIONS CAUSED BY OR ASSOCIATED WITH HYPERTENSIVE EMERGENCIES

Etiology	Goal of Treatment*	Usual Drug of Choice†	Comments
Cerebrovascular			
Hypertensive encephalopathy	20–25% reduction in MAP	Nitroprusside	Failure to improve within hours of blood pressure reduction should suggest alternative diagnosis
Stroke or intracerebral hemorrhage	Blood pressure ≈ 180/105	Nitroprusside or labetalol	Other agents are preferred over nitroprusside when diastolic blood pressure is < 140 mm Hg
Subarachnoid hemorrhage	20–25% reduction in blood pressure, but not lower than 170–180/100	Nimodipine	If CNS deterioration occurs, discontinue therapy and consider the possibility of a rebleeding episode
Cardiovascular			
Acute left ventricular failure	Empiric	Nitroprusside or nitroglycerin	Avoid agents that increase heart rate; avoid β-blocking agents in systolic dysfunction

Unstable angina or acute myocardial infarction	Pain resolution; MAP < 80 mm Hg	Nitroglycerin or labetalol	Tolerance may develop during nitroglycerin therapy; avoid agents that increase heart rate
Acute aortic dissection	Systolic blood pressure 100–120 mm Hg; MAP < 80 mm Hg	Nitroprusside along with a β-blocking agent, labetalol, or trimethaphan camsylate	See Chapter 32 in this book
Pheochromocytoma	Normotension	Phentolamine mesylate	β-adrenergic blocking agents are contraindicated
Sympathomimetic Drug Effect	Normotension	Labetalol or phentolamine mesylate	Antihypertensive drug withdrawal syndromes require alternative control of blood pressure before reintroduction of the withdrawn drug
Eclampsia	Diastolic blood pressure < 105 mm Hg	Hydralazine or labetalol	Avoid fluid restriction

*MAP = mean arterial pressure.

†Nitroprusside is indicated for initial, temporary use only. Other parenteral or oral antihypertensive agents should be introduced and nitroprusside discontinued as soon as possible.

Patients in hypertensive crisis are commonly volume depleted. Overzealous diuresis or fluid restriction should be avoided, particularly during the first few days of treatment. Volume expansion may be necessary to optimize the response to antihypertensive drugs and to avoid precipitating hypotension. Finally, cardiac output is typically reduced secondary to marked increases in systemic vascular resistance. Therefore, pure β-adrenergic blocking agents should not be used in isolation because they promote peripheral vasoconstriction.

Oral Antihypertensive Therapy. Sublingual, oral, or enteral administration of antihypertensive agents is usually appropriate for patients with hypertensive urgency. Commonly used representative oral drugs include:

- **Clonidine.** The loading dose is 0.1–0.2 mg, followed by 0.05–0.1 mg, repeated as frequently as every hour initially, to a maximum dose of 0.8 mg/day. Dosage should be reduced by 25 to 50% in the elderly. The usual duration of action is 6–12 hours. The average decrease in MAP is approximately 40 mm Hg at 3 hours. Associated hypotension occurs in less than 1% of cases. The drug should be avoided in patients with bradycardia, sick sinus syndrome, and atrioventricular block. Its sedating effects limit its application in patients with associated neurologic complications.
- **Nifedipine.** Typically, this agent is administered by having the patient bite or swallow a 10- or 20-mg capsule. Onset and peak action occur at 5 and 15 minutes, respectively, after sublingual use, and at 20 and 30 minutes, respectively, after oral ingestion. The dose can be repeated after 30 minutes. Most patients achieve a 25% reduction in MAP. The maximum suggested dose is 30 mg every 6 hours. Usual duration is 4 to 6 hours. Reflex tachycardia can occur.
- **Captopril.** Experience using this angiotensin-converting enzyme inhibitor for the treatment of hypertensive urgency is limited, but doses of 6.25–25 mg usually produce a significant decline in MAP. The peak effect occurs at 30–90 minutes. Hypotension can occur, particularly in volume-depleted patients. Associated reflex tachycardia does not occur. Patients with low renin hypertension may not respond well to this class of drugs.
- **Labetalol.** This agent antagonizes both α- and β-adrenergic receptors. The initial oral dose is based on the severity of the hypertension; e.g.,
  - 100 mg for diastolic blood pressure 100–120 mm Hg.
  - 200 mg for diastolic blood pressure 120–130 mm Hg.
  - 300 mg for diastolic blood pressure 130–140 mm Hg.
  - 400 mg for diastolic blood pressure more than 140 mm Hg.

  Onset of effect is typically approximately 2 hours, followed by a peak effect at approximately 4 hours. This agent shares contraindications common to most β-adrenergic blocking agents.

- **Minoxidil.** Initial dose is 5–20 mg. One repeat dose of 2.5–20 mg may be given at 4 hours, followed by 12- or 24-hour interval dosing. This agent is usually combined with a loop diuretic and a β-adrenergic blocking agent to counter the expected compensatory sodium retention and reflex tachycardia. It can be combined with other agents in refractory cases. Hypertrichosis occurs in one-fourth of long-term recipients.

Intravenous Antihypertensive Therapy. Parenteral therapy is indicated for patients who cannot take oral medications, or in whom more urgent blood pressure reduction is indicated. Among the IV agents commonly used for this purpose are:

- **Nitroprusside.** Given as a continuous infusion, the initial dose is 0.1–0.5 μg/kg/min, titrated according to blood pressure response, to a maximum rate of 10 μg/kg/min. Peak effect occurs in 1–2 minutes, with a duration of effect of 3–10 minutes. Cyanide toxicity can occur with high-dose or prolonged infusion. Thiocyanate toxicity can also occur, particularly in patients with renal failure. Toxicity risk is reduced by coinfusion of thiosulfate (500 mg sodium thiosulfate 50 mg sodium nitroprusside) or hydroxocobalamin and by discontinuing nitroprusside as soon as feasible.
- **Diazoxide** is best administered as a minibolus IV injection of 1–3 mg/kg (50–150 mg) every 5–30 minutes. After initial titration, the dose may be repeated at 4–24 hours, but other agents are usually used beyond that point. Formerly, rapid injection of a single 300-mg dose was recommended, but hypotension frequently occurred. Nausea and hyperglycemia may also occur. This drug is not recommended for patients with angina pectoris, myocardial infarction, or aortic dissection.
- **Hydralazine.** Intermittent IV doses range from 10–20 mg, usually given at intervals of 4–6 hours. Peak action occurs within 20–40 minutes. It may also be given as a continuous IV infusion (0.2 mg/min), by intermittent IM injection (10–50 mg), or PO. The principal side effect is reflex tachycardia; therefore, this drug is avoided in patients with myocardial ischemia or dissecting aortic aneurysm.
- **Labetalol** possesses mixed α- and β-adrenergic blocking activity, with the former predominating during IV use. It is usually given as a 20-mg IV bolus over 2 minutes, with subsequent escalating doses of 20–80 mg at 10-minute intervals as necessary. Alternatively, it may be given as a continuous infusion at 0.5–2 mg/min. The maximum recommended dose is 300 mg/day, al-

though doses as large as 2400 mg/day have been reported. Like other β-blocking agents, labetolol can cause bronchospasm, heart failure, and cardiac conduction disturbances.

- **Nitroglycerin** is predominantly a venodilator when used topically, PO, or at low IV doses. At high IV doses, usually exceeding 100 μg/min, it can have direct arterial vasodilating effects. The initiating IV dose is 10 μg/min by continuous infusion. It is a drug of choice for patients with hypertensive crisis and signs of ongoing cardiac ischemia. Prolonged or high-dose infusions may cause methemoglobinemia. Tolerance can develop rapidly with continued exposure.
- **Methyldopa** is usually given as 125–1000 mg by intermittent IV infusion over 30–60 minutes every 6 hours. The peak effect is often delayed for 3–6 hours. The maximum daily dose is 3000 mg. Short-term adverse effects include sedation, bradycardia, carotid sinus hypersensitivity, and first-degree heart block. It can also be given orally.
- **Trimethaphan camsylate** is administered by continuous IV infusion at 0.5–5 mg/min. Onset of action is 1–5 minutes, with a duration of effect of approximately 10 minutes. The antihypertensive effect of this ganglionic blocking agent is often substantially enhanced by raising the head of the bed. Its major role is in the treatment of aortic dissection when β-blocking agents are contraindicated. Tachyphylaxis can develop in 24–72 hours, but sensitivity may be restored with diuresis. It is associated with paralytic ileus, urinary retention, and mydriasis. In patients with renal insufficiency, the drug may reduce renal blood flow and precipitate renal failure. Respiratory arrest has been reported with doses more than 5 mg/min.
- **Phentolamine mesylate** blocks α_1- and α_2-adrenergic receptors. It is useful for treating hypertensive crisis caused by pheochromocytoma, hypertensive reactions caused by cocaine use or coingestion of tyramine-containing foods and monoamine oxidase inhibitors, and withdrawal reactions after abrupt discontinuation of α_2-adrenergic agonists. The dose is 5–15 mg, IM or IV bolus, or 0.2–5 mg/min by continuous IV infusion. Its onset of action is within 1 minute, and duration is approximately 10 minutes. Nausea, vomiting, and reflex tachycardia may occur.

Suggested Readings

Gifford RW. Management of hypertensive crises. *JAMA* 1991; 266:829–835.

Rationale and guidelines for antihypertensive therapy in a variety of settings.

McDonald AJ, Yearly DM, Jacobson S. Oral labetalol versus oral nifedi-

pine in hypertensive urgencies in the ED. *Am J Emerg Med* 1993;11:460–463.
Small comparative trial along with a review of the literature assessing the efficacy of labetalol in hypertensive urgencies.
Nibbelink DN. Cooperative Aneurysm Study: Antihypertensive and antifibrinolytic therapy following subarachnoid hemorrhage from ruptured intracranial aneurysm. In: Whisnant JP, Sandok BA, eds. *Cerebral vascular diseases.* New York: Grune and Stratton, 1975, pp 155–165.
Presents interesting data on the U-shaped relationship between blood pressure and outcome in subarachnoid hemorrhage.
Phillips SJ. Pathophysiology and management of hypertension in acute ischemic stroke. *Hypertension* 1994;23:131–136.
Explains how hypertension causes cerebral infarction and how to manage blood pressure in the setting of acute ischemic stroke (80 references).
Robin ED, McCauley R. Nitroprusside related cyanide poisoning: Time (long past due) for urgent, effective interventions. *Chest* 1992; 102:1842–1845.
Contrary view of safety of nitroprusside emphasizing the difficulty in diagnosing toxicity.

CHAPTER 32

Aortic Dissection

(See Chapter 98)

Vivian L. Clark and James A. Kruse

Aortic dissection is a medical emergency. It occurs when there is a tear in the aortic intima with extravasation of blood between the intimal and medial layers, resulting in the creation of a false lumen. The extravasated blood may remain within the false lumen, with eventual thrombosis, or it may rupture through the outer wall of the aorta. The most common point of origin is in the ascending aorta, followed by the descending aorta just distal to the left subclavian artery. There are many risk factors for dissection, including hypertension, connective tissue disease, congenital bicuspid aortic valve, coarctation of the aorta, pregnancy, and trauma secondary to catheterization. There may be a higher incidence in men and in African-American patients.

Classification

Dissections can be classified as either proximal (type A) or distal (type B). This differentiation has important therapeutic implications. A proximal dissection begins in the ascending aorta. It may be limited to that portion of the

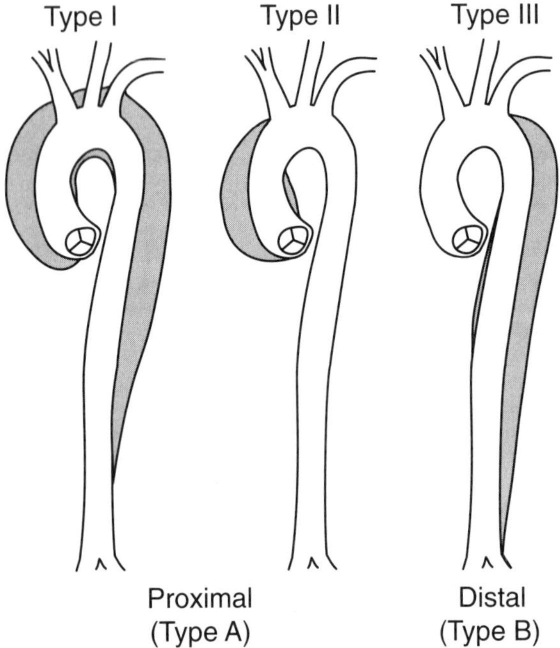

Figure 32–1. Classification of aortic dissection. For comparison, the older DeBakey classification is also shown.

aorta, or it may extend into the descending aorta. Proximal, or type A, dissections comprise DeBakey types I and II (see Figure 32–1). Distal, or type B (synonymous with DeBakey type III), aortic dissections begin beyond the origin of the left subclavian artery and extend into the descending aorta.

Diagnosis

The diagnosis of aortic dissection requires a high index of suspicion. It is sometimes misdiagnosed as acute myocardial infarction. This misdiagnosis can have disastrous consequences if treatment with anticoagulants or thrombolytic agents is initiated. The presenting symptoms, physical findings, and clinical setting provide clues to the possibility of dissection, but a definitive diagnosis usually requires some type of imaging study.

History. Pain is the most common symptom. It has the following characteristics:

- It occurs in the chest, abdomen, or both, depending on the site of origin and the extent of the dissection.

- It is severe and tearing in character, and it is usually of maximal intensity at onset.
- It is frequently localized to the back, although anterior pain can occur as well. The pain may migrate as the dissection spreads.
- The discomfort may mimic ischemic cardiac pain. Painless dissections also occur.

In addition to pain, a number of other symptoms can occur. These are usually secondary to hemorrhage or related to compromise of branches arising from the aorta. For example, a dissection that results in carotid occlusion may lead to syncope or neurologic symptoms of hemispheric stroke. Left subclavian artery involvement can lead to symptoms of ischemic peripheral neuropathy. Compromise of aortic branches to the spinal cord can cause paraplegia.

Physical examination often provides important clues to the diagnosis and may suggest the level of the dissection.

- **Hypertension** and tachycardia are present in most patients at presentation. Hypotension and circulatory shock can occur, and are usually related to hemorrhage or pericardial tamponade.
- **Pulse deficits** and blood pressure differential between the two upper extremities, or between the upper and lower extremities, may be present as a result of compromise of the origin of aortic branches.
- **Diastolic heart murmur** indicates aortic insufficiency and is often detectable in proximal aortic dissections.
- **Pulmonary findings** may include decreased breath sounds and dullness if there is hemothorax, or rales if there is concomitant heart failure.
- **Neurologic deficits** are frequently present. They are related to the secondary neurologic problems described above.

Laboratory and Imaging Studies

- **Routine blood tests** are rarely helpful in the diagnosis of dissection, but this information can help to identify alternative diagnoses or complications. Anemia may be present, and the white blood cell count may be elevated. Cardiac enzyme levels will be increased if there is involvement of the coronary ostium, with resulting myocardial infarction.
- **Electrocardiography** typically shows sinus tachycardia. Because underlying hypertension is common, left ventricular hypertrophy is also typical. There may be evidence of acute myocardial infarction or ischemia if the dissection results in compromise of coronary blood flow.
- **Chest radiography** findings may provide clues to the presence of dissection, but are not definitive. Mediasti-

nal widening may be present, but it is common in supine chest radiographs taken with a portable unit. The aortic contour may be abnormal. Separation of aortic intimal calcification from the outer aortic shadow (> 0.5 cm) as a result of blood in the false lumen is occasionally seen, and suggests dissection. A left pleural effusion is sometimes present.

- **Aortography** has conventionally been considered the criterion standard for definitive diagnosis. However, some of the newer imaging techniques may obviate the need for this procedure. Aortic root angiography requires invasive catheterization and radiocontrast dye injection. It may not identify a false lumen that is thrombosed.
- **Transthoracic echocardiography** has a sensitivity of 80 to 100% and a specificity of approximately 90%. Sensitivity decreases with distal dissections. The key finding is an abnormal intraluminal linear echo representing an intimal flap. Doppler color flow mapping often allows identification of the true and false lumens. Acute aortic insufficiency and possible hemopericardium can be easily identified.
- **Transesophageal echocardiography** has a sensitivity of nearly 100% and a specificity of 70–100% for the diagnosis of thoracic aortic dissection. It offers high accuracy and bedside capability. As with transthoracic echocardiography, it can identify pericardial effusion and aortic valve incompetence as well as provide other important information about cardiac function. Potential disadvantages include the invasive nature of the procedure and the need for a physician skilled in the technique, which may limit its availability.
- **Computed tomography** (CT) scanning has a diagnostic accuracy of nearly 100% for aortic dissection. The extent of the dissection can often be identified, which is a potential advantage over transesophageal echo. However, the lack of portability and need for radiocontrast injection are disadvantages.
- **Magnetic resonance imaging** (MRI) has sensitivity and specificity of nearly 100% for the diagnosis of aortic dissection. As with CT scanning, the extent of the dissection can often be identified. Logistic, timing, transport, and monitoring problems may occur if MRI scanning is performed in unstable, critically ill patients who require the use of ferromagnetic appliances and close monitoring.

Treatment

Medical therapy should be initiated in any suspected dissection before diagnostic studies are obtained. This therapy consists chiefly of IV administration of antihypertensive drugs to lower mean arterial pressure to 60 to 75 mm Hg, if possible. In some cases, this level of reduction may not be well tolerated, e.g., in subjects with chronic severe hypertension and severe atherosclerotic cerebrovascular disease. The lowest level that is compatible with adequate systemic perfusion should be the goal. The most commonly used agents are:

- **Sodium nitroprusside,** given by continuous infusion (initiated at 0.5 μg/kg/min and titrated to the desired blood pressure response) is commonly used as a first-line agent. However, this drug can increase the rate of pressure change within the aorta (dp/dt), which could lead to extension of the dissection. To counter this effect, it should only be used in combination with a β-adrenergic receptor blocking drug.
- **Propranolol** has been conventionally recommended for use with nitroprusside to reduce myocardial contractility and aortic wall stress. It can be given at 0.5–1.0 mg by IV injection every 5 minutes until the desired effect is achieved, up to 0.15 mg/kg, followed by maintenance doses.
- **Esmolol** is an attractive alternative to propranolol because it can be titrated rapidly. However, experience in using this drug for treating dissection is limited. It may have a role in patients with a relative contraindication to β-blockade.
- **Trimethaphan,** initiated at 1 mg/min, is a ganglionic blocker that is the conventional alternative to combination therapy with nitroprusside and β-blockade. It does not increase dp/dt, but has disadvantages related to its effects on the autonomic nervous system, such as causing urinary retention, and tachyphylaxis.
- **Labetalol,** 20 mg by IV injection over 2 minutes, followed by a continuous infusion of 0.5–2 mg/min, is a mixed α- and β-adrenergic antagonist that has been successfully used alone to treat aortic dissection (see Chapter 31 in this book for further information on these drugs).

Other agents that can be employed in refractory cases or for longer-term therapy include metoprolol, α-methyldopa, clonidine, and verapamil. Sedatives may be helpful as an adjunct to controlling blood pressure. Narcotic analgesics may be necessary to control pain. Careful clinical and hemodynamic monitoring of the patient is essential to detect extension of the dissection or compromise of vital organs. An arterial catheter should be used to monitor blood pressure. In patients who are hypotensive or in whom rupture is suspected, volume loading should be initiated.

After stabilization and diagnostic evaluation, definitive surgical treatment of dissection is indicated in most proximal dissections. It may be indicated in certain complicated distal dissections, such as those associated with extension into the ascending aorta, progression of the dissection with arterial compromise of an extremity or vital organ, rupture or impending rupture, or Marfan's syndrome. Appropriate medical therapy should be initiated promptly, even if urgent operation is anticipated.

Suggested Readings

DeSanctis RW, Doroghazi RM, Austen WG, et al. Aortic dissection. *N Engl J Med* 1987;317:1060–1067.
Excellent general review of aortic dissection.

Hashimoto S, Kumada T, Osakada G, et al. Assessment of transesophageal Doppler echography in dissecting aortic aneurysm. *J Am Coll Cardiol* 1989;14:1253–1262.
Describes use of echocardiography in diagnosis of dissection.

Masuda Y, Yamada Z, Morooka N, et al. Prognosis of patients with medically treated aortic dissection. *Circulation* 1991;84(suppl III):III-7–III-13.
In this study of 228 patients with aortic dissection, survival rates at 24 hours, 2 weeks, and 10 years were 72%, 43%, and 28%, respectively, for type A dissections. Rates were 100%, 92%, and 56%, respectively, for type B dissections.

Nienaber CA, von Kodolitsch Y, Nicolas V, et al. The diagnosis of thoracic aortic dissection by noninvasive imaging procedures. *N Engl J Med* 1993;328:1–9.
In this study, diagnostic sensitivities of magnetic resonance imaging, transthoracic echocardiography, transesophageal echocardiography, and computed tomography for detecting aortic dissection were 98.3%, 97.7%, 93.8%, and 59.3%, respectively. Respective specificities were 97.8%, 76.9%, 87.1%, and 83%.

Pinet F, Froment JC, Guillot M, Gourdal Y, et al. Prognostic factors and indications for surgical treatment of acute aortic dissections: A report based on 191 observations. *Cardiovasc Intervent Radiol* 1984;7:257–266.
Reviews the surgical treatment of aortic dissection.

Spittell PC, Spittell JA, Joyce JW, et al. Clinical features and differential diagnosis of aortic dissection: Experience with 236 cases (1980 through 1990). *Mayo Clin Proc* 1993;68:642–661.
Large series of cases seen at one institution.

CHAPTER 33

Pericardial Tamponade

(See Chapter 92)

Vivian L. Clark and James A. Kruse

Pericardial tamponade is defined as fluid in the pericardium to a degree that results in impaired cardiac filling and inadequate cardiac output. The occurrence of pericardial tamponade is dependent not only on the volume of fluid, but also on the rapidity with which it accumulates.

Any process that causes pericardial effusion can lead to tamponade. Etiologies of pericardial effusion include:

- Infectious pericarditis.
- Malignancy.
- Trauma, blunt or penetrating.
- Uremia.
- Dressler's syndrome.
- Hypothyroidism.
- Postpericardiotomy.
- Aortic dissection.
- Collagen vascular disease.
- Idiopathic causes.

The most common causes of pericardial effusion leading to tamponade are malignancy, trauma, and complications of cardiac surgery.

Clinical Findings

Symptoms associated with tamponade tend to be nonspecific, and can occur with a number of other cardiac and noncardiac conditions. The most common symptoms are fatigue, dyspnea, and chest pain, which can be pleuritic or pressure-like. Symptoms are often exacerbated by the supine position and relieved by sitting upright.

The classic triad of physical findings is tachycardia, neck vein distension, and a quiet precordium. The patient with tamponade usually appears anxious and in distress, and may be tachypneic. Hypotension is a common finding, and there is often pulsus paradox of more than 12 mm Hg. A pericardial friction rub may be present, and there may be dullness to percussion over the back just medial to and below the left scapula (Ewart's sign). The lungs are usually clear to auscultation, although there may be dullness at the bases if there is associated pleural effusion or atelectasis.

Laboratory and Imaging Studies

The ECG reading often shows sinus tachycardia and diffuse ST segment elevation consistent with pericarditis. There may also be a reduction in QRS voltage and electrical alternans (beat-to-beat variability in QRS amplitude).

The chest radiograph may show an enlarged, globular, or water bottle–shaped cardiac silhouette. However, normal heart size does not exclude tamponade, particularly in cases of trauma or other causes of rapidly accumulating effusions. The pulmonary vasculature usually appears normal. Pleural effusions are sometimes present.

When tamponade is suspected, an echocardiogram should be obtained. It will help to support the diagnosis and exclude other cardiac causes of hypotension. It may also be useful in identifying impending tamponade and loculated effusions. Echocardiographic findings include a large pericardial clear space and collapse of the right ventricular and right atrial walls during inspiration. Central venous or pulmonary artery catheterization can be diagnostic. There is low cardiac output in addition to elevation and equalization of right atrial, right ventricular diastolic, pulmonary artery diastolic, and pulmonary artery occlusion pressures.

Differential Diagnosis

The differential diagnosis of cardiac tamponade includes the following clinical entities:

- **Right ventricular myocardial infarction,** which can usually be differentiated by the history and ECG findings. Hemodynamically, however, it can be difficult to distinguish from tamponade.
- **Pulmonary embolism** can present with similar history and physical findings, but can usually be distinguished by the chest radiograph and hemodynamic findings.
- **Severe biventricular failure** may cause symptoms similar to those of pericardial tamponade, but significant pulmonary congestion may be evident on physical examination and by chest radiography.
- **Constrictive or restrictive disease** of the myocardium may cause similar symptoms and physical findings. However, the onset is usually more insidious than that of tamponade. In addition, the chest radiograph generally does not show an enlarged cardiac silhouette, but may provide other clues, such as pericardial calcification in the case of constriction.

Echocardiography is particularly useful in excluding the above conditions.

Treatment

Volume loading may temporarily improve hemodynamic parameters in pericardial tamponade by augmenting cardiac filling; however, the definitive treatment is drainage of pericardial fluid, either percutaneously or by surgical placement of a pericardial window (see Chapter 12 in this book). Often, removal of only a small volume of fluid will result in dramatic clinical improvement. The removed pericardial fluid should be sent for diagnostic studies, including cell counts, microbiologic stains and cultures, and cytologic analysis, to determine the etiology of the effusion. If percutaneous drainage is undertaken, a small catheter may be left in place for continuous drainage.

Surgical placement of a pericardial window, although more invasive, has several potential advantages over percutaneous fluid drainage:

- It allows continuous drainage of fluid and prevents re-accumulation.
- Direct visualization of the pericardium facilitates recognition and drainage of loculated pericardial effusions.
- A biopsy of the pericardium can be obtained and may aid in determining the etiology.

Suggested Readings

Ameli S, Shah PK. Cardiac tamponade: Pathophysiology, diagnosis and management. *Cardiol Clin* 1991;9:665–674.
In-depth review of pericardial tamponade (50 references).

Berge KH, Lanier WL, Reeder GS. Occult cardiac tamponade detected by transesophageal echocardiography. *Mayo Clin Proc* 1992;67:667–670.
Case report of pericardial tamponade that was not detectable by transthoracic echocardiography or hemodynamic measurements, but was found by transesophageal echocardiography.

Brown J, MacKinnon D, King A, et al. Elevated arterial blood pressure in cardiac tamponade. *N Engl J Med* 1992;327:463–466.
Of 18 consecutive patients with tamponade, six had elevated arterial blood pressure. All six had preexisting hypertension.

Levine MJ, Lorell BH, Diver DJ, et al. Implications of echocardiographically assisted diagnosis of pericardial tamponade in contemporary medical patients: Detection before hemodynamic embarrassment. *J Am Coll Cardiol* 1991;17:59–65.
In a study of 50 consecutive patients thought to have tamponade, the presence of right atrial and ventricular diastolic collapse did not identify a more hemodynamically decompensated group compared with patients without that echocardiographic finding.

Wall TC, Campbell PT, O'Connor CM, et al. Diagnosis and management (by subxiphoid pericardiotomy) of large pericardial effusions causing cardiac tamponade. *Am J Cardiol* 1992;69:1075–1078.
Of 57 consecutive patients with new, large pericardial effusions, 44% had tamponade.

Wolf MW, Edelman ER. Transient systolic dysfunction after relief of cardiac tamponade. *Ann Intern Med* 1993;119:42–44.
Case reports of patients experiencing ventricular dysfunction after treatment of pericardial tamponade by pericardiocentesis.

CHAPTER 34

Cardiovascular Pharmacotherapy

(See Chapters 94 and 113)

John P. Dervan

Pharmacologic agents that affect cardiac function and vasomotor tone are frequently used in the care of the critically ill patient. Among these are drugs that activate or

Text continued on page 228

TABLE 34–1

INOTROPIC AND VASOACTIVE DRUGS*

Drug	Mechanism	Indications	Contraindications†	Usual Dose	Adverse Effects
Dopamine	Low dose: renal vasodilator; intermediate dose range: stimulates β-receptors; high dose: stimulates α-receptors	Cardiogenic, septic, and anaphylactic shock; particularly useful in patients with renal insufficiency	Ventricular dysrhythmias; pheochromocytoma; associated use of cyclopropane or halogenated hydrocarbon anesthetics; use of monoamine oxidase inhibitors	Low dose: ≤ 3 μg/kg/min; intermediate dose: 3–10 μg/kg/min (β range); high dose: > 10 μg/kg/min (α range)	Myocardial ischemia; tachycardia, dysrhythmias; subcutaneous extravasation can cause skin sloughing
Dobutamine	Stimulates β-receptors; augments myocardial contractility with minimal effects on systemic vascular resistance	Heart failure, cardiogenic shock; also useful in right ventricular infarctions	Relative: tachycardia, ventricular dysrhythmias	Range 2.5–15 μg/kg/min	Tachycardia, dysrhythmias
Epinephrine	Stimulates predominantly α_1- and β_1-adrenergic receptors	Cardiac arrest; supplement to other inotropic agents for profound hypotension; anaphylaxis; status asthmaticus	Myocardial ischemia Relative: ventricular dysrhythmias	1 mg in 10-ml ampule IV or endotracheally; infusion rates of 1–6 μg/min	Dysrhythmias, tachycardia; hypertension; headache; cerebral hemorrhage; pulmonary edema

Norepinephrine	Potent vasoconstrictor; stimulates α_1-, α_2-, and β_1-receptors	Cardiac arrest, cardiogenic or septic shock	Myocardial ischemia; late pregnancy	2–12 μg/min	Impaired renal and splanchnic circulation; subcutaneous extravasation can cause skin sloughing
Phenylephrine	Potent α agonist; vasoconstriction with minimal cardiac effect	Hypotension in patients with hypertrophic cardiomyopathy	Hypertension; severe peripheral vascular disease	Initial doses of 100–200 μg/min for a rapid response, followed by a maintenance dose of 20–80 μg/min	Reflex bradycardia; subcutaneous extravasation can cause skin sloughing
Amrinone	Phosphodiesterase inhibitor; positive inotropic agent with vasodilating activity	Congestive heart failure	Myocardial ischemia; aortic stenosis; hypertrophic cardiomyopathy	Initial dose of 0.75 mg/kg IV bolus over 3 minutes; then 5–10 μg/kg/min maintenance	Dysrhythmias, hypotension; hepatotoxicity; hypersensitivity reactions; thrombocytopenia
Digitalis Glycosides digoxin, digitoxin	Inhibits sodium pump; digoxin ($t_{1/2}$ 24–36 hours) is excreted by the kidney; digitoxin ($t_{1/2}$ 6–7 days) is excreted by the liver	Congestive heart failure as a result of systolic dysfunction, particularly when associated with atrial dysrhythmias	AV block; Wolff-Parkinson-White syndrome; diastolic dysfunction	Digoxin: load with 0.75–1.0 mg over 24 hours; then 0.125–0.375 mg daily; Digitoxin: load with 0.8–1.2 mg over 24 hours; then 0.05–0.20 mg daily	Dysrhythmias, nausea, vomiting, visual disturbances, AV block; interactions with quinidine, verapamil, amiodarone, ACE inhibitors

*Also see Chapters 91 and 113 in the main text.

†Some contraindications are relative.

AV = atrioventricular; ACE = angiotensin-converting enzyme.

TABLE 34–2

VASODILATING DRUGS*

Drug	Mechanism	Indications	Contraindications†	Usual Dose	Adverse Effects
Nitrates Nitroglycerin, isosorbide dinitrate, isosorbide-5-mononitrate	Direct venodilator; at high doses, causes arterial dilatation	Unstable angina, acute myocardial infarction, congestive heart failure, perioperative patients with increased ischemic risk; stable angina	Relative: hypotension; diastolic dysfunction; hypertrophic cardiomyopathy; aortic stenosis	IV: begin at 5–10 µg/min, titrate according to response and MAP; blunted response with infusion rates > 100 µg/min; sublingual: 0.3–0.4 mg, peak effect in about 2 minutes; PO: 2.5–40 mg every 6–8 hours; transdermal: paste 0.5–1.5 inches every 4 hours; patches 7.5–20 mg applied 12 hr/day	Hypotension; headache; methemoglobinemia; nitrate tolerance: occurs with IV infusion over 1–2 days, resulting in the need for higher doses; transdermal nitrates should be applied for 12 hours only to prevent tolerance
Sodium Nitroprusside	Direct-acting vasodilator; equally affects veins and arteries; reduces afterload and preload	Severe hypertension; heart failure, especially with associated hypertension; bacute mitral and	Hypotension	Begin at 0.25–1 µg/kg/min, with titration to achieve desired hypotensive effect; short $t_{1/2}$; va-	Cyanide and thiocyanate toxicity, especially in patients with renal insufficiency or with

		aortic regurgitation, with hemodynamic compromise		sodilation can be reversed within 5–10 minutes	prolonged use; coronary steal in patients with ischemic heart disease
Hydralazine	Direct arteriolar smooth muscle vasodilator	Hypertension; afterload reduction in heart failure	Hypotension	IV: begin with 5 mg; increase to 10–20 mg IV every 4 to 6 hours; PO: 25–50 mg every 6 hours	Hypotension; reflex tachycardia; drug-induced lupus
Angiotensin-Converting Enzyme (ACE) Inhibitors Captopril, enalapril, lisinopril, ramipril	Blocks formation of angiotensin II, enhancing vasodilation and decreasing aldosterone; captopril has shortest $t_{1/2}$	Afterload reduction in heart failure; hypertension; after myocardial infarction, particularly with low ejection fraction	Hypotension; renal artery stenosis	Captopril: begin with 6.25 mg PO every 6 hours; up to 50 mg PO every 6 hours; other ACE inhibitors: 2.5–20 mg PO every 12 hours; IV (enalaprilat): 1.25–2.5 mg initially, with maintenance dose of 2.5–5.0 mg every 6 hours	Reduced renal blood flow; may aggravate azotemia and hyperkalemia, thus, creatinine and potassium levels should be monitored; rash; cough is common with long-term use

*Also see Chapter 31 in this book and Chapters 91 and 114 in the main text.
[†]Some contraindications are relative.
AV = atrioventricular; MAP = mean arterial pressure.

TABLE 34–3

ANTIANGINAL DRUGS*

Drug	Mechanism	Indications	Contraindications†	Usual Dose	Adverse Effects
β-receptor Antagonists					
Propranolol, atenolol, metoprolol, timolol, pindolol, acetbutolol, labetolol, nadolol (also see antiarrhythmic drugs)	Inhibit β_1- and β_2-receptors; cardioselective agents (e.g., metoprolol) have little β_2 effect; some (e.g., pindolol) have intrinsic sympathomimetic activity; labetolol has α blocking action	Angina pectoris; acute myocardial infarction (especially atenolol and metoprolol); prophylaxis after myocardial infarction; hypertension	AV block, bradycardia; hypotension, heart failure caused by systolic dysfunction, peripheral vascular disease; brittle diabetes; asthma, obstructive lung disease	For acute myocardial infarction: 5–10 mg atenolol IV or 5–15 mg metoprolol IV; PO: dosage varies with specific agent	Hypotension; bradycardia, AV block; exacerbation of heart failure; depression; fatigue; impotence; bronchospasm

Calcium Channel Antagonists					
Verapamil, dihydropyridines (nifedipine, nicardipine, amlodipine), diltiazem	Inhibit inward movement of calcium across cell membranes, resulting in smooth muscle relaxation; dihydropyridines have more vasodilator activity; verapamil has greater effects on conduction; and diltiazem has a combination of effects	Angina pectoris, hypertension, non-Q wave infarction, with preserved left ventricular function, and supraventricular dysrhythmias (see below)	AV block, severe bradycardia; hypotension; acute myocardial infarction with poor ventricular function	PO: verapamil 40–120 mg every 6–8 hours; nifedipine 10–30 mg every 8 hours (extended release form: 30–90 mg every 24 hours); diltiazem 30–120 mg every 6–8 hours (for IV dosing, see Table 34–4); amlodipine 5–10 mg every 24 hours	AV block, asystole, or significant hypotension; exacerbation of heart failure; constipation (verapamil); headache; rash; fluid retension (dihydropyridines)

*Also see Chapter 90 in the main text.
†Some contraindications are relative.
AV = atrioventricular.

TABLE 34–4

ANTIARRHYTHMIC DRUGS

Drug	Mechanism	Indications	Contraindications[†]	Usual Dose	Adverse Effects
Digoxin (also see Table 34–1)	Blocks AV node	PSVT; atrial fibrillation or atrial flutter with rapid response	Sick sinus; bradycardia; second- or third-degree AV block; WPW with wide QRS tachycardia; hypertrophic cardiomyopathy	0.50 mg IV followed by 1–2 additional doses of 0.25 to a total of 0.75–1.0 mg over 24 hours; maintenance dose of 0.125–0.375 mg daily	Bradycardia or AV block; dysrhythmias; nausea and vomiting; visual disturbances
Adenosine	Blocks AV node; extremely short $t_{1/2}$	PSVT; may temporarily slow atrial fibrillation or atrial flutter with rapid response	VT; WPW with wide QRS tachycardia; high-degree AV block; sick sinus syndrome; bronchospasm	6 mg IV bolus; 12 mg after 1–2 minutes if no response (may be repeated once)	Hypotension; dyspnea, flushing, headache; bradycardia or AV block; transient dysrhythmias

Calcium Channel Antagonists Verapamil, diltiazem (also see Table 34–3)	Blocks AV node	PSVT; atrial fibrillation or flutter with rapid response	VT; WPW with wide QRS tachycardia; high-degree AV block; sick sinus syndrome; digoxin toxicity; hypotension; severe heart failure; Relative: use of other AV nodal blockers	Verapamil: 5 mg IV over 3–5 minutes; 10 mg after 15 minutes if no response; diltiazem: 0.25 mg/kg IV over 2 minutes; after 15 minutes, a second dose of 0.35 mg/kg; then an infusion of 5–15 mg/hr	Hypotension; dyspnea, flushing, headache; bradycardia or AV block
β-receptor Antagonists Esmolol, propranolol	Inhibit β_1- and β_2-receptors; block AV node	PSVT; atrial fibrillation or flutter with rapid response; multifocal atrial tachycardia	VT; WPW with wide QRS tachycardia; high-degree AV block; sick sinus syndrome; hypotension; severe heart failure; bronchospasm	Esmolol: 0.50 mg/kg loading dose followed by an infusion of 50–200 μg/kg/min propranolol: 1–10 mg IV over 3–5 minutes	Hypotension; bradycardia; AV block, especially if other AV blocking agents used; heart failure caused by systolic dysfunction; bronchospasm

Table continued on following page

TABLE 34–4 *Continued*

ANTIARRHYTHMIC DRUGS

Drug	Mechanism	Indications	Contraindications[†]	Usual Dose	Adverse Effects
Atropine	Inhibits vagal tone through muscarinic receptor antagonism	Bradycardia secondary to SA or AV nodal dysfunction, or asystole	Glaucoma; obstructive uropathy; intestinal obstruction; myasthenia gravis	0.6–1.0 mg IV, can be given to total dose of 2.0 mg IV; $t_{1/2}$ 2–3 hours	Paradoxical bradycardia if given in doses < 0.5 mg; tachycardia; blurred vision; urinary retention
Isoproterenol	β-adrenergic agonist	Bradycardia secondary to SA or AV nodal dysfunction or asystole; overdrive torsades de pointes	Myocardial ischemia; tachydysrhythmias	0.5–10 mg/min as an infusion; $t_{1/2}$ is 2 minutes	Tachycardia, dysrhythmias; headache; sweating

Lidocaine	Inhibits fast sodium channels	VT; may be used in WPW for wide QRS tachydysrhythmias	Bradycardia	Loading dose of 1 mg/kg IV; repeat with 0.5 mg/kg in 20–30 minutes; maintenance dose 1–4 mg/min; reduce maintenance dose with heart failure or liver disease	Dysrhythmias; toxicity usually manifests with CNS symptoms (e.g., confusion, obtundation, seizures); nausea, vomiting
Procainamide	Blocks active sodium channel, blocks potassium channel	VT and PSVT; WPW with wide QRS tachydysrhythmias; pharmacologic conversion of atrial fibrillation or flutter (after rate is slowed)	Prolonged QT interval; torsades de pointes; congestive heart failure	IV 6–13 mg/kg given slowly at 0.2–0.5 mg/kg/min; maintenance dose of 2–5 mg/min	Dysrhythmias; hypotension; exacerbation of heart failure; drug-induced lupus-like syndrome with chronic use

Table continued on following page

TABLE 34–4 *Continued*

ANTIARRHYTHMIC DRUGS

Drug	Mechanism	Indications	Contraindications†	Usual Dose	Adverse Effects
Quinidine	Blocks active sodium channel, blocks potassium channel, also has α-receptor antagonist effects	VT; pharmacologic conversion of atrial fibrillation or flutter (only after rate is controlled); WPW	Same as procainamide	PO: load with 300 mg every 3 hours for 3 doses; maintenance dose of 600–1000 mg/day; gluconate formulation will require a slightly higher dosage	Dysrhythmias; long QT; hypotension; nausea, vomiting, diarrhea
Disopyramide	Blocks active sodium channel, blocks potassium channel, also affects muscarinic receptors	VT and SVT; also used to decrease left ventricular contractility in hypertrophic cardiomyopathy	Same as procainamide Relative: glaucoma	No IV preparation; PO maintenance dose of 100–400 mg every 6 hours	Dysrhythmias, prolonged QT interval; heart failure; parasympathetic side effects causing urinary hesitancy, blurred vision

Bretylium	Blocks potassium channel, α- and β-receptors are initially stimulated and subsequently inhibited	VT in patients who do not respond to lidocaine; refractory VF during cardiac arrest	Relative: hypotension	Load with 5–10 mg/kg at 1–2 mg/kg/min; give more quickly with cardiac arrest; maintenance dose of 0.5–2 mg/min	Hypotension; nausea/vomiting
Amiodarone	Inhibits sodium, calcium, and potassium channels, also has α- and β-receptor antagonism; $T_{1/2}$ 25–110 days	VT; also used increasingly for atrial dysrhythmias	High-degree AV block	IV available only for investigational basis; PO: 800–1600 mg/day for 1–3 weeks; then maintenance dose of 200–400 mg daily	Dysrhythmias; AV block, particularly if combined with calcium channel or β-receptor antagonists; pulmonary pneumonitis/fibrosis; hyper- or hypothyroidism; tremor; nausea; corneal microdeposits; interaction with warfarin and digoxin

*Also see Chapters 90, 91, and 94 in the main text.

†Some contraindications are relative.

AV = atrioventricular; SA = sinoatrial; PSVT = paroxysmal supraventricular tachycardia; SVT = supraventricular tachycardia; VF = ventricular fibrillation; VT = ventricular tachycardia; WPW = Wolff-Parkinson-White syndrome.

inhibit adrenergic, parasympathetic, and calcium channel receptors, direct-acting vasodilators, inotropic agents, and antiarrhythmic drugs.

General Principles

Several principles to remember when administering these agents to critically ill patients are:

- Congestive heart failure and circulatory shock may alter drug metabolism. Serial monitoring of serum drug levels or their effects may be necessary to prevent toxicity.
- Hepatic and renal function are frequently impaired in critically ill patients, thus requiring reductions in drug dosages (see Chapter 58 in this book). In addition, a number of agents may lead to further compromise of hepatic or renal function (e.g., aminoglycosides).
- Critically ill patients often require treatment with multiple drugs; therefore, drug–drug interactions may occur.
- Some pharmaceutical agents may be incompatible with certain IV solutions or other coadministered drugs, necessitating additional venous access.
- IV administration of some drugs requires large volume loads, which could worsen or precipitate congestive heart failure. In addition, a number of drugs are given as sodium or potassium salts, and these may contribute to fluid and electrolyte imbalances.
- Drug toxicity may be confused with worsening of the patient's underlying illness.
- Correction of underlying precipitating factors may eliminate the need for pharmacologic therapy. For example, correction of acid–base or electrolyte disturbances may obviate the need for antiarrhythmic drug therapy.

Specific Agents

- **Inotropic and vasoactive agents** (see Tables 34–1 and 27–2) are among the most commonly used drugs in the ICU. These include catecholamines, phosphodiesterase inhibitors, and digitalis glycosides, which are frequently used in the treatment of circulatory shock and cardiac failure.
- **Vasodilators** (Table 34–2) affect the vasomotor tone of the veins, arteries, or both. They are used for preload and afterload reduction and, in the case of nitrates, to increase coronary blood flow. It is important to know which vascular bed is affected when using these agents, because some actions may be beneficial in one situation

and deleterious in another. Calcium channel blocking agents, which all have at least some vasodilator activity, are discussed with antianginal drugs.

- **Antianginal drugs** (Table 34–3) include vasodilators (e.g., nitrates and calcium channel blockers) and drugs that block β-adrenergic receptors. Many antianginal drugs also have negative inotropic effects, but still may be of value in the treatment of cardiac failure caused by diastolic dysfunction. In addition, a number of these agents are useful in the treatment of cardiac dysrhythmias.
- **Antiarrhythmic drugs** (Table 34–4) act through a variety of mechanisms. Some agents are used in the treatment of supraventricular dysrhythmias, others in the treatment of ventricular dysrhythmias, and a number are effective for both types of dysrhythmia.

Suggested Readings

Akhtar M, Breithardt G, Camm AJ, et al. CAST and beyond. Implications of the Cardiac Arrhythmia Suppression Trial. *Circulation* 1990;81:1123–1127.

Discusses risk of antiarrhythmic drugs in light of the mortality findings of the CAST.

Opie LH, ed. *Drugs for the heart,* 3rd ed. Philadelphia: WB Saunders, 1991.

Excellent reference on cardiac drugs.

Opie LH. Interactions with cardiovascular drugs. *Curr Probl Cardiol* 1993;18:529–584.

Good, up-to-date review of cardiac drug interactions.

Task Force of the Working Group on Arrhythmias of the European Society of Cardiology. The Sicilian gambit: A new approach to the classification of antiarrhythmic drugs based on their actions on arrhythmogenic mechanisms. *Circulation* 1991;84:1831–1851.

Review and revision of the classification of antiarrhythmic agents based on a mechanistic approach.

The Fifth Report of the Joint National Committee on Detection, Evaluation, and Treatment of High Blood Pressure. *Arch Intern Med* 1993;153:154–183.

Compendium of doses, interactions, and side effects of drugs used in the treatment of hypertension. Many of these agents are also used for other cardiac disorders.

Tzivoni D, Banai S, Schuger C, et al. Treatment of torsades de pointes with magnesium sulfate. *Circulation* 1988;77:392–397.

Reminder of the importance of the use of magnesium in the acute care setting for the management of dysrhythmias.

Zaloga GP, Prielipp RC, Butterworth IV JF. Pharmacologic cardiovascular support. *Crit Care Clin* 1993;9:335–362.

Overview of inotropic drugs.

Neurologic Disorders

CHAPTER 35
Coma

(See Chapter 55)

Alan B. Ettinger

Coma is defined as a state of profoundly depressed consciousness and is characterized by an absence of awareness of the self or environment. Patients in coma do not show psychologically understandable responses to external stimuli or internal needs.

Etiology

Coma occurs as a result of extensive bilateral hemispheric injury or from a disturbance of the reticular formation of the brainstem. The cause may be structural, toxic, or metabolic. A structural cause should be suspected in the presence of focal or lateralizing signs on examination, such as unilateral pupillary dilation. Structural causes include intracranial hemorrhage, brain infarction, abscess, and neoplasm. The examination is usually, but not uniformly, nonlocalizing in toxic or metabolic causes of coma. Toxic causes include barbiturate, opiate, and other sedative-hypnotic or narcotic drug overdoses as well as intoxication with ethanol, methanol, salicylates, and a variety of other drugs and poisons. Metabolic causes include hypoglycemia, severe hyperglycemia, uremia, hepatic failure, myxedema, and hypoxia. Generalized seizures, including subclinical seizures, can cause coma, either during the seizure or postictally. Other nonstructural causes include hyperthermia, hypothermia, sepsis, and anoxia.

Clinical Assessment

A brief history and physical examination should be performed while life-saving interventions are initiated. Important historical information includes medical and psychiatric disorders, recent drug use, and how the patient was found. Family and bystanders should be interviewed. If available, medical records should be carefully reviewed.

The physical examination provides clues to the etiology of coma and to the potential sites and severity of neuronal injury. Salient features of the examination and examples of findings include:

Vital Signs

- **Body temperature** may show fever pointing to infection, hypothalamic lesions, or hyperthermia. Hypothermia can occur as a result of barbiturate or alcohol intoxication, hypothyroidism, sepsis, and environmental exposure.

- **Pulse:** Dissociation between the heart rate and blood pressure is sometimes observed in intracranial hypertension. Cardiac dysrhythmias may be detected.
- **Blood pressure:** Hypotension can occur as a result of hemorrhage, sepsis, hypoadrenalism, cardiac disease, aortic dissection, and intoxication with alcohol, barbiturate, or other agents.
- **Respiration** should be evaluated with respect to rate, depth, and pattern. Several patterns may be observed in neurologic abnormalities associated with coma, including:
    - **Hypopnea,** which can occur in drug intoxication, metabolic alkalosis, and hypothyroidism.
    - **Tachypnea,** which can occur with a variety of respiratory disorders, any cause of metabolic acidosis, and hepatic failure.
    - **Cheyne-Stokes** respiration, which is a form of periodic breathing in which the amplitude gradually increases and then decreases, sometimes to the point of apnea. It is observed in early rostral-caudal herniation and other bihemispheric disturbances.
    - **Central neurogenic hyperventilation,** which is a form of rapid hyperventilation seen in association with some midbrain lesions and in the upper pontine phase of rostral-caudal herniation.
    - **Apneustic** breathing, which consists of a midinspiratory arrest alternating with end-expiratory pauses. It is seen in the pontine phase of rostral-caudal herniation.
    - **Ataxic** or chaotic respiration, which occurs in the medullary phase of rostral-caudal herniation.

General appearance may show poor hygiene in patients with dementia and in chronic drug abusers. Evidence of incontinence suggests the possibility of a seizure.

Breath odor may be characteristic of ethanol, hepatic failure, or ketoacidosis.

Skin inspection may show cyanosis (caused by hypoxia), jaundice (in hepatic failure), moist pallor and cool temperature (in circulatory shock), rubor (in carbon monoxide poisoning), petechiae (in bleeding disorders), or dry skin (in heat stroke, anticholinergic poisoning, or diabetic ketoacidosis).

Head and neck examination may show ecchymoses, contusions, lacerations, or other evidence of cranial or cervical trauma. Meningismus is frequently detectable in meningitis or subarachnoid hemorrhage.

Fundi: Papilledema occurs in some cases of increased intracranial pressure. Arteriolar narrowing indicates hypertensive disease, and cotton-wool spots indicate diabetes.

Pupils: Small, but preserved, pupillary reactivity is characteristic of narcotic exposure or pontine hemorrhage. Dilated and unreactive pupils are seen with anticholinergic intoxication. A unilaterally dilated pupil can be caused by third-nerve palsy seen in uncal herniation as a result of intracranial mass lesions and intracranial hypertension. The classic sequence of rostral-caudal herniation follows the following stages:

- **Diencephalic stage:** small, but reactive pupils.
- **Mesencephalic stage:** large or midposition, unreactive pupils.
- **Pontine stage:** pinpoint pupils.
- **Medullary stage:** fixed, dilated pupils.

Horner's syndrome (miosis, ptosis, and anhydrosis) occurs in lateral pontine, medullary, and ventrolateral cervical cord lesions.

Eye movements may be spontaneous or provoked. Spontaneous roving movements are seen in metabolic disturbances and disorders that spare the brainstem. Downward deviation suggests a thalamic lesion. Vertical dysconjugation suggests a posterior fossa lesion. Lateral conjugate deviation can be observed in structural cortical lesions or seizures. Ocular bobbing points to a pontine lesion; ocular dipping suggests a diffuse anoxic injury. Eye movements may be provoked by quickly turning the head (oculocephalic reflex or "doll's eyes" phenomenon) or by otic irrigation with cold water (caloric testing). Inability to achieve conjugate deviation of eyes ipsilateral to the cold-water stimulus occurs in brainstem disorders.

Motor examination: A graded assessment of spontaneous movements and responses to nonnoxious and noxious stimuli should be performed.

- **Asymmetric movements** suggest a structural cause for coma.
- **Adventitious movements,** such as tremor, asterixis, or multifocal myoclonus, suggest metabolic conditions. Focal tonic, focal clonic, or generalized myoclonic activity points to seizures.
- **Posturing** may be decorticate (flexor) in the diencephalic stage of rostral-caudal herniation, or it may be decerebrate (extensor) in lower stages.

Laboratory Studies

- **Routine screening,** such as complete blood count with differential and platelets, serum electrolytes, renal and liver function tests, routine coagulation studies, urinalysis, ECG, chest radiograph, should be performed.

- **Special tests,** such as neuroimaging (e.g., computed tomography), toxicologic screen, electrophysiologic tests (e.g., electroencephalogram, evoked potentials), lumbar puncture for cerebrospinal fluid tests, and intracranial pressure monitoring, should be performed as indicated.

Management

- **Vital functions** are stabilized, e.g., institution of endotracheal intubation and mechanical ventilation, establishment of IV access, monitoring of cardiac rhythm.
- **Hypoglycemia** is treated with 50% dextrose IV. Dextrose should be administered routinely, in case there is hypoglycemia, while results of serum glucose test results are awaited. Thiamine is routinely given immediately before concentrated dextrose is administered.
- **Specific treatments** depends on the underlying cause or associated problems. Examples include therapeutic hyperventilation for increased intracranial pressure, naloxone for opiate overdose, gastric lavage or activated charcoal for poisoning, antibiotic therapy for meningitis, and neurosurgical evacuation for subdural hematoma.
- **Nonvital supportive care** includes prophylaxis against venous thrombosis and gastric stress ulcers, frequent turning to prevent decubitus ulcers, pulmonary toilet, and the use of methylcellulose eye drops and taping of the eyelids to prevent corneal damage. Other measures to be considered in patients with long-term coma include tracheostomy, jejunostomy feeding tube placement, and splinting of extremities.

Suggested Readings

Krieger D, Adams HP, Schwarz S, et al. Prognostic and clinical relevance of pupillary responses, intracranial pressure monitoring, and brainstem auditory evoked potentials in comatose patients with acute supratentorial mass lesions. *Crit Care Med* 1993;21:1944–1950.

Concludes that pupillary abnormalities may serve as a reliable parameter, superior to brainstem auditory evoked potential testing and intracranial pressure monitoring, for predicting outcome in patients with coma as a result of supratentorial mass lesions.

Levy DE, Bates D, Caronna JJ, et al. Prognosis in nontraumatic coma. *Ann Intern Med* 1981;94:293–301.

Landmark study of 500 patients showing features of the examination that are most predictive of prognosis in coma. Within hours of the onset of coma, only 1 of 120 patients who lacked two of corneal, pupillary, and oculovestibular responses ever regained independent function.

Plum F, Posner JB. *The diagnosis of stupor and coma,* 3rd ed. Philadelphia: FA Davis, 1982.

Authoritative text on coma discussing pathophysiology, etiologies, examination, and prognosis (377 pages).

Sacco RL, VanGool R, Mohr JP, et al. Nontraumatic coma: Glasgow

coma score and coma etiology as predictors of 2-week outcome. *Arch Neurol* 1990;47:1181–1184.
Glasgow coma scores were determined within 72 hours of onset of coma in 188 patients. The 2-week outcome for patients with scores of 3 to 5 was 15% awake and 85% dead or in a persistent coma.

Samuels MA. A practical approach to coma diagnosis in the unresponsive patient. *Cleve Clin J Med* 1992;59:257–261.
Brief review including an algorithmic diagnostic and treatment protocol.

CHAPTER 36

Cerebrovascular Accidents

(See Chapter 57)

Oded Gerber

Brain Infarction

Timely management of ischemic cerebrovascular accidents necessitates early recognition and rapid differentiation from other conditions. The major categories of ischemic stroke are thrombotic, embolic, hemodynamic, and vasculopathic (see Table 57–2 in the main text). In-hospital ischemic strokes generally occur for one of the following reasons:

- **Systemic hypotension,** e.g., associated with hemorrhage or anesthesia.
- **Severe hypertension.**
- **Thromboembolism** associated with thrombosis, atrial fibrillation, cardioversion, myocardial infarction, mitral valve replacement, mural thrombus, bacterial endocarditis, catheterization, cardiac disease (including cardiac arrest), and air or fat embolism.

Clinical Assessment. Rapid assessment is intended to:

- Exclude nonvascular conditions, such as seizures, hypoglycemia, and other metabolic or toxic brain dysfunction; brain infection; osmotic demyelination syndrome; neuromuscular junction abnormalities; and the neuropathies and myopathies of critical illness.
- Anatomically localize the stroke.
- Determine the responsible vascular lesion.

History. In addition to the routine history, the clinician should emphasize the following points:

- **General risk factors for stroke,** e.g., hypertension, diabetes, cigarette smoking, hyperlipidemia, atrial fibrillation.
- **Risk factors specific to ICU patients,** e.g., hypoperfu-

sion (caused by shock, pump failure, dysrhythmias, etc.), risk factors for embolism, hypercoagulability.

- **Previous cerebrovascular events,** such as transient ischemic attack (TIA) or stroke.
- **Tempo and evolution of stroke,** e.g., sudden or gradual onset, stepwise or fluctuating.
- **Blood pressure fluctuations** before stroke.
- **Seizures,** e.g., partial or generalized, or behavior suggestive of seizures.

Physical Examination. The emphasis should be on:

- **Auscultation for murmurs** that may be associated with embolic phenomena.
- **Signs of emboli,** e.g., petechiae or funduscopic lesions.
- **Vascular examination,** to assess pulses, search for bruits.
- **Neurologic assessment,** including evaluation of cognitive and language function, cranial nerves (including visual field assessment), motor strength, sensation, and coordination.

Clinical features of the various stroke syndromes by location are:

- **Left hemispheric:** any combination of aphasia, right-sided weakness, right-sided sensory loss, right visual field loss, and left eye deviation.
- **Right hemispheric:** any combination of left-sided weakness, left-sided sensory loss, left visual field loss, and right eye deviation.
- **Brainstem:** any combination of dysarthria, bilateral weakness or ataxia, vertigo, nystagmus, and diplopia.

In addition, stroke can occur without motor manifestations, as with isolated visual loss or isolated language dysfunction.

Laboratory Studies. After the clinical diagnosis of stroke is established, further tests are performed to determine the type and cause of the event if this information is not obvious from the clinical data (see Table 57–5 in the main text).

- **Routine blood tests,** including complete blood cell count with differential, platelet count, automated serum chemistry panel, prothrombin time (PT), partial thromboplastin time (PTT), and arterial blood gases, if indicated.
- **Special blood tests** may be indicated in specific situations, e.g., in young patients or those with no other cause for stroke protein S, protein C, and antithrombin III assays. Patients with a propensity to thrombotic events (venous or arterial) or miscarriages should have assays for antiphospholipid antibodies.
- **Chest radiograph.**

- **12-lead ECG.** In addition, 24-hour ECG monitoring may be indicated if a cardiac dysrhythmia is suspected.
- **Echocardiography** is indicated if there is suspicion of a cardiac source. If suspicion of a cardiac source remains high despite a normal transthoracic echocardiogram reading, a transesophageal echocardiogram should be performed.
- **Computed tomography** (CT) of the brain is performed early in the course of a stroke, without contrast, to exclude a hemorrhagic etiology. Infarcts generally are not obvious for the first 24 hours. The scan is repeated later in the course to assess the size and location of stroke. Contrast infusion is frequently unnecessary unless there is a question of a neoplastic or inflammatory lesion. CT scanning may not detect small cerebral infarctions or brainstem infarctions.
- **Magnetic resonance imaging** (MRI) demonstrates ischemia earlier than CT scanning, and is therefore better for imaging small infarcts, brainstem infarcts, and venous thromboses. However, it is much more difficult to perform than CT scanning, it limits the ability to monitor the patient during the study, and it therefore may be impractical in ICU patients.
- **Magnetic resonance angiogram** (MRA) is useful for detecting gross lesions in the large extracranial vessels and the larger intracranial vessels. This procedure is still in its infancy, but it may obviate cerebral angiography for gross occlusions, stenoses, and other large vascular lesions.
- **Cerebral angiography** is performed in unexplained strokes in which vascular lesions are subtle, need clearer characterization than is possible with noninvasive techniques, or involve smaller vessels. It is also performed before vascular surgical intervention.
- **Duplex Doppler scanning** of the extracranial carotid arteries and vertebral arteries is a useful, noninvasive, and accurate method for detecting hemodynamically significant extracranial lesions.
- **Transcranial Doppler** studies may be useful for diagnosing diminished flow in the larger intracranial vessels. It is also useful for sequentially following vasospasm in subarachnoid hemorrhages.

General management considerations include:

- **Performing frequent neurologic assessments** in an ICU setting, until the patient is stable, so that any progression is detected rapidly.
- **Ensuring adequate oxygenation** by assessing oxygenation with pulse oximetry or arterial blood gas determination and administering supplemental oxygen if necessary.

- **Considering endotracheal intubation** in obtunded patients to provide adequate pulmonary toilet.
- **Considering continuous ECG monitoring.**
- **Monitoring blood pressure.** Moderate elevations should not be treated, but more extreme elevations (e.g., > 190/120 mm Hg) should be treated gently without lowering the blood pressure to the normal range. Labetalol or angiotensin-converting enzyme inhibitors are useful agents to consider.
- **Assessing and maintaining fluid and electrolyte balance.**
- **Avoiding hyperglycemia.** Hyperglycemia may have adverse CNS consequences in the setting of acute ischemic stroke.
- **Preventing decubitus ulcer development** with conventional techniques.
- **Preventing aspiration pneumonitis,** e.g., elevating the head of the bed, considering endotracheal intubation in obtunded or comatose patients.
- **Preventing deep venous thrombosis** with low-dose subcutaneous heparin (if not contraindicated) or lower-extremity pneumatic compression devices.
- **Preventing bladder infections.** In-dwelling bladder catheters are used only when necessary.

Specific therapies include:

Anticoagulation is indicated in most cases of cardioembolic stroke unless specifically contraindicated (e.g., in bacterial endocarditis). A continuous IV heparin infusion is initiated, without a loading dose, with the goal of achieving a PTT of 1.5–2 times the control time. Heparinization should be withheld or deferred in certain cases, e.g.,

- **Hemorrhagic infarctions**—anticoagulation is generally delayed if this complication is shown by CT scanning.
- **Large infarctions**—anticoagulation is delayed for several days or more.
- **Coma.**
- **Severe hypertension,** if uncontrolled.

Once effective heparinization has been achieved and the patient is stable, warfarin can be used in place of heparin. The duration of anticoagulation subsequent to the acute phase depends on the embolic source.

Antiplatelet Agents. Antiplatelet agents, either aspirin or (if aspirin cannot be used or is ineffective) ticlopidine, are administered to patients with strokes who are not anticoagulated.

Surgery. In large cerebellar infarctions, there may be brainstem compression or obstruction to the flow of cerebrospinal fluid. In these cases, surgery may be indicated to relieve the obstruction or decompress the infarcted cerebellum.

Investigational Treatments. Calcium channel blocking agents and fibrinolytic drugs are undergoing clinical trials.

Intracerebral Hemorrhage

Intracerebral hemorrhages constitute approximately 10% of all strokes. The etiologies can be categorized as follows:

- **Hypertension,** usually long-standing and poorly controlled.
- **Vascular anomalies,** e.g., arteriovenous malformations.
- **Bleeding diatheses,** e.g., severe coagulopathy or thrombocytopenia.
- **Drugs,** e.g., cocaine or amphetamines.
- **Vasculopathies,** e.g., cerebral amyloid angiopathy, systemic lupus erythematosus, polyarteritis nodosa, and primary CNS vasculitis.
- **Brain tumors,** primary or metastatic.
- **Others,** e.g., moyamoya disease, venous thrombosis, mycotic aneurysms.

Clinical Manifestations. The general features of intracerebral hemorrhage include onset of neurologic dysfunction that is usually severe within minutes, variably accompanied by headache, nausea, and vomiting, and less frequently by seizures or nuchal rigidity. If a large enough hematoma is present, altered mentation occurs. Characteristic signs and symptoms by location are as follows:

- **Putaminal hemorrhage** is the most common location of hypertensive hemorrhage. Signs and symptoms are those of major hemispheric dysfunction, with obtundation, depending on the size of the hematoma and the amount of edema.
- **Thalamic hemorrhage.** Signs may include hemisensory or hemisensorimotor disturbances, small pupils, upward gaze restriction, and downward and inward eye deviation. Changes in consciousness depend on the size of the lesion and the amount of edema.
- **Lobar hemorrhage,** by definition, occurs out in the hemispheres. Symptoms and signs depend on the specific location within the hemispheres.
- **Brainstem hemorrhage** primarily occurs in the pons. It usually has a rapid onset, with catastrophic brain stem dysfunction accompanied by coma, commonly with decerebration and pinpoint pupils. Rarely, the neurologic findings are more confined.
- **Cerebellar hemorrhage.** Hemiataxia, truncal ataxia, or both may be present. If hemorrhage is sufficiently large or is accompanied by edema, obstructive hydrocephalus and brainstem compression can develop.

Diagnostic Evaluation. The diagnosis may be apparent from the history and physical examination. CT imaging is diagnostic. Hematomas are readily visible without the use of contrast material. Lumbar puncture should be avoided. It would be indicated only if an infectious or inflammatory etiology is suspected, but is contraindicated if there is brainstem compression, increased intracranial pressure with shift of midline structures, or noncommunicating hydrocephalus.

Management. General management considerations are the same as for brain infarction (see above). Coagulopathy or thrombocytopenia should be corrected by administration of blood products. Seizures and cerebral edema should be treated conventionally (see Chapters 37 and 39 in this book). There is no consensus as to the advantage of surgical evacuation as opposed to medical management for most hypertensive hematomas. Most are treated medically; however, surgical decompression is indicated for cerebellar hematomas with potential or actual brain stem compression. Surgical placement of a ventriculostomy catheter may also be necessary for hydrocephalus.

Subarachnoid Hemorrhage

Nontraumatic subarachnoid hemorrhages are most often caused by rupture of congenital or acquired saccular aneurysms, usually occurring at bifurcations off the circle of Willis. The incidence of multiple aneurysms is 10 to 20%. Less common causes include extension of an intracerebral hemorrhage, arteriovenous malformation, bleeding diathesis, vasculopathy, and cocaine or sympathomimetic drug use.

Clinical Manifestations. The onset of rupture of an aneurysm may be during exertion or performance of the Valsalva maneuver. It is heralded by a sudden, severe headache. Neck stiffness, photophobia, nausea, vomiting, and back pain may be present. The sensorium can range from normal to comatose.

Cerebral vasospasm occurs in 40% of patients with subarachnoid hemorrhage, but only about half of these patients are symptomatic. It usually begins no earlier than day 3 or 4, and it peaks by day 7 to 10. Symptoms of vasospasm may be focal or global, and they are correlated with the amount of blood in the basal cisterns.

Laboratory Diagnosis

- **Blood tests.** In addition to routine tests, PT, PTT, and platelet counts should be obtained. If findings are abnormal, fresh-frozen plasma or platelet transfusions should be given.
- **CT scanning** shows subarachnoid blood in approximately 90% of cases if performed within 72 hours.

- **Lumbar puncture** shows subarachnoid blood in 99% of cases. Xanthochromia appears after 6 to 8 hours.
- **Angiography** is mandatory for visualizing the aneurysm and searching for multiple aneurysms. Angiographic imaging also documents vasospasm.

Management includes transfer to an ICU, complete bed rest, use of stool softeners, pain control, and prophylactic use of pneumatic or elastic stockings to prevent deep vein thrombosis. Low-dose heparin should not be used. Routine prophylactic use of anticonvulsants is controversial, as is routine use of corticosteroids to treat chemical meningitis. Systemic hypertension is treated cautiously; hypotension must be avoided.

Nimodipine is given for prophylaxis against vasospasm. Other measures for preventing vasospasm include providing adequate hydration, avoiding hypotension, avoiding hyponatremia, and considering early neurosurgical intervention. Therapy includes intravascular volume expansion and induced hypertension. However, the latter procedure can be performed safely only after surgical clipping.

Although there has been some controversy regarding the timing of surgical clipping of aneurysms, patients with grade 1, 2, or 3 subarachnoid hemorrhage (see Table 57–11 in the main text) are usually candidates for early operation, before the onset of vasospasm, to decrease the risk of rebleeding. Hydrocephalus may occur at any point during the course of subarachnoid hemorrhage, and ventricular drainage may be necessary, depending on the clinical manifestations and extent of hydrocephalus.

Suggested Readings

Fisher M, Bogousslavsky J. Evolving toward effective therapy for acute ischemic stroke. *JAMA* 1993;270:360–364.

Current summary of potential therapies, imaging techniques, and trial designs in acute stroke.

Kopitnik TA, Samson DS. Management of subarachnoid haemorrhage. *J Neurol Neurosurg Psychiatry* 1993;56:947–959.

Summarizes clinical aspects of subarachnoid hemorrhage.

Marshall RS, Mohr JP. Current management of ischaemic stroke. *J Neurol Neurosurg Psychiatry* 1993;56:6–16.

Good summary of therapeutic modalities available for treating patients with stroke.

Powers WJ. Acute hypertension after stroke: The scientific basis for treatment decisions. *Neurology* 1993;43:461–467.

Timely and concise discussion of hypertension in acute stroke and its management.

Welch KMA, ed. Cerebrovascular diseases: 18th Princeton Conference. *Stroke* 1993;24(suppl):I93–I108.

Up-to-date discussion of medical and surgical treatment of intracerebral hemorrhage.

CHAPTER 37

Seizures and Status Epilepticus

(See Chapter 58)

Alan B. Ettinger

Seizures are the clinical manifestation of excessive and hypersynchronous neuronal activity in the cerebral cortex. Seizures are classified as either partial or generalized, and are either convulsive or nonconvulsive. In contrast to status epilepticus (SE), most seizures are self-limited and associated with little morbidity. However, new-onset seizures may be symptomatic of a serious condition, such as brain tumor or infection; therefore, potential etiologies should be thoroughly investigated. In patients with known underlying epilepsy, seizure recurrences are secondary to inadequate compliance with anticonvulsant therapy, the refractory nature of the epileptic condition, or a new condition that lowers the seizure threshold.

SE is a condition characterized by persistent seizure activity or recurrent seizures intermixed with periods of persistently depressed consciousness that last 30 minutes or longer. However, because SE is a medical emergency, protocols to treat it are often initiated substantially before 30 minutes have passed.

SE may be characterized by any type of partial or generalized seizure, but generalized convulsive types are associated with the highest rates of morbidity and mortality. Tonic-clonic SE may produce systemic complications that result in peripheral organ damage as well as cerebral injury. Examples of systemic complications include hypoxia, rhabdomyolysis with secondary renal failure, severe autonomic system failure, aspiration pneumonia and pulmonary edema, cardiac dysrhythmias, and electrolyte disturbances. Local CNS effects of SE also cause neuronal injury independent of systemic factors. These complications are related to the type of SE, the duration of seizures, and the underlying etiology. Reported mortality rates for combined early and late complications average 40%.

SE is an example of a condition in which initial treatment precedes detailed diagnostic evaluation.

Treatment

The immediate objectives of treatment are to:

- Maintain adequate airway, ventilation, and circulation.

- Stop the seizure as quickly as possible.
- Prevent seizure recurrence.
- Establish and treat underlying conditions.
- Prevent systemic complications.

Immediate management includes the following:

- Establishing an airway and providing supplemental oxygenation and ventilation by bag-valve mask. If it is clear that the seizure activity is prolonged, or if the patient is hemodynamically unstable, endotracheal intubation is necessary.
- Monitoring and stabilizing vital signs, securing IV access, and obtaining blood specimens for glucose level, blood counts, serum electrolyte levels, routine chemistry assays (including renal function tests), arterial blood gas evaluation, and anticonvulsant drug levels.
- Giving concentrated dextrose (50 mL of 50% dextrose in water) and thiamine (100 mg) by IV injection to empirically treat possible hypoglycemia.
- Administering IV lorazepam ($\leq$ 0.15 mg/kg at $\leq$ 2 mg/min) or diazepam ($\leq$ 0.3 mg/kg at $\leq$ 5 mg/min). These are first-line agents because of their effectiveness and rapid onset of action.
- Administering phenytoin. For patients who have not already received the drug, an IV loading dose of 18 mg/kg is given at a rate no faster than 50 mg/min.
- For patients already receiving phenytoin, who have not received phenobarbital, the latter may be given at a loading dose of 10–20 mg/kg IV, no faster than 50 mg/min.

IV midazolam as a continuous infusion has also been successful in controlling SE. Benzodiazepines may be titrated according to seizure manifestations and side effects, namely hypotension. Drug-induced hypotension may respond to vigorous fluid resuscitation, but in some cases may limit the rate or total dose of benzodiazepine administration. Respiratory depression is treated by bag-valve ventilation with a face mask or endotracheal intubation, rather than by withholding benzodiazepine administration. Because of their short half-life, benzodiazepine administration should be immediately followed by a loading dose of phenytoin or phenobarbital.

Phenytoin is typically administered before phenobarbital because of the lower risks of respiratory depression (especially in combination with benzodiazepines), sedation, and depression of consciousness after seizures are terminated. To prevent precipitation, phenytoin should be given through a saline IV rather than through a dextrose-containing IV. ECG and blood pressure should be monitored during the initial infusion because hypotension and dysrhythmias may occur.

For refractory SE that continues despite these measures, pentobarbital (5 mg/kg initially, infused up to 20 mg/kg until seizure activity stops, then 1–3 mg/kg/hr) can be used to induce barbiturate coma in SE that is refractory to the above measures. Hypotension may limit the dose; hemodynamic monitoring and the use of fluids or inotropic or vasoactive drugs may be necessary. Continuous EEG monitoring or serial intermittent EEG studies should be obtained to allow titration of the anticonvulsant regimen. The infusion can be decreased every 6 hours to determine whether seizures have stopped. Other drugs that have been employed in refractory SE include thiopental, paraldehyde, lidocaine, valproic acid, and general anesthetic agents (see Chapter 58 in the main text). In the patient who remains unresponsive, but who has no clinically apparent seizure activity, EEG testing should be performed to exclude subclinical SE. Subclinical SE warrants additional pharmacologic treatment.

Maintenance therapy of anticonvulsant drugs is initiated after SE is terminated. Typical maintenance dosing regimens are phenytoin (300–600 mg/day), phenobarbital (60–300 mg/day), carbamazepine (600–2400 mg/day), or valproic acid (750–3000 mg/day). Dosing must be titrated according to serum drug levels. The clinician should be aware of potential drug interactions (including metabolic induction or inhibition and competition for protein binding) that can alter levels of anticonvulsants or concomitant medications.

Diagnostic Considerations

The etiology of the seizure should be evaluated by reviewing the history, physical examination findings, and laboratory test results. Common, correctable factors that may cause or precipitate seizures in the ICU setting include hypoxemia, extreme alkalemia or acidemia, and severe electrolyte derangements, such as hyponatremia or hyocalcemia. When the etiology is unclear, the possibility of CNS infarction, hemorrhage, or other mass lesion should be considered, and appropriate imaging studies performed. CNS infection may also be a consideration.

Suggested Readings

Browne TR. The pharmacokinetics of agents used to treat status epilepticus. *Neurology* 1990;40(suppl 2):28–32.

Discusses the application of pharmacokinetic concepts, including half-life, volume of distribution, and elimination of drugs used in the management of status epilepticus.

DeLorenzo R, Towne A, Pellock J, et al. Status epilepticus in children, adults and the elderly. *Epilepsia* 1992;33:S15–S25.

Hauser WA. Status epilepticus: Epidemiologic considerations. *Neurology* 1990;40:9–12.

Reviews the etiologies, causes of brain pathology, and mortality rate in patients with status epilepticus.
Leppik IE. Status epilepticus: The next decade. *Neurology* 1990;40(suppl 2):4–9.
General review of definitions, etiologies, treatment, and prognosis.
Meldrum BS, Brierley JB. Prolonged epileptic seizures in primates: Ischemic cell change and its relation to ictal physiological events. *Arch Neurol* 1973;28:10–17.
Landmark study of the adverse effects of status epilepticus on the brain.
Wijdicks EF, Parisi JE, Sharbrough FW. Prognostic value of myoclonus status in comatose survivors of cardiac arrest. *Ann Neurol* 1994; 35:239–243.
Of 107 consecutive patients who remained in a coma after cardiac resuscitation, 37% had myoclonic status, and all of these patients died. Concludes that myoclonic status should be considered an agonal phenomenon indicating devastating neocortical damage.

CHAPTER 38

Brain Injury After Cardiac Arrest: ICU Management and Outcome, Including Brain Death

(See Chapter 56)

Oded Gerber

During cardiac arrest, there is cessation of brain perfusion, resulting in the following sequence of events:

- After approximately 10 seconds, loss of consciousness occurs.
- After approximately 20 seconds, loss of cortical electroencephalogram (EEG) activity occurs.
- After 4 to 8 minutes, permanent brain injury develops. Longer periods of cardiac arrest can cause infarction of the entire brain.

Other causes of brain damage that result in a clinical syndrome resembling cardiac arrest are:

- Prolonged, severe hypotension.
- Profound hypoxemia.
- Hypoglycemia.
- Status epilepticus.

- Certain forms of poisoning (e.g., carbon monoxide or cyanide).

Management of Patients During and After Cardiac Arrest

Optimal resuscitation efforts should achieve effective brain perfusion and oxygenation during the arrest. Efforts after the arrest should be directed toward maintaining adequate arterial oxygen tension (PaO_2), normal blood glucose concentration, and adequate cerebral perfusion. Systemic complications should be identified and treated promptly. Drugs that depress brain function should be avoided, if possible. Hypercapnia may cause increased intracranial pressure and tissue acidosis. Hypocapnia causes intracranial vascular constriction and impairs neuronal function. Hyperglycemia aggravates ischemic brain injury. High fever increases brain metabolism and intracranial pressure. Evidence of intracranial hypertension, such as papilledema or cerebral edema by computed tomography (CT), should prompt treatment directed at lowering intracranial pressure (see Chapter 39 in this book and Chapter 18 in the main text).

Postresuscitation Diagnostic Evaluation

If the prearrest clinical findings are atypical, or if the arrest is unexpected, the patient should be examined for conditions in which cardiac arrest may have occurred as a secondary event, such as intracranial hemorrhage or drug overdose. To assess the degree of neurologic injury, serial neurologic examinations should be performed, with the following points emphasized:

- **Level of consciousness.** Observations are recorded on a standardized form, such as the Glasgow Coma Scale (see table in Chapter 6 in this book).
- **Brainstem reflexes,** including pupillary light reaction, extraocular muscle movements, and corneal reflexes.
- **Motor responses,** such as evidence of posturing, facial movements, roving eye movements, eyelid opening, grimacing, and chewing movements, either spontaneously or in response to noxious stimulation.

It is important to look particularly for evidence of focality, i.e., asymmetry in the brainstem, motor, or reflex examination. Focal signs may indicate a watershed infarction as a result of cardiac arrest.

CT may be performed if an underlying lesion is suspected as the cause of cardiac arrest. A CT scan may also identify brain swelling or infarction that may have resulted from the cardiac arrest. An EEG is useful for confirming suspected seizures. Lumbar puncture is rarely useful, and is necessary only in the uncommon instance of suspected meningitis or when subarachnoid hemorrhage is suspected but not seen on CT.

Seizures After Cardiac Arrest

(also see Chapter 37 in this book and Chapter 58 in the main text)

Generalized seizures, focal seizures, and multifocal myoclonus occur frequently after cardiac arrest. These complications may appear separately or in combination, and may be accompanied by an abnormal EEG that shows multifocal or periodic epileptiform discharges. An effective treatment for such phenomena does not exist. A loading dose of phenytoin given IV as 15–18 mg/kg in 250 mL saline (no faster than 50 mg/min), followed by intermittent maintenance doses (typically initiated at 100 mg every 8 hours and guided by serum drug levels), is a useful strategy. Sodium valproate or clonazepam may be used for myoclonus. The use of more aggressive measures, such as inducing pentobarbital coma, is predicated on the patient's overall prognosis; therefore, these measures are rarely used.

Neurologic Outcome from Cardiac Arrest

Patients who remain in coma for more than 6 hours after cardiac arrest have a mortality rate of 64% at 1 week and a rate of 90% at 1 year. The severity of neurologic sequelae depends on the duration of ischemia to the brain which, in turn, depends on the time required to reestablish adequate cerebral perfusion. For clarity and simplicity, brain dysfunction after cardiac arrest can be categorized into five levels of severity. These stages are not discreet, but rather are on a continuous spectrum.

- After a brief loss of cardiac rhythm or blood pressure, there is a short period of unconsciousness and, consequently, amnesia of the events of the arrest.
- More protracted brain ischemia may result in minutes to hours of postarrest unconsciousness, followed by a confusional state that can last for several days. Amnesia is common, both anterograde and retrograde. Patients often have a decreased ability to recall new information.
- After more severe global brain ischemia, patients may awaken after 12 hours of coma or longer, but in a state of global and severe confusion. These patients may have hyperreflexia, hypertonia, ataxia, weakness, and signs

of parkinsonism. They rarely regain independent function.

- Even more prolonged ischemia results in a vegetative state that is usually persistent. Patients with this syndrome eventually may be capable of spontaneous eye opening and blinking, but they remain unresponsive. There are rare reports of patients with late recovery of some mental function.
- The most severely brain damaged patients have no signs of eye opening or other wakening. Some progress to brain death, and others die of medical complications.

Brain Death

Brain death is irreversible cessation of all function of the entire brain, including the brainstem. Common causes include severe head trauma, cerebrovascular disease, and anoxic encephalopathy. Less common causes include tumor, infection, certain poisonings, and various metabolic disorders.

Clinical Diagnosis. The diagnosis of brain death implies no possibility of any recovery of brain function. The presence of a single brainstem reflex precludes the diagnosis. There must be complete coma, with no response to multiple stimuli, such as loud noises, calling the patient's name, and application of painful stimuli to the fingernails or face. There can be no decorticate or decerebrate posturing. Formal apnea testing should be performed (see below and Table 56–9 in the main text). Patients may have some persistent movements as a result of spinal reflex activity, such as the triple flexion response to pain, but this finding requires careful interpretation by an experienced observer. All brainstem reflexes should be tested, including pupillary reaction, corneal reflexes, oculocephalic reflexes, and cold-water caloric testing; all must be absent.

The clinician confirming the diagnosis of brain death should be satisfied that the following conditions are met:

- The cause or extent of brain injury should be known and should be consistent with brain death.
- Reversible medical conditions, such as hypothermia, severe metabolic disorders, hypoxia, hypotension, sedative drug overdose, and muscle paralysis, should be excluded.
- The absence of clinical signs of brain function should be confirmed during a period of observation. This period depends on the physician's judgment, institutional policies and, in some jurisdictions, legal statutes. It typically ranges from 12–24 hours after the first observation of brain death. In obvious cases, such as severe head trauma or physical destruction of most of the brain, a shorter period of observation may be appropriate.

An apnea test should be part of the institutional protocol. Typically, it is performed as follows:

- The apnea test is performed after all other portions of the clinical examination for brain death have been completed.
- If the patient is hypocapnic, eucapnia is achieved by adjusting minute ventilation and documenting that arterial carbon dioxide tension ($Paco_2$) is normal by arterial blood gas analysis.
- The patient is hyperoxygenated with a fraction of inspired oxygen (Fio_2) of 1.0 for at least 10 minutes. A cannula suitable for introduction through the endotracheal tube is connected to an oxygen source delivering an Fio_2 of 1.0 at 8 L/min.
- Mechanical ventilation is discontinued, the oxygen cannula is quickly inserted into the trachea by way of the endotracheal tube, and the time is noted.
- The patient should be uncovered and observed carefully for any signs of ventilatory or other movement. If such movement occurs, the test is halted and ventilation is immediately reinstituted.
- During the apnea test, the patient is monitored with continuous ECG and pulse oximetry. Blood pressure is also monitored. Development of significant dysrhythmias, hypotension, or hypoxemia may necessitate halting the apnea test prematurely.
- After 3 to 10 minutes (as long as the patient is hemodynamically stable and pulse oximetry shows adequate oxygenation), an arterial blood specimen is quickly obtained for blood gas analysis. Mechanical ventilation is reinstituted immediately after the blood specimen is drawn.
- To confirm brain death, the $Paco_2$ at the end of the apnea test should have reached 50–60 torr.

Confirmatory Laboratory Tests. Although some local policies mandate routine EEG testing to confirm the diagnosis of brain death, this testing is not generally recognized in the medical literature as a requirement. Confirmatory tests are used when an adequate examination cannot be performed, such as when there is severe facial trauma that precludes full assessment of brain stem reflexes. In addition to EEG testing, cerebral arteriography, radionuclide perfusion scanning, transcranial Doppler flow studies, and xenon flow cranial CT scanning have been used to confirm the diagnosis of brain death by showing no blood flow to the brain.

Suggested Readings

Al Jumah M, McLean DR, Al Rajeh S, et al. Bulk diffusion apnea test in the diagnosis of brain death. *Crit Care Med* 1992;20:1564–1567.

Describes experience with apnea testing with an alternative oxygenation technique.

Bates D. Defining prognosis in medical coma. *J Neurol Neurosurg Psychiatry* 1991;54:569–571.

Reviews clinical and laboratory methodologies and studies for predicting outcome after cardiac arrest.

Kirsch JR, Dean JM, Rogers MC. Current concepts in brain resuscitation. *Arch Intern Med* 1986;146:1413–1419.

Discusses pathophysiologic treatment of global cerebral ischemia.

Madl C, Grimm G, Kramer L, et al. Early prediction of individual outcome after cardiopulmonary resuscitation. *Lancet* 1993;341:855–858.

Interesting study of the utility of sensory evoked potentials for predicting outcome after cardiac arrest.

Mullie A, Verstringe P, Buyalert W, et al. Predictive value of Glasgow coma score for awakening after out-of-hospital cardiac arrest: Cerebral Resuscitation Study Group of the Belgian Society for Intensive Care. *Lancet* 1988;8578:137–140.

Discusses value of Glasgow Coma Score for predicting neurologic outcome.

Snyder BD, Tabbaa MA. Assessment and treatment of neurological dysfunction after cardiac arrest. *Stroke* 1988;19:269–273.

Contains good discussion of prognosis, laboratory techniques, and proposed treatments of anoxic encephalopathy.

CHAPTER 39

Neurophysiological Monitoring and Intracranial Hypertension

(See Chapters 18, 54, and 63)

Magdy S. Shady and Alan B. Ettinger

A variety of neurophysiologic testing modalities are available as clinical tools to evaluate neurologic conditions commonly encountered in the ICU setting. One goal of brain monitoring is to decrease morbidity and mortality rates by providing the clinician with quantitative physiologic information that can be integrated into a therapeutic plan. Brain monitors can be used to assess cerebral perfusion, brain metabolism, or cerebral function. They may be used to localize sites of neurologic injury, provide physiologic data, and help to predict prognosis. Although less anatomically precise than neuroimaging, neurophysiologic testing can provide more dynamic assessments and can be readily performed at the patient's bedside.

Cerebral Blood Flow Monitoring

Cerebral ischemia is a state of inadequate oxygen delivery to the brain. The cerebellum, basal ganglia, and watershed zones between major branches of the intracranial vessels appear to be selectively more vulnerable to ischemic injury than other areas of the brain. The severity of brain damage secondary to cerebral ischemia is proportional to the magnitude and duration of the injury. Cerebral ischemia may be focal or global and complete or incomplete. Cerebral blood flow is affected by three important factors:

- **Metabolic demands** that vary with body temperature and level of brain activity (e.g., fever, seizures, pain).
- **Cerebral perfusion pressure** that affects cerebral blood flow only when it is outside the range of autoregulation (normally approximately 50–130 mm Hg).
- **Arterial carbon dioxide tension (P_{CO_2}),** which is a potent regulator of cerebral vascular resistance over a range of 20–80 torr.

Cerebral blood flow measurement has produced significant descriptive data in patients with head injury, but has not been routinely used for management. Low regional cerebral blood flow is a poor prognostic indicator in patients with severe head trauma. Cerebral blood flow may be measured by ^{133}Xe clearance or transcranial Doppler ultrasonography. The latter technique can be used to measure the arterial blood flow velocity in intracranial vessels. Its main value is in detecting occlusion or severe stenosis (> 65%) in basal intracranial arteries, assessing the patterns and extent of collateral circulation, detecting arteriovenous malformation, and evaluating and following vasospasm in subarachnoid hemorrhage from aneurysms. It can also be used to evaluate patients with suspected brain death.

Near-infrared spectroscopy dynamically monitors cerebral oxygenation and blood flow by measuring the absorbance of light by circulating deoxyhemoglobin and oxyhemoglobin. This potentially promising technique is currently in the research stages.

Evoked Potential Monitoring

Evoked potentials, also known as evoked responses, are time-locked changes in the electrical activity of the nervous system in response to an electrical stimulus. Responses are measured as a set of waveforms produced at sites distant from the stimulus. Distortions in waveform amplitude, morphology, or latency (conduction time) can help localize areas of neuronal disturbance in specific sensory or motor pathways. These studies are influenced by sedatives, narcotics, and anesthetics as well as by trauma, hypoxia, and ischemia.

Visual evoked potentials are waveforms recorded in occipital scalp electrodes in response to exposing the retina to flashing lights or alternating checkerboard patterns. Brain stem auditory evoked potentials generate electrical potentials in the auditory pathways. Somatosensory evoked potentials generate potentials at scalp electrodes in response to an electrical stimulus administered to a peripheral nerve, such as the median nerve. Motor evoked potentials are generated by magnetically or electrically stimulating proximal portions of motor pathways in the cerebral cortex and measuring conduction to distal muscle groups.

Electroencephalogram

The cortical electroencephalogram (EEG) detects cerebral anatomic or physiologic abnormalities as shown by alterations in the electrical patterns recorded by scalp electrodes. It has several uses:

- **Epileptic disorders** can be identified, including subclinical seizure activity.
- **Brain death** can be corroborated as an adjunctive test to clinical examination and apnea testing.
- **Monitoring during surgery,** e.g., during carotid endarterectomy and cardiac surgery.
- **Etiology of encephalopathy** may be suggested. Certain EEG patterns are characteristic of hepatic disease, uremia, anoxia, or drug effects. The severity of encephalopathy can also be assessed.
- **Monitoring during sedation** or in a chemically induced coma to provide early evidence of seizures or cerebral ischemia.
- **Prognostication** for patients in coma.
- **Detection of structural lesions.** In unusual cases, EEG may even show abnormalities that are poorly identified on neuroimaging.

Computer-Enhanced EEG Methods. Digital EEG recordings may supplement the routine EEG by:

- Displaying data in easily interpreted formats, such as colorful topographic maps.
- Providing precise frequency quantification.
- Extracting information that cannot be obtained by routine visual inspection.
- Detecting paroxysmal events, such as epileptiform activity.

Computer-enhanced EEG monitoring does not preclude the need for a trained electroencephalographer to exclude artifact from the analysis. Compressed spectral array monitoring, which records single-channel EEG readings and displays them graphically, should be supplemented by careful interpretation of simultaneously recorded routine EEG readings.

Peripheral Nervous System Neurophysiologic Techniques

Nerve conduction studies measure the amplitude and velocity of nerve impulse conduction through sensory and motor nerves. These studies can show the integrity of axonal and myelin components of nerves, and can provide clues to the presence of neuropathic disorders.

Electromyography (EMG) measures electrical activity in selected muscles as recorded by a needle electrode inserted into the muscle. The nature of the signal and the identification of affected muscle groups help to localize the site of peripheral nervous system disease (e.g., myopathy vs. radiculopathy).

Repetitive stimulation measures the integrity of the neuromuscular junction by repetitively stimulating a nerve and recording potentials from the corresponding muscle. For example, this test can confirm the diagnosis of myasthenia gravis.

Specialized techniques include single-fiber EMG testing, used to assess neuromuscular junction disorders, and blink reflex studies, used to assess the integrity of trigeminal nerve–facial nerve pathways (see Chapter 54 in the main text for a discussion of the application of neurophysiologic testing in specific disorders).

Intracranial Pressure Monitoring

Normal intracranial pressure (ICP) is less than 20 mm Hg, but it fluctuates with position and activity. Cerebral perfusion pressure can be calculated as mean arterial pressure minus ICP. Severe increases in ICP therefore can reduce cerebral perfusion pressure and cerebral blood flow. The use of ICP monitoring may improve the outcome of patients with closed head trauma by preventing or prompting treatment of intracranial hypertension to avoid hypoperfusion or cerebral herniation. It also allows the treatment of intracranial hypertension to be optimally titrated. Among the available methods of ICP monitoring are:

- **Intraventricular catheter** placement, which is the criterion standard method. It allows waveform analysis and measurement of brain compliance, elastance, and pressure–volume index. Cerebrospinal fluid can be removed through the catheter if necessary. Its chief disadvantages are its invasiveness and a higher infection rate than other methods. The ventricular cannula may become obstructed, especially when there is intraventricular hemorrhage. Its use may increase cerebral edema or cause intracerebral hemorrhage. Placement can be difficult to perform if the lateral ventricles are small.

- **Subarachnoid screw** placement, which is easy to apply and remove. The infection rate is lower than with an intraventricular catheter. The technique occasionally results in erroneous measurements; there is no access for cerebrospinal fluid; and pressure volume index, compliance, and elastance cannot be measured.
- **Fiberoptic devices,** which are available for placement within the epidural space, subdural space, brain parenchyma, or ventricular system. There is no lumen to become obstructed.

Treatment of Intracranial Hypertension. The goals of treatment are to ensure adequate cerebral metabolism by maintaining adequate cerebral blood flow and oxygenation. Basic measures include controlling seizures, avoiding hypoxemia, and maintaining adequate arterial blood pressure, an adequate hemoglobin level, and a normal electrolyte balance (particularly the serum sodium level). Nonsurgical measures to reduce intracranial pressure include:

- **Elevating the patient's head** 15–30 degrees is commonly recommended.
- **Diuretics,** e.g., furosemide 10–40 mg IV may be considered, especially if there is evidence of fluid overload despite mannitol administration.
- **Mannitol,** e.g., 0.25–1.0 g/kg IV is given to reduce cerebral edema. The dose may be repeated at half the initial dose at 4–8-hour intervals. Serum osmolality should be monitored to avoid inducing a hyperosmolar state (> 320 mOsm/kg H_2O). Dehydration, electrolyte imbalance, renal failure, and rebound intracranial hypertension can occur.
- **Induced hyperventilation** with mechanical ventilation to an arterial carbon dioxide tension ($Paco_2$) of 25–30 torr (assuming normal underlying acid–base balance) induces mild cerebral vasoconstriction. More extreme reduction of $Paco_2$ may worsen cerebral ischemia by compromising cerebral blood flow.
- **Barbiturate-induced coma** is a controversial method that is recommended by some to reduce cerebral metabolism. Pentobarbital has been used IV at a loading dose of 5–30 mg/kg followed by continuous infusion or hourly maintenance doses. Endpoints are control of ICP and burst suppression on EEG.
- **Hypothermia** may reduce cerebral metabolism, especially in children. Fever is controlled with antipyretics or a cooling blanket.

- **Corticosteroids** are useful in decreasing cerebral edema secondary to tumor, but their value has not been proven for head injury or ischemic stroke.
- **Cerebrospinal fluid drainage** can be accomplished if there is an intraventricular catheter in place.

Suggested Readings

Cascino GD. Neurophysiological monitoring in the intensive care unit. *J Intensive Care Med* 1988;3:215–223.

Cruz J. Combined continuous monitoring of systemic and cerebral oxygenation in acute brain injury: Preliminary observations. *Crit Care Med* 1993;21:1225–1232.

Young adults with acute brain trauma were monitored with jugular bulb and pulmonary artery oxyhemoglobin saturations. The systemic–cerebral oxygenation and systemic–cerebral ventilatory indexes were calculated as new variables and were potentially useful for the combined assessment of global systemic and cerebral oxygenation.

Facco E, Munari M, Baratto F, et al. Multimodality evoked potentials (auditory, somatosensory and motor) in coma. *Neurophysiol Clin* 1993;23:237–258.

Discusses complementary roles of different types of evoked potentials in predicting prognosis in comatose patients.

Louis PT, Goddard-Finegold J, Fishman MA, et al. Barbiturates and hyperventilation during intracranial hypertension. *Crit Care Med* 1993;21:1200–1206.

Prospective, randomized study of hyperventilation versus hyperventilation plus barbiturate therapy in a canine model of increased intracranial pressure. The addition of barbiturates was not more effective than hyperventilation alone in controlling intracranial pressure.

Lyons MK, Meyer FB. Cerebrospinal fluid physiology and the management of increased intracranial pressure. *Mayo Clin Proc* 1990;65:684–707.

(126 references.)

CHAPTER 40

Neuromuscular Diseases

(See Chapter 59)

Mark A. Kaufman

Patients with abnormalities of the motor neurons, the peripheral motor and sensory nerves, the neuromuscular junction, or the muscle itself, frequently require treatment in the ICU. These illnesses can be categorized as follows:

- Clinical worsening of a known neuromuscular disease.
- Fulminant acute neuromuscular disease.

- Neuromuscular consequences of systemic disease or treatment.

The initial care for any of these conditions requires ensuring an adequate airway and providing oxygenation or ventilation as necessary. In addition, any cardiovascular abnormalities should receive immediate attention.

Patients with Known Neuromuscular Disease

Motor Neuron Disease. These patients have marked weakness with muscle wasting. In addition, there is a striking increase in deep tendon reflexes (DTRs). Bilateral Babinski signs may be present when upper motor neurons are involved. There should be no sensory loss. Problems with bulbar functions, such as articulation, chewing, and swallowing, may be prominent, but extraocular movements are spared until late in the course. Common causes of deterioration of pulmonary status include:

- Progressive loss of motor neurons to muscles of respiration.
- Infection of the respiratory tract or other organ system.
- Fluid and electrolyte imbalance.
- Debilitation caused by poor nutritional status.

Patients with motor neuron disease, particularly amyotrophic lateral sclerosis, are at greatest risk for compromised respiratory function. Many of these patients have advance directives regarding their wishes for intubation and cardiopulmonary resuscitation.

Myasthenia Gravis. This disorder is the most common disease of the neuromuscular junction. It is caused by antibodies to the nicotinic muscle receptor for acetylcholine and is therefore postsynaptic in location. Extraocular movement abnormalities (with normally reactive pupils), along with bulbar and extremity weakness, are present. DTRs are preserved. Weakness has a pattern of worsening throughout the day or with repetitive muscle strength testing. Patients with myasthenia gravis are also at great risk for respiratory demise. A vital capacity of less than 15 mL/kg signals the requirement for endotracheal intubation and mechanical ventilation. Clinical worsening of patients with myasthenia gravis can be caused by:

- Increased severity of neuromuscular blockade (myasthenic crisis).
- Compromised pulmonary function as a result of concomitant respiratory infection.
- Cholinergic excess because of treatment with acetylcholinesterase inhibitors (cholinergic crisis).

- Fluid and electrolyte imbalance, particularly hypocalcemia or hypermagnesemia.
- Infection or condition affecting other organ systems.
- Treatment with medications that affect neuromuscular transmission (e.g., aminoglycosides or penicillamine).

In general, edrophonium chloride testing is not useful in the setting of acute worsening of a patient with myasthenia gravis. Cholinergic crisis is less common than myasthenic crisis, and may be associated with muscarinic receptor-mediated effects, such as sweating, lacrimation, salivation, or GI cramping. The effect of medication is best evaluated by following objective clinical features of the illness, such as muscle strength, eye movement, or vital capacity, while medication is withheld. Electrodiagnostic testing, particularly the finding of a decremental response of the compound muscle action amplitude to repetitive nerve stimulation at low rates of speed (2–5 Hz), is useful for confirming the diagnosis of myasthenia gravis. Elevated levels of serum acetylcholine receptor antibodies provide additional confirmation.

Treatment of myasthenic crisis includes the use of acetylcholinesterase inhibitors (pyridostigmine or neostigmine) in divided doses, and plasmapheresis or plasma exchange. The dosing of acetylcholinesterase inhibitors is determined by disease severity and patient response to treatment. Pyridostigmine 60 mg PO every 2 to 3 hours or neostigmine 15 mg PO every 3 to 4 hours is often required. The necessity of thymectomy and treatment with corticosteroids or azathioprine is determined on an individual basis.

Myopathies. Primary diseases of muscle involving the muscles of respiration or caused by overall severity of weakness necessitate admission to an ICU. In Duchenne muscular dystrophy, for example, respiratory insufficiency can be precipitated by an infection in the respiratory tract or elsewhere in the body. In the absence of infection or other acute illness, progression of the muscle disease itself is responsible.

Polymyositis and dermatomyositis are inflammatory diseases of muscle associated in the early active stages with significant elevation of the muscle enzyme creatine phosphokinase (CPK). Weakness is generally confined to muscles of the extremities, more so proximally than distally. Severe cases restrict patients to bed rest, and involvement of the muscles of the neck and posterior pharynx can make swallowing impossible. Dermatomyositis is associated with malignancy. Both polymyositis and dermatomyositis can respond dramatically to corticosteroids, but high doses may be required (80 to 100 mg prednisone daily), often for long periods.

Fulminant Acute Neuromuscular Disease

Guillain-Barré Syndrome (GBS), also known as acute inflammatory demyelinating polyneuropathy, is the most common condition acutely involving peripheral nerves that requires ICU treatment. Salient features include:

- Antecedent infectious illness, usually respiratory, 1–3 weeks earlier (seen in 40% of cases).
- Progressive muscle weakness, with or without paresthesias, worsening over several days or as long as 4 weeks.
- Diminished or absent DTRs.
- Increase in cerebrospinal fluid protein concentration without elevated numbers of inflammatory cells.

Weakness and sensory symptoms are caused by a loss of myelin from segments of the peripheral nerves. Classically, weakness ascends from the legs to the arms over time. The nerves to the muscles of respiration are frequently involved, necessitating endotracheal intubation and mechanical ventilation. Intubation should be considered before it is emergently required.

Treatment for GBS should be initiated as soon as the diagnosis is made, before the need for intubation, if possible. Plasmapheresis shortens both the mean time of ventilator dependency and the interval for improving one grade on a disability scale. There are reports of clinical worsening 1 to 2 weeks after plasmapheresis. This rebound must be distinguished from chronic inflammatory demyelinating polyneuropathy, which may progress in severity from onset or wax and wane over long periods. It is unclear whether intravenous gammaglobulin is as effective as plasmapheresis in GBS, but it is clear that corticosteroids are not of benefit in this condition.

Involvement of the autonomic nervous system, with persistent tachycardia or fluctuations in blood pressure, worsen the prognosis, as do prominent axonal degeneration and demyelination. Overall, approximately 10% of patients with GBS have a significant amount of disabling weakness after recovery.

Acute Intermittent Porphyria (AIP), a genetic disorder of heme synthesis, carries the potential for neurologic symptoms. There is no cutaneous involvement in AIP. Neurologic involvement occurs in attacks that are typically induced by drugs such as barbiturates, analgesics, sulfonamides, or anticonvulsants. Unlike GBS, AIP is a systemic disorder. Symptoms may include:

- Abdominal pain caused by autonomic neuropathy.
- CNS symptoms, ranging from delirium and psychosis to seizures.
- Progressive peripheral axonal neuropathy, primarily involving the motor nerves.

The diagnosis is confirmed by the laboratory finding of precursors of heme (δ-aminolevulinic acid and porphobilinogen) in urine. The cerebrospinal fluid protein level is not elevated. Treatment includes hematin (e.g., 1–4 mg/kg/day for 3–14 days) to suppress activity in the synthetic pathway for heme, along with anticonvulsants and symptomatic treatment for pain.

Infections. Poliomyelitis and rabies (see Chapter 74 in this book) are infections that have profound neuromuscular effects. Although an effective vaccination program has dramatically reduced the incidence of poliomyelitis, there are still rare cases of disease from this virus or other members of the enterovirus group. Destruction of motor neurons can include prominent bulbar involvement as well as involvement of motor neurons to the respiratory muscles.

Rabies usually occurs as a febrile illness, with headache and drowsiness followed by convulsions, delirium, hypersalivation, and laryngeal spasms. A paralytic variety of rabies is highlighted by initial weakness. Preventing illness with rabies vaccine is important after any suspicious animal bite.

Toxins. Botulism and tetanus are both mediated by toxins caused by infection. Tetanus toxin presynaptically blocks inhibitory spinal synapses to alpha motor neurons. Symptoms include:

- Spasms of the muscles of the face, jaw, and back.
- Generalized seizures.
- Rhabdomyolysis, with possible myoglobinuria and renal failure.
- Autonomic dysfunction.

Treatment of tetanus includes tetanus immune globulin (3,000–6,000 units IM) as well as penicillin or appropriate substitution in cases of penicillin allergy. Anticonvulsant therapy for seizures and even neuromuscular blockade are included when indicated.

Botulism or, more specifically, its toxins, inhibit the presynaptic release of acetylcholine. Symptoms follow the ingestion of contaminated food from one to several days and include, in order:

- Initial nausea and vomiting (not always present).
- Diplopia caused by weakness of the extraocular muscles.
- Visual disturbances caused by dilated, nonreactive pupils, with associated loss of accommodation.
- Weakness of other cranial nerve–innervated muscles.
- Weakness of the limb muscles and the muscles of respiration.
- Systemic autonomic manifestations (e.g., ileus, urinary retention, cardiac rhythm disturbances).

Treatment includes antitoxin (20,000–40,000 units two or

three times daily) for the three common types of toxin. Treatment with guanidine hydrochloride is controversial because of its effects on bone marrow and renal function.

Neuromuscular Consequences of Systemic Disease and Treatment

Patients with disease at any point along the motor unit will become more symptomatic as a result of any other systemic illness. The more impaired the patient initially, the greater the effect of additional illness. Treatments that target part of the pathway from motor neuron to muscle may have dramatic effects on already compromised function. Some general treatment guidelines include:

- Maintenance of fluid and electrolyte balance, particularly avoiding or correcting abnormalities in serum calcium, magnesium, potassium, and phosphorus levels.
- Avoidance of drugs with neuromuscular blocking effects (aminoglycoside, penicillamine) in patients with myasthenia gravis.
- Avoidance of drugs that are toxic to the peripheral nerves in patients with neuropathy.
- Avoidance of barbiturates in patients with porphyria.

An important neurologic problem associated with sepsis and multiple systemic illness is the neuropathy of critical illness. This severe generalized axonal neuropathy is often the cause of severe weakness, including the inability to wean from mechanical ventilatory support. Recovery requires improvement in the precipitating illness.

A fulminant form of acute myopathy has been described in association with the use of nondepolarizing paralytic agents, particularly vecuronium. Prolonged neuromuscular blockade may persist for a week or more after discontinuation of the paralytic agent. Weakness can be as severe as complete paralysis of all limbs. Serum CPK levels are mildly or severely elevated, and histologic examination shows muscle fiber atrophy.

Suggested Readings

McKhann GM, Griggin JW, Cornblath DR, et al. Plasmapheresis and Guillain-Barré syndrome: Analysis of prognostic factors and the effect of plasmapheresis. *Ann Neurol* 1988;23:347–353.

Importance of timing for the initiation of plasmapheresis and its effect on the outcome of Guillain-Barré syndrome are discussed.

Munsat TL, Andres PL, Finison L, et al. The natural history of motoneuron loss in amyotrophic lateral sclerosis. *Neurology* 1988;38:409–413.

Describes rate of disease progression, with emphasis on bulbar, respiratory, and limb muscles.

So YT, Olney RK. AAEM Case report #23: Acute paralytic poliomyelitis. *Muscle Nerve* 1991;14:1159–1164.

Illustrative case and review of neurophysiology of poliomyelitis.

Spitzer AR, Giancarlo T, Maher L, et al. Neuromuscular causes of prolonged ventilator dependency. *Muscle Nerve* 1992;15:682–686.
Reviews 21 patients who could not be weaned from ventilator support, and underlying neuromuscular causes.
Zochodne DW, Bolton CF, Wells GA, et al. Critical illness polyneuropathy: A complication of sepsis and multiple organ failure. *Brain* 1987;110:818–842.
Excellent review of the subject. Early initiation of treatment is essential.

Gastrointestinal Disorders

CHAPTER 41

The Acute Abdomen

(See Chapter 129)

Lonnie W. Frei and Jean M. Ferber

A definition of the acute abdomen is difficult because it represents a diffuse group of diseases that share similarities in signs and symptoms. The hallmark of the clinical entities that make up the acute abdomen is acute abdominal pain. The nature and location of the pain are helpful in the differential diagnosis. The primary mechanisms for pathology in the acute abdomen include infection, inflammation, ischemia, and obstruction. Because the acute abdomen encompasses conditions that are managed both surgically and nonsurgically, differential diagnosis is an important part of management.

Evaluation

The history and physical examination are the starting points in diagnosing the acute abdomen. The onset of pain, its pattern and duration, and its location are all important factors. The presence or absence of nausea, vomiting, abnormal bowel movements, and distension are also pertinent. A history of similar pain is important. The patient's intercurrent diseases may also provide clues about the diagnosis, and may constitute an important piece of information. Age, sex, location of the pain, and other factors identified during the evaluation help to narrow the differential diagnosis. Pain in the right upper quadrant is likely to be biliary, whereas pain in the left lower quadrant is more likely to be diverticulitis, especially in the elderly patient.

The physical examination supplements the history. Pain may be localized more specifically, masses may be detected, or guarding, rebound, or rigidity may be detected. The presence or absence of bowel sounds and the nature of those sounds may help in the diagnosis.

Diagnostic studies aid in differentiating causes and establishing the diagnosis. General laboratory studies include complete and differential blood cell counts, a serum chemistry profile, and urinalysis. Specific laboratory tests are dictated by findings from the history and physical examination. They frequently include serum amylase, lipase, and liver function studies and, in women of childbearing age, a pregnancy test. The basic imaging study is the plain abdominal radiograph. Other potentially useful modalities include abdominal ultrasound and computed tomography (CT).

In a few instances, the diagnosis may still be elusive. In some cases, the diagnosis is established only by more invasive means, such as diagnostic peritoneal lavage, endoscopy, laparoscopy, or laparotomy.

Diagnostic Categories

Peritonitis is often caused by perforation of a hollow viscus or intra-abdominal hemorrhage. Findings include diffuse abdominal pain that may be sudden in onset, but is frequently not well localized. The pain is severe and unremitting. Guarding and rigidity are seen. The white blood cell count is usually elevated, with a marked shift to the left. Radiography may show free-air collections if perforation is present. However, the amount of air may be small, and decubitus films may be necessary to show the collection. An ileus pattern may also be present on the abdominal radiograph. Hemorrhage is not easily diagnosed by plain films; findings of hypotension, tachycardia, and anemia are more helpful. Surgical consultation is necessary for patients with peritonitis caused by perforation or hemorrhage.

Peritonitis can also be caused by inflammatory or infectious processes. In these cases, the signs and symptoms may be similar, with diffuse abdominal pain and leukocytosis. However, other signs may point to the diagnosis. Fever may suggest infectious causes, as may a lack of specific radiologic findings. A common infectious cause of peritonitis in ICU patients is *Clostridium difficile* enterocolitis. Stool should be analyzed for the presence of the associated toxin. When the *Clostridium difficile* enterocolitis is severe, it can produce a fulminant picture of peritonitis, but it is usually treated medically unless a complication, such as megacolon or perforation, occurs.

Inflammatory processes that cause peritonitis may be difficult to differentiate from processes that cause peritonitis and require surgery. The best example is pancreatitis, which is usually a medically treated disease that requires surgery only when complications arise. Sometimes the disease may be so overwhelming that the picture is more of a diffuse peritoneal process and the diagnosis is made only at laparotomy. Usually, the amylase level is elevated. Although this test is nonspecific, it should be included in the laboratory evaluation of the acute abdomen with peritonitis.

Appendicitis is the most common acute disorder of the GI tract causing an acute abdomen. It usually results from obstruction of the appendiceal lumen or perforation of the appendix. The classic picture is periumbilical pain that moves to the right lower quadrant. The pain is typically gradual in onset. Localized guarding or rigidity may occur, and rebound pain may also be present. The patient is anorectic in most cases. The white blood cell (WBC) count is usually elevated, and there may be a low-grade fever. Elderly patients more commonly have perforation and diffuse peritonitis, but may not have the classic symptoms.

The differential diagnosis of acute appendicitis is extensive. It includes gynecologic problems, such as pelvic inflammatory disease, tubo-ovarian abscess, ectopic pregnancy, ovarian cyst, and torsion. Renal calculi and urinary tract infection occasionally masquerade as appendicitis. Crohn's disease may be difficult to differentiate from appendicitis, and sometimes the diagnosis is established at laparotomy. Mesenteric lymphadenitis in young patients may also be indistinguishable on examination from appendicitis. Gastroenteritis is common, and may pose as appendicitis. Studies that are useful for excluding these entities include vaginal examination and culture, pregnancy test, urinalysis, and ultrasound of the pelvis and abdomen.

Diverticulitis is another common cause of acute abdomen. It can develop while the patient is in the ICU for other reasons. It may be caused by the inactivity of the colon secondary to lack of feeding or the use of agents that retard bowel motility. It also may occur simply because this disease is common among the elderly and they constitute a large proportion of the patients in most adult ICUs. The pain is usually gradual in onset, and is localized to the segment of colon involved, most commonly the sigmoid colon. A mass is often palpable. It may represent the phlegmon of the involved segment or, in more complicated cases, an abscess. The WBC count is elevated. Plain films of the abdomen are often not helpful. Contrast studies of the colon should be performed with caution because they may lead to perforation or leakage of contrast material into the peritoneal cavity, with potentially lethal consequences. Uncomplicated diverticulitis may be treated with antibiotics and bowel rest. Complications such as perforation or abscess formation require surgical intervention. The complication of hemorrhage from diverticulitis occurs as lower GI bleeding rather than as acute abdomen.

Intestinal obstruction is a relatively common cause of acute abdomen. The clinical picture varies depending on the level of the obstruction. Low obstructions usually are associated with a gradual onset and abdominal distension. High obstruction is associated with nausea and vomiting, but distension is not common. Adhesions from previous surgery, hernia, tumor, or an inflammatory process are the usual causes. The patient describes obstipation or constipation. The clinical history and the radiographic picture of distended or dilated loops of bowel usually confirm the diagnosis. Surgery may be necessary to relieve the obstruction, but it should take place after resuscitation. These patients are frequently hypovolemic and metabolically deranged. Decompression of the GI tract with nasogastric suction is also part of the management.

Cholecystitis and other biliary tract problems usually cause colicky right upper quadrant pain. The diagnosis is often established by finding stones, pericholecystic fluid collections, wall thickening, and sludge on ultrasound imaging. Acalculous cholecystitis is increasingly seen in the ICU setting, and can be difficult to diagnose. The diagnosis is often one of exclusion in the critically ill patient who continues to deteriorate or does not improve and who seems to have an abdominal source for the problem. Cholecystectomy is the treatment of choice. However, in the critically ill patient who is too sick to withstand general anesthesia, cholecystostomy or percutaneous drainage of the gallbladder may be feasible.

Peptic ulcer disease of the stomach and duodenum occurs with high frequency both before and after admission to the ICU. The use of H_2-receptor blocking agents for the control of gastric acid production has decreased the incidence of bleeding complications. The complication of ulcer disease that is most likely to produce acute abdomen is perforation. The pain is sudden in onset, and is localized to the epigastrium if the perforation is contained. If not contained, a perforated ulcer may lead to generalized peritonitis. Free air is usually seen on plain films of the abdomen; however, perforations into the lesser sac may not show free air. Both ulcer disease and cholecystitis must be differentiated from pancreatitis.

Pancreatitis can be caused by biliary tract disease, infection, ischemia, or drugs (most commonly, alcohol). In addition to stones, biliary sludge can lead to pancreatitis. Serum amylase and lipase levels are usually elevated, sometimes to extreme levels. Ultrasound or CT is useful in evaluating the pancreas and biliary system, and can be used to follow the course of the disease. Pancreatitis may follow a benign course or may cause life-threatening complications, including pancreatic abscess, hemorrhagic pancreatitis, pseudocyst formation, or intercurrent respiratory failure caused by adult respiratory distress syndrome. The criteria developed by Ranson may be used to evaluate the severity of the disease (see Chapter 42 in this book). The presence of three or more criteria indicates severe disease, with an increased likelihood of complications. The management of pancreatitis is supportive, consisting of bowel rest and fluid and electrolyte support. If complications develop, ventilatory support, antibiotics, nutritional support, and possibly surgery may be necessary.

Gynecologic disorders may cause acute abdomen; they are not commonly seen in the ICU setting. On occasion, patients with severe infectious complications from pelvic inflammatory disease or a tubo-ovarian abscess may require treatment in the ICU. The pain associated with these conditions is usually lower abdominal or pelvic in location. Performing a pelvic examination is crucial in the diagnosis of gynecologic tract disease. The patients at risk are usually young, frequently in their childbearing years. The most useful laboratory tests are a pregnancy test, cervical culture, and routine studies, such as the complete blood cell (CBC) count. Ultrasound is usually the preferred imaging modality, although CT may be used. The treatment varies with the abnormality, and may be medical or surgical.

Abdominal vascular disorders, such as ruptured abdominal aneurysm and mesenteric ischemia, produce severe abdominal pain that may be sudden in onset. With aneurysm rupture, the pain is frequently centered in the back and is usually associated with signs of hemodynamic instability. Mesenteric ischemia is classically described as severe pain associated with minimal findings on physical examination, or pain out of proportion to the physical findings. Mesenteric ischemia is often associated with bloody stools. Plain abdominal radiographs may be nonspecific or may show the calcific rim of an aneurysm or the thumbprinting of mesenteric ischemia. Mesenteric ischemia is more likely to develop in patients who are already in the ICU, especially patients with atrial fibrillation, recent myocardial infarction, a hypercoagulable state, or recent cardiopulmonary bypass or aneurysm surgery. Patients who have low-flow hemodynamics may also have mesenteric ischemia, especially if they have evidence of vascular occlusive disease elsewhere. Both of these entities are surgical emergencies. They are associated with a high mortality rate. This rate may be slightly improved with early diagnosis and treatment.

Other Considerations

Although the causes of acute abdomen described above do not constitute all possibilities, they account for most cases. Nevertheless, there remain some important caveats and considerations regarding acute abdomen that are especially pertinent to patients in the ICU setting. The first is that not all of the causes of acute abdomen are intra-abdominal entities. Pneumonia in the lower lobe can produce acute abdominal pain that may be confused with biliary tract disease. Pulmonary embolism with infarction may cause a similar type of pain. Acute myocardial infarction may cause pain that simulates gastritis or acute cholecystitis. A thorough history and physical examination and inclusion of an ECG and chest radiograph in the evaluation may help to exclude some of these possibilities.

Special consideration must be given to certain patient populations seen in the ICU or hospital setting. Patients with leukemia and lymphoma may have acute abdomen secondary to infiltration of the bowel by tumor cells or secondary to chemotherapy-induced neutropenia. Splenic rupture may also occur in this patient population, and may occur as an abdominal catastrophe.

Patients with acquired immune deficiency syndrome (AIDS) may have abdominal pain that may be surgically or medically treated. The pain may be mild or severe, localized or generalized, and is often associated with abnormal physical findings, such as rebound tenderness, guarding, or rigidity. There may be associated findings such as diarrhea or nausea. The possible causes of acute abdominal pain in patients with AIDS include enterocolitis resulting from opportunistic organisms or lymphoma. Cytomegalovirus enterocolitis may resemble ulcerative colitis, with colonic distension that leads to ischemia and perforation. In these patients, the diagnosis may be aided by radiographic studies, including plain films and CT scans. Patients with AIDS may have acute abdomen from common causes as well.

Numerous drugs and toxins may cause acute abdomen, such as mercury, arsenic, and iron, in addition to acid or alkali ingestion. The disorder produced may include intestinal ischemia, hepatic necrosis, pancreatitis, and antibiotic-associated colitis.

The acute abdomen poses one of the most challenging diagnostic problems in clinical medicine. Accurate diagnosis is crucial to proper treatment, and it relies on a knowledge of the diversity of problems that may produce abnormalities within and adjacent to the peritoneal cavity.

Suggested Readings

Gottlieb JE, Menashe PI, Cruz E. Gastrointestinal complications in critically ill patients: The intensivist's overview. *Am J Gastroenterol* 1986;81:227–238.

Reviews GI disorders in the critically ill whose initial problem involved another organ system. Focuses on stress ulcers, acute hepatic dysfunction, and intestinal ischemia (93 references).

Kiernan GJ, Cales RH, eds. Acute abdominal disorders. *Emerg Med Clin North Am* 1989;7:437–747.

This issue is devoted to various topics on the acute abdomen. It includes monographs on evaluation of abdominal pain, AIDS and the acute abdomen, appendicitis, toxicologic causes, ascites, and abdominal catastrophes.

Sawyers JL, Williams LF, eds. The acute abdomen. Surg Clin North Am 1988;68:233–476.

Issue contains 15 review articles on specific aspects of the acute abdomen, including peritonitis; urologic, gynecologic, and vascular causes; imaging studies; early postoperative period; and immunocompromised host.

Silen W, ed. *Cope's early diagnosis of the acute abdomen,* 18th ed. New York: Oxford University Press, 1991.

Classic text on the acute abdomen.

Wilson SE, Robinson G, Williams RA, et al. Acquired immune deficiency syndrome (AIDS): Indications for abdominal surgery, pathology and outcome. *Ann Surg* 1989;210:428–433.

Report of 36 abdominal operations on 35 patients with AIDS. The operative findings were related to AIDS in 94%, with cytomegalovirus and mycobacterial infections being the most common infectious processes and non-Hodgkin's lymphoma being the most common malignancy.

CHAPTER 42

Acute Pancreatitis

(See Chapter 132)

Lonnie W. Frei

Pancreatitis is seen in the ICU setting as both a primary problem for admission and a secondary problem that develops during the course of hospitalization. Its diagnosis and subsequent treatment depend on the course of the disease, which may proceed in several ways. This chapter reviews the disease and its course and provides a brief guide to its management and treatment.

Etiology

Major causes of pancreatitis include:

- Alcohol abuse.
- Biliary tract disease.
- Trauma.
- Ischemia.
- Drugs.
- Infections.
- Hyperlipidemia.
- Idiopathic causes.

Pancreatitis can also occur in the postsurgical patient (e.g., after coronary bypass or aneurysm surgery). In most cases, the cause is clear. In the United States, approximately two-thirds of cases are caused by either alcohol or concomitant biliary tract disease. Alcohol is directly toxic to the pancreas, and it produces marked inflammatory changes in the gland. Most patients with biliary pancreatitis have cholelithiasis. However, a form of pancreatitis is seen with increasing frequency in the hospitalized patient whose gallbladder is not stimulated and who accumulates sludge in the gallbladder, subsequently developing pancreatitis.

The patient who is admitted with a diagnosis of pancreatitis is most likely to have biliary or alcohol-associated pancreatitis. The patient who has the disease during hospitalization will most likely have disease secondary to biliary problems caused by drugs, ischemia, infection, or idiopathic causes.

Diagnosis

The diagnosis of pancreatitis should be suspected in any patient with upper abdominal pain. The pain is usually centered in the midepigastrium, radiates to the back, and is severe and unremitting. The pain may be so severe that it appears to be diffuse peritonitis with involvement of the entire abdomen. There is usually abdominal guarding, and there may be rigidity. Ileus may be present, so bowel sounds can be absent or decreased. Associated jaundice can occur if the etiology of the pancreatitis is secondary to biliary tract disease.

The differential diagnosis of pancreatitis includes cholecystitis, hepatitis, and peptic ulcer disease. The leading possibilities may all be associated with the development of pancreatitis, and thus not only may have to be differentiated from pancreatitis but also may need treatment. If abdominal pain is diffuse, the differential diagnosis of peritonitis is pertinent.

The main diagnostic test for pancreatitis is the serum amylase level. This test is sensitive, but is nonspecific, and amylase levels are elevated in most cases of acute pancreatitis. The absolute level of hyperamylasemia is not predictive of the course of the disease; however, amylase levels may be elevated in other abdominal abnormalities, such as perforated viscus or ovarian disease. Salivary amylase is differentiated by means of isoenzyme analysis. An elevated serum lipase level adds specificity to the amylase level.

Other diagnostic studies include liver function studies and routine blood tests, including a CBC count and a serum chemistry profile. Radiologic studies include plain films of the abdomen, which may show sentinel loop in the right upper quadrant or an ileus pattern. These findings are nonspecific, however, and do not confirm the diagnosis. Calcifications in the region of the pancreas are seen in chronic pancreatitis, but this condition is different from acute pancreatitis. Computed tomography (CT) scanning of the abdomen may be used to confirm the disease and to evaluate the patient for complications such as infection, abscess, or pseudocyst. Ultrasonography is also a useful modality in acute pancreatitis, and it is useful for following the course of known disease.

Occasionally, the diagnosis is established only by more invasive means, such as surgical exploration. The need for surgery arises when the disease occurs as acute abdomen with diffuse abdominal findings. Endoscopic retrograde cholangiopancreatography (ERCP) may also be used in the diagnosis of pancreatitis, but care must be exercised because it may lead to pancreatitis or may exacerbate the episode. In most cases, however, standard noninvasive diagnostic studies confirm the diagnosis.

Acute versus Chronic Pancreatitis

Most cases of pancreatitis seen in the hospital are acute pancreatitis. This disease is reversible and self-limited in its course. On resolution, it leaves no sequelae of pancreatic dysfunction. Chronic pancreatitis is an irreversible disease that occurs as a chronic pain syndrome associated with evidence of pancreatic exocrine insufficiency and, occasionally, pancreatic endocrine insufficiency (i.e., diabetes mellitus). In chronic pancreatitis, serum amylase levels are minimally elevated, if at all. Abdominal radiography shows pancreatic calcifications, one of the signs of the irreversibility of the disease. The predominant findings are those associated with pancreatic insufficiency, e.g., fat malabsorption, with diarrhea and bulky stool. Diabetes associated with chronic pancreatitis may be brittle and difficult to control.

Prognosis

Once acute pancreatitis develops, its course can be variable. It may run a brief, benign course, or it may become fulminant and unremitting, ending in the death of the patient. Criteria have been established to help in assessing the severity and course of the disease. The best-known and probably most widely applied is Ranson's criteria. These 11 criteria consider factors at admission and 48 hours afterward. The admission criteria are:

- Patient age > 55 years.
- WBC count > 16,000 mm^{-3}.
- Serum glucose level > 200 mg/dL.
- Serum glutamic-oxaloacetic transaminase level more than six times the upper normal limit.
- Serum lactate dehydrogenase level more than twice the upper normal limit.

The 48-hour criteria are:

- Estimated fluid sequestration > 6 L.
- Decrease in hematocrit > 10%.
- Increase in serum urea nitrogen level > 5 mg/dL.
- Total serum calcium concentration < 8 mg/dL.
- Base deficit > 4 mEq/L.
- Arterial oxygen tension (Pa_{O_2}) < 60 torr.

Severe disease is present when three or more criteria are met. Additionally, the risk of complication from pancreatitis increases as the number of criteria increases.

A newer way to assess the course of the disease uses the APACHE II scoring system (see Chapter 6 in this book). APACHE scores of less than 10 are associated with a favorable outcome, whereas scores of greater than 20 are associated with severe disease that is likely to have a fatal outcome.

Management

The management of acute pancreatitis depends on the course of the disease. However, certain elements of management are standard no matter what the extent of disease, e.g., the provision of IV fluids for resuscitation and maintenance. Patients with pancreatitis often sequester large amounts of fluid in the soft tissues of the retroperitoneum and also freely in the peritoneal cavity. They may also have diffuse capillary leaks that lead to edema formation and further intravascular dehydration.

The patient with pancreatitis should not be permitted to eat to allow the GI tract to rest and to prevent further stimulation of the pancreas. Parenteral nutrition may be necessary during this time. The patient with pancreatitis should have nothing by mouth, but there is no confirmed role for nasogastric suction. Likewise, there is no confirmed role for antibiotics in acute pancreatitis; rather, the use of antibiotics may lead to colonization with resistant organisms or the development of other problems, such as antibiotic-associated colitis.

Other treatment modalities depend on individual differences in the disease. For example, if a patient has adult respiratory distress syndrome secondary to the disease, then ventilatory support must be provided. In biliary pancreatitis, the treatment usually includes cholecystectomy once the disease has subsided, or ERCP-guided extraction of obstructing stones and biliary drainage when the disease persists or worsens.

The role of surgery in the management of acute pancreatitis is usually supportive because the disease is primarily medically treated. Surgery becomes necessary when the cause is biliary tract disease, when the diagnosis is unclear in the setting of diffuse peritonitis, and when complications such as abscess, hemorrhage, or pseudocyst occur.

Pancreatitis-associated abscesses occur in patients with severe disease. These patients display a septic picture with spiking fevers, elevated white blood cell count and, occasionally, positive blood culture findings. The diagnosis is supported by CT scanning that shows collections of multiple small air bubbles in or around the pancreas. Although CT-guided drainage may be attempted, it is not likely to be successful, and these abscesses are best managed by surgical debridement. Often these abscesses require multiple surgical procedures to fully drain and debride the area.

Hemorrhagic pancreatitis is often a lethal disease, even when treated surgically. Because the pancreatic bed sits in an area rich in blood supply, not only to the pancreas but also to surrounding tissues and organs, it is not surprising that hemorrhage may complicate this disease. Surgical exploration with ligation of bleeding points may offer the only hope for patients with this form of the disease.

Pancreatic pseudocysts herald their development by persistent elevations of serum amylase levels. They may occur anywhere in the pancreas. Their treatment depends on the course they follow, which may vary from complete resolution to persistence or spontaneous rupture. They may also erode into surrounding structures or become infected. They are easily followed with ultrasound. The treatment options for patients with pseudocysts include drainage (internal or external, surgical or nonsurgical) and resection. Approximately one-third of all pseudocysts spontaneously resolve.

Suggested Readings

Fan ST, Lai EC, Mok FP, et al. Early treatment of acute biliary pancreatitis by endoscopic papillotomy. *N Engl J Med* 1993;328:228–232.

From this study of 195 patients, the authors conclude that emergency endoscopic retrograde cholangiopancreatography is indicated in treatment of patients with acute biliary pancreatitis.

Lee SP, Nicholls JF, Park HZ. Biliary sludge as a cause of acute pancreatitis. *N Engl J Med* 1992;326:589–593.

Study and discussion of biliary sludge as a cause of pancreatitis separate from biliary stone disease.

Ranson JH, Rifkind KM, Turner JW. Prognostic signs and nonoperative peritoneal lavage in acute pancreatitis. *Surg Gynecol Obstet* 1976; 143:209–219.

Original report on development of the now-classic criteria used to assess severity of acute pancreatitis.

Wilson C, Heath DI, Imrie CW. Prediction of outcome in acute pancreatitis: A comparative study of APACHE II, clinical assessment, and multiple-factor scoring systems. *Br J Surg* 1990;77;1260–1264.

Offers an alternative means for evaluating severity and possible outcome of pancreatitis.

CHAPTER 43

Acute Mesenteric Ischemia

(See Chapter 130)

Kara H. V. Kvilekval and
Slobodan Jazarevic

Acute mesenteric ischemia (AMI) is a catastrophic event that may occur at any age; however, it most commonly occurs in the elderly. The mortality rate remains at 60% to 90%, and has not significantly changed since a mortality rate of 70% was reported in 1933. This lack of improvement in survival despite improved surgical techniques may be attributed to:

- Delay in diagnosis until after intestinal gangrene has begun.
- Progression of bowel infarction even after the initiating event has resolved.
- Vasospasm.
- Poor state of health of patients with AMI.
- Propensity to multiple organ system failure.

Etiology

The mechanism of injury is mechanical occlusion or functional limitation resulting in restriction of blood flow, secondary to arterial or venous occlusive disease or vasospasm.

Arterial Occlusion. An embolus to the superior mesenteric artery (SMA) is the most common cause of AMI (approximately 50%). Ninety percent of SMA emboli are from a cardiac (left atrial) source and are associated with atrial dysrhythmias, the presence of atrial or ventricular thrombi, or atrial myxoma. Macroemboli usually lodge at the bifurcation of the SMA, distal to the middle colic artery, and result in ischemia of the distal jejunum, entire ileum, and ascending colon, with sparing of the proximal jejunum and distal colon. Another source of emboli is an atheromatous aorta that may shower microemboli, resulting in patchy, segmental infarcts.

Thrombosis of the SMA is less common, and patients often have a history of symptoms of chronic intestinal ischemia, such as postprandial pain or weight loss. Thrombosis generally occurs at the origin of the SMA, at the site of preexisting arterial occlusive disease. The entire small bowel and ascending colon are involved.

Other etiologies include blunt and penetrating trauma, vasculitides, and iatrogenic causes.

Venous Occlusion. Approximately 20% of cases of AMI are secondary to venous occlusion. The cause may be a hypercoagulable state, such as pregnancy, oral contraceptive use, polycythemia vera, protein C or S deficiency, or antithrombin III deficiency. Other conditions associated with mesenteric venous thrombosis are sickle cell anemia, splenectomy, migratory thrombophlebitis, inflammatory bowel disease, portal hypertension, intra-abdominal infections, and carcinomatosis.

Nonocclusive Ischemia. In this situation, the functional reduction of oxygen delivery below critical levels leads to subsequent tissue ischemia. Etiologies include circulatory shock, low-flow states, drug-induced vasoconstriction, and arterial–venous fistula. Predisposing factors include atherosclerotic disease, diabetes mellitus, and vasculitis. There can be asymptomatic flow limitations that become critical in the face of hypotension.

Diagnosis

AMI envelops a broad spectrum of syndromes, ranging from reversible ischemic changes to complete necrosis of the bowel wall. The injury, initially mucosal, may extend to involve the full thickness of the bowel wall. AMI must be differentiated from other intra-abdominal processes, such as strangulated or perforated viscus, pancreatitis, or ischemic colitis.

Clinical Findings. AMI usually occurs in a sick, elderly patient (older than age 50) with underlying cardiac disease. It is characterized by a paucity of symptoms and a lack of specific laboratory findings. Potential signs and symptoms include:

- Severe abdominal pain out of proportion to the physical findings.
- Unexplained abdominal distension or GI bleeding.
- Gut emptying, i.e., vomiting or defecation.
- Abdominal tenderness.
- Peritoneal signs.
- Nonspecific findings, such as tachycardia, mental confusion, and tachypnea.

Patients with embolic occlusion tend to have acute, unremitting, poorly localized pain that becomes more localized over time. In contrast, patients with mesenteric venous occlusion tend to have a more insidious onset that may develop over a period of days to weeks. Those with nonocclusive mesenteric ischemia also tend to have a longer prodromal phase, which occurs over several days to a week. On the other hand, any of these patient groups may have no pain at all.

Laboratory Findings. Leukocytosis greater than 15,000 mm^{-3} and metabolic acidosis are the most consistent laboratory abnormalities. They occur in 75% and 50% of cases, respectively. Another possible abnormality is elevated serum and peritoneal amylase level. Hematocrit and blood urea nitrogen levels may be elevated secondary to hemoconcentration.

Diagnostic Studies

- **Abdominal radiography** is important to exclude other causes of abdominal pain. Thumbprinting and portal venous gas are late and ominous signs of AMI.
- **Angiography** is the criterion standard diagnostic test. A selective mesenteric angiogram must be performed to establish the diagnosis. In addition, it will differentiate embolus from thrombosis, arterial from venous involvement, and occlusive from nonocclusive disease. It may also be used therapeutically for selective infusion of vasodilator agents.
- **Computed tomography** (CT) may be useful to detect air in the bowel wall and thrombosis in the portal and superior mesenteric vein.
- **Duplex Doppler ultrasound** scanning has limited use because of the usually associated ileus. However, its use may allow visualization of arterial and venous thrombosis.
- **Magnetic resonance imaging** (MRI) may have a role, but it remains to be defined.

Management

General. Patients with AMI frequently have associated cardiac and metabolic disease. In addition, with significant third spacing into the bowel, they may be profoundly hypovolemic. Initial management should be directed at limiting the extent of intestinal injury and systemic sequelae. Treatment includes:

- Correction of the underlying or precipitating cause, e.g., cardiac dysrhythmia, congestive heart failure, or circulatory shock.
- Fluid resuscitation, which may require the use of invasive hemodynamic monitoring to assist with maintaining adequate cardiac output.
- Correction of electrolyte abnormalities.
- Broad-spectrum antibiotic coverage.
- Avoidance of mesenteric vasoconstrictors, such as digitalis and norepinephrine.
- Decompression of the GI tract with nasogastric aspiration.

Emergency selective splanchnic angiography is performed as soon as initial stabilization is completed and the patient is hemodynamically stable.

Arterial Embolic Occlusion. Preoperatively, the diagnosis is established by angiography. Operative intervention includes embolectomy with revascularization and subsequent bowel resection as necessary, unless the emboli are very distant. In this case, resection alone is performed. Operative assessment of bowel viability is accomplished by inspection of bowel color, palpation of mesenteric pulses, and observation of peristalsis and bleeding. Other aids to determine bowel viability intraoperatively include the use of fluorescein dye, surface oximetry, and Doppler ultrasonography. A second-look operation (within 24 hours) should be planned if areas of questionable viability are found. Postoperatively, the patient should be heparinized after 48 hours. Long-term anticoagulation with warfarin should be planned if the source of the embolus is cardiac because recurrent embolization can occur in as many as 15% of these patients.

Arterial Thrombotic Occlusion. Preoperative angiography establishes the diagnosis. The treatment is revascularization, with saphenous vein bypass grafting. Bowel viability is assessed as described above, and resection performed as needed. Because of anorexia and weight loss, the nutritional state of the patient is usually poor. These patients tend to have a poor long-term prognosis, even if they survive the perioperative period, as a result of their significant underlying atherosclerotic and coronary vascular disease.

Venous Occlusion. Initial treatment involves aggressive resuscitation and anticoagulation to prevent thrombosis extension. For patients who do not display any peritoneal signs, nonoperative intervention may be adequate. However, early surgical intervention is important when there are signs of transmural infarction and peritoneal irritation. Operative intervention consists of wide resection of infarcted bowel. A low threshold for performing a second-look operation is advisable. Long-term anticoagulation is necessary, and assessment for a hypercoagulable state should be performed. If treatment is initiated early, the prognosis is good.

Nonocclusive mesenteric ischemia usually occurs in the presence of a generalized illness resulting in a low-flow state and splanchnic vasoconstriction. Treatment is essentially nonoperative, and is aimed at restoring mesenteric flow to the appropriate levels. This goal requires aggressive optimization of fluids and cardiac output. Additionally, selective superior mesenteric artery infusion of papaverine may be beneficial. Operative intervention is required in the face of peritoneal signs. Papaverine infusion may be continued throughout the perioperative period.

Suggested Readings

Benjamin E, Oropello JM, Iberti TJ. Acute mesenteric ischemia: Pathophysiology, diagnosis and treatment. *Dis Mon* 1993;39:131^210.
Comprehensive review (293 references).

Boley SJ, Kaleya RN, Brandt LJ. Mesenteric venous thrombosis. *Surg Clin North Am* 1992;72:183^201.
Discusses diagnosis, clinical features, and treatment of this uncommon cause of intestinal ischemia.

Fisher DF Jr, Fry WJ. Collateral mesenteric circulation. *Surg Gynecol Obstet* 1987;164:487–492.
Reviews basic and pathologic anatomy of the mesenteric arterial system.

Kaleya RN, Sammartano RJ, Boley SJ. Aggressive approach to acute mesenteric ischemia. *Surg Clin North Am* 1992;72:157–182.
Clear and concise review that includes algorithms for the diagnosis and management of acute mesenteric ischemia.

Taylor LM, ed. Mesenteric ischemia. *Semin Vasc Surg* 1990;3:141–175.

Williams LF Jr. Mesenteric ischemia. *Surg Clin North Am* 1988;68:331–353.
Good review of pathogenesis, useful diagnostic tests, and therapy (64 references).

CHAPTER 44

Spontaneous Bacterial Peritonitis

(See Chapters 42 and 133)

Peter F. Ells

Spontaneous bacterial peritonitis (SBP) is bacterial infection of pre-existing ascitic fluid in the absence of any other intra-abdominal source of infection. Clinically, this syndrome differs from other forms of bacterial peritonitis. Abdominal findings and symptoms are much more subtle; peritoneal signs are almost always absent. In fact, their presence should raise the suspicion of other causes of peritonitis. Most patients (60%) have either fever or abdominal pain. Consideration of the setting for the condition is crucial. SBP can complicate ascites caused by any condition, but it is much more common when the ascitic fluid protein level is low. Thus, it is much more likely to occur in cirrhotic or nephrotic ascites than in ascites secondary to malignancy or heart failure. Given the relatively high prevalence of cirrhosis, the typical patient has cirrhosis with ascites. The only clue might be unexplained hepatic encephalopathy, hypotension, or hypothermia. Typically,

12% of patients undergoing paracentesis on admission have SBP.

Diagnosis

Because the diagnosis requires examination of the ascitic fluid, paracentesis must be performed whenever the clinical situation suggests the diagnosis. Because many of these patients have cirrhosis with prolonged prothrombin times and low platelet counts, the issue of the safety of performing paracentesis is often raised. Diagnostic paracentesis is unlikely to cause significant hemorrhage, even in the face of coagulopathy and thrombocytopenia. A small-gauge needle should be used, and care should be taken to avoid abdominal scars, which may harbor large portal–systemic collateral vessels. When SBP is suspected, ascitic fluid should be obtained for examination as soon as possible. In general, the procedure need not be delayed by attempts to correct coagulopathy or thrombocytopenia.

Laboratory Analysis. A number of diagnostic laboratory tests can be performed on ascitic fluid. Although some assume that the most crucial finding is the culture result, the ascitic fluid polymorphonuclear (PMN) cell count is of central importance.

- **Absolute PMN cell count** $> 250\ mm^{-3}$ in ascitic fluid is generally sufficient to make the diagnosis. This finding may be the most useful predictor of the need for treatment. Patients with low PMN cell counts who have a positive culture finding (bacterascites) do not usually benefit from therapy. In contrast, those who have a negative culture result despite an elevated PMN cell count seem to benefit from therapy. The latter situation has been called *culture-negative* neutrocytic ascites.
- **Gram stain and culture** of peritoneal fluid is essential. Identification of the responsible organism allows the most appropriate antibiotic to be used, and occasionally suggests a secondary etiology. Current recommendations suggest that bedside inoculation of 10 mL of fluid into each of two blood culture bottles maximizes the culture yield.
- **Chemistry assays,** including peritoneal fluid protein, albumin, amylase, lactate dehydrogenase (LDH), glucose, lactate, and pH, have been variously recommended. In SBP, ascitic fluid protein concentrations are usually < 1 g/dL, glucose concentrations roughly parallel those of serum, and the LDH level is generally not higher than the normal level for serum. In contrast, peritonitis caused by bowel perforation is usually associated with protein levels > 1 g/dL, glucose concentrations < 50 mg/dL, and LDH levels that exceed the normal limit for serum.

Treatment

The choice of antibiotic is reasonably straightforward given the range of organisms isolated. The major causes are enteric bacilli, such as *Escherichia coli* and *Klebsiella pneumoniae. Streptococcus* species are also relatively common. Anaerobic organisms are uncommon. Because many of these patients have cirrhosis and are likely to have complicating renal failure, aminoglycosides are best avoided. Third-generation cephalosporins, such as cefotaxime, cover most causative organisms and are currently recommended as first-line therapy. Repeat paracentesis should be performed after 48 hours of therapy to document a favorable response. The PMN cell count should be 50% or less of the pretreatment level. A lack of clinical response or appropriate decrease in PMN cell count suggests peritoneal inflammation secondary to an underlying intra-abdominal cause, i.e., secondary bacterial peritonitis. Other findings that suggest a secondary etiology include isolation of more than one organism and isolation of an anaerobic organism. In general, therapy should be continued for at least 5 days, but should be guided by the results of repeated paracenteses. Therapy may be stopped when the PMN cell count is less than 250 mm^{-3}.

Although prompt recognition and treatment of SBP improves the survival rate significantly, the occurrence of SBP in a patient with cirrhosis and ascites is a poor prognostic sign. It may indicate the need to consider definitive therapy, such as hepatic transplantation.

Suggested Readings

Fong T-L, Akriviadis EA, Runyon BA, et al. Polymorphonuclear cell count response and duration of antibiotic therapy in spontaneous bacterial peritonitis. *Hepatology* 1989;9:423–426.

Compares duration of therapy based on clinical response with use of a polymorphonuclear cell count of less than 250 mm^{-3} as an endpoint for antibiotic therapy. Using the polymorphonuclear cell endpoint method allowed shorter duration of therapy without increase in mortality rate or recurrent infection rate.

Hoefs JC. Spontaneous bacterial peritonitis: Prevention and therapy. *Hepatology* 1990;12:776–781.

Good review of pathogenetic concepts. Addresses use of prophylactic antibiotics to prevent recurrent infection. Counsels further study of costs and benefits before widespread use of this modality is adopted.

Pelletier G, Lesur G, Ink O, et al. Asymptomatic bacterascites: Is it spontaneous bacterial peritonitis? *Hepatology* 1991;14:112–115.

Compares the features and outcome of cirrhotic patients with asymptomatic bacterascites with those with spontaneous bacterial peritonitis. Peritonitis rarely develops in patients with asymptomatic bacterascites, and antibiotic therapy is not required for most of these patients.

Runyon BA. Spontaneous bacterial peritonitis: An explosion of information. *Hepatology* 1988;8:171–175.

Good review of pathogenesis that also emphasizes safety of paracentesis in patients with coagulopathy. Describes appropriate culture techniques in detail.

Toledo C, Salmerón J-M, Rimola A, et al. Spontaneous bacterial peritonitis in cirrhosis: Predictive factors of infection resolution and survival in patients treated with cefotaxime. *Hepatology* 1993;17:251–257. *Cefotaxime was effective in resolving infection in 77% of cases. In many of the remaining 23%, efficacy could not be ascertained because of early deaths caused by GI hemorrhage or terminal liver failure.*

CHAPTER 45

Upper Gastrointestinal Tract Hemorrhage

(See Chapters 124 and 125)

Brian E. Pinard

Upper gastrointestinal tract (UGI) hemorrhage is defined as bleeding originating proximal to the duodenojejunal flexure. More than 250,000 people are hospitalized annually in the United States with this diagnosis. Upper and lower GI tract bleeding together account for 2% of all medical and surgical admissions in the United States. Surgery is required in approximately 15% of patients with UGI hemorrhage. However, treatment outcome is better than is statistically evident. Because of improved medical care and longevity, there is a larger pool of older patients. In these patients, bleeding is more likely and the prognosis is more adversely affected.

Factors Indicating Severity

The rate of bleeding determines the likely presenting signs and symptoms as well as the outcome. Factors affecting survival include:

- **Severity of bleeding** as judged by the number of units of packed red blood cells transfused.
- **Episode of rebleeding,** which is indicative of poor prognosis.
- **Advanced age,** which results in a survival rate in patients older than 60 years approximately 30% lower than that in younger patients.
- **Vital organ system disease,** such as underlying congestive heart failure; dysrhythmias; or pulmonary, hepatic, or renal dysfunction. All are associated with increased risk of death.
- **Bright red blood** evident from the rectum or nasogas-

tric tube, which is associated with a nearly fourfold increase in mortality rate.

Other factors associated with worse outcome include a bleeding vessel visible by endoscopy, intracranial hemorrhage, and delay in therapy. Nearly one in three patients who bleed while in the hospital do not survive. Hemorrhage from esophageal varices carries a high mortality rate; it is the second most common cause of death among patients with cirrhosis.

General Principles of Management

A general management plan for the acutely bleeding patient is described below.

- **Pertinent history** is obtained, including any previous bleeding episodes, prescribed and nonprescribed drugs, and a review of systems to determine significant underlying organ system disease.
- **Directed physical examination** is performed to identify signs of hypovolemia (e.g., tachycardia, orthostatic hypotension), signs of poor peripheral circulation, stigmata of liver disease, etc.
- **Routine laboratory tests** are done, including prothrombin time, partial thromboplastin time, liver function tests, and a complete blood count with platelet count.
- **Nasogastric intubation** should be performed to evaluate the gastric aspirate, prevent aspiration, monitor ongoing bleeding, and evacuate enzyme-activating clot. An Ewald tube may be necessary to effectively evacuate clots for later esophagogastroduodenoscopy.
- **Airway protection** with endotracheal intubation may be necessary in patients who are at significant risk for aspiration (e.g., those with an altered sensorium) and those in whom esophageal balloon tamponade is anticipated.
- **Volume resuscitation** should be aggressive. Isotonic fluids are infused to replace intravascular volume, packed red blood cells are transfused to correct anemia, fresh-frozen plasma is transfused to correct coagulopathy, and platelets are transfused to maintain the platelet count $> 50{,}000\ mm^{-3}$.
- **Close monitoring** of vital signs, serial hemoglobin or hematocrit assays, blood gases, and physiologic parameters is performed in a critical care setting. At least one large-bore venous access site is required. Central venous or pulmonary artery catheterization may be indicated to monitor intravascular pressures. Urinary bladder catheterization is performed to monitor urine output.
- **Antacid treatment** or use of H_2-receptor antagonists or sucralfate is used for therapy and prophylaxis.
- **Surgical consultation** should be obtained immediately.

- **Esophagogastroduodenoscopy** should be considered early, along with measurement of intra-esophageal venous pressure. Repeat upper endoscopy may be performed if the first attempt is nondiagnostic.
- **Visceral angiography** may be considered if the bleeding is massive and the source is undiagnosed. Sensitivity of this test requires bleeding > 0.5–1 mL/min.
- **Radionuclide scanning** with ^{99m}Tc-labeled sulfur colloid or ^{99m}Tc-labeled red blood cells can detect and grossly localize acute bleeding < 0.5 mL/min. If necessary, tagged-cell scanning can be repeated serially to identify intermittent bleeding.

Management of Specific Bleeding Sources

Peptic ulcer disease accounts for approximately one-half of the cases of UGI bleeding. If a specific vessel is visualized endoscopically, injection and bipolar therapy should be attempted. This treatment is usually successful. Angiographic injection or embolization techniques can be considered in patients who are at high surgical risk. Surgery is indicated for life-threatening hemorrhage in patients who do not respond to multimodality medical therapy.

Acute Gastric Mucosal Hemorrhage. Gastric erosions are especially common among patients with preexisting critical illness, often severe sepsis. Treatment of the underlying critical illness is paramount. In addition, H_2-receptor antagonist therapy may be given by continuous IV infusion. Selective angiography with left gastric artery infusion of vasopressin has been used in extreme cases in which the patient has persistent bleeding and is at high surgical risk. Surgery may be necessary as a last resort.

Esophageal Varices. A nonvariceal bleeding site should be considered, even if the patient has previously diagnosed varices. With endoscopic identification of bleeding varices, sclerotherapy is the first choice and the most effective intervention. If it is unsuccessful initially, it may be repeated. Pharmacologic management consists of IV infusion of vasopressin (beginning at 1–2 units/min) along with nitroglycerin, given either topically or by IV infusion (e.g., at 5 mg/min). The reason for the latter agent is to offset the risk of inducing coronary vasoconstriction and myocardial ischemia. Balloon tamponade, with a Sengstaken-Blakemore tube or similar device, may be used as a supportive measure if sclerotherapy is unsuccessful (see Chapters 14 and 125 in the main text). Surgical procedures for variceal bleeding include transesophageal ligation and various portal–systemic shunting procedures (e.g., portal–caval shunt or splenorenal shunt). Portal–systemic shunt creation controls bleeding by lowering portal blood flow and pressure. It may be considered in patients in whom endoscopic and medical control of bleeding is unsuccessful, but it is risky in those with advanced liver disease, such as patients meeting Child's class C criteria (see Chapter 6 in this book). A relatively new procedure, transjugular intrahepatic portal–systemic shunt placement (TIPS), is comparatively safer and shows significant promise as an effective nonsurgical alternative.

Patients with esophageal varices often have elevated coagulation times because of their underlying liver disease. Aggressive use of fresh-frozen plasma is necessary to attempt correction of the coagulopathy, but is frequently unsuccessful. Delerium tremens or hepatic encephalopathy may develop and complicate the management of these patients. Prophylactic treatment may be indicated in some cases; however, sedative drugs should be used with caution because they may blunt the patient's ability to protect the airway.

Mallory-Weiss injury may be observed after violent retching or vomiting. It accounts for approximately 10% of cases of UGI hemorrhage in the United States. It typically occurs in association with alcohol abuse, but also can occur in other settings, such as pregnancy. Volume repletion should be followed by diagnostic and possibly therapeutic endoscopy using injection or electrocoagulation techniques. This entity is usually self-limiting, but surgical intervention should be considered if significant bleeding persists (e.g., need for > 10 units of packed red blood cells over 24 hours).

Suggested Readings

Adams L, Soulen MC. TIPS: A new alternative for the variceal bleeder. *Am J Crit Care* 1993;2:196–201.

Reviews a collective multicenter experience with this procedure in more than 300 cases. Technical success was achieved in 95% of cases, with a procedural mortality rate of 3%. Early shunt patency was >90%, ascites resolved in >80% of patients, and rates of encephalopathy and rebleeding were <15%. This procedure will probably become a primary treatment of choice as a bridging option in the patient awaiting heterotopic liver transplantation.

Chen YL. Mechanical gastritis as cause of upper gastrointestinal hemorrhage. *Scand J Gastroenterol* 1993;28:512–514.

From endoscopic evaluation of five patients with Mallory-Weiss syndrome, the author concludes that friction and compression of the gastric mucosa prolapsing through a constriction ring of the diaphragm into a hiatal hernia during retching and vomiting causes mechanical trauma to the gastric mucosa, resulting in gastritis, erosions, and hemorrhage.

Cook DJ, Fuller HD, Guyatt GH, et al. Risk factors for gastrointestinal bleeding in critically ill patients. *N Engl J Med* 1994;330:377–381.

Only 1.5% of 2,252 ICU patients had clinically significant bleeding. The authors conclude that stress ulcer prophylaxis can be safely withheld from critically ill patients unless they have coagulopathy or require mechanical ventilation.

Cook DJ, Guyatt GH, Salena BJ, et al. Endoscopic therapy for acute nonvariceal upper gastrointestinal hemorrhage: A meta-analysis. *Gastroenterology* 1992;102:139–148.

Thirty randomized controlled trials evaluating hemostatic endoscopic treatment showed that this therapy, including monopolar, bipolar, and heater probe maneuvers, significantly reduced the rate of further bleeding and the necessity of surgery. This decrease became statistically significant only for laser therapy. Rebleeding was not reduced, however, in the patient with flat, pigmented spots in the ulcers or in ulcers with adherent clots.

Graham DY, Hepps KS, Ramirez FC, et al. Treatment of *Helicobacter pylori* reduces the rate of rebleeding in peptic ulcer disease. *Scand J Gastroenterol* 1993;28:939–942.

This 31-patient group had major upper GI hemorrhage from peptic ulcers. Patients were randomized for treatment either with tetracycline, metronidazole, and bismuth subsalicylate for 2 weeks, or with ranitidine, which was continued until ulcer healing or for 16 weeks. Significant rebleeding occurred in 30% of the ranitidine treatment group and in none of the triple-therapy group.

Jenkins SA. Somatostatin in acute bleeding oesophageal varices: Clinical evidence. *Drugs* 1992;44(suppl 2):36–55, 70–72.

Somatostatin may have an effect as good as or better than that of vasopressin, either alone or combined with nitroglycerin therapy. Fewer side effects were noted as well. The average control rate in controlled trials was 69%. Its efficacy is comparable to that of balloon tamponade, H_2-receptor antagonists, and injection sclerotherapy.

Pescovitz MD, Satterberg TL, Shearen JG. Endoscopic control of bleeding ulcers: The Minnesota experience with several methods. In: Najarian JS, Delaney JP, eds. *Progress in gastrointestinal surgery*. Chicago: Year Book, 1989, pp 247–254.

Stark ME, Gostout CJ, Balm RK. Clinical features and endoscopic management of Dieulafoy's disease. *Gastrointest Endosc* 1992;38:545–550.

Identifies the disease in 19 of 1,124 patients with upper GI bleeding. Thirty-seven percent of these patients required repeat endoscopy to make the diagnosis. Eighty percent of the lesions were identified in the proximal stomach. Therapeutic maneuvers included combination of epinephrine injection, heater probe and bipolar coagulation, and laser photocoagulation. There were no deaths, and there was one treatment failure in which surgery was required.

Teres J, Bosch J, Bordas JM, et al. Propranolol versus sclerotherapy in preventing variceal rebleeding: A randomized controlled trial. *Gastroenterology* 1993;105:1508–1514.

This study involved 116 patients with cirrhosis who were admitted for variceal bleeding. They were randomized to receive continuous propanolol (to reduce resting heart rate by 25%) or weekly intravariceal sclerotherapy (until varices disappeared). No differences were found in rebleeding index, hospitalization requirements, survival, or cause of death. The actuarial probability of rebleeding was lower in the sclerotherapy group. Complications and lack of beneficial effects on parameters other than rebleeding suggest that the use of sclerotherapy as long-term therapy should be restricted.

CHAPTER 46

Lower Gastrointestinal Tract Hemorrhage

(See Chapter 126)

Brian E. Pinard

Lower gastrointestinal tract (LGI) hemorrhage causes the passage of bright red or maroon stool from the rectum. However, the color and quantity of blood is not a specific index of either location or etiology of GI bleeding. Because of the cathartic effect of blood, a brisk upper gastrointestinal (UGI) hemorrhage sometimes results in hematochezia. In fact, UGI sources are the most common causes of melena and hematochezia. In patients older than 65 years, vascular ectasia and malignancy are common LGI causes of bleeding, whereas intestinal polyps and inflammatory bowel disease are more common in younger adults. Diverticulosis is common in both age ranges.

Diagnosis

Initial evaluation should include a directed history and physical examination: the former to determine predisposing factors or a history of bleeding, the latter to assess the significance of this bleeding episode. A variety of methods are available to determine the specific site of hemorrhage. In addition to these methods, esophagogastroduodenoscopy may be necessary to exclude a UGI source of bleeding.

Colonoscopy in the face of ongoing hemorrhage is generally considered nondiagnostic and impractical. Regional localization of the site of bleeding (right colon vs. left colon) may be helpful in limiting the extent of colonic resection if the patient requires surgery. In less actively bleeding subjects, the specific site of bleeding can be identified after bowel preparation. Occasionally, the site of bleeding can be identified in the patient whose massive bleeding has stopped. Diagnostic accuracy is reportedly as high as 70–90%.

Angiography. The rate of active bleeding must exceed 0.5 to 1 mL/min to be detected by contrast angiography. LGI hemorrhage is frequently intermittent, making detection by this method problematic. It is therefore imperative that the patient be studied while actively bleeding, with resuscitation ongoing. The site is identified in 70% of cases if the bleeding is rapid enough.

Radionuclide Studies. Less vigorous bleeding can be more frequently localized with radionuclide scanning than with radiocontrast angiography. The minimal bleeding rate for ^{99m}Tc sulfur colloid scan or ^{99m}Tc-labeled red blood cell scan to be helpful may be as low as 0.1 mL/min. Although these tests are more sensitive than angiography, they have poor site specificity and may be confusing and misleading if used as the sole means to direct colonic resection. The isotope-labeled red blood cell study has the advantage of retaining its diagnostic use for 12 hours or more, at which time rescanning may provide more information.

Therapeutic Options

Most episodes of colonic bleeding are self-limiting; only approximately 10% of patients require emergency surgery. In addition, many patients with GI bleeding are elderly or have concomitant cardiac, pulmonary, or other diseases that increase the risk of surgery. Therefore, prompt nonsurgical localization and therapy are desirable.

Angiographic Procedures. In more than 90% of patients, the bleeding stops after direct intra-arterial infusion of vasopressin (Pitressin). Unfortunately, 80–90% of these patients will rebleed. This procedure significantly reduces the operative mortality rate during subsequent surgical resection. However, in the elderly, regional arterial infusion of vasopressin carries a significant risk of causing ischemia and subsequent infarction of the colon. Angiographically directed therapeutic embolization is effective, but it too carries a risk of inducing bowel ischemia.

Endoscopic Procedures. In highly experienced hands, as many as 25% of cases of active LGI hemorrhage may be amenable to endoscopic electrocoagulation or laser ablation. Patients with bleeding as a result of vascular ectasia or after polypectomy are the best candidates for this therapeutic modality. There is a risk of bowel perforation; on the other hand, rebleeding from untreated vascular ectasia occurs in approximately 80% of cases.

Surgery. If nonoperative management of bleeding (generally defined as the use of more than 6 units packed red cells over a period of 24 hours) is unsuccessful or unavailable, operative management is the treatment of choice. A well-directed segmental colon resection carries less than a 10% incidence of rebleeding. If the bleeding site is unidentifiable, or if there is a significant rebleed after segmental colon resection, subtotal colectomy with ileorectal anastomosis is indicated.

Suggested Readings

Browder W, Cerise EJ, Litwin MS. Impact of emergency angiography in massive lower gastrointestinal bleeding. *Ann Surg* 1986;204:530–536.

Angiography successfully localized the site of bleeding in this series, allowing segmental colectomy. The operative mortality rate was significantly improved compared with historical control subjects (9% vs. 37%) undergoing emergency subtotal colectomy without angiography.

DeMarkles MP, Murphy JR. Acute lower gastrointestinal bleeding. *Med Clin North Am* 1993;77:1085–1100.

Dusold R, Burke K, Carpentier W, et al. The accuracy of technetium-99m-labeled red cell scintigraphy in localizing gastrointestinal bleeding. *Am J Gastroenterol* 1004;89:345–348.

Retrospective study of 153 patients. Ninety had positive scans, with 44 going on to have corrective surgery. Of those 44, the bleeding site had been correctly identified by the radionuclide scan in 75%.

Guy GE, Shetty PC, Sharma RP, et al. Acute lower gastrointestinal hemorrhage: Treatment by superselective embolization with polyvinyl alcohol particles. *AJR* 1992;159:521–526.

This small group of 10 patients underwent this modified embolization procedure with polyvinyl alcohol particles (approximately 300 μm in diameter). All cases but one were controlled, and no cases of intestinal infarction occurred.

Setya V, Singer JA, Minken SL. Subtotal colectomy as a last resort for unrelenting, unlocalized, lower gastrointestinal hemorrhage: Experience with 12 cases. *Am Surg* 1992;578:295–299.

This 12-case experience resulted in a 33% mortality rate, whereas only 25% of patients survived to be discharged home. Diverticulosis was the cause of bleeding in 83% of this patient group.

Voeller GR, Bunch G, Britt LG. Use of technetium-labeled red blood cell scintigraphy in the detection and management of gastrointestinal hemorrhage. *Surgery* 1991;110:799–804.

Comparison of scintigraphy with arteriography, endoscopy, and surgery for the determination of bleeding site. In this study of 103 patients, sensitivity for the radionuclide procedure was only 23%; it did not direct surgical intervention, nor did it adequately screen patients for arteriography.

CHAPTER 47

Diarrhea in the ICU Patient

(See Chapter 127)

Margaret M. Wojnar and Jean M. Ferber

Diarrhea is an increase in the frequency of stools or an increase in stool volume (or weight) of more than 250 mL (or grams) over a 24-hour period. Acute diarrhea lasts less than 2 or 3 weeks; chronic diarrhea is present for a longer period. The distinction is important because acute diarrhea is usually infectious, except in the ICU setting, where iatrogenic causes (such as enteral feedings or drug-induced causes) are more common. The mechanisms of diarrhea involve:

- Increased luminal osmolality.
- Decreased nutrient or electrolyte absorption.
- Increased secretion of electrolytes.

Diarrhea frequently complicates the course of the ICU patient by interfering with fluid and electrolyte balance and administration of enteral nutrition (see Chapter 127 in the main text for a review of the pathophysiology of diarrhea).

Etiology

Diarrheal states can be grouped mechanistically, by acuity or chronicity, or by inciting event. Common causes among ICU patients include:

- **Drugs,** e.g., antibiotics, laxatives, magnesium-containing antacids, colchicine, quinidine, digoxin, angiotensin-converting enzyme inhibitors, β-adrenergic blocking agents, diuretics, lactulose, sorbitol, theophylline, levothyroxine, aspirin, nonsteroidal anti-inflammatory drugs, cimetidine, cyclophosphamide (Cytoxan), methotrexate, 5-fluorouracil.
- **Infections,** e.g., bacterial causes (*Shigella, Salmonella, Yersinia, Campylobacter, Mycobacterium* species); enterotoxins (from *Vibrio cholerae, Clostridium difficile, Staphylococcus aureus*); traveler's diarrhea; viral causes (Norwalk-like agents, enteroviruses, cytomegalovirus); parasitic or protozoal causes *(Giardia, Amoeba,* tapeworm, *Cryptosporidium, Schistosoma).*
- **Enteral feeding formulas.**
- **Malabsorption,** e.g., pancreatitis; small bowel malabsorption (celiac sprue, tropical sprue, Whipple's disease, amyloidosis); postsurgical causes (gastrectomy, pancreatectomy, cholecystectomy); short-bowel syndrome.
- **Immunosuppressive disease,** e.g., human immunodeficiency virus (HIV), organ transplant, graft-versus-host disease.
- **Hormonal causes,** e.g., diabetes mellitus (caused by autonomic neuropathy or secretory defect); thyrotoxicosis; adrenal insufficiency; VIPoma.
- **Malignancy-related** causes, e.g., radiation therapy, paraneoplastic syndromes, drug-related problems (with or without neutropenia).
- **Exudative or inflammatory causes,** e.g., ulcerative colitis, Crohn's disease, small bowel fistula, gastrocolonic fistulas.
- **Miscellaneous** causes, e.g., lactose intolerance, sepsis, fecal impaction, bacterial overgrowth, heavy metal poisoning, vascular disease, vasculitis.

Multiple etiologies may underlie the cause of diarrhea in ICU patients (e.g., a septic postoperative patient who is receiving antibiotics, has been receiving parenteral nutrition with nothing by mouth for a week, and was recently administered jejunal enteric feedings).

Diagnosis

History. Factors that help to narrow the differential diagnosis include acute versus chronic presentation, pre-existing illness or surgery, travel history, antibiotic use (within 6 to 8 weeks of presentation), other drug use, treatment or diagnosis of cancer (including radiation of the abdomen or pelvis), current and previous food intake, and the presence of fever or pain.

Physical Examination. A general examination is performed to identify underlying or intercurrent illness. The abdominal examination focuses on the presence or absence of pain, tenderness, distension, and surgical scars. A rectal examination is performed to determine the presence of stool, its consistency, presence of blood (occult vs. gross), presence of masses, and muscle tone.

Laboratory Examination. Stool should be examined for the presence of gross or occult blood, fecal leukocytes, and mucus. If an infectious cause is suspected, stool is examined for ova and parasites, *C. difficile* toxin, and enteric pathogens, depending on the patient's history. Immunocompromised patients may need a more extensive evaluation for opportunistic infections. Sudan stain for fecal fat is used when malabsorption is suspected. Bowel rest will help to differentiate secretory versus osmotic diarrhea. Changes in stool volume are observed during a 24- to 48-hour period of complete bowel rest. Stool volume does not change in secretory diarrhea, whereas it decreases in osmotic diarrhea. The stool osmole gap can also aid in this distinction. It is calculated from fecal sodium (Na_f) and potassium (K_f) concentrations and stool osmolality (osm_f) as:

$$\text{Stool osmole gap} = osm_f - 2 \times (Na_f + K_f)$$

A value greater than 50 mOsm/kg H_2O indicates an osmotic cause. Other tests that may be helpful in some circumstances are plain abdominal radiographs, sigmoidoscopy, small or large bowel biopsy, breath hydrogen test for bacterial overgrowth, and visceral angiography.

Treatment

- **Fluid and electrolyte** replacement is central to initial therapy. Sodium, potassium, magnesium, and phosphorus levels should be periodically assessed. Central venous monitoring may be needed for titration of fluid replacement, especially in elderly patients or those with cardiac disorders.

- **Offending and unnecessary drugs** are discontinued.
- **Tube feedings** can be stopped, diluted, or changed to an isotonic formula, and the effect on diarrhea observed. If after several changes, the diarrhea continues, another source of the diarrhea should be sought. Diarrhea that starts shortly after tube feedings are initiated is usually associated.
- **Antibiotic treatment** constitutes specific therapy for *C. difficile* infection. Oral vancomycin (125 mg PO every 6 hours for 10–14 days) or metronidazole (250 mg PO every 6 hours for 10–14 days) is usually sufficient. The triple combination of IV vancomycin, IV metronidazole, and vancomycin by nasogastric tube or high rectal enema is recommended for seriously ill patients with bowel obstruction or ileus. For recurrent *C. difficile* infection, biotherapy with *Lactobacillus* or *Saccharomyces* species has been used successfully.
- **Directed therapy** for an enteric pathogen should be initiated once the pathogen is identified. Enteric isolation procedures should be instituted. For a given pathogen, the type and duration of therapy may differ in immunocompromised versus immunocompetent patients.
- **Underlying diseases** that can cause or exacerbate diarrhea, e.g., thyrotoxicosis, sepsis, or diabetes mellitus, should be treated. Tighter glucose control of diabetes may help, but probably will not eliminate diarrhea. The use of the somatostatin analog octreotide (50 μg subcutaneously twice a day) is effective, as is clonidine.

Suggested Readings

Borlase BC, Bell SJ, Lewis EJ, et al. Tolerance to enteral tube feeding diets in hypoalbuminemic critically ill, geriatric patients. *Surg Gynecol Obstet* 1992;174:181–188.

Prospective, randomized trial of elemental versus free amino acid diets in 16 critically ill, elderly patients with hypoalbuminemia. Tolerance to enteral feeding was similar in the two groups.

Edwards IR, Coulter DM, Macintosh D. Intestinal effects of captopril. *Br Med J* 1992;304:359–360.

Brief report of six patients with diarrhea and constipation that promptly resolved after captopril was discontinued.

Fekety R, Shah AB. Diagnosis and treatment of *Clostridium difficile* colitis. *JAMA* 1993;269:71–75.

Excellent review of diagnosis and management of C. difficile *colitis, including an algorithm for evaluation and treatment.*

Kelly TWS, Patrick MR, Hillman KM. Study of diarrhea in critically ill patients. *Crit Care Med* 1983;11:7–9.

In this prospective study of patients admitted to an ICU for more than 48 hours during a 12-month period, 41% had diarrhea. Major factors associated with development of diarrhea were the use of enteric feedings and cimetidine.

Surawicz CM, McFarland LV, Elmer G, et al. Treatment of recurrent *Clostridium difficile* colitis with vancomycin and *Saccharomyces boulardii*. *Am J Gastroenterol* 1989;84:1285–1287.

Thirteen patients were treated with vancomycin (10 days) and S. boulardii *(a nonpathogenic yeast, given for 30 days) for recurrent* C. difficile *colitis. Eleven had resolution without further recurrence.*

Walker JJ, Kaplan DS. Efficacy of the somatostatin analog octreotide in the treatment of two patients with refractory diabetic diarrhea. *Am J Gastroenterol* 1993;88:765–767.

CHAPTER 48

Hepatic Failure and Encephalopathy

(See Chapters 30, 133, 134, and 135)

Peter F. Ells

Hepatic failure may be the end stage of chronic liver disease, or it may result from acute fulminant disease. Because diagnostic and therapeutic approaches vary, it is useful to consider these two syndromes separately.

Fulminant Hepatic Failure

Fulminant hepatic failure (FHF) is defined as hepatic failure with encephalopathy occurring within 8 weeks of the onset of illness in a patient without previous liver disease. Determining the cause is important because the prognosis is partly determined by the etiology. Causes include:

Viral hepatitis, the most common cause of FHF.

- **Hepatitis A,** which accounts for approximately 5% of cases.
- **Hepatitis B,** the most common viral etiology of FHF, accounting for 30–65% of cases.
- **Hepatitis C** (non-A, non-B hepatitis).
- **Hepatitis D** (or delta hepatitis), a coinfection that can occur with hepatitis B and results in increased severity.
- **Other viruses,** including herpes simplex, cytomegalovirus, and Epstein-Barr virus, which can cause FHF, particularly in immunocompromised patients. These causes are rare.

Toxin or drug-induced causes may be mediated by idiosyncratic reactions or dose-dependent, direct hepatotoxicity.

- **Acetaminophen** overdose is the most common form of drug-induced FHF. An active metabolite of the drug has intrinsic dose-dependent hepatotoxicity. Early presentation after overdosage allows therapeutic intervention with *N*-acetylcysteine to prevent injury (see Chapter 89 in this book).

- **Other drugs:** Most other drug-induced cases of FHF are idiosyncratic reactions. In some cases, the mechanism is a true allergic reaction, and it may be accompanied by features suggestive of allergy, such as fever, rash, or eosinophilia. The classic example is halothane. Other drugs and toxins that cause FHF include carbon tetrachloride, isoniazid, methyldopa, sodium valproate, and monoamine oxidase inhibitors.
- **Mushroom poisoning:** Ingestion of certain toxic mushrooms, notably *Amanita phalloides,* causes liver injury by a direct hepatotoxic effect. There is an asymptomatic, latent phase that ranges from 6–24 hours. The second phase is a short period (12–24 hours) of GI symptoms, including abdominal pain, nausea, vomiting, and profuse watery diarrhea. Liver disease, the third phase, usually occurs after recovery from the GI symptoms. The mortality rate without liver transplantation is approximately 25%.

Uncommon causes

- **Wilson's disease** occasionally presents as FHF. This type of FHF is associated with severe hemolysis, and there may be characteristic eye findings known as Kayser-Fleischer rings. Diagnosis is made by measuring serum copper levels because ceruloplasmin is synthesized by the liver and will be low in all causes of FHF.
- **Fatty liver of pregnancy** is an uncommon disorder that occurs in the third trimester of pregnancy. The mortality rate is approximately 25%. Early diagnosis and definitive treatment, which consists of expeditious delivery, decreases maternal and fetal mortality rates.
- **Reyes syndrome:** Except for rare cases in young adults, this uncommon syndrome is limited to children.

The history, clinical setting, and results of serologic tests are important for differentiating the above etiologies. Percutaneous liver biopsy is unlikely to be safe because of coagulopathy. When available, a transjugular biopsy may be useful; however, the small tissue sample obtained is a serious limitation.

Treatment.

Encephalopathy is necessary for the diagnosis of FHF. Encephalopathy can be divided into four grades:

- **Grade I:** The patient is mildly confused, thought processes are slowed, and speech may be slurred. Mild asterixis may be present.

- **Grade II:** The patient is drowsy, may behave inappropriately, is often incontinent, and has asterixis.
- **Grade III:** The sensorium may range from stuporous to somnolent, but arousable. Speech is incoherent, confusion is significant, and asterixis is present.
- **Grade IV:** The patient is deeply comatose and may be completely unresponsive to noxious stimuli. Asterixis is absent.

There is no proof of efficacy for most treatments for chronic encephalopathy when used in patients with FHF. Lactulose in a dose tailored to result in two to three loose stools may be useful. Overtreatment with lactulose can cause excessive free-water loss and hypernatremia. Neomycin should be avoided because of its potential nephrotoxicity and ototoxicity.

Although encephalopathy is to be expected in FHF, a variety of other treatable factors can occur as complications, and may potentially worsen mental status. These include:

- Hypoglycemia.
- Hemorrhage.
- Hypotension.
- Acid–base imbalances.
- Hypoxemia.
- Infection.
- Drug-induced sedation.
- Electrolyte disturbances.

Cerebral edema is the major cause of death in patients with FHF. It usually occurs in grade IV encephalopathy. Because it does not occur in the encephalopathy of chronic liver disease, its occurrence suggests a difference in the pathogenesis of the two disorders. Brain swelling leads to increased intracranial pressure (ICP). As ICP increases, cerebral perfusion pressure (mean arterial pressure minus ICP) tends to decrease. The use of ICP pressure monitoring in FHF has expanded our knowledge about cerebral edema and its therapy. Inability to maintain cerebral perfusion pressure greater than 40 mm Hg can result in brainstem herniation. Simple turning of the patient's head may increase ICP because of increased resistance to venous flow in the neck. Therapy should be initiated when ICP reaches 30 mm Hg (see Chapter 39 in this book). The routine clinical use of ICP monitors in FHF is controversial because ICP monitoring has not been shown to improve survival rates in FHF and because of the potential complications associated with the procedure. Although the risk of bleeding during or after insertion is relatively low and can be reduced by fresh-frozen plasma (FFP) infusion, ICP monitoring should be reserved for cases in which cerebral edema is difficult to control.

Coagulopathy is a multifactorial process that is often severe. There is decreased hepatic production of clotting factors. Thrombocytopenia is common, and results from hypersplenism, decreased production, and increased consumption. In addition, low-grade disseminated intravascular coagulation is often present.

- Abnormal coagulation parameters should be monitored closely.
- Vitamin K should be administered parenterally for the first 3 days. This treatment is sufficient to replenish stores, so there is no value to continuing this administration on a daily basis.
- Prophylactic FFP may be unnecessary. FFP can be given with platelet transfusion when surgical procedures are planned.
- GI bleeding as a result of stress-related mucosal disease is common. It may be severe because of the hemostatic abnormalities. H_2-receptor antagonists are effective in decreasing GI bleeding.

Hypotension is common and is often associated with low systemic vascular resistance and high cardiac output. This pattern is probably related to poor hepatic clearance of endogenous vasodilators, but may be difficult to differentiate from a septic pattern. Hypotension can occur in the absence of sepsis, but it is appropriate to be vigilant for complicating infection. The presence of hypotension does not necessitate volume expansion. This treatment should be reserved for patients in whom volume depletion is evident or systolic blood pressure is consistently less than 90 mm Hg.

Pulmonary complications are common. Patients with grade IV encephalopathy should be endotracheally intubated prophylactically to protect the airway.

Hypoglycemia can result from impaired hepatic gluconeogenesis. Infusion of a 5% or 10% dextrose solution is usually sufficient to prevent hypoglycemia, but it is important to monitor glucose levels closely to facilitate titration of the infusion.

Transplantation. Because deterioration can be rapid and there are no specific therapies available, patients with FHF should be transferred to a liver transplant center as early as possible. The decision to transplant acutely is a difficult one. In general, transplant survival decreases with worsening clinical status. However, some patients recover without specific intervention. Overall, the survival rate of patients who undergo transplantation for FHF is significantly lower than the 80% survival rate seen with elective transplantation.

Etiology is of some prognostic value. Patients with FHF secondary to hepatitis A, hepatitis B, or acetaminophen poisoning have a survival rate of approximately 50%.

Those with FHF secondary to non-A and non-B hepatitis, halothane, or other drug reactions have survival rates of approximately 15%.

Contraindications to transplantation include:

- Extrahepatic malignancy.
- Active extrahepatic sepsis.
- Extensive mesenteric venous thrombosis.
- Irreversible brain damage.

FHF secondary to hepatitis B is not a contraindication because the hepatitis B surface antigen usually clears after transplantation. In contrast, the recurrence of hepatitis B is nearly universal after transplantation for chronic hepatitis B infection.

Chronic Hepatic Failure

Chronic hepatic failure usually develops and progresses over a period of many months to years. Essentially all patients with this syndrome have irreversible hepatic damage, and the etiology is usually cirrhosis. Patients with evidence of ongoing hepatic injury related to recent alcohol use may benefit from corticosteroid therapy (see Chapter 133 in the main text).

Encephalopathy. Most cases of encephalopathy in patients with chronic liver disease are related to some precipitating factor and not to an acute decrease in hepatic function. Prompt recognition of and attention to the precipitant can result in rapid improvement. Common precipitants include:

- **Azotemia,** which is sometimes diuretic-induced.
- **GI hemorrhage,** which can occur as a result of stress-related gastritis, esophageal varices, or other causes.
- **Constipation,** which may lead to increased absorption of ammonia produced by gut flora.
- **Hypokalemia,** which is known to stimulate renal ammonia production.
- **Sedative-hypnotic use,** e.g., benzodiazepines.
- **Infection:** There may be no obvious signs; therefore, a careful search is necessary.

Diagnosis. Hepatic failure in the setting of chronic liver disease is a diagnosis of exclusion. Patients with cirrhosis are susceptible to all of the usual causes of stupor and coma.

- Asterixis is not specific for portal-systemic encephalopathy, but can be seen with other etiologies of metabolic encephalopathy.
- Measurement of the plasma ammonia level may be useful for suggesting a hepatic cause in encephalopathy of unknown etiology. If used, it should be measured in the

arterial blood. It is not useful for following the response to treatment; that is best done with clinical parameters. Thus, there is no need for serial determinations.

- Appropriate testing to exclude meningitis, subdural hematoma, or other etiologies may be necessary in certain patients.

Therapy

- **Precipitating factors** that may have precipitated the encephalopathy should be identified, and appropriate treatment initiated.
- **Low-protein diet:** At the time of acute encephalopathy, it is appropriate to stop protein intake and administer IV glucose. Treatment should allow prompt reintroduction of dietary protein. It is necessary to consider the patient's nutritional state in a risk–benefit analysis of protein restriction.
- **Lactulose** (30 mL 2–4 times daily) is often effective. The dose should be adjusted to result in two to three loose stools per day. There may be a delay in onset after oral use. A common error is to give multiple large oral doses and cause intractable diarrhea, which can complicate fluid management. Lactulose enemas (300 mL lactulose syrup in a total volume of 1 L) may be useful in comatose patients.
- **Neomycin** is effective because it decreases the colonic flora that are responsible for urea metabolism. Because of the risk of ototoxicity and nephrotoxicity, it is usually reserved as a second-line agent. It is effective in combination with lactulose because the two agents apparently affect different bacterial flora. It should be reserved for those rare patients with chronic encephalopathy that cannot be treated with lactulose alone.
- **Metronidazole** is as effective as neomycin, and it might be useful as an adjunct in occasional patients or in patients who cannot tolerate lactulose.

Suggested Readings

Donaldson BW, Gopinath R, Wanless IR, et al. The role of transjugular liver biopsy in fulminant liver failure: Relation to other prognostic indicators. *Hepatology* 1993;18:1370–1376.

Summarizes use of transjugular liver biopsy in 61 patients with fulminant hepatic failure. Appears safe and effective as an adjunct for determining etiology and prognosis.

Emond JC, Aran PP, Whitington PF, et al. Liver transplantation in the management of fulminant hepatic failure. *Gastroenterology* 1989; 96:1583–1588.

Summarizes use of liver transplantation for treatment of fulminant hepatic failure. Addresses survival with and without transplantation.

Harrison PM, Keays R, Bray GP, et al. Improved outcome of paracetamol-induced fulminant hepatic failure by late administration of acetylcysteine. *Lancet* 1990;335:1572–1573.

Suggests that patients with fulminant hepatic failure secondary to acetamino-

phen use will benefit from N-acetylcysteine treatment, even when treatment is delayed more than 36 hours after ingestion.
Lee WM. Acute liver failure. *N Engl J Med* 1993;329:1862–1872.
Comprehensive review of the subject with long reference list.
O'Grady JG, Alexander GJ, Hayllar KM, et al. Early indicators of prognosis in fulminant hepatic failure. *Gastroenterology* 1989;97:439–445.
Analyzes predictors of survival in 588 patients treated over a 12-year period at a single specialized unit. Survival rate varies with etiology, but has improved for all causes with time.
William R, Gimson AES. Intensive liver care and management of acute hepatic failure. *Dig Dis Sci* 1991;36:820–826.
Good review of overall therapeutic strategies from the world's most experienced center, King's College Hospital.

CHAPTER 49

Enteral Alimentation and Nutritional Assessment

(See Chapter 136)

Dane J. Nichols

Nutritional assessment and support is an integral part of the care of the critically ill patient. Organ system function, immune competence, and the metabolic response to injury are all influenced by the overall nutritional status of the patient. The primary goals of nutritional therapy in the ICU are to provide a source of metabolic energy, protect visceral protein stores, maintain GI function, and meet the specific needs of patients with single or multiple organ system failure.

Nutritional Assessment

By some estimates, as many as half of hospitalized patients have protein-calorie malnutrition. An assessment of nutritional status aids in identifying patients who are at risk for serious complications and in designing support strategies. Unfortunately, conventional assessment tools are imprecise and have not been adequately validated. Conventional tools include:

- **Measurement of body weight,** with comparison of current body weight (CBW) with ideal body weight (IBW; see Chapter 58 in this book) or usual body weight (UBW; Table 49–1):

TABLE 49–1

USEFUL INDICATORS FOR ASSESSING THE DEGREE OF MALNUTRITION

Indicator	Mild	Moderate	Severe	Comments
Physical Examination				
Percentage of ideal weight	80–90	70–79	< 70	Based, e.g., on Metropolitan Life Insurance tables or calculated from formulas (see Chapter 58)
Percentage of usual weight	85–95	75–84	< 75	Recent weight change shows better correlation with adverse outcome
Subcutaneous fat	Normal	↓	↓↓	Ideally, triceps skin-fold thickness measured with calipers
Muscle mass	Normal	↓	↓↓	Deltoids and quadriceps femoris evaluated for bulk and tone
Edema or ascites	None	+	++	May be present in more advanced states of malnutrition
Immune Competence				
Absolute lymphocyte count (mm^{-3})	1200–2000	800–1200	< 800	May also perform skin tests to common antigens
Serum Protein values (half-life)				
Albumin (20 days), g/dL	2.8–3.5	2.1–2.7	< 2.1	Reflects synthesis, redistribution, and catabolism of albumin
Transferrin (8–10 days), mg/dL	150–200	100–150	< 100	Derived level routinely underestimates value; altered by iron deficiency
Thyroxine-binding prealbumin (2 days), mg/dL	10–15	5–10	< 5	An acute-phase reactant; therefore, baseline level may be elevated in certain inflammatory conditions
Retinol-binding protein (10–12 hours), mg/dL	Normal	< 3	< 3	An acute-phase reactant; also elevated in renal failure

$$\text{Percentage of IBW} = (\text{CBW}/\text{IBW}) \times 100\%$$

$$\text{Percentage of UBW} = (\text{CBW}/\text{UBW}) \times 100\%$$

$$\text{Percentage of recent weight change} = [(\text{UBW} - \text{CBW})/\text{UBW}] \times 100\%$$

- **Subjective global assessment** by physical examination (see Table 49–1), when coupled with weight assessment, provides a reasonable estimate in most patients.
- **Serum protein evaluation,** including albumin, prealbumin, transferrin, thyroxine-binding protein, and retinol-binding protein (see Table 49–1); transferrin level can be estimated from serum total iron-binding capacity (TIBC) according to the formula:

  $$\text{Estimated serum transferrin level} = (0.8 \times \text{TIBC}) - 43$$

- **Excretion studies,** e.g., creatinine–height index, urinary 3-methylhistidine excretion, or 24-hour urinary nitrogen excretion.
- **Nitrogen balance,** calculated as:

  $$N_{BAL} = (P_{IN}/6.25) - \text{UUN} - 4$$

  where N_{BAL} is nitrogen balance (g/day), P_{IN} is protein intake (g/day), UUN is urinary urea nitrogen (g/day), and 4 is estimated nonurinary nitrogen loss (g/day).
- **Indicators of immune competence,** such as total lymphocyte count (see Table 49–1) and results of skin testing for delayed hypersensitivity reactions.

The appropriate level of testing is debatable. Minimal assessment should include weight loss history, physical examination, serum albumin evaluation, estimated transferrin level, and total lymphocyte count.

Estimating Energy Requirements

Nutritional requirements vary from patient to patient, and are influenced by age, sex, body habitus, activity level, and underlying illness. Estimates based on the Harris-Benedict equations provide reasonably accurate values in adult patients who are not critically ill:

$$\text{Male: REE} = 66.47 + 13.75 \times \text{weight} + 5.00 \times \text{height} - 6.76 \times \text{age}$$

$$\text{Female: REE} = 655.1 + 9.56 \times \text{weight} + 1.85 \times \text{height} - 4.68 \times \text{age}$$

where REE is resting energy expenditure expressed in kilocalories per day, weight is expressed in kilograms, height is expressed in centimeters, and age is expressed in years. To obtain the estimated energy expenditure in a critically ill patient, the above results are then multiplied by a correction factor in the range of 0.7–1.8, depending on the disease state and severity (see Table 136–3 in the main text). The Harris-Benedict equations tend to overestimate energy expenditure in ICU patients, sometimes by as much as 25%.

Resting energy expenditure can also be measured indirectly with either expired gas analysis or measurements obtained by pulmonary artery catheterization. In indirect calorimetry, expired gas is analyzed to determine oxygen consumption ($\dot{V}O_2$) and carbon dioxide production ($\dot{V}CO_2$). Energy expenditure can then be estimated with the simplified Weir equation:

$$\text{Energy expenditure} = 3.9 \times \dot{V}O_2 + 1.1 \times \dot{V}CO_2$$

where $\dot{V}O_2$ and $\dot{V}CO_2$ are expressed in liters per minute and energy expenditure is expressed in kilocalories per day. With the Fick method, a thermodilution pulmonary artery catheter is used to obtain measurements of cardiac output and mixed venous oxygen tension and saturation. Mixed venous ($C\bar{v}O_2$) oxygen content is then calculated from the equation:

$$C\bar{v}O_2 = (1.39 \times Hb \times S\bar{v}O_2) + (0.0031 \times P\bar{v}O_2)$$

where Hb is hemoglobin concentration (g/dL), and $S\bar{v}O_2$ and $P\bar{v}O_2$ are mixed venous blood oxygen saturation (fraction) and tension (torr), respectively. An arterial blood specimen is also obtained, and arterial oxygen content (CaO_2) is calculated with the same formula, substituting arterial oxygen saturation and tension. $\dot{V}O_2$ can then be obtained from the equation:

$$\dot{V}O_2 = \text{cardiac output} \times (CaO_2 - C\bar{v}O_2) \times 14{,}400$$

where cardiac output is expressed in liters per minute and $\dot{V}O_2$ is expressed in liters per day. Multiplying $\dot{V}O_2$ by the known caloric value of oxygen (4.8 kcal/L) yields the estimated daily energy expenditure.

Enteral Nutrition

In the absence of contraindications, enteral nutrition (EN) is the preferred method of nutrient delivery. EN buffers gastric acids, stimulates bile secretion, and helps to preserve the integrity of the GI wall. Indications include a recent nonvolitional loss of 10% or more of usual body weight, serum albumin concentration of less than 3.3 g/dL, and food intake that meets less than half of the nutritional requirements of the patient. The GI tract must be functional. Contraindications include vomiting, intestinal obstruction, severe ileus, and upper GI bleeding. Marked hemodynamic instability and severe multiple organ system failure are relative contraindications.

Formula Selection

In selecting an enteral nutrition formula, the patient's protein and calorie requirements, GI tract digestive (absorptive) capacity, and fluid and electrolyte restrictions should be considered (see Figure 136–3 in the main text). Typically, enteral alimentation formulas have a caloric density of 1 to 2 kcal/mL.

Enteral dietary formulations may be classified as:

- **Polymeric formulas** containing complex forms of the three basic nutrients. They are typically isotonic and lactose free, and have a caloric density of 0.6–2.0 kcal/mL.
- **Elemental formulas** containing basic nutrients supplied in monomeric form (e.g., crystalline amino acids, medium-chain triglycerides, dextrose and oligosaccharides). They are typically hypertonic and unpalatable.
- **Specialized formulas** containing alterations in nutrient content to meet specific needs.

Specialized formulas have been formulated for specific disease states, including:

- **Hepatic encephalopathy** formulas, which contain decreased content of aromatic amino acids.
- **Renal failure** formulas, which have low levels of potassium and in which the nitrogen source is restricted to essential amino acids.
- **Hypercatabolic state** formulas, which have increased content of branched-chain amino acids and a high protein–calorie ratio.
- **Respiratory failure** formulas, which have a high lipid and a low carbohydrate content.
- **Immune-enhanced** formulas, which provide high levels of immunomodulating nutrients (e.g., ribonucleic acid, medium-chain triglycerides, omega-3 fatty acids, glutamine, arginine).

The indications and efficacy of many of these specialized formulations are under evaluation.

GI Access and Delivery

Short-term GI tract access (< 4 weeks) is generally accomplished by placement of a nasogastric or nasoenteric tube. Although not always feasible, cannulation of the small bowel is preferred in critically ill patients because of the increased frequency of gastroparesis and aspiration. Intestinal placement can be facilitated by placing the patient in the right lateral decubitus position during and after tube passage. Administration of prokinetic agents, such as metaclopramide, has also been advocated. Fluoroscopic or endoscopic techniques are sometimes employed in difficult cases.

Continuous feeding offers several advantages over bolus methods. Tolerance is improved, residual volumes tend to be smaller, and the risk of aspiration may be decreased. It has also been associated with improved weight gain and nitrogen balance in selected populations. Hyperosmolar solutions are generally well tolerated when delivered to the stomach. For small bowel delivery, isotonic formulas are often better tolerated. Alternatively, tonicity can be adjusted by simply diluting hypertonic solutions. Continuous infusion can be initiated at 30 mL/hr and increased by 10 to 15 mL/hr daily as tolerated until nutritional goals are met. As GI tolerance develops, hypertonic solutions can be introduced.

Monitoring and Complications

After tube placement has been performed, tube position is confirmed by instillation of air, aspiration of GI contents, and radiography. Monitoring protocols (see Table 136–8 in the main text) help to avoid complications and achieve nutritional goals. Complications arising from enteral nutrition can be classified into the following categories:

- **GI,** such as delayed gastric emptying with associated distension (occasionally ameliorated by metaclopramide 10 mg IV every 6 hours), and diarrhea (often of multifactorial etiology), which may occur in half of critically ill patients.
- **Metabolic,** such as hyperglycemia and fluid and electrolyte imbalances, including hypernatremia, hyponatremia, hypokalemia, hypophosphatemia, and hypomagnesemia.
- **Aspiration,** with incidence ranging from 1% to 44%. Risk is reduced by elevating the head of the bed 30 degrees, feeding beyond the pylorus, and maintaining low residual volumes. Occult aspiration is detected through the addition of food coloring to formula and by testing tracheal aspirates for glucose.
- **Mechanical,** such as local tissue erosion, luminal obstruction, sinusitis, otitis media, and tube placement outside the GI tract. The risk of placement in the tracheobronchial tree and pleural space is increased in obtunded patients.

Suggested Readings

Baskin WN. Advances in enteral nutrition techniques. *Am J Gastroenterol* 1992;87:1547–1553.

Excellent review of various devices and techniques for providing long-term enteral nutrition.

Benya R, Mobarhan S. Enteral alimentation: Administration and complications. *J Am Coll Nutr* 1991;10:209–219.
Comprehensive overview of benefits and hazards of enteral nutrition.
Boyes RJ, Kruse JA. Nasogastric and nasoenteric intubation. *Crit Care Clin* 1992;8:865–878.
Detailed description of techniques for inserting nasogastric and nasoenteric feeding tubes.
Liggett SB, St. John RE, Lefrak SS. Determination of resting energy expenditure utilizing the thermodilution pulmonary artery catheter. *Chest* 1987;91:562–566.
Provides comparison of resting energy expenditure estimates derived from cardiac output versus indirect calorimetry. Formula derivations are included.
McMahon MM, Farnell MB, Murray MJ. Nutritional support of critically ill patients. *Mayo Clin Proc* 1993;68:911–920.
Details metabolic response to circulating cytokines and hormones. Provides guidelines for developing nutritional support strategies.
Montecalvo MA, Steger KA, Farber HW, et al. Nutritional outcome and pneumonia in critical care patients randomized to gastric versus jejunal tube feedings. *Crit Care Med* 1991;10:1377–1387.
Examines effect of feeding tube location on incidence of nosocomial pneumonia.
Murray MJ, Marsh HM, Wochos DN, et al. Nutritional assessment of intensive-care patients. *Mayo Clin Proc* 1988;63:1106–1115.
Evaluates many nutritional assessment tools and their relation to outcome.

CHAPTER 50

Parenteral Alimentation

(See Chapter 136)

Dane J. Nichols

Parenteral nutrition is frequently indicated for critically ill patients in whom enteral alimentation is contraindicated or does not meet established nutritional goals. These formulas can be prepared in the hospital pharmacy from concentrated dextrose and amino acid solutions to which electrolytes, vitamins, and trace elements are added.

Total Parenteral Nutrition

Total parenteral nutrition (TPN) is appropriate for severely malnourished, hypercatabolic, or volume-restricted patients who are expected to require long-term nutritional support. Infusion into the central venous circulation allows for rapid mixing and dilution of mixtures with high osmolarity and caloric density. Central venous cannulation should be performed as a sterile procedure with the use of cap, mask, sterile gown and gloves. Once placed, the line should be used solely for TPN administration;

coinfusion of drugs, blood products, and other fluids should be avoided. In-line stopcocks and monitoring systems should also be avoided.

Formula Calculations. Nutritional requirements can either be estimated or measured by indirect calorimetry (see Chapter 49 in this book). The caloric density of TPN solutions can be calculated from the following relationships:

- Dextrose contains 3.4 kcal/g.
- Amino acids contain 4.0 kcal/g.
- 10% lipid emulsion contains 1.1 kcal/mL.
- 20% lipid emulsion contains 2.0 kcal/mL.

For most patients, providing 25 to 30 nonprotein kcal/kg/day along with 1.0–1.5 g/kg/day of amino acids (both based on lean body weight) meets nutritional goals. Severely stressed and septic patients should receive 1.5–2.5 g/kg/day of amino acids. Lipid administration should be restricted to less than 60% of total nonprotein calories or less than 2.5 g/kg/day. Fluid requirements (mL/day) may be estimated with any of the following formulas:

$$30 \text{ to } 35 \times \text{body weight (kg)}.$$

1000 mL for the first 10 kg body weight
+ 500 mL for the next 10 kg
+ 20 mL for every 10 kg thereafter.

$$1500 \times \text{body surface area } (m^2).$$

Body surface area may be determined from a nomogram or with the following formula:

$$\text{Body surface area} = \text{weight}^{0.425} \times (\text{height} \times 2.54)^{0.725} \times 0.007184$$

where weight is in kilograms and height is in inches. Typical electrolyte and trace element requirements are shown in Tables 50–1 and 50–2. One single-dose ampule of a multivitamin preparation is generally provided on a daily basis. Vitamin K (10 mg) can be administered once per week by subcutaneous injection. Supplemental iron is generally not required. The addition of heparin (e.g., 6000 units/day) to TPN solutions has been advocated to prevent fibrin sleeve formation and to enhance the clearance of lipids.

Initiating and Monitoring Total Parenteral Nutrition. The rate of delivery of TPN solutions is guided by the glucose and fluid tolerance of the patient. The initial infusion rate can begin at 20 to 40 mL/hr and be increased by 10 to 20 mL/hr/day until nutritional goals are met. In patients with underlying renal and cardiac disease, maximum solution concentrations of glucose and amino acids are often used to allow fluid restriction to 1.5 L/day or less.

TABLE 50–1

TYPICAL REQUIREMENTS FOR TOTAL PARENTERAL NUTRITION ELECTROLYTES

Electrolyte	Typical Concentration	Typical Concentration Range	Comments
Sodium	35 mmol/L	0–150 mmol/L	Amount dictated by intravascular volume requirements and total body water and sodium balance
Potassium	30 mmol/L	0–80 mmol/L	Provide 5–6 mmol/g N; requirements may exceed 200 mmol/day
Chloride	40 mmol/L	0–150 mmol/L	Relative proportions of chloride and acetate are dictated by patient's acid–base status
Acetate	70 mmol/L	70–220 mmol/L	
Calcium	2 mmol/L	0–8 mmol/L	Also may provide 0.25 mg/kg/day (as calcium gluconate)
Magnesium	4 mmol/L	0–8 mmol/L	Also may provide 1 mmol/g N; decreased requirements in renal failure
Phosphate	15 mmol/L	0–20 mmol/L	Provide 7–9 mmol/1000 nonprotein kcal; fat emulsions contain phosphate (7.5 mmol/500 mL)

TABLE 50–2

TYPICAL REQUIREMENTS FOR TOTAL PARENTERAL NUTRITION TRACE ELEMENTS

Trace Element	Typical Daily Dose	Typical Daily Dosage Range	Comments
Zinc	3.0 mg	2.5–4.0 mg	Increased requirements with diarrhea, ethanol abuse; dose decreased in renal failure unless receiving dialysis
Copper	1.2 mg	0.5–1.5 mg	Dose decreased in biliary tract obstruction
Chromium	12 μg	5–15 μg	Dose decreased in renal failure
Manganese	0.3 mg	0.15–0.80 mg	Dose decreased in biliary tract obstruction
Iodine	100 μg	1–2 μg/kg	Inorganic iodide is handled like chloride by GI tract, so enteral absorption occurs even in the face of malabsorption
Selenium	100 μg	40–200 μg/day	Usually added after 4 weeks of total parenteral nutrition

The intensity of monitoring is determined by the stability of the patient, but at a minimum, should include:

- Daily weight and fluid balance.
- Urine glucose and ketone assays every 6 hours (diabetic and metabolically unstable patients may require serum or capillary blood glucose determinations instead).
- Complete blood count and serum levels of sodium, potassium, chloride, CO_2, calcium, phosphorus, magnesium, urea nitrogen, and creatinine measured at baseline and then daily for at least the first 5 days.
- Liver function tests, albumin, total protein, triglycerides, and prothrombin time measured at baseline and then twice weekly.
- 24-hour urine urea nitrogen monitoring may be performed 1 to 2 times per week.
- Scrupulous catheter maintenance, with routine site inspection, dressing, and IV tubing changes.

Electrolyte derangements and hyperglycemia are the most frequently encountered metabolic problems. In patients with known diabetes or glucose intolerance, a sliding-scale insulin regimen is used initially for control. Critically ill patients may require 200% or more of their prehospital daily insulin dose. Once insulin needs are determined, two-thirds to an equal amount of the daily insulin requirement may be added to the daily TPN solution. The infusion rate should not be advanced until adequate glycemic control has been demonstrated.

Parenteral Nutrition in Specific Conditions

Acute Renal Failure. TPN formulation in this setting is dictated by fluid restrictions, electrolyte and trace element excretion limitations, the degree of blood urea nitrogen level elevation, and the use of dialysis. In patients with oligoanuria, the total TPN volume is generally limited to 1–1.5 L/day. Administration of amino acids is reduced in patients with advanced renal insufficiency who are not undergoing dialysis. Because amino acids are removed by dialysis, their administration should be increased to approximately 1 g/kg/day once dialysis is initiated. Increasing the amount of acetate in the formula can be useful for countering metabolic acidosis. Trace elements are withheld for the first 2 weeks, but thereafter, may be given every other day (on nondialysis days). Patients undergoing hemodialysis have increased requirements for folate and other water-soluble vitamins.

Hepatic Dysfunction. Requirements for folate and zinc are often increased in this population, but certain trace elements (copper and manganese) are normally excreted by the liver and therefore may be contraindicated. Protein restriction is generally not indicated unless encephalopathy is present. Branched-chain amino acid formulations allow for delivery of larger protein loads, but do not affect mortality rate.

Pulmonary Insufficiency. Consumption of calories in excess of requirements can elevate the respiratory quotient and increase CO_2 production. This change can potentially precipitate or worsen hypercapnia, and may interfere with weaning from mechanical ventilation. Avoidance of overfeeding and increasing the fraction of nonprotein calories delivered as lipid will mitigate this effect. Weaning may also be facilitated in some patients by reducing calories to somewhat below the resting energy expenditure. Increased nitrogen losses occur in patients who are taking high-dose steroids for airway disease or other reasons.

Neurologic Injury. Energy expenditure is typically 40 to 50% greater than normal, and is inversely related to Glasgow Coma Scale score. Pentabarbital-induced coma reduces energy expenditure and nitrogen excretion below that predicted. In patients with acute spinal cord injury, energy requirements are similar to those of patients with head injury. Because of the expected metabolic responses, positive nitrogen balance may not be achievable in the first week after injury. Resting energy expenditures for chronically paraplegic and quadriplegic patients typically average 27 and 23 kcal/kg/day, respectively.

Pancreatitis. TPN is indicated in situations associated with protracted abdominal pain, ascites, and high GI fistula drainage. Nutritional support is not indicated for acute and chronic relapsing cases that are mild and last less than 1 week. Lipid emulsion may be safely given if patients are not hyperlipidemic. Triglyceride levels should be maintained at less than 400 mg/dL during lipid infusion and at less than 250 mg/dL after infusion.

Peripheral Parenteral Nutrition

Peripheral parenteral nutrition (PPN) can be an effective means of delivering nutritional support in selected ICU patients. It is appropriate for patients who require parenteral nutrition for a limited period (< 2 weeks) and are not severely malnourished, do not have excessive metabolic requirements (are not hypercatabolic), and can tolerate the large fluid volume necessary in PPN. Advantages of PPN include avoidance of mechanical and infectious complications associated with central vein catheterization.

Osmolarity Considerations. The thrombophlebitic potential of highly osmolar solutions necessitates lower concentrations of dextrose and amino acids when delivered into the peripheral circulation. In general, concentration should be limited to 600–800 mOsm/L, roughly estimated as follows:

$$\text{Osmolarity} \approx (50\ \text{mOsm/L} \times \%\ \text{dextrose}) + (100\ \text{mOsm/L} \times \%\ \text{amino acids})$$

Final osmolarity also depends on the concentration of electrolytes in the formula. Because of these osmolar constraints, conventional PPN has a low caloric density and usually does not completely meet energy goals, even when relatively high infusion volumes are used. A typical mixture consists of equal volumes of 3 to 5% amino acid and 5 to 10% dextrose solutions, with required electrolytes, vitamins, and trace elements. Lipid emulsion has been given through the same IV catheter as the PPN solution or through a separate peripheral IV catheter. Lipid emulsion has also been directly combined with the dextrose–amino acid solution during preparation (triple mixture); however, this practice may increase the risk of calcium phosphate precipitate formation and secondary respiratory complications.

Catheter Maintenance. Several reports have suggested methods to reduce the thrombotic complications associated with PPN. Factors leading to the development of peripheral venous thrombosis include:

- **Cannula size.** Larger, longer, and more rigid catheters are associated with a higher incidence of thrombosis.
- **Particulate matter.** Use of an in-line filter is recommended.
- **Mixture pH.** Incidence is lower when pH is adjusted to 7.2–7.4; however, the stability of buffered solutions is not well established.
- **Trauma of venipuncture.** Significant reduction in flow rate ($\leq$ 50%) occurs secondary to catheter placement alone; topical nitroglycerin administration may prolong vein patency.
- **Osmolarity.** Increased risk is noted with solution strengths of $\geq$ 600 mOsm/L.

Suggested Readings

ASPEN Board of Directors. Guidelines for the use of parenteral and enteral nutrition in adult and pediatric patients. *JPEN* 1993; 17(suppl):1SA–52SA.

Detailed, expert recommendations on role of nutrition in various disease states (e.g., malignancy, renal failure, respiratory failure).

Hongsermeier T, Bistrian BR. Evaluation of a practical technique for determining insulin requirements in diabetic patients receiving total parenteral nutrition. *JPEN* 1993;17:16–19.

Guide to management of hyperglycemia in patients receiving total parenteral nutrition.

Payne-James JJ, Khawaja HT. First choice for total parenteral nutrition: The peripheral route. *JPEN* 1993;17:468–478.

Comprehensive review of indications, techniques, and complications associated with peripheral parenteral nutrition.

Raad II, Bodey GP. Infectious complications of indwelling vascular catheters. *Clin Infect Dis* 1992;197–210.

Provides guidelines for management of the febrile patient with vascular catheters.

Sax HC, Bower RH. Hepatic complications of total parenteral nutrition. *JPEN* 1988;12:615–618.

Describes mechanisms leading to hepatic dysfunction associated with total parenteral nutrition, along with practical means of avoidance.

Renal and Electrolyte Disorders

CHAPTER 51

Hyponatremia and Hypernatremia

(See Chapter 100)

Michael J. Freeland
and James A. Kruse

Disturbances of serum sodium concentration (Na_s) become clinically important only insofar as they reflect disturbances in effective osmolality, or tonicity, and thus the volume of the intracellular fluid (ICF) compartment, which is in osmotic equilibrium with the extracellular fluid (ECF) compartment. Normally, tonicity homeostasis is maintained independently of sodium and volume homeostasis (see Chapter 99 in the main text). Water balance is achieved through osmoregulatory mechanisms that affect water intake by stimulating thirst and influence renal water excretion through the action of antidiuretic hormone (ADH). However, there are also nonosmotic stimuli of ADH release that may result in hyponatremia in a variety of pathophysiologic states. Similarly, hypernatremia may result from deficient ADH secretion or renal hyporesponsiveness to this hormone.

Hyponatremia

Clinical Manifestations. Cerebral edema appears to be the major factor leading to the neurologic disturbances that dominate the clinical manifestations of hyponatremia, which include:

- Headache, malaise, anorexia, nausea, vomiting.
- Lethargy, irritability, confusion, stupor, coma.
- Asterixis, myoclonus, muscle weakness, areflexia.
- Seizures, respiratory arrest.

Most patients do not become symptomatic until Na_s is less than 120 mmol/L, but the severity of symptoms correlates poorly with the degree of hyponatremia. Manifestations of hyponatremia are more dependent on the rapidity with which the Na_s decreases. Although symptoms generally resolve with treatment, hyponatremia can be fatal, and permanent neurologic sequelae can occur among survivors.

Differential Diagnosis. A practical approach to determining the etiology of hyponatremia is to determine serum osmolality or tonicity and then, if necessary, to evaluate the ECF volume status (Figure 51–1). Isotonic hyponatremia is recognized by the finding of apparent hyponatremia in the presence of normal serum osmolality (Osm_s). The additional serum space occupied by excess lipids or proteins interferes with volumetric laboratory determinations, resulting in a spuriously decreased assay result. However, the physiologically important concentration of sodium per liter of plasma water remains normal. Because the low sodium concentration is only artifactual, it is sometimes called pseudohyponatremia. The discovery of elevation of serum lipid or protein levels confirms the diagnosis. Because there is no true disturbance in sodium activity, no treatment is required to correct the sodium value. Nonspurious isotonic hyponatremia can occur after IV infusions of isotonic glucose or mannitol.

Hypertonic hyponatremia is caused by the accumulation in the plasma of effective osmoles other than sodium. This accumulation results in shifting of water from the ICF to the ECF compartment, with dilution of all plasma solutes, including sodium. The most common offending osmole is glucose. Therapeutic administration of hypertonic solutions of osmotically active substances, such as mannitol, is another cause. Hypertonic hyponatremia can be excluded by measuring Osm_s or, in patients who have not received osmotherapy, by measuring serum glucose level. Treatment of hyperglycemia or discontinuation of mannitol therapy will result in correction of the hyponatremia.

Hypotonic (hypo-osmolar) hyponatremia is responsible for most cases of hyponatremia. In this form of hyponatremia, Na_s is low because of an excess of plasma water relative to sodium, resulting in dilutional hyponatremia. (Unless otherwise qualified, the term hyponatremia will be used below to describe situations in which low Na_s is indicative of hypotonicity.) The differential diagnosis is long, but can usually be narrowed by clinical assessment of the patient's ECF volume status:

- **Hypovolemic hyponatremia** caused by volume-depletion states, e.g., salt-wasting nephropathies, Addison's disease, vomiting, nasogastric suctioning, diarrhea, diuretic or laxative use, third-space fluid losses (e.g., pancreatitis, peritonitis, ileus).
- **Hypervolemic hyponatremia** (edematous states) caused by cirrhosis, nephrosis, congestive heart failure, renal failure.
- **Euvolemic hyponatremia** caused by hypothyroidism, the syndrome of inappropriate antidiuretic hormone secretion (SIADH), reset osmostat syndrome, psychogenic polydipsia.

Hypovolemia is suggested by the presence of physical findings such as tachycardia, orthostatic hypotension, and low central venous pressure. On the other hand, neck-vein

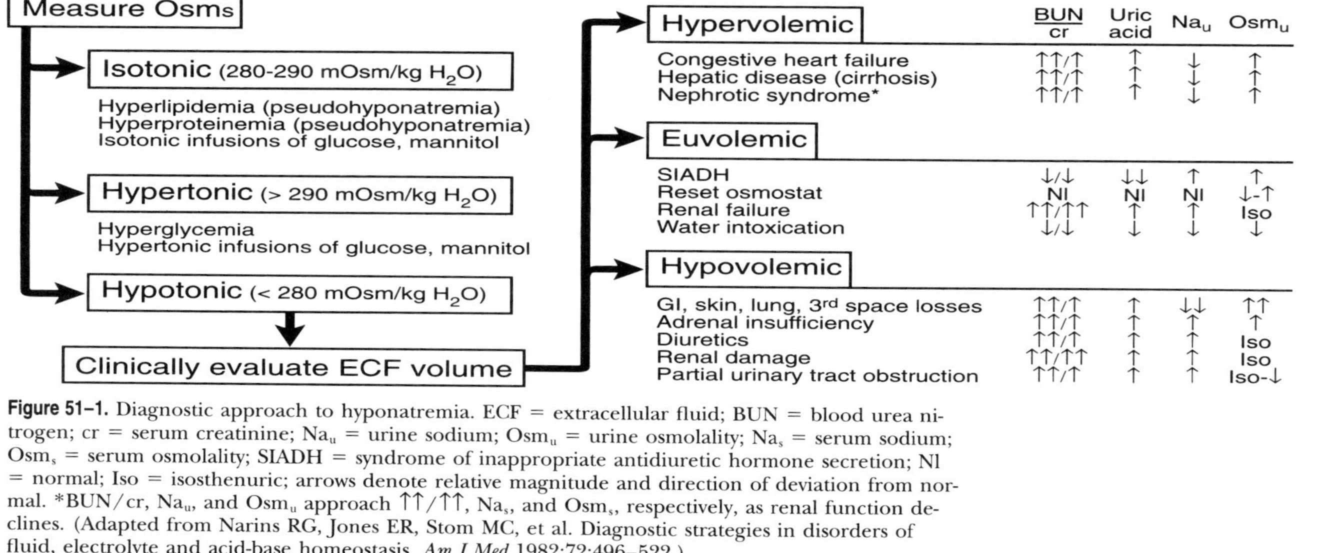

Figure 51–1. Diagnostic approach to hyponatremia. ECF = extracellular fluid; BUN = blood urea nitrogen; cr = serum creatinine; Na_u = urine sodium; Osm_u = urine osmolality; Na_s = serum sodium; Osm_s = serum osmolality; SIADH = syndrome of inappropriate antidiuretic hormone secretion; Nl = normal; Iso = isosthenuric; arrows denote relative magnitude and direction of deviation from normal. *BUN/cr, Na_u, and Osm_u approach ↑↑/↑↑, Na_s, and Osm_s, respectively, as renal function declines. (Adapted from Narins RG, Jones ER, Stom MC, et al. Diagnostic strategies in disorders of fluid, electrolyte and acid-base homeostasis. *Am J Med* 1982;72:496–522.)

distension and pitting edema suggest hypervolemia. The absence of any of these findings suggests a clinically euvolemic state. The causes of hypovolemic and hypervolemic hyponatremia are often obvious from the patient's clinical history and physical findings. The presence of other electrolyte and acid–base disturbances may provide additional clues. For example, hyponatremia caused by diuretic use, vomiting, diarrhea, or adrenal insufficiency is frequently associated with characteristic derangements in potassium and acid–base balance.

SIADH is the most common form of hypotonic hyponatremia associated with a clinically euvolemic state. It is most often the result of central nervous system (CNS) disorders, pulmonary diseases that stimulate ADH release, or neoplasms that synthesize and secrete ADH:

- **CNS causes** include head trauma, intracranial hemorrhage, encephalitis, brain tumor, stroke, Guillain-Barré syndrome, and acute intermittent porphyria.
- **Pulmonary causes** include bacterial, viral, or fungal pneumonia; tuberculosis; lung abscess; cystic fibrosis; and bronchiectasis.
- **Neoplastic causes** include oat cell carcinoma of the lung, carcinoma of the duodenum, carcinoma of the pancreas, thymoma, and lymphoma.

A variety of endocrine disorders, including hypothyroidism and glucocorticoid and mineralocorticoid deficiency, are also associated with SIADH. Non–ADH-mediated mechanisms may be operative with some of the drug- and endocrine-related causes. A number of drugs may impair renal water excretion through several ADH-mediated mechanisms:

- **ADH analogues** include oxytocin and desamino-D-arginine vasopressin.
- **Stimulants of ADH release** include chlorpropamide, clofibrate, carbamezapine, cyclophosphamide, vincristine, neuroleptics, antidepressants, and narcotics.
- **Potentiators of ADH action** include chlorpropamide, cyclophosphamide, and nonsteroidal anti-inflammatory drugs.

Clinically, SIADH is a diganosis of exclusion. A urine osmolality (Osm_u) greater than 100 mOsm/kg H_2O is necessary to exclude primary water intoxication. Nonosmotic stimuli of ADH release must also be excluded. These include ECF volume depletion, hypotension, severe pain, and acute psychosis. The criteria for diagnosis of SIADH can be summarized as follows:

- $Na_s < 135$ mmol/L and $Osm_s < 280$ mOsm/kg H_2O.
- Clinical euvolemia.
- $Osm_u > 100$ mOsm/kg H_2O

- Normal renal, cardiac, hepatic, adrenal, pituitary, and thyroid function.
- Absence of drugs that impair renal water excretion.
- Absence of severe emotional or physical stress.
- $Na_u > 20$ mmol/L in the absence of restricted sodium intake.

Although it is not a criterion for diagnosis, hypouricemia is common in SIADH, and reflects the increased GFR and decreased net reabsorption of uric acid that accompanies chronic hypervolemia.

Some patients appear to have SIADH but show normal renal water handling while maintaining a low Na_s. This finding suggests that their osmostat mechanism is set at a lower level as opposed to having excess ADH.

Treatment. Hypertonic saline administration should be considered in the patient with neurologic manifestations, such as seizures. Considerable controversy exists regarding the ideal rate and magnitude of correction of Na_s. A syndrome of osmotic demyelination may complicate too rapid or excessive correction. This rare, but catastrophic complication is associated with demyelinating CNS lesions, particularly in the pons, and is manifested by delayed neurologic deterioration, including flaccid quadriplegia, pseudobulbar palsy, and alterations in mental status. Chronic debilitating illness, underlying liver disease, structural lesions of the CNS, diuretic use, a hypoxic episode, and female gender are believed to be predisposing factors. Although the distinction is often not easily made, patients with chronic hyponatremia (> 48 hours) are believed to be at greater risk for this syndrome than those with acute hyponatremia.

Although consensus is lacking, the following approach to treating severe hyponatremia seems prudent:

- Increase the Na_s by no more than 1–2 mmol/L/hr.
- Increase the Na_s by no more than 10–12 mmol/L acutely and no more than 12–20 mmol/L/day or 25 mmol/L over the initial 48 hours.
- Do not completely correct the Na_s acutely, but aim for a target Na_s of 120–130 mmol/L.
- Avoid overcorrection of the Na_s.

Hypovolemic hyponatremia is treated with isotonic saline, discontinuation of diuretics and, in the case of adrenal insufficiency, hormone replacement. In the asymptomatic patient, isotonic saline should be used to restore the effective circulating volume and normalize the Na_s. The severely symptomatic patient, however, may require hypertonic saline. The required volume of 3% saline (in liters) and infusion rate can be calculated as follows:

$$\text{Volume of 3\% saline} = \frac{0.6 \times \text{Weight(kg)} \times (\text{Desired } Na_s - \text{Current } Na_s)}{513 \text{ mmol/L}}$$

$$\text{Infusion rate} = \frac{\text{Volume of 3\% saline}}{(\text{Desired Na}_s - \text{Current Na}_s)/\text{Rate of correction}}$$

Patients with clinically hypervolemic hyponatremia rarely become severely symptomatic. This situation is fortunate because treatment with hypertonic saline would exacerbate the volume overload. Asymptomatic patients can often be managed with water restriction alone or in combination with a loop diuretic. Restriction of water intake to 500 mL less than urine output and combined enteral losses usually provides for a negative water balance of 700–900 mL/day from insensible loss. These patients usually require sodium as well as water restriction. In addition to diuretic therapy, those with decreased effective circulating volume on the basis of heart failure may benefit from afterload reduction or inotropic support. Those with cirrhosis and nephrosis may temporarily improve with administration of IV albumin. Low-dose dopamine has also been employed in the management of these patients.

Asymptomatic hyponatremia due to water intoxication, SIADH, or fluid overload associated with renal failure should be managed by water restriction. However, patients with SIADH who cannot dilute their urine to less than 300 mOsm/kg H_2O may be poorly compliant with the severe restriction sometimes required to achieve negative water balance. These patients can be treated with low doses of a loop diuretic (e.g., furosemide 20 mg PO twice daily) in combination with a high-salt diet to prevent volume depletion or with administration of an agent that inhibits ADH action. Demeclocycline at a dose of 300–600 mg PO twice daily is the drug most frequently used. Lithium has also been used, but has the potential for significant toxicity. Thiazide diuretics, because they do not interfere with urinary concentrating ability, should not be used.

In the treatment of the severely symptomatic patient with SIADH, hypertonic saline is usually combined with a loop diuretic. The loop diuretic promotes water excretion, and the hypertonic saline is used to replace urinary sodium losses. Potassium chloride supplementation is sometimes required as well. As a guide to this therapy, the following formula can be used to estimate excess body water in liters from the patient's current body weight and Na_s:

$$\text{Excess body water} = 0.6 \times \text{Weight (kg)} \times \left(1 - \frac{\text{Current Na}_s}{\text{Desired Na}_s}\right)$$

The urine flow needed to excrete this excess water and increase the Na_s at any desired rate can be estimated by:

$$\text{Urine flow} = \frac{\text{Excess body water}}{\text{Desired Na}_s - \text{Current Na}_s} \times \text{Desired rate of Na}_s \text{ correction}$$

Furosemide is administered to produce a diuresis slightly in excess of this calculated excretion of free water, and 3% saline is infused at a rate necessary to replace urinary sodium losses based on the measure of urine sodium concentration (Na_u):

$$\text{Infusion rate} = \frac{\text{Na}_u \times \text{Urine flow}}{513 \text{ mmol/L}}$$

As an initial estimate, Na_u after furosemide administration approximates that of 0.45% saline (i.e., approximately 77 mmol/L). Beyond the initial period of therapy, however, treatment should be guided by frequent monitoring of serum and urine electrolytes as well as hourly urine flow. Treatment with hypertonic saline alone may be relatively ineffective in patients with a high Osm_u. The treatment of drug-induced SIADH should include discontinuation of the offending agent. Drugs that impair water excretion should be avoided. Patients with reset osmostat, sometimes said to have essential hyponatremia, usually do not require any treatment.

Hypernatremia

Clinical Manifestations. Cellular dehydration and loss of brain volume are believed to be the primary causes of the neurologic symptoms that also dominate the clinical picture of severe hypernatremia. These manifestations may include:

- Fever, nausea, vomiting, irritability.
- Lethargy, stupor, coma.
- Muscle weakness, fasciculations, spasticity.
- Seizures (unusual before institution of therapy).

Brain shrinkage may place enough traction on the intracerebral veins to cause them to rupture. In response to chronic hypernatremia, idiogenic osmoles are postulated to accumulate in the brain cells to help minimize cerebral dehydration.

Differential Diagnosis. Hypernatremia can develop by only two mechanisms, either alone or in combination: pure water loss or gain of hypertonic sodium salts. Thirst is a strong defense against hypernatremia. Patients with an intact thirst mechanism and the ability to access water do not become hypernatremic. Therefore, hypernatremia is always associated with either impairment of thirst or impaired access to water. For this reason, hypernatremia is most likely to occur in patients at the extremes of age or in those with intercurrent illness.

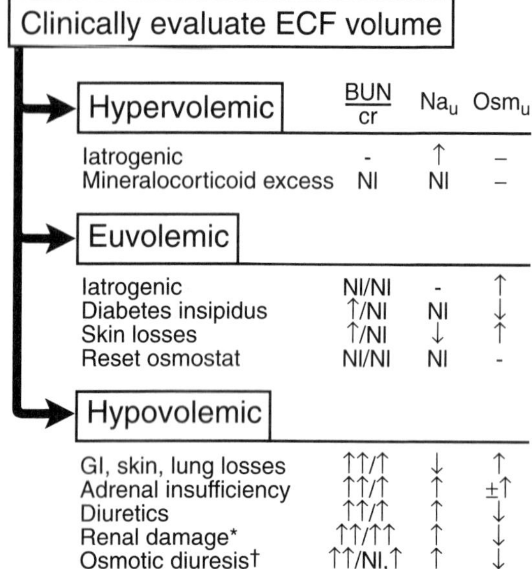

Figure 51–2. Differential diagnosis of hypernatremia. ECF = extracellular fluid; BUN = blood urea nitrogen; cr = serum creatinine; Na_u = urine sodium; Osm_u = urine osmolality; Nl = normal; – = variable; arrows denote relative magnitude and direction of deviation from normal. *Includes polyuric renal failure, partial urinary tract obstruction. †For example, glycosuria, treatment with mannitol, urea diuresis. (Adapted from Narins RG, Jones ER, Stom MC, et al. Diagnostic strategies in disorders of fluid, electrolyte and acid-base homeostasis. *Am J Med* 1982;72:496–522.)

As with hyponatremia, the diagnostic approach to hypernatremia is simplified by categorizing patients according to clinical assessment of their ECF volume (Figure 51–2). Hypovolemic hypernatremia indicates a loss of both water and sodium, but water to a greater degree.

Hypervolemic hypernatremia indicates a gain of both sodium and water, but sodium to a greater degree. In hospitalized patients, this condition is most often iatrogenic, caused by overtreatment with hypertonic saline or sodium bicarbonate. Endogenous or exogenous mineralocorticoid excess causes sodium retention and ECF volume expansion. The expanded ECF space suppresses or resets the threshold for ADH release.

Clinically, euvolemic hypernatremia indicates pure water loss (e.g., as a result of diabetes insipidus), replacement of hypotonic losses with isotonic saline, or a reset osmostat (sometimes referred to as essential hypernatremia or primary hypodipsia).

Treatment. All forms of hypernatremia require free-water replacement to lower Na_s. Replacement may be accomplished by either the IV or enteral route. As with hyponatremia, rapid correction of hypernatremia can result in rapid fluid shifts in the brain, with potentially serious consequences. The same idiogenic osmoles that preserve brain water and conserve intracellular brain volume in chronic hypernatremia increase the risk of cerebral edema during correction of the hypertonic state. It is generally accepted that initial water repletion should proceed more rapidly in the treatment of symptomatic acute hypernatremia than in the treatment of symptomatic chronic hypernatremia. In either case, the free-water deficit (in liters) may be estimated from the patient's current body weight and Na_s as follows:

$$\text{Water deficit} = 0.6 \times \text{Weight} \times \left(\frac{\text{Current Na}_s}{\text{Desired Na}_s} - 1\right)$$

where "weight" represents the patient's current body weight in kilograms. Guidelines for replacement of this deficit and lowering of Na_s include:

- In acute hyponatremia, replace approximately half of the calculated water deficit over the first 12–24 hours.
- Avoid reduction of Na_s by >2 mmol/L/hr in acute hyponatremia.
- In chronic hypernatremia, lower the Na_s initially at a rate of 1–2 mmol/L/hr.

Deterioration in neurologic status after initial improvement in symptoms suggests the development of cerebral edema and requires discontinuation of water replacement until neurologic status improves. When symptoms have resolved, more gradual replacement, over several days, is appropriate. The method by which these above goals are achieved varies based on the ECF volume status of the patient.

In hypovolemic hypernatremia, treatment is directed at restoration of the ECF volume deficit as well as replacement of the free-water deficit. Isotonic (0.9%) saline should be used initially to correct any circulatory compromise. Free-water replacement is then instituted by a change to hypotonic saline, 5% dextrose in water, or enteral water administration. Reduction of excessive free-water losses may require treatment of fever, control of hyperglycemia, reduction of osmotic load (e.g., decreased protein in parenteral nutrition formula), evaluation of and appropriate intervention directed toward the cause of diarrhea, or attempts at reduction of enteric fistula or nasogastric drainage (e.g., by administering somatostatin or an H_2-receptor blocking agent). Insensible losses are estimated to be 0.6 mL/kg/hr in an afebrile patient, increasing by 20% for each 1°C rise in body temperature.

Patients with hypervolemic hypernatremia require removal of the source of sodium and water gain (e.g., discontinuation of hypertonic saline or sodium bicarbonate administration) followed by removal of the excess sodium. Volume expansion and hypernatremia induce natriuresis. Nevertheless, in the setting of acute hypernatremia, it may be necessary to enhance urinary sodium loss through the use of a loop diuretic. Urine losses are then replaced with an equal volume of 5% dextrose in water. Patients with renal failure or an inadequate response to diuretics may require dialysis.

See Chapter 62 in this book for a discussion of the treatment of euvolemic hypernatremia caused by diabetes insipidus.

Suggested Readings

Anderson RJ. Hospital-associated hyponatremia. *Kidney Int* 1986; 29:1237–1247.

Case report and review of clinical approach to and outcome determinants of hyponatremia.

Arieff AI, Ayus JC. Treatment of symptomatic hyponatremia: Neither haste nor waste. *Crit Care Med* 1991;19:748–751.

Editorial on controversy surrounding the rapid versus slow therapeutic approach to hyponatremia.

Berl T. Treating hyponatremia: Damned if we do and damned if we don't. *Kidney Int* 1990;37:1006–1018.

Discusses therapeutic dilemma of deciding on optimal rate of correction of hyponatremia.

Martinez-Maldonado M. Inappropriate antidiuretic hormone secretion of unknown origin. *Kidney Int* 1980;17:554–567.

Narins RG, Jones ER, Stom MC, et al. Diagnostic strategies in disorders of fluid, electrolyte and acid-base homeostasis. *Am J Med* 1982;72:496–522.

Classic and extensive review of disorders of sodium, other serum electrolytes, and acid–base balance.

Oh MS, Carroll HJ. Disorders of sodium metabolism: Hypernatremia and hyponatremia. *Crit Care Med* 1992;20:94–103.

Covers pathogenesis, diagnosis, and treatment of these two electrolyte disorders (34 references).

Sterns RH. Severe hyponatremia: The case for conservative management. *Crit Care Med* 1992;20:534–539.

Weisberg LS. Pseudohyponatremia: A reappraisal. *Am J Med* 1989; 86:315–318.

Explains in detail why pseudohyponatremia occurs and why the sodium assay result depends on the particular laboratory methodology employed.

CHAPTER 52

Hypokalemia and Hyperkalemia

(See Chapter 101)

James A. Kruse

Hypokalemia

Hypokalemia is one of the most common electrolyte disturbances among ICU patients. Severe hypokalemia that occurs during hospitalization can often be prevented by anticipating GI and renal potassium (K^+) losses, providing adequate amounts of K^+ in maintenance IV fluids, and monitoring serum potassium concentration (K_s) at appropriate intervals.

Clinical Manifestations. Hypokalemia is often not recognized clinically, except by measurement of K_s. Its potential manifestations involve the following systems:

- **Cardiac,** such as ventricular dysrhythmias, ECG abnormalities (flattened T waves, prominent U waves, ST segment depression, conduction defects; see Figure 52–1).
- **Neuromuscular,** such as weakness, paralysis (with respiratory failure), gastroparesis, paralytic ileus, rhabdomyolysis.
- **Metabolic,** such as glucose intolerance, negative nitrogen balance.
- **Renal,** such as polyuria, polydipsia, increased ammonium production (leading to exacerbation of hepatic encephalopathy), metabolic alkalosis.

Etiologies. Causes of hypokalemia include:

- **Inadequate K^+ intake,** e.g., starvation, anorexia nervosa, chronic alcoholism, inadequate K^+ supplementation, insufficient K^+ added to parenteral nutrition formulas.
- **Pharmacologic agents,** e.g., thiazide and loop diuretics, insulin, glucose, sodium bicarbonate, β-adrenergic agonists, carbenoxolone, cisplatin, certain antibiotics (e.g., sodium penicillin, carbenicillin, ticarcillin, gentamicin, amphotericin B, rifampicin), corticosteroids, L-dopa, granulocyte–macrophage colony-stimulating factor.
- **Transcellular distribution,** e.g., insulin (and treatment of diabetic ketoacidosis), alkalemia, refeeding syndrome, treatment of megaloblastic anemia, familial hypokalemic periodic paralysis, barium poisoning.
- **GI K^+ loss,** e.g., diarrhea, vomiting, nasogastric suction, villous adenoma, laxative abuse.

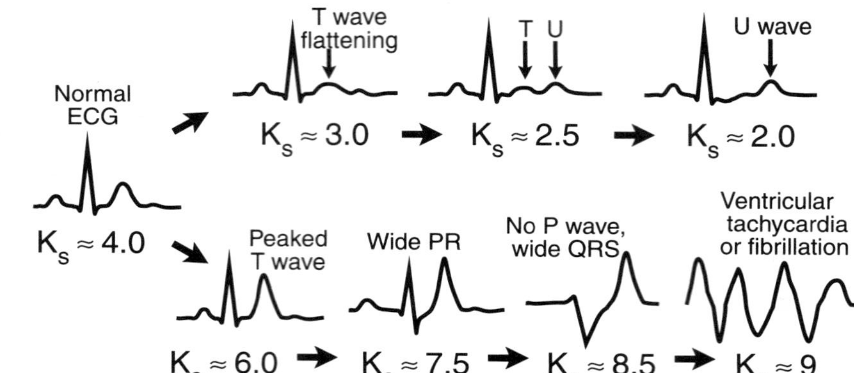

Figure 52–1. Representative ECG manifestations of hypokalemia and hyperkalemia. K_s = serum potassium concentration in mmol/L.

- **Renal K^+ loss,** e.g., proximal and distal renal tubular acidosis, ureterosigmoidostomy, diuretic phase of acute tubular necrosis, postobstructive diuresis, polyuria of any cause.
- **Mineralocorticoid excess,** e.g., primary (Conn's syndrome) and secondary hyperaldosteronism, Cushing's syndrome, congenital adrenal hyperplasia, ectopic ACTH (adrenocorticotropic hormone) syndrome, licorice ingestion.
- **Miscellaneous causes,** e.g., post-resuscitation, post-myocardial infarction, hypercalcemia, hypomagnesemia, Bartter's syndrome, Liddle's syndrome.

The most common cause of hypokalemia among patients who have been in the hospital for more than a day is probably inadequate supplementation.

Treatment. K_s decreases by approximately 0.3 mmol/L for every 100 mmol of total body K^+ deficiency, assuming the hypokalemia is caused by deficiency and not transcellular redistribution. Therefore, total body K^+ level is often deficient by 200 mmol or more before hypokalemia becomes apparent. Mild degrees of hypokalemia in stable patients often can be treated with oral K^+ supplements. In critically ill patients, oral supplementation is often not possible and parenteral supplementation is necessary. IV administration is also mandatory for severe degrees of hypokalemia. K^+ must not be administered by rapid IV injection (i.e., IV push) because life-threatening hyperkalemia can result. Hypokalemic patients undergoing continuous ECG monitoring in an ICU setting can be safely given 20 mmol KCl (diluted, for example, in 100 mL saline) by controlled IV infusion over at least 1 hour. A series of infusions may be administered in this manner, with the number of infusions determined by the severity of the hypokalemia. It is prudent not to exceed 60 mmol without reevaluating K_s. Although there can be considerable individual variation, the average increase in K_s with this method of replacement is 0.25 mmol/L per 20 mmol infusion. The amount of replacement needed depends not only on the total body deficit, but also on ongoing K^+ losses and any concomitant factors that affect the internal distribution of K^+ between tissues and plasma. Profound degrees of hypokalemia may require rates of administration exceeding 20 mmol/hr; however, this must be done cautiously, with frequent monitoring of K_s. Dangerous levels of hyperkalemia can occur during parenteral K^+ replacement. This situation is particularly likely to occur in patients who have underlying renal dysfunction, who are receiving drugs that can cause hyperkalemia, and who are receiving K^+ supplementation by multiple routes (e.g., by intermittent K^+ infusions along with concomitant oral supplements, K^+-containing parenteral nutrition formulas, or K^+-containing maintenance IV infusions).

Hyperkalemia

Although hyperkalemia is much less common than hypokalemia in hospitalized patients, it is not rare. Even mild degrees of hyperkalemia should alert the clinician to the possibility of further elevations into the life-threatening range. Thus, frequent monitoring of K_s concentration is mandatory in patients with any degree of hyperkalemia. A K_s level greater than 6 mmol/L should be considered an emergency that requires immediate treatment.

Clinical Manifestations. Hyperkalemia primarily affects the heart. Life-threatening ventricular dysrhythmias can occur, including ventricular tachycardia, flutter, and fibrillation. Usually, the earliest ECG finding is the appearance of tall, peaked T waves (see Figure 52–1). Other ECG abnormalities may include prolongation of PR or QRS intervals and absence of P waves, despite underlying sinus rhythm (sinoventricular rhythm). Dangerous degrees of hyperkalemia can occur despite a normal ECG appearance, and the first ECG manifestation may be ventricular fibrillation. Neuromuscular effects of hyperkalemia may include weakness, paresthesias, and paralysis. As with hypokalemia, hyperkalemia is often not recognized clinically, except by measurement of K_s.

Etiologies. Measuring K_s at appropriate intervals and recognizing the various etiologies of hyperkalemia will decrease the risk of hyperkalemia in critically ill patients. Causes of hyperkalemia include:

- **Excessive K^+ intake,** such as oral or IV K^+ supplements, parenteral nutrition formulas, salt substitutes, K^+ salts of drugs (e.g., potassium penicillin), blood transfusions, cardioplegic solutions, renal allograft preservatives.
- **Primary renal causes,** such as acute or chronic renal failure, intrinsic K^+ secretory defects (e.g., tubulointerstitial renal disease, sickle cell disease, systemic lupus erythematosus, amyloidosis, renal transplantation, obstructive uropathy).
- **Transcellular distribution,** such as cell lysis syndromes (e.g., rhabdomyolysis, tumor lysis, massive hemolysis, extensive burns, reabsorption of hematoma, GI hemorrhage, mesenteric infarction), hypertonicity (e.g., glucose, saline, mannitol), insulin deficiency, inorganic metabolic acidosis, respiratory acidosis, malignant hyperthermia, hyperkalemic periodic paralysis.
- **Mineralocorticoid deficiency,** such as Addison's disease, hyporeninemic hypoaldosteronism (e.g., caused by diabetes, lead nephropathy, acquired immune defi-

ciency syndrome [AIDS], systemic lupus erythematosus), hyperreninemic hypoaldosteronism, pseudohypoaldosteronism.

- **Pharmacologic agents,** such as amiloride, spironolactone, triamterene, angiotensin-converting enzyme inhibitors, nonsteroidal anti-inflammatory drugs, succinylcholine, β-adrenergic antagonists, α-adrenergic agonists, digitalis intoxication, lithium, heparin, pentamidine, cyclosporin, arginine or lysine hydrochloride.
- **Pseudohyperkalemia,** such as caused by laboratory error, prolonged tourniquet application, in vitro hemolysis, thrombocytosis, or leukocytosis.

Treatment. K^+ supplements should be discontinued and the cause of the hyperkalemia investigated. Severe hyperkalemia must be considered an emergency requiring immediate therapy. Continuous ECG monitoring is mandatory. However, prompt initiation of treatment should not be delayed because of lack of typical ECG changes. Emergency treatment of hyperkalemia is designed to antagonize the potential cardiac effects of K^+; as a temporizing measure, to lower K_s by redistributing K^+ into the cells; and to lower K_s by promoting K^+ elimination from the body. These goals can be accomplished with the following treatments:

- **Calcium gluconate.** Usual dose is 10–20 mL of a 10% solution IV; acts as membrane antagonist (cardioprotective effect); onset is in seconds to minutes, with a duration of 30–60 minutes.
- **Sodium bicarbonate.** Usual dose is 50–100 mmol IV; onset is within 15 minutes; duration is several hours; acts as membrane antagonist and drives K^+ into cells; lest precipitation occurs, do not administer calcium and bicarbonate through the same IV line unless the tubing is flushed between infusions.
- **Insulin and glucose.** Typical dose is 10 units of regular insulin IV plus 25 g glucose IV; onset is within minutes, and effect can last several hours; affects redistribution of K^+; can be repeated every 2–3 hours if necessary.
- **Albuterol.** 10–20 mg given by nebulized aerosol; onset is within minutes, and duration may be several hours; affects redistribution of K^+.
- **Hypertonic saline,** e.g., 3% sodium chloride; onset is within minutes; duration is up to several hours; acts by membrane antagonism; sodium bicarbonate is usually employed instead, but hypertonic saline may be useful in patients with combined hyperkalemia, hyponatremia, and alkalemia; necessitates caution in selecting dose to avoid hypernatremia and fluid overload.
- **Cation exchange resin.** Typically initiated with 20–50 g sodium polystyrene sulfonate (Kayexalate) given PO, by nasogastric tube, or per rectum, along with sorbitol; on-

set is approximately 2 hours; duration is 4–6 hours; affects elimination of K^+ from GI tract by exchanging sodium and potassium; repeated dosing is usually necessary (e.g., every 3–8 hours).

- **Diuretics,** e.g., furosemide (typical dose is 40 mg IV, but depends on renal functional level); increases renal K^+ excretion; onset and duration parallel diuresis.
- **Dialysis** removes K^+ from the body; onset is immediate on initiation of hemodialysis (slower for peritoneal dialysis).

Mild cases of hyperkalemia can often be treated with cation exchange resin alone. Severe cases require calcium gluconate, followed by glucose and insulin, sodium bicarbonate, or both, and administration of cation exchange resin. Exchange resin treatment is more effective if given orally compared with rectal retention enemas. Each gram of administered resin typically removes approximately 0.5 (if given rectally) to 1 (if given orally) mmol of K^+. Dialysis is often necessary in patients with hyperkalemia and underlying renal failure.

Suggested Readings

Allon A, Dunlay R, Copkney C. Nebulized albuterol for acute hyperkalemia in patients on hemodialysis. *Ann Intern Med* 1989;110:426–429.
A significant decrease in serum potassium concentration was evident by 30 minutes and was sustained for at least 2 hours after treatment with this β_2-adrenergic agonist. Mean maximal decrease in serum potassium concentration was 0.62 mmol/L after administration of 10 mg albuterol and was 0.98 mmol/L after administration of 20 mg.

Kruse JA, Carlson RW. Rapid correction of hypokalemia using concentrated intravenous potassium chloride infusions. *Arch Intern Med* 1990;150:613–617.
Retrospective study reporting the effects of consecutive 20-mmol K^+ infusions, given by central or peripheral IV over 1 hour, to a large group of ICU patients. Among 495 sets of infusions, there were 10 instances of hyperkalemia.

Kruse JA, Clark VL, Carlson RW, et al. Concentrated potassium chloride infusions in critically ill patients with hypokalemia. *J Clin Pharmacol* 1994;34:1077–1082.
Prospective study examining effects of a single 20-mmol K^+ infusion given over 1 hour on plasma potassium levels and ECG findings. Mean change in plasma potassium concentration at the end of the 1-hour infusion was 0.48 mmol/L, and mean change 1 hour later was 0.25 mmol/L. The frequency of premature ventricular beats significantly decreased during infusion period, compared with the 1-hour preinfusion period.

Weisberg LS, Szerlip HM, Cox M. Disorders of potassium homeostasis in critically ill patients. *Crit Care Clin* 1987;5:835–854.
Concise review (75 references).

Wrenn KD, Slovis CM, Slovis BS, et al. The ability of physicians to predict hyperkalemia from the ECG. *Ann Emerg Med* 1991;20:1229–1232.
Demonstrates low sensitivity of using ECG analysis to estimate severity of hyperkalemia. Specificity is higher, but initiating empiric therapy for hyperkalemia based on ECG findings alone will lead to inappropriate treatment in at least 15% of patients.

CHAPTER 53

Disturbances of Calcium, Magnesium, and Phosphorus

(See Chapters 102 and 103)

Michael J. Freeland

Calcium

Calcium exists in plasma in three forms: a free ionized fraction, constituting 45–50%; a protein-bound (primarily to albumin) fraction, constituting 40%; and a nonionized fraction, complexed to a variety of anions and constituting 10–15%. The ionized fraction is physiologically active. Hypoalbuminemia reduces the total calcium measurement and the bound fraction, but does not change the ionized fraction. On the other hand, changes in pH may lower the ionized fraction (alkaline pH) or increase it (acid pH) without changing the total calcium measurement. Direct measurement of ionized calcium is necessary to accurately evaluate the physiologically active fraction.

The extracellular ionized calcium level is maintained within a narrow range through regulation of calcium absorption from the gut, calcium exchange between bone and the extracellular fluid, and calcium reabsorption or excretion by the kidneys. Three calcium-regulating hormones participate in the control of these processes: parathyroid hormone (PTH), calcitonin, and vitamin D sterols.

Hypocalcemia. Although low total and calculated ionized calcium levels have been found in 70–90% of ICU patients, the incidence of measured ionized hypocalcemia is much more variable, occurring in 10–70% of patients, depending on the type of ICU population studied. Causes of hypocalcemia include:

- **Sepsis and septic shock.**
- **Circulatory shock and cardiac arrest.**
- **Renal failure,** e.g., decreased production of calcitriol.
- **Acid–base disorders,** e.g., alkalemia, lactic acidosis.
- **Chelation,** e.g., hyperphosphatemia, blood transfusion, lipids.
- **Pancreatitis,** e.g., calcium soap formation, free fatty acids.
- **Miscellaneous causes,** e.g., burns, primary hypoparathyroidism, pseudohypoparathyroidism, anticonvulsants (increased metabolism of calciferol), plicamycin

(mithramycin), colchicine (inhibition of bone resorption).

Neuromuscular irritability and muscle weakness dominate the clinical presentation of symptomatic hypocalcemia, although cardiovascular and psychiatric disturbances may also be present. Neuromuscular findings include paresthesias, tetany, muscle cramps, seizures, depression, dementia, movement disorders, and proximal myopathy. Cardiovascular findings include QT and ST interval prolongation, bradycardia, heart block, congestive heart failure, and hypotension. These findings are rare unless the ionized calcium level is less than 0.8 mmol/L, but their appearance depends not only on the absolute concentration, but also on the rapidity with which the calcium level decreases.

Evaluation of the hypocalcemic patient should routinely include determination of serum magnesium and phosphorus levels. Severe hypomagnesemia (< 0.4 mmol/L) results in inhibition of PTH secretion as well as skeletal resistance to PTH. Increases in serum magnesium level (> 2.2 mmol/L) may also suppress PTH release as well as reduce renal calcium reabsorption. Acute hyperphosphatemia can lead to hypocalcemia by chelation with ionized calcium, resulting in ectopic calcification of soft tissues. Chronic hyperphosphatemia reduces the synthesis of calcitriol, the most active form of vitamin D. The risk of soft-tissue calcification is greatly increased when the product of the serum phosphorus and total calcium concentrations exceeds 5.6 $mmol^2/L^2$ (70 mg^2/dL^2).

Because of concerns that routine calcium supplementation may be detrimental in the critically ill patient, the clinician should employ replacement therapy judiciously, even when measured ionized hypocalcemia has been shown. Symptomatic and severe ionized hypocalcemia should be treated with IV infusion of 100–300 mg elemental calcium over 10 to 15 minutes. This dose represents 1–3 g calcium gluconate (93 mg elemental calcium/g) or 1 g calcium chloride (272 mg elemental calcium/g). Calcium gluconate may be preferable to calcium chloride because it is less irritating to the veins. Except in emergent situations, calcium should be diluted before IV administration (e.g., 100–200 mg elemental calcium in ≥ 100 mL 5% dextrose in water). Highly concentrated solutions can be toxic to tissues, and are most safely administered through a central vein. Rapid administration may result in hypertension, nausea, vomiting, flushing, bradycardia, heart block, or chest pain, and may induce digitalis-toxic dysrhythmias. Bolus doses of calcium increase the ionized level for only a short period (sometimes only 1–2 hours), and may necessitate repeated boluses or a continuous infusion. If symptoms are severe or do not resolve, a continuous infusion of calcium should be administered at a rate of 0.3–2.5 mg/kg/hr, with ionized calcium level determinations taken every 2 to 4 hours. After the ionized calcium level has normalized (usually requiring several hours), the infusion rate should be decreased to 0.3–0.5 mg/kg/hr. Resolution of symptoms, not normalization of the ionized calcium level, should be the endpoint in patients with severe hyperphosphatemia. If magnesium depletion is suspected and renal function is intact, magnesium sulfate may be administered empirically and continued if a serum magnesium level obtained before therapy is low. Once the ionized calcium level is stable, calcium may be given by the enteral route. Most patients require 1–4 g elemental calcium daily, which is best given in divided doses between meals. Vitamin D supplementation may be required as well.

Hypercalcemia. Hypercalcemia is encountered far less frequently in critically ill patients than is hypocalcemia. Causes of hypercalcemia include:

- **Malignancy-associated hypercalcemia,** such as solid tumors with or without bone metastases, hematologic malignancies.
- **Primary hyperparathyroidism.**
- **Thyrotoxicosis.**
- **Vitamin D and A intoxication.**
- **Granulomatous disorders.**
- **Adrenal insufficiency.**
- **Thiazide diuretics.**
- **Recovery phase of acute tubular necrosis,** especially if caused by rhabdomyolysis.
- **Renal transplant.**

The clinical manifestations of acute hypercalcemia can involve multiple organ systems. Central nervous system (CNS) symptoms include confusion, memory loss, stupor, coma, and neurogenic muscle weakness. Renal disorders include polyuria secondary to acquired nephrogenic diabetes insipidus, decreased glomerular filtration secondary to renal vasoconstriction, and tubular obstruction as well as interstitial nephritis consequent to calcium deposition. Cardiovascular disorders include hypertension, ventricular arrhythmias, and heart block. The ECG reading often shows shortening of the QT interval, ST coving, T wave broadening, and first-degree heart block. GI manifestations include anorexia, nausea, vomiting, constipation, and pancreatitis.

Treatment should be directed toward the underlying cause, but the goal of acute therapy is to lower the circulating calcium level by increasing renal calcium excretion, inhibiting gut absorption of calcium, or inhibiting calcium mobilization from bone. Volume expansion and forced saline diuresis are the mainstays of therapy. From 3–5 L/day, and in some cases 10 or more L/day, saline may be required. Furosemide, 40–200 mg/day, is administered after initial volume expansion to enhance renal calcium excretion and protect against volume overload. Potassium and magnesium supplementation is usually required to replace urinary losses.

A number of agents decrease calcium mobilization from bone through inhibition of osteoclastic bone resorption. Salmon calcitonin is safe, and rapidly lowers circulating calcium levels in 50–70% of patients when given at a dose of 4 MRC units/kg subcutaneously every 12 hours. However, the action is short lived (2–3 days), and resistance caused by antibody formation is often limiting. Prednisone in a dose of 20–40 mg daily may delay resistance. Corticosteroids alone are most likely to be effective in patients with granulomatous disease or hematologic malignancies. They are less effective in hyperparathyroid states and solid tumor-associated hypercalcemia.

Biphosphonates are also effective and lower the circulating calcium level for as long as several weeks, but take several days to reach maximum effect. Both etidronate and the more potent pamidronate can be given orally or parenterally, but the former must be given parenterally in the treatment of hypercalcemia of malignancy, whereas the latter is associated with a high level of GI side effects when given PO. Etidronate, given at a dose of 7.5 mg/kg/day, diluted in 250 mL or more saline and infused over 2 hours or more for 2 to 4 days (5–7 days, if necessary), can be followed by as much as 20 mg/kg/day PO. Pamidronate is a newer biphosphonate that has been used IV and PO as effective therapy for hypercalcemia. The dose of pamidronate must be adjusted in the setting of renal insufficiency.

Plicamycin is a chemotherapeutic agent that effectively inhibits osteoclastic activity beginning within 6 to 12 hours and lasting 5 to 14 days, but it is not as easy to use as the previously described agents. It must be administered IV, and is particularly hazardous in patients with impaired renal function. In addition to direct nephrotoxicity, it can lead to hepatic dysfunction, thrombocytopenia, and a hemorrhagic diathesis. The usual recommended dose is 25 μg/kg/day for 3 or 4 days.

Oral phosphates, which bind calcium in the gut, are effective therapy in patients with a serum phosphorus level of less than 1.2 mmol/L, but are dangerous in patients with impaired renal function because of the risk of soft-tissue calcium deposition. Doses of 500–1500 mg elemental phosphorus daily in divided doses with meals are most often limited by diarrhea.

Magnesium

Like calcium, extracellular magnesium exists in three forms: free ionized (60%), protein bound (30–35%), and complexed (5–10%). Unfortunately, ionized magnesium levels are not routinely available in most centers. Hypomagnesemia often coexists with other electrolyte derangements, including hypokalemia, hypocalcemia, hypophosphatemia, and hyponatremia. Hypokalemia that is refractory to potassium supplementation caused by failure of the renal tubules to reabsorb potassium in the absence of magnesium is being recognized more frequently.

Hypomagnesemia. Most studies report a 10–20% incidence of hypomagnesemia in patients admitted to the ICU, but some report a rate as high as 65%. As with severe hypocalcemia, neuromuscular irritability, muscle weakness, cardiac dysrhythmias, and neuropsychiatric manifestations dominate the clinical presentation of severe magnesium deficiency.

Neuromuscular symptoms include tremor, facial grimaces, myoclonic jerks, tetany, seizure, nystagmus, ataxia, dysphagia, and gut hypomotility. Dysrhythmias include premature ventricular contractions, ventricular tachycardia, torsades de pointes, and ventricular fibrillation. These symptoms usually require a magnesium level of less than 0.5 mmol/L, but may be absent despite severe hypomagnesemia. However, patients with acute myocardial infarction complicated by dysrhythmias, digitalis intoxication with dysrhythmias, refractory hypokalemia, and hypocalcemia may benefit from magnesium supplementation, despite normal serum levels.

Hypomagnesemia may be caused by inadequate intake, malabsorption, renal wasting, or increased metabolism as a result of the following conditions:

- **Starvation and refeeding.**
- **Alcoholism.**
- **Diabetic ketoacidosis.**
- **Pancreatitis.**
- **Intestinal loss.**
- **Renal loss** (e.g., due to diuretics, aminoglycosides, amphotericin B, cisplatin).

Except in the presence of renal insufficiency, magnesium may be given with relative safety either PO, IM, or IV. Because approximately 50% of a parenterally administered dose will be excreted in the urine, twice the estimated deficit should be provided. Because cellular exchange is slow and magnesium is rapidly removed from the extracellular space by the kidneys, a continuous infusion or repeated boluses is usually necessary. When renal function is compromised, dose adjustment is indicated.

Magnesium sulfate is the most commonly used parenteral formulation, and is available in 10%, 20%, and 50% solutions. One gram (4.1 mmol) of $MgSO_4$ contains 96 mg elemental magnesium. A 70-kg patient may require 8 to 10 g $MgSO_4$ in the first day. For true emergencies such as seizures or life-threatening dysrhythmias, 2–3 g of a 10% or 20% solution may be administered by slow IV injection over several minutes. Because of its sclerosing effect, the 50% solution should be diluted in a small volume of 5% dextrose in water and administered over 5 to 10 minutes. This dose should be followed by a continuous infusion of 4–6 g over the next several hours. In less urgent situations, 2 g $MgSO_4$ as the 50% solution (i.e., 4 mL) can be given IM (usually divided between two sites) every 2 to 4 hours. Then 4–6 g $MgSO_4$ may be administered daily for the next 2 to 5 days. Oral replacement is best accomplished with magnesium gluconate or oxide. These agents are better tolerated than other oral formulations but can require a long time to correct large deficits.

Frequent (every 4–6 hours) determinations of serum magnesium levels as well as monitoring of deep tendon reflexes should guide therapy in patients with impaired renal function or those treated emergently with large doses of parenteral magnesium.

Hypermagnesemia. Severe hypermagnesemia most often occurs in the setting of renal insufficiency and excessive intake of magnesium, usually in the form of magnesium-based antacids or purgatives. Mild hypermagnesemia may be seen with acute acidosis, pheochromocytoma, Addison's disease, and hyperparathyroidism.

Diminution of deep tendon reflexes may be seen at magnesium levels greater than 2 mmol/L. Loss of patellar reflexes usually occurs at levels of 3.3–4.2 mmol/L, respiratory depression at still higher levels, and paralysis of voluntary and respiratory muscles at levels greater than 5.8–6.7 mmol/L. Intraventricular conduction delay, followed by first-degree heart block and a prolonged QT interval, is often seen with moderately severe hypermagnesemia. At levels greater than 5 mmol/L, heart block worsens. Complete heart block and asystole occur at levels greater than 12 mmol/L. Variable degrees of hypotension may also be seen.

Patients with respiratory depression or life-threatening cardiac disturbances may be treated with IV administration of 200–300 mg elemental calcium (2–3 g calcium gluconate or 1 g calcium chloride by slow injection) as an antagonist and with glucose and insulin to promote the intracellular shift of magnesium. Those with milder symptoms may be treated with forced saline diuresis to enhance magnesium excretion. Patients with advanced renal failure may require hemodialysis.

Phosphorus

Phosphorus plays a fundamental role in cellular integrity and metabolism. Dietary intake is an important determinant of the amount of phosphorus absorbed. Although the GI tract secretes a relatively fixed amount of phosphorus, the kidneys play the most important role in the regulation of serum phosphorus concentration. Urinary phosphate excretion is influenced by the filtered load as well as the action of PTH, which depresses tubular reabsorption of phosphate. Transcellular shift of phosphate is also an important determinant of the serum phosphorus concentration.

Hypophosphatemia. Severe hypophosphatemia (< 0.48 mmol/L) has been implicated as a factor in a number of clinical conditions, including erythrocyte and leukocyte dysfunction, metabolic acidosis, osteomalacia, peripheral neuropathy, CNS dysfunction, myocardial dysfunction, and diaphragmatic muscle weakness. Depletion of intracellular adenosine triphosphate and decreased levels of 2,3-diphosphoglycerate may underlie some of the clinical manifestations of hypophosphatemia. Etiologies of hypophosphatemia include:

- **Decreased intestinal absorption** because of malnutrition, starvation, phosphate binders, vitamin D deficiency.
- **Renal loss** as a result of hyperparathyroidism (primary or secondary), hypercalcemia of malignancy, glycosuria, renal tubular transport defects (including Fanconi's syndrome, oncogenic osteomalacia, familial hypophosphatemic rickets), idiopathic hypercalciuria.
- **Transcellular shift** caused by glucose infusion, refeeding, respiratory alkalosis, sepsis, chronic liver disease, hyperadrenergic state, hungry bone syndrome, metabolic acidosis.
- **Multifactorial** causes, such as alcoholism, burns, diabetic ketoacidosis, diuretic phase of acute tubular necrosis, postobstructive diuresis, renal transplantation.

In most patients, the cause of hypophosphatemia is apparent from the history or clinical setting. Glucose infusion, insulin treatment of hyperglycemia, and respiratory alkalosis are the most common causes in ICU patients. In patients in whom the cause is less obvious, determination of the daily urinary phosphorus excretion and the serum calcium level can suggest the appropriate diagnoses to be considered. In the absence of a reduced glomerular filtration rate, low urinary phosphorus excretion (< 3 mmol/day) suggests decreased intestinal absorption or transcellular shift. A higher urinary phosphorus excretion (> 3 mmol/day) suggests renal loss. Serum calcium level is elevated with primary hyperparathyroidism and hypercalcemia of malignancy, but low or normal with the other conditions associated with renal phosphate loss.

Mild to moderate hypophosphatemia (0.48–0.8 mmol/L) is usually asymptomatic, and can be treated with correction of the underlying disorder and restoration of adequate dietary intake. Patients with severe hypophosphatemia (< 0.32 mmol/L), or those with a more modest degree of hypophosphatemia in circumstances in which the contribution of hypophosphatemia to a given clinical finding is uncertain (e.g., inability to wean from ventilatory support), should be treated more aggressively. Oral therapy is the preferred route for asymptomatic patients who are not critically ill. Nonfat milk is an excellent source of phosphorus (approximately 1 g/L), and a variety of sodium or potassium phosphate salts are available. These preparations differ substantially in their phosphate, sodium, or potassium content. Enteral replacement therapy is typically initiated with 1 to 2 g phosphorus daily in two to four divided doses and titrated to maintain the desired phosphorus level. Dose-dependent diarrhea frequently limits enteral therapy.

IV administered phosphate salts are frequently used in patients with deficiency manifestations or those who cannot take oral supplements. Guidelines for safe rate or venous route (i.e., central or peripheral) are disparate, and often are as much limited by the potassium content as by the phosphate content. Although larger doses are commonly administered at more rapid rates in monitored settings without adverse consequences, a prudent recommendation is to administer a dose of 0.08–0.2 mmol/kg over 6 hours, with determinations of the serum phosphorus level at 3 and 6 hours. The infusion should be discontinued after the phosphate concentration rises to more than 0.5 mmol/L. With severe hypophosphatemia (< 0.2 mmol/L), the dose may be increased to 0.4 mmol/kg administered over 6 hours. If severe hyper- or hypocalcemia is present, IV phosphate should be used cautiously, if at all, until the abnormal calcium level is corrected. Serum calcium determinations should be obtained frequently. A precipitous decrease in the calcium level or a calcium–phosphate product exceeding 5.6 $mmol^2/L^2$ (70 mg^2/dL^2) necessitates discontinuation of the phosphate infusion. Correction of severe hypomagnesemia is also recommended as adjunctive therapy.

Hyperphosphatemia. Increased intestinal absorption, impaired renal excretion (or enhanced renal tubular reabsorption), or translocation of phosphate from the intracellular to extracellular compartment leads to hyperphosphatemia. Causes include:

- **Renal failure.**
- **Increased intestinal absorption** because of excessive intake (including phosphate-containing laxatives, enemas), vitamin D excess.
- **Enhanced renal reabsorption** because of hypoparathyroidism (primary or secondary), PTH resistance (pseudohypoparathyroidism), acromegaly, thyrotoxicosis, sickle cell anemia, tumoral calcinosis.

- **Transcellular shift** caused by tumor lysis, rhabdomyolysis, respiratory acidosis, increased catabolism.
- **IV phosphate therapy.**

The clinical manifestations are primarily related to secondary changes in calcium metabolism and ectopic calcification of soft tissues. Ectopic calcification may involve the blood vessels, periarticular tissue, cornea, lung, and skin. The cause of hyperphosphatemia is often apparent from the history and clinical setting. When the cause is not apparent, determination of urinary phosphorus excretion should suggest appropriate diagnoses to be considered. Values greater than 32 mmol/day are consistent with increased intestinal absorption or transcellular shift; values less than 32 mmol/day suggest enhanced renal tubular absorption.

Treatment of severe hyperphosphatemia with symptomatic hypocalcemia is difficult in the patient with advanced or end-stage renal disease in whom urinary phosphate excretion cannot be enhanced with the use of isotonic saline or sodium bicarbonate and acetazolamide to force diuresis. Hemodialysis is inefficient at removing phosphate, but can achieve significant removal if the dialysis treatment is extended and repeated more frequently. Hemodialysis can simultaneously correct hypocalcemia. When prompt lowering of the phosphorus level is necessary, the infusion of glucose and insulin will promote the intracellular shift of phosphate. Patients with advanced renal failure, hypoparathyroidism, or tumoral calcinosis may benefit from dietary phosphate restriction and phosphate binders (e.g., antacids containing aluminum, magnesium, or calcium) taken with meals. Aluminum- and magnesium-containing antacids should be avoided in patients with advanced renal failure. Calcium-containing antacids should similarly be avoided in patients with tumor-related calcinosis.

Suggested Readings

Agus ZS, Wasserstein A, Goldfarb S. Disorders of calcium and magnesium homeostasis. *Am J Med* 1982;72:473–488.

Lengthy review of causes, manifestations, and therapy of disturbances of calcium and magnesium (110 references).

Bilezikian JP. Management of acute hypercalcemia. *N Engl J Med* 1992;326:1196–1203.

Detailed review of treatment options for hypercalcemia (102 references).

Desai TK, Carlson RW, Geheb MA. Hypocalcemia and hypophosphatemia in acutely ill patients. *Crit Care Clin* 1987;3:927–941.

Ratcliffe WA, Hutchesson CJ, Bundred NJ, et al. Role of assays of parathyroid hormone-related protein in investigation of hypercalcemia. *Lancet* 1992;339:164–167.

Stoff JS. Phosphate homeostasis and hypophosphatemia. *Am J Med* 1982;72:489–495.

Whang R. Magnesium deficiency: Pathogenesis, prevalence, and clinical implications. *Am J Med* 1987;8(suppl 3A):24–29.

Zaloga GP. Hypocalcemia in critically ill patients. *Crit Care Med* 1992;20:251–262.
Reviews incidence, causes, and effects of hypocalcemia and implications of acute replacement therapy.

CHAPTER 54

Acid–Base Disorders

(See Chapter 104)

Michael J. Freeland and James A. Kruse

The hydrogen ion concentration ($[H^+]$), or pH, of the extracellular fluid (ECF) and intracellular fluid (ICF) compartments is normally maintained within a narrow range despite widely variable acid and alkaline loads. This stability is necessary for the proper functioning of numerous metabolic processes that use enzymes that are optimally active at a specific pH. Drastic changes in $[H^+]$ are prevented by the presence of chemical buffers (chiefly HCO_3^- in the ECF compartment), by control of the arterial partial pressure of carbon dioxide ($Paco_2$) through changes in alveolar ventilation, and by control of the serum bicarbonate concentration ($[HCO_3^-]$) through changes in renal H^+ excretion and reclamation of HCO_3^-.

Most acid–base disturbances can be readily characterized with a graphic nomogram (Figure 54–1) developed from empirically derived clinical and experimental data. The black elliptic region in the center of the graph represents the composite normal range for arterial blood gas values. The other black regions represent each of the primary acid–base disturbances, portrayed as a statistical confidence interval. The first step is to plot the patient's $[HCO_3^-]$ and $Paco_2$ values on the nomogram. If the values lie within one of the black confidence bands, it can be concluded that the findings are consistent with a single (i.e., simple) acid–base disturbance, defined by the label of the band. If the values lie between any of the confidence bands, more than one (i.e., a mixed) disturbance is present, defined by the labels on the adjacent bands. If the values lie in close proximity to the central ellipse, it is frequently difficult to characterize the disorder from the

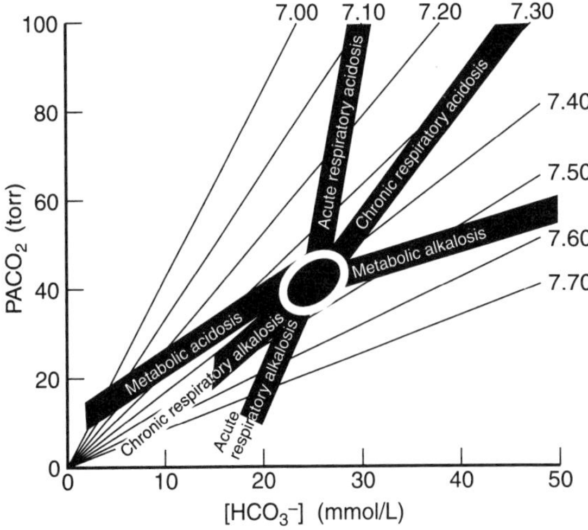

Figure 54–1. Acid–base nomogram showing confidence bands for simple acid–base disturbances. (From Kruse JA. Acid–base interpretations. In: Prough DS, Traystman RJ, eds. *Critical care state of the art.* Anaheim, CA: Society of Critical Care Medicine, 1993;14:275–297.)

blood gas results alone. When this situation occurs, the associated disturbances are usually mild.

Simple disturbances can be discerned from directional changes in blood gas (pH, $Pa{CO_2}$, and $[HCO_3^-]$) results. Mixed disorders, which are common among patients in the ICU, cannot be fully characterized by examining directional changes. They require quantitative assessment of the relationship between the blood gas values. This assessment can be accomplished with the graphic nomogram or with simple regression equations that describe the lines of the nomogram:

Metabolic acidosis: Expected $Pa{CO_2} \approx 1.5 \times [HCO_3^-] + 8$

Metabolic alkalosis: Expected $Pa{CO_2} \approx 0.9 \times [HCO_3^-] + 15$

Acute respiratory acidosis: Expected $\Delta\ [HCO_3^-] \approx 0.1 \times \Delta Pa{CO_2}$

Chronic respiratory acidosis: Expected $\Delta\ [HCO_3^-] \approx 0.35 \times \Delta Pa{CO_2}$

Acute respiratory alkalosis: Expected $\Delta\ [HCO_3^-] \approx 0.2 \times \Delta Pa{CO_2}$

Chronic respiratory alkalosis: Expected $\Delta\ [HCO_3^-] \approx 0.4 \times \Delta Pa{CO_2}$

Each of these equations allows calculation of an expected value (the dependent variable) of one blood gas parameter from another blood gas parameter that was actually measured (the independent variable). If the expected value closely approximates the corresponding measured value, then the patient's blood gas findings are consistent with the disturbance described by the equation. If the actual value deviates significantly from the expected value, then a different primary disturbance is present, or there is a mixed disorder.

For example, a patient has a [HCO_3^-] of 12 mmol/L and a $Paco_2$ of 27 torr. Using the equation for metabolic acidosis, the expected value for $Paco_2$ is 26 torr. Therefore, because the expected $Paco_2$ approximates the measured $Paco_2$ (within ± 2 torr), this patient probably has simple metabolic acidosis. In other words, the level of respiratory compensation ($Paco_2$) in this case is consistent with that expected for this degree of metabolic acidosis ([HCO_3^-]). If the measured $Paco_2$ had been lower (e.g., 20 torr), then a concomitant respiratory alkalosis would likely be present. On the other hand, if the measured $Paco_2$ had been higher (e.g., 33 torr), then a concomitant respiratory acidosis would be likely. In the latter case, there is respiratory acidosis, even though the $Paco_2$ is lower than normal because metabolic acidosis normally provokes hyperventilation. If hyperventilation is not present, or is present to an inadequate degree, the condition qualifies as respiratory acidosis. Recognition of a second disturbance alerts the clinician to the possibility of an otherwise unrecognized disease process.

Respiratory Acidosis

Simple respiratory acidosis results from relative hypoventilation that causes hypercapnia and a decrease in pH. This situation may occur as a consequence of central nervous system (CNS) depression, pleural disease, lung disease, or musculoskeletal disorder. In the ICU, it can also occur as a result of iatrogenic hypoventilation, particularly in patients undergoing mechanical ventilation and receiving sedatives or neuromuscular-blocking drugs. Acutely, the compensatory response consists of a rapid, mild increase in [HCO_3^-] because of the formation of HCO_3^- by:

$$CO_2 + H_2O \rightleftharpoons H_2CO_3 \rightleftharpoons H^+ + HCO_3^-$$

A slower, but quantitatively more important, compensatory mechanism consists of HCO_3^- formation by the kidney. This activity is mediated at the level of the renal tubular cells by the presence of hypercapnia. Renal compensation begins within a matter of hours, and reaches maximum effect within 3 to 5 days.

Treatment of respiratory acidosis is directed at the underlying cause (e.g., naloxone for CNS depression caused by opiate overdose, tube thoracostomy for pneumothorax, drug therapy for cardiogenic pulmonary edema). Such therapy may suffice in some cases, but other cases will require endotracheal intubation and mechanical ventilation.

Respiratory Alkalosis

The primary disturbance in simple respiratory alkalosis is hyperventilation, resulting in hypocapnia and an increase in pH. This situation is most commonly caused by acute pain or anxiety, but it also occurs as a consequence of catastrophic CNS disorders (e.g., intracerebral hemorrhage), decreased lung compliance (even in the absence of hypoxemia), drugs that stimulate the respiratory center in the brain stem (e.g., salicylates, progesterone), sepsis, hepatic failure, and pregnancy.

As with respiratory acidosis, a slight change in [HCO_3^-] is expected during acute respiratory alkalosis because of a shift in the equilibrium reaction of bicarbonate and CO_2. Subsequently, the kidney responds to hypocapnia by diminished renal H^+ excretion, which results in loss of HCO_3^- in the urine. Because full renal compensation takes several days to reach its maximal effect, the expected changes in [HCO_3^-], as given by nomogram or equation, are different in acute compared with chronic respiratory acid–base disturbances. Arterial blood gas results that lie between confidence bands for the acute and corresponding chronic disturbance usually signify that the respiratory disturbance, whether acidosis or alkalosis, has been of intermediate duration.

Spontaneously breathing patients with respiratory alkalosis usually do not require specific therapy beyond that directed at the underlying cause. In some cases, severe respiratory alkalosis is a harbinger of impending respiratory failure. Respiratory alkalosis in patients receiving mechanical ventilation may be caused by the underlying disease or may be iatrogenic as a result of inappropriate ventilator settings. The latter condition can be remedied by adjusting the ventilator controls, but the former situation is frequently more difficult to treat, short of deeply sedating the patient.

Metabolic Acidosis

Simple metabolic acidosis is characterized by acidemia, a decrease in [HCO_3^-], and compensatory hypocapnia. The decrease in [HCO_3^-] may reflect loss of HCO_3^- from the kidneys or GI tract or loss as a result of buffering an acid load (other than carbonic acid).

TABLE 54–1

CAUSES OF METABOLIC ACIDOSIS

Normal Anion Gap	High Anion Gap
Diarrhea and small bowel loss	Lactic acidosis
Renal tubular acidoses	Diabetic ketoacidosis
Type 1 (distal)	Alcoholic or starvation ketoacidosis
Type 2 (proximal)	Advanced renal failure
Type 4 (hypoaldosteronism)	Certain toxic ingestions
Ureterosigmoidostomy	Salicylate
Ileal loop conduit	Methanol
Inorganic acid ingestion (HCl, NH_4Cl)	Ethylene glycol
Parenteral amino acids (as HCl salts)	Paraldehyde
Ingestion of $CaCl_2$ or $MgCl_2$	Toluene
Significant volume expansion with saline	

The Serum Anion Gap. If metabolic acidosis is present, the serum anion gap should be determined to establish if it is increased or normal. The anion gap is equal to the difference between the serum concentrations of the major measured cation, sodium ($[Na^+]$), and the major measured anions, chloride ($[Cl^-]$) and $[HCO_3^-]$:

$$\text{Serum anion gap} = [Na^+] - ([Cl^-] + [HCO_3^-])$$

The conventional normal range of the anion gap is 8 to 16 mEq/L. Calculation of the anion gap assists with the differential diagnosis of metabolic acidosis (Table 54–1).

Knowing the anion gap, the clinical setting, and the results of specific biochemical measurements (e.g., serum creatinine, lactate, ketones) usually allows identification of the underlying cause of the metabolic acidosis. However, the limitations of the anion gap must be recognized.

Several factors can independently lower the serum anion gap, including:

- Hypoalbuminemia (because of the decrease in the unmeasured anion, albumin).
- Severely elevated levels of unmeasured cations (e.g., Mg^{++}, Ca^{++}, K^+, or Li^+).
- Multiple myeloma; immunoglobulin G is also an unmeasured cation.
- Bromide or iodide intoxication (because of interference with serum chloride assay).

Occasionally, an elevated anion gap may be the only biochemical evidence of metabolic acidosis in a patient with mixed metabolic acidosis and alkalosis. This situation occurs when metabolic alkalosis, a process that tends to increase [HCO_3^-], develops simultaneously with metabolic acidosis, a process that tends to decrease [HCO_3^-]. If both primary disturbances are of equal severity, [HCO_3^-] may remain within normal limits, despite the presence of two severe acid–base disorders.

Δgap/Δ[HCO_3^-]. If the anion gap is increased, the ratio of the increase in the anion gap to the decrease in [HCO_3^-] should be calculated. If the patient initially has a normal [HCO_3^-] of 24 mmol/L and a normal anion gap of 12 mEq/L, this ratio is calculated as:

$$\frac{\Delta\text{gap}}{\Delta[\text{HCO}_3^-]} = \frac{\text{Anion gap} - 12}{24 - [\text{HCO}_3^-]}$$

In pure anion gap acidosis, this quotient is usually close to unity (0.8–1.2). In pure non–anion gap acidosis, it should be zero. Intermediate values (0.3–0.7) signify either the concomitant presence of both types of metabolic acidosis, mixed high anion gap acidosis and chronic respiratory alkalosis, or high anion gap acidosis that is partially masked by preexisting low anion gap (e.g., as a result of hypoalbuminemia). Values substantially greater than unity (> 1.2) indicate the presence of superimposed metabolic alkalosis in addition to anion gap acidosis or mixed high anion gap acidosis and chronic respiratory acidosis.

The Urine Anion Gap. Analogous to the serum anion gap, this calculated value is the difference between the commonly measured urine cations Na^+ and K^+ and the lone commonly measured urine anion Cl^-:

$$\text{Urine anion gap} = [\text{Na}^+] + [\text{K}^+] - [\text{Cl}^-]$$

The urine anion gap is normally a positive value or is near zero. It becomes negative in metabolic acidosis caused by GI HCO_3^- loss, mediated by increased renal ammonium production. The same situation occurs in metabolic acidosis caused by hydrochloric acid or acetazolamide administration and also in proximal renal tubular acidosis (RTA). However, the urine anion gap remains positive in distal RTA as a result of impaired renal ammonium generation. Thus this calculation can sometimes assist in discriminating these etiologies of normal anion gap metabolic acidosis.

$NaHCO_3$ Therapy. As with all acid–base disturbances, treatment of metabolic acidosis is directed toward correction of the underlying cause where possible. Severe acidemia (pH < 7.10) may warrant treatment with supplemental HCO_3^-, particularly in metabolic acidosis caused by renal failure or RTA. Cogent arguments have been raised against the use of alkali therapy for the treatment of lactic and ketoacidosis, even when the degree of acidemia is severe, but this area remains controversial. When treatment with $NaHCO_3$ is used, it is rarely appropriate to correct the serum $[HCO_3^-]$ completely. Initial therapy should be aimed at increasing $[HCO_3^-]$ to greater than 10 mmol/L over several hours. The dose of $NaHCO_3$ (mmol) required to achieve the desired plasma bicarbonate level can be estimated with the following formula:

$$NaHCO_3 \text{ dose} = \left(0.4 + \frac{2.4}{[HCO_3^-]_{current}}\right) \times \text{Weight (kg)} \times ([HCO_3^-]_{desired} - [HCO_3^-]_{current})$$

Because the rate of H^+ production or HCO_3^- loss is not included in this calculation, arterial blood gas levels must be monitored frequently to assess the adequacy of therapy. Patients who cannot tolerate the Na^+ load and consequent ECF volume expansion may require hemodialysis to correct their acidosis.

Metabolic Alkalosis

Simple metabolic alkalosis is characterized by an elevation in $[HCO_3^-]$ and an increase in pH. The degree of respiratory compensation (hypercapnia) observed in this primary disturbance is more variable and hence less predictable than that seen in metabolic acidosis. However, low arterial carbon dioxide tension ($PaCO_2$) in metabolic alkalosis is clearly inappropriate, and indicates concomitant respiratory alkalosis. Except in some severe cases of metabolic alkalosis, it is unusual to see $PaCO_2$ greater than 55 torr.

Common etiologies and mechanisms of metabolic alkalosis include:

- **Gastrointestinal H^+ loss** as a result of vomiting, nasogastric suction, certain villous adenomas, and other causes.
- **Renal H^+ loss** as a result of diuretics, mineralocorticoid excess, posthypercapnia, nonreabsorbable anion administration, and other causes.
- **Retention of HCO_3^-** as a result of bicarbonate administration, massive blood transfusion, milk–alkali syndrome, and other causes.
- **Contraction alkalosis** as a result of diuretic administration, gastric loss with achlorhydria, sweat loss in cystic fibrosis, and other causes.

When the etiology of the metabolic alkalosis is not clear from the history, measurement of urine Cl^- concentration can sometimes be helpful in narrowing the differential diagnosis (Table 54–2).

Treatment of metabolic alkalosis in the ICU patient is often accomplished by discontinuation of diuretics and nasogastric suction, correction of ECF volume contraction, and repletion of chloride and potassium deficits. In

TABLE 54–2

URINE CHLORIDE CONCENTRATION IN METABOLIC ALKALOSIS

< 10 mmol/L	> 20 mmol/L
Vomiting or nasogastric suction	Mineralocorticoid excess
Diuretics (after discontinuation)	Diuretics (during use)
Post-hypercapnia	Alkali loading
Low chloride intake	Severe hypokalemia

rare circumstances, severe alkalemia may require rapid correction by the infusion of hydrochloric acid. This treatment is sometimes necessary if the arterial pH is high (pH > 7.60) and there are associated life-threatening dysrhythmias or seizures. HCl at a concentration of 100–200 mmol/L can be infused into a central vein. The dose (mmol) of HCl that is needed to achieve a specific [HCO_3^-] can be estimated by:

$$H^+ \text{ deficit} = 0.5 \times \text{Weight(kg)} \times ([HCO_3^-]_{current} - [HCO_3^-]_{desired})$$

Some authors advocate a more conservative formula, substituting 0.2 for 0.5 in the above equation. The maximal rate of infusion should not exceed approximately 0.2 mmol/kg/hr. This rate, however, is rarely necessary beyond the initial several hours of therapy, after which correction can proceed over a 24- to 48-hour period. Once again, frequent arterial blood gas determinations should guide treatment.

Suggested Readings

Friedman BS, Lumb PD. Prevention and management of metabolic alkalosis. *J Intensive Care Med* 1990;5(suppl):522–527.

Gabow PA. Disorders associated with an altered anion gap. *Kidney Int* 1985;27:472–483.

Comprehensive review that includes detailed explanations of causes of a decreased anion gap.

Halperin ML, Richardson RMA, Bear RA, et al. Urine ammonium: The key to the diagnosis of distal renal tubular acidosis. *Nephron* 1988;50:1–4.

Detailed explanation of urine anion gap.

Koch SM, Taylor RW. Chloride ion in intensive care medicine. *Crit Care Med* 1992;20:227–240.

Despite the title's suggestion to the contrary, this is a comprehensive review of metabolic acid–base disturbances.

Kruse JA. Acid-base interpretations. In: Prough DS, Traystman RJ, eds. *Critical care state of the art.* Anaheim, CA: Society of Critical Care Medicine, 1993;14:275–297.

Clear explanation of empiric and statistical bases of nomogram confidence bands. Gives multiple alternative formulas for estimating appropriate levels of compensation.

Narins RG, Cohen JJ. Bicarbonate therapy for organic acidosis: The case for its continued use. *Ann Intern Med* 1987;106:615–618.

One side of argument surrounding the use of $NaHCO_3$ treatment of metabolic acidosis.
Stacpoole PW. Lactic acidosis: The case against bicarbonate therapy. *Ann Intern Med* 1986;105:276–279.
Other side of argument regarding $NaHCO_3$ treatment of lactic acidosis.

CHAPTER 55
Lactic Acidosis

(See Chapter 105)

James A. Kruse

Lactic acidosis arises chiefly from pathologic conditions that interfere with tissue perfusion and oxygenation. Inadequate delivery of oxygen to peripheral tissues leads to oxygen debt and partial reliance on anaerobic metabolism. The end product of anaerobic metabolism is lactate, accompanied by the obligatory production of hydrogen ions. Increased concentrations of blood lactate serve as a clinical marker for circulatory shock or more subtle degrees of perfusion impairment. Much less commonly, lactic acidosis is observed in association with certain systemic disorders and a variety of intoxications, but without evidence of tissue hypoxia.

Etiologies

The metabolism of lactate and the pathologic mechanisms underlying the various etiologies of lactic acidosis are described in Chapter 105 in the main text. These etiologies have been conventionally divided into two categories: types A and B. The former includes etiologies that involve systemic or regional tissue hypoxia or a pathologic imbalance between oxygen demand and the supply of available oxygen at the tissue level. In this classification system, lactic acidosis caused by other or unknown mechanisms is known as type B.

Type A Lactic Acidosis. Tissue hypoxia and lactic acidosis result when systemic oxygen delivery is inadequate to meet systemic oxygen demands. Circulatory shock is the most common cause of lactic acidosis. Decreased cardiac output, such as in cardiogenic or hypovolemic shock, leads to a reduction in oxygen delivery. Peripheral tissues are normally able to increase oxygen extraction from the circulation and thus compensate for this impairment in oxygen delivery. If oxygen delivery decreases beyond the point at which this compensatory mechanism is maximized, hypoxic tissues are forced to rely on anaerobic metabolism, and net production of lactate occurs. Besides impairment in cardiac output, oxygen delivery is compromised in anemia and hypoxemia. However, lactic acidosis is uncommonly due solely to these conditions unless they are of profound severity or there is concomitant cardiac dysfunction. This situation is rare because oxygen delivery is maintained in hypoxemia and anemia by a compensatory increase in cardiac output.

Seizures are another common cause of type A lactic acidosis. In this case, the tremendous increase in oxygen demand by contracting skeletal muscles cannot be met by the available oxygen supply. This situation is akin to the lactate accumulation that occurs physiologically during strenuous exercise.

Status asthmaticus is occasionally accompanied by lactic acidosis. The problem is both an increase in oxygen demand, because of increased work of breathing, and a decrease in oxygen supply, because of hypoxemia and because of impaired cardiac output secondary to limitations in venous return imposed by large variations in intrathoracic pressure.

Type A lactic acidosis can occur on a regional basis as well as a systemic basis. For example, mesenteric arterial occlusion caused by thromboembolic disease may lead to isolated splanchnic hypoxia and accompanying lactate accumulation.

Type B Lactic Acidosis. This category includes all etiologies that ostensibly do not involve an imbalance between oxygen supply and demand as the underlying mechanism. It is conventionally divided into three subcategories: type B_1 includes a heterogenous group of illnesses that are associated with lactic acidosis; type B_2 is caused by certain drugs and toxins that can lead to lactic acidosis; and type B_3 encompasses the congenital etiologies that are caused by inborn errors in metabolism. Representative etiologies for each of these categories include:

- **Type B_1** sepsis, malignancy, hepatic disease, diabetes mellitus, short-bowel syndrome, thiamine deficiency, alkalemia, pheochromocytoma.
- **Type B_2** phenformin, isoniazid, cyanide, salicylates, acetaminophen, methanol, ethylene glycol, propylene glycol, iron, fructose, catecholamines, sorbitol, sodium bicarbonate.
- **Type B_3** type I glycogen storage disease, hereditary fructose intolerance, fructose-1,6-biphosphate deficiency, pyruvate carboxylase deficiency, mitochondrial encephalopathy with lactic acidosis and stroke (MELAS) syndrome.

The mechanism for some type B causes has been elucidated and shown not to involve tissue hypoxia (see Chapter 105 in the main text). However, some of the type B etiologies may involve tissue hypoxia as the underlying mechanism. For example, although severe hepatic disease has long been believed to lead to lactate accumulation, there is evidence that this situation occurs only in the setting of hypoperfusion or circulatory shock. Similarly, the lactic acidosis observed in severe iron poisoning is probably secondary to the accompanying seizures or circulatory shock.

Detection and Measurement

Detection and confirmation of lactic acidosis is readily performed by direct assay of lactate. With modern analytic methods, lactate assays can be performed in minutes on fractional milliliter quantities of plasma, serum, or whole blood. The specimen should be placed on ice and promptly delivered to the laboratory for immediate analysis; otherwise, ongoing in vitro metabolism will result in a falsely elevated lactate level. Alternatively, the blood specimen can be collected in a special tube containing a glycolytic inhibitor, such as fluoride (designated by a gray rubber stopper on some commercially available vacuum blood sampling tubes). An arterial or mixed venous specimen is preferred over blood from a peripheral vein.

Traditionally, lactic acidosis has been recognized clinically by finding metabolic acidosis by blood gas analysis, along with an elevated serum anion gap. Once other causes of high anion gap acidosis are excluded, these findings are indirectly diagnostic of lactic acidosis. The converse, however, is not true. That is, absence of a high anion gap or lack of blood gas findings consistent with metabolic acidosis does not exclude the possibility of clinically significant elevations of blood lactate levels. The relative insensitivity of blood gases and the anion gap to changes in blood lactate is partly caused by the normal degree of variability in acid–base and electrolyte values. In addition, concomitant respiratory or metabolic alkalosis is not uncommon in these patients. Thus, routine measurement of lactate level is desirable in critically ill patients who are at risk for lactic acidosis. This measurement is especially important in monitoring the severity or recovery from lactic acidosis.

Clinical Significance

Lactic acidosis is a common and expected complication of critical illness that has progressed to the point of severe and global tissue hypoxia. In clinical situations in which frank circulatory shock is indicated by hypotension and obvious evidence of organ dysfunction, the presence and severity of lactic acidosis underscore the severity of the hypoperfusion state. However, the detection of milder degrees of lactic acidosis, or hyperlactatemia without acidemia, may alert the clinician to more subtle degrees of hypoperfusion. This information allows early institution of therapeutic interventions that may improve tissue oxygen delivery, halt or reverse vital organ ischemia, and avert progression to frank or irreversible circulatory shock. Therefore, even relatively mild degrees of lactate elevation may be of clinical importance. This observation is supported by findings from many clinical investigations that blood lactate concentrations in excess of 2.5–3.0 mmol/L are associated with increased mortality rates.

Although lactic acidosis can occur in a number of conditions other than shock, many of these other conditions are infrequently encountered or result in only minor elevation of blood lactate levels. Therefore, inadequate tissue oxygenation should be the first consideration when a patient with lactic acidosis is encountered. In addition to serving as a marker for detecting inadequate perfusion, serial blood lactate levels can be helpful in monitoring the response to therapeutic interventions designed to improve systemic oxygen delivery. For patients with systemic hypoperfusion and elevated lactate concentrations, the effect of augmenting cardiac output with fluid infusions, inotropic agents, or intra-aortic balloon counterpulsation, for example, can be assessed by following sequential changes in blood lactate level. In conjunction with other clinical indicators of organ perfusion (such as urine output and changes in sensorium) and, in selected cases, with invasive hemodynamic measurements, this simple blood test provides a physiologically sound endpoint for titrating such therapies.

Treatment

The treatment of lactic acidosis is directed toward alleviating the underlying cause. Because the most common cause is circulatory shock, the primary aim of treatment in most cases is to restore adequate systemic perfusion and oxygenation. This goal is frequently accomplished by using supplemental oxygen, IV fluids, vasoactive drugs, blood transfusions, and other measures that improve oxygen delivery and mitigate tissue hypoxia. More specific therapy depends on the underlying cause. For example, antibiotic treatment and abscess drainage may be indicated in septic shock.

Sodium bicarbonate has conventionally been used as an adjunct to treat lactic acidosis associated with significant acidemia that is not otherwise immediately reversible. The rationale for its use is based chiefly on the observation that acidemia itself impairs cardiac function and potentially worsens hypoperfusion. This cardiac depression further decreases peripheral oxygen delivery and increases the severity of the lactic acidosis. Correcting the acidemia may break this cycle by improving cardiac function. However, more recent studies, both experimental and clinical, either have not shown beneficial effects or have shown adverse effects of administering bicarbonate in lactic acidosis. These adverse effects include mixed venous hypercarbia, hyperosmolality, fluid overload, worsening intracellular acidosis, increased lactate production, and an unfavorable effect on the affinity of hemoglobin for oxygen. On this basis, cogent arguments have been raised against the use of this alkalinizing agent. Routine administration of sodium bicarbonate to treat lactic acidosis remains controversial.

Sodium dichloroacetate is an experimental agent that stimulates pyruvate dehydrogenase and hastens lactate use. It has been shown to lower blood lactate levels in animals and patients with lactic acidosis. Although it is effective at decreasing blood lactate level, a randomized clinical trial did not show any positive effects on survival in patients with lactic acidosis.

Suggested Readings

Cooper DJ, Walley KR, Wiggs BR, et al. Bicarbonate does not improve hemodynamics in critically ill patients who have lactic acidosis. *Ann Intern Med* 1990;112:492–498.

Controlled, crossover study of the effects of sodium bicarbonate on hemodynamics in patients with lactic acidosis. Hemodynamic effects after sodium bicarbonate administration were no different from those seen after sodium chloride administration.

Kruse JA. The cellular basis of conventional and experimental pharmacotherapies for circulatory shock. *Anaesth Pharmacol Rev* 1994;2:115–127.

Details mechanisms of cellular injury in shock and the effects of a variety of pharmacologic agents used to treat shock and lactic acidosis. Proposed mechanisms for adverse effects of sodium bicarbonate are reviewed.

MacDonald L, Kruse JA, Levy DB, et al. Lactic acidosis and acute ethanol intoxication. *Am J Emerg Med* 1994;12:32–35.

Of 60 patients treated for acute ethanol intoxication in an emergency department, none had blood lactate levels greater than 5 mmol/L. Of seven patients with lactate levels greater than 2.4 mmol/L, another explanation for lactate level elevation (e.g., hypoxia, seizures, hypoperfusion) was present in each case. Ethanol intoxication is an uncommon cause of lactic acidosis.

Stacpoole PW, Wright EC, Baumgartner TG, et al. A controlled clinical trial of dichloroacetate for treatment of lactic acidosis in adults. *N Engl J Med* 1992;327:1564–1569.

This multicenter, placebo-controlled, randomized trial examined the effect of dichloroacetate therapy in 252 patients with blood lactate levels of 5 mmol/L or greater and arterial blood pH of 7.35 or less. Dichloroacetate was effective in lowering blood lactate levels but without any significant associated improvement in hemodynamics or survival rate.

CHAPTER 56

Acute Renal Failure

(See Chapters 107 and 108)

Michael J. Freeland

Acute renal failure (ARF) is an acute deterioration in the glomerular filtration rate (GFR) characterized by the accumulation of metabolic waste products normally excreted by the kidneys. Attempts to define ARF as an absolute rise in serum creatinine (Cr_s) or blood urea nitrogen (BUN) concentration are limited by the inherent inaccuracy of these parameters in reflecting GFR. Similarly, attempts to define ARF by urine volume, although sometimes useful in the diagnostic approach, also have limitations. If information about the patient's previous renal functional status is not available, the distinction between acute and chronic renal failure (CRF) may be difficult. Clinical history, physical examination, urinalysis, urinary indices, and other laboratory and imaging studies may be helpful.

GFR can decrease as a consequence of systemic disease or primary diseases of the kidney or its collecting system. A simplified approach to the differential diagnosis of ARF divides the potential causes into three broad functional categories: prerenal ARF, resulting from a reduction in renal blood flow (RBF); intrarenal ARF, resulting from disease of or injury to the renal parenchyma; or postrenal ARF, resulting from obstruction of urine flow.

Prerenal Acute Renal Failure

Causes of this form of ARF include:

- **Hypovolemia** as a result of diuretics, GI losses, third-space losses, skin losses, hemorrhage, renal salt wasting, and other causes.
- **Decreased cardiac output** as a result of myocardial infarction, decompensated congestive heart failure, cardiac tamponade, pulmonary embolism, and other causes.
- **Peripheral vasodilatation** as a result of sepsis, antihypertensive medications, shock, drug overdoses, liver failure, and other causes.
- **Renal vascular obstruction** as a result of renal artery stenosis, dissecting aneurysm, embolism, thrombosis, compression, vasculitis, and other causes.
- **Disruption of renal autoregulation** as a result of angio-

tensin-converting enzyme inhibitors, nonsteroidal anti-inflammatory drugs (NSAIDs), and other causes.
- **Hepatorenal syndrome** as a result of end-stage cirrhosis, fulminant hepatic failure, and other causes.

Autoregulatory mechanisms normally maintain RBF across a wide range of systemic arterial pressures. Because maintenance of GFR is highly dependent on RBF, severe or persistent hypoperfusion results in a decline in GFR. Renal hypoperfusion is usually part of a systemic process involving hypoperfusion of other organs and tissue beds. This condition most commonly occurs as a result of intravascular volume depletion, but it also occurs as a result of diminished effective circulating volume caused by decreased cardiac output or peripheral vasodilation. Renal vascular obstruction and drugs that disrupt renal autoregulation may, however, cause renal hypoperfusion in the absence of otherwise significant hypovolemia or decreased effective circulating volume. Hepatorenal syndrome is a form of prerenal ARF that occurs in the setting of severe hepatic disease. In hepatorenal syndrome, there is no clinical, laboratory, or anatomic evidence of any alternative recognized cause of renal failure. The severe renal vasoconstriction that occurs in this condition may be caused by an unidentified humoral factor, and it is associated with alterations in renal prostaglandin levels. The diagnosis of hepatorenal syndrome is one of exclusion of other causes of prerenal ARF.

Diagnosis. Hypovolemia and conditions associated with decreased cardiac output or peripheral vasodilation are usually apparent from the history and clinical examination. A history of difficult to control or recently accelerated hypertension in a patient older than 50 years with arteriosclerotic disease should lead the clinician to suspect atheromatous renovascular disease. An abrupt deterioration in renal function after the institution of treatment with an angiotensin-converting enzyme inhibitor is an important clue to the presence of bilateral renal artery stenosis (or stenosis involving a single functioning kidney). The medication history should also include specific questions about the use of over-the-counter pain relievers because nonprescribed NSAID use may not be volunteered.

With prerenal ARF, the BUN:Cr_s (mg/dL) ratio usually exceeds 20:1 (normal range, 10–15:1). Other urinary indices (Table 56–1), particularly the fractional excretion of sodium (FE_{Na}), are more useful in distinguishing between ARF with prerenal causes and ARF caused by acute tubular necrosis (ATN). A low FE_{Na} typically reflects avid sodium and water reabsorption—the expected physiologic response to renal hypoperfusion. In the absence of impaired renal sodium or water handling (e.g., because of diuretics or CRF), a FE_{Na} that is not low is supportive of a diagnosis

TABLE 56–1

URINARY INDICES IN ACUTE RENAL FAILURE

Index	Prerenal Azotemia	Acute Tubular Necrosis
Specific gravity	> 1.020	< 1.010
Urine osmolality (mOsm/kg H_2O)	> 500	< 350
Urine sodium (mmol/L)	< 20	> 40
Urine to serum urea nitrogen	> 8	< 3
Urine to serum creatinine	> 40	< 20
Fractional excretion of sodium (%) $\frac{Na_u/Na_s}{Cr_u/Cr_s} \times 100$	< 1	> 1
Renal failure index $= \frac{Na_u}{Cr_u/Cr_s}$	< 1	> 1

of ATN. However, while the FE_{Na} and other indices are helpful, it is important to recognize that prerenal ARF may be superimposed on ATN. The urine sediment with prerenal ARF is classically bland or remarkable only for sparse hyaline and fine granular casts.

Treatment. The goal of therapy in prerenal ARF is to improve renal perfusion. Intravascular volume depletion should be corrected with isotonic fluids. Cardiac failure should be treated with afterload reduction and inotropic support, if necessary. Septic shock often requires a combination of volume expanders, vasopressors, and inotropes in addition to therapy directed at the underlying cause. Renal artery stenosis requires either renal artery bypass surgery or angioplasty. Hepatorenal syndrome usually marks the terminal stage of advanced liver disease, and therapy directed toward improving renal function alone is usually ineffective. Low-dose dopamine is often used, but proof of its efficacy is lacking. Hemodialysis may be indicated as a supportive measure in patients who are believed to have potentially reversible liver disease. Drugs that disrupt renal autoregulation should be discontinued, if feasible, in any patient with prerenal ARF.

Intrarenal Acute Renal Failure

Most cases of hospital-acquired ARF that are not the result of prerenal causes are caused by ATN resulting from an ischemic or nephrotoxic injury. The latter can be caused by:

- **Antibiotics,** e.g., aminoglycosides, amphotericin B, cephalosporins.
- **Radiocontrast media.**
- **Endogenous toxins,** e.g., myoglobin, myeloma light chains.

- **Chemotherapeutic agents,** e.g., cisplatin, doxorubicin (adriamycin).
- **Immunosuppressive agents,** e.g., cyclosporine.
- **Anesthetic agents,** e.g., enflurane, methoxyflurane.
- **Organic solvents,** e.g., carbon tetrachloride, ethylene glycol.
- **Heavy metals,** e.g., lead, mercury, arsenic, cadmium, bismuth.

Often, both an ischemic and a nephrotoxic injury are operative simultaneously. The deterioration in renal function may be abrupt after an episode of profound hypotension or exposure to a radiocontrast agent, or may be more insidious, as with aminoglycoside nephrotoxicity. The administration of large volumes of fluid or blood products during the resuscitative stages of shock or during the intra- and postoperative periods may dilute and mask an increase in BUN and Cr_s. These factors, in addition to failure to recognize the normal decline in GFR with aging and the relationships between muscle mass and Cr_s and between protein malnutrition and BUN, often result in delayed recognition of a decline in renal function. Thus, ATN sometimes becomes a diagnosis of exclusion. The clinician must consider acute interstitial nephritis (AIN), atheroembolic disease, renal artery occlusion, and acute or rapidly progressive glomerulonephritis (AGN or RPGN) as well as postrenal causes (see below).

Nonoliguric ATN (urine volume > 500 mL/day) probably reflects a lesser degree of renal damage, and probably has a better prognosis than oliguric ATN because of a lesser incidence of hyperkalemia and volume overload requiring dialysis. Renal excretory failure lasts an average of 7 to 21 days in the typical setting of ATN. Cr_s may continue to increase, even during the recovery phase. A decrease in the rate of rise usually portends the diuretic phase of ATN.

Diagnosis. After prerenal and postrenal (see below) causes of ARF have been excluded, intrarenal causes are left. The utility of urinary indices has already been discussed; however, certain causes of intrarenal ARF may be associated with a low FE_{Na}. Among these are radiocontrast-induced ARF and ARF associated with rhabdomyolysis. Additionally, AGN or RPGN may be associated with a low FE_{Na} as long as tubular function remains intact. The urine sediment in ATN is characterized by numerous granular and epithelial cell casts as well as renal tubular epithelial (RTE) cells. A urine dipstick test result that is strongly positive for blood in the absence of red blood cells (RBCs) on microscopy is consistent with hemoglobinuria (i.e., intravascular hemolysis) or myoglobinuria (i.e., rhabdomyolysis).

AIN may be caused by a multitude of drugs and by infectious and autoimmune diseases. Frequent offending drugs include phenytoin, allopurinol, furosemide, α-interferon, NSAIDs, and many antibiotics. Although fever, rash, and eosinophilia may occur with drug-induced AIN, their absence does not preclude the diagnosis. Infection with a variety of bacteria, viruses, or fungi may cause AIN. Streptococcal and staphylococcal infections are associated with AGN as well. Sarcoidosis and Sjögren's syndrome are the most common autoimmune processes associated with AIN. Interstitial disease is usually evidenced by white blood cells, (WBCs), WBC casts, eosinophiluria (in the case of drug-induced AIN), RBCs, and RTE cells on urine microscopy.

The sudden onset of flank pain and hematuria suggests renal emboli (septic, bland, or atheroemboli), renal infarction (e.g., caused by a dissecting aortic aneurysm), or renal vein thrombosis (most common in the setting of nephrotic syndrome). Other signs and symptoms of embolization, organ or tissue ischemia, or infarction are often present. Renal failure from atheroembolic disease may be associated with an active urine sediment (i.e., cellular casts), hypocomplementemia, and eosinophilia.

AGN is suggested by the sudden onset of edema, hematuria, and hypertension, especially after upper respiratory or skin infections. RPGN may be immune complex induced (e.g., poststreptococcal or lupus associated), antiglomerular basement membrane antibody induced (e.g., Goodpasture's syndrome), or idiopathic, associated with systemic vasculitis (e.g., Wegener's granulomatosis, polyarteritis, or hypersensitivity vasculitis). Evidence of multisystem disease and positive serologic findings often suggest the proper diagnosis. Urinary findings include heavy proteinuria, RBCs and RBC casts, WBCs, oval fat bodies, free fat droplets, and fatty casts.

Certain clinical settings suggest other diagnoses. Malignant hypertension or preeclampsia suggests malignant nephrosclerosis. ARF in late pregnancy or the puerperium, especially when associated with abruptio placentae, should lead to the consideration of acute cortical necrosis. In the appropriate cancer patient, the clinician should consider uric acid nephropathy complicating tumor lysis syndrome, urinary obstruction caused by abdominal or pelvic masses, myeloma kidney, ARF caused by malignancy-associated hypercalcemia, and infiltrative disease of the kidney. Uric acid and urate crystals may be present in the urine of patients with acute uric acid nephropathy. The presence of other types of crystals may also be helpful diagnostically. Calcium oxalate crystalluria may be seen in the setting of ARF accompanying ethylene glycol intoxication.

Finally, a renal biopsy may be considered in patients with intrarenal disease when the etiology is unclear and less invasive studies cannot establish the diagnosis, or when the severity and activity of injury must be assessed directly to determine the appropriate therapy.

Treatment. Treatment of intrarenal ARF should begin with prevention. Intravascular volume depletion and hypotension or overaggressive control of hypertension should be avoided in patients who are exposed to nephrotoxic agents or drugs that disrupt renal autoregulation and in those with renovascular obstruction. Drugs should be appropriately dosed for underlying renal as well as hepatic dysfunction. Patients undergoing radiocontrast studies should be well hydrated before the procedure. Forced diuresis with saline, with or without administration of a loop diuretic or mannitol, should be begun before and continued for several hours after the study in patients who are at high risk. However, intravascular volume depletion should be avoided. Ischemic time during major abdominal vascular procedures should be kept to a minimum. The nephrotoxicity of hemoglobin and myoglobin pigment should be considered in the treatment of patients with severe intravascular hemolysis or rhabdomyolysis. When washout of myoglobin can be expected from the release of compartment pressures by fasciotomy or arterial embolectomy of ischemic limbs, the above prophylactic measures are most beneficial when instituted early. Calcium channel blocking agents and low-dose dopamine may help to preserve renal perfusion, but they are second-line agents after adequate hydration is ensured. Patients with leukemia, lymphoma, or large tumor burdens should be treated with allopurinol before cytotoxic therapy.

Once established, the treatment of ATN is primarily supportive. Although a judicious fluid challenge may be warranted in the patient suspected of having volume depletion superimposed on ATN, large-volume fluid administration and large doses of intravenous mannitol may contribute to intravascular volume overload. High IV doses of loop diuretic (e.g., $\leq$ 1 g/day furosemide) can be administered in an attempt to convert oliguric to nonoliguric ARF and facilitate fluid management, but this treatment carries the risk of ototoxicity, and should not be continued if there is little or no response.

The role of corticosteroids in the treatment of drug-induced AIN is not well defined. They may provide for more rapid and complete resolution of the renal injury, but are usually reserved for patients with more severe disease because spontaneous recovery is the rule once the inciting drug is removed.

Dialysis has the greatest effect on survival when it is instituted before the development of symptomatic uremia. Although patients may become uremic at variable levels of BUN, it is reasonable to consider dialysis at a BUN level of 100 mg/dL, especially when the level is increasing rapidly and recovery is not expected soon. Pericarditis is a generally accepted indication for urgent dialysis. Dialysis is also necessary to treat severe hypervolemia, hyperkalemia, and metabolic acidosis refractory to or not amenable to medical therapy with high-dose IV loop diuretics, cation-exchange resin (i.e., sodium polystyrene sulfonate), or sodium bicarbonate, respectively. Intensive dialysis (e.g., daily to maintain BUN < 60 mg/dL and $Cr_s < 5$ mg/dL) provides no further improvement in survival rate. Adequate nutritional support should not be withheld to decrease dialysis requirements.

Postrenal Acute Renal Failure

Urinary tract obstruction (UTO) may occur at the level of the renal pelvis, ureter, bladder trigone, bladder neck, or urethra:

- **Renal pelvis,** as a result of stones, sloughed papillae, stricture, aberrant vessel.
- **Ureter,** as a result of stones, sloughed papillae, blood clot, retroperitoneal carcinoma or fibrosis, pelvic carcinoma, gravid uterus, uterine fibroids, stricture, edema, accidental surgical ligation.
- **Bladder or urethra,** as a result of prostatic hypertrophy or carcinoma, bladder carcinoma, urethral valve or stricture, meatal stenosis, neurogenic bladder.

Anuria is sufficiently rare in association with other conditions that it can usually be attributed to complete UTO until proven otherwise. Notable exceptions include severe glomerulonephritis or vasculitis, bilateral vascular occlusion, or renal cortical necrosis. Complete UTO of the upper tract must be bilateral or involve a single functioning kidney. More common is incomplete, or partial, UTO. This condition may be associated with low, normal, or increased urine volume. Because the obstruction can often be readily relieved, and unrecognized obstruction can result in irreversible injury, UTO should be considered and promptly excluded in any patient with ARF in whom other causes are not obvious.

Diagnosis. Pain caused by renal colic or distension of the bladder, collecting system, or renal capsule are common symptoms with acute UTO. However, pain may be absent or vague if obstruction is gradual or partial. Its location may be a clue to the site of obstruction. Physical examination may show flank or suprapubic tenderness. The bladder may be palpably distended. Urinalysis findings are frequently unremarkable, although hematuria is common with stone disease, a sloughed papilla, and malignancy. The urine tends to be isosthenuric because of impaired sodium and water reabsorption.

Bladder catheterization should be performed if bladder

neck obstruction or a neurogenic bladder is suspected. If this treatment does not result in prompt diuresis, and obstruction is still suspected, further evaluation is indicated. A plain film of the abdomen may show a radiopaque stone. Renal and bladder ultrasonography can show hydronephrosis, and can often establish its cause. It also confirms the presence of two kidneys and allows for determination of their size and echogenicity. This information is useful in establishing the existence of underlying CRF and nonsurgically amenable renal disease. However, dilation of the collecting system may not be evident, despite the presence of UTO in the setting of early or mild obstruction, or when the collecting system is encased by retroperitoneal tumor or fibrosis.

Computed tomography or intravenous pyelography may be indicated if visualization with ultrasonography is inadequate or is unable to identify the level of obstruction. These techniques, however, carry the risk associated with radiocontrast. Antegrade pyelography can also be performed through a percutaneous nephrostomy. Retrograde pyelography can be performed during cystoscopy.

Treatment. Bladder outlet obstruction that cannot be relieved by insertion of a urethral catheter can be treated with a suprapubic cystostomy tube. More proximal obstruction can be relieved by percutaneous nephrostomy and external drainage or by internal drainage through an antegrade-placed ureteral stent. Cystoscopy may allow for retrograde placement of a ureteral stent or basket extraction of a stone.

Depending on the cause, surgical interventions might include resection of the prostate gland, ureteral reimplantation, urinary diversion, ureterolysis, or stone removal. Shock wave lithotripsy can be used to fragment suitably located stones that are not expected to pass spontaneously because of their size.

A neurogenic bladder is effectively managed by intermittent catheterization or discontinuation of anticholinergics or drugs with α-adrenergic properties (e.g., levodopa), which may be exacerbating the functional obstruction.

Relief of complete UTO is characteristically followed by postobstructive diuresis, which may be massive. The cause of this diuresis is believed to be multifactorial, resulting from volume expansion during the period of obstruction, an osmotic diuresis from retained urea, or tubular resistance to antidiuretic hormone. Milliliter-for-milliliter replacement of urinary output may become the driving force for persistent polyuria; therefore, it should not be routinely instituted. Massive diuresis may be associated with the need for potassium and magnesium replacement.

Suggested Readings

Badr KF, Ichikawa I. Prerenal failure: A deleterious shift from renal compensation to decompensation. *N Engl J Med* 1988;319:623–629.
Clear review of mechanisms involved in real adaptation and prerenal failure.
Corwin HL, Bonventre JV. Acute renal failure in the intensive care unit. *Intensive Care Med* 1988;14:10–16,86–96.
Hricik DE, Dunn MJ. Angiotensin-converting enzyme inhibitor-induced renal failure: Causes, consequences, and diagnostic uses. *J Am Soc Nephrol* 1990;1:845–858.
Mandal AK, Hebert LA, eds. Renal disease. *Med Clin North Am* 1990;74(4):859–1083.
Contains several individual articles covering various forms of acute renal failure, including acute tubular necrosis, glomerulonephritis, urinary tract obstruction, drug-induced renal injury, and hepatorenal syndrome.
Myers BD, Moran SM. Hemodynamically mediated acute renal failure. *N Engl J Med* 1986;314:97–105.
Reviews mechanisms of tubular injury related to acute renal hypoperfusion (54 references).
Zarich S, Fang LST, Diamond JR. Fractional excretion of sodium: Exceptions to its diagnostic value. *Arch Intern Med* 1985;145:108–112.
Describes diagnostic utility and limitations of FE_{Na} and other common urinary indices.

CHAPTER 57

The Renal Transplant Patient

(See Chapter 110)

Michael J. Freeland

The increasing number of kidney transplants performed annually and improved graft survival has resulted in more frequent encounters between physicians and renal transplant recipients. As selection criteria broaden and older patients and those with more complex medical problems come to transplant, more physicians than the transplant surgeon and nephrologist are becoming involved in their care. Additionally, more long-term complications are being reported.

It is unusual for a patient to die as a direct result of kidney transplantation. When death does occur and is not attributable to the transplant surgery or the extrarenal health of the recipient, it is most often caused by complications of immunosuppression. For this reason, patient survival rates show trends similar to those of allograft survival, and are highly dependent on the antigen match. In addition to an awareness of the medical and surgical complications of renal transplantation, knowledge of the side effects, toxicities, and drug interactions of commonly used immunosuppressive agents is vital for the care of transplant recipients.

Postoperative Care and Complications

Although most patients are extubated in the operative suite or postanesthesia care unit, all patients require ICU support in the first 24 to 48 hours. This support is necessary for the careful monitoring of vital signs and fluid and electrolyte status, especially in patients with delayed graft function. Hourly urine output should be replaced milliliter-for-milliliter for the first 24 hours unless central venous or pulmonary artery pressures suggest otherwise. Oliguria should lead to reevaluation of fluid status and challenges, with administration of either colloid or crystalloid as indicated. If the response to volume resuscitation is unsatisfactory, a loop diuretic should be administered.

Potassium, calcium, phosphorus, magnesium, and bicarbonate levels should be checked frequently, and replacement provided as needed. As many as one-third of patients become hypercalcemic at some point after successful transplantation. This condition may occur within days, and is common within the first month. Severe hypophosphatemia may develop rapidly if normal renal function is restored quickly.

A decrease in urine output or persistent oliguria in the early postoperative period requires a systematic search for the cause before it is attributed to delayed graft function. The bladder catheter should be manually irrigated to exclude mechanical obstruction from blood clots. A change to a large, multihole catheter may be helpful if there is hematuria with clots. Continuous bladder irrigation is contraindicated because of the recent bladder anastomosis. Persistent oliguria or anuria should prompt consideration of more proximal obstruction or arterial or venous thrombosis. In addition to blood clots, more proximal obstruction may be caused by torsion or necrosis of the ureter or extrinsic compression of the ureter by fluid collections. Urinary extravasation may occur at the cystostomy site. Hematomas, seromas, urinomas, and lymphoceles all may compromise renal blood or urine flow. Ultrasonography may show hydronephrosis, and it allows for evaluation of the perinephric bed. Serial renograms should be performed to assess renal blood flow and tubular function. Most urologic complications occur in the first few weeks after transplant.

If serial renograms show deterioration in uptake or flow,

or there is no clinical improvement in 10 to 14 days in a patient with delayed graft function, a percutaneous renal biopsy should be considered to exclude rejection (see below).

The incidence of wound complications has significantly decreased in recent years, but vigilance is still required to decrease the risk of postoperative infection in the immunosuppressed transplant recipient. The most common infections in the first month after transplant are bacterial infections, including urinary tract infection (UTI), wound infection, pneumonia, sepsis, and endocarditis. Infections that occur during this period may be caused by preexisting UTI, pneumonia, hepatitis, or herpes simplex, or may result from infections transmitted by the renal allograft, such as hepatitis B, human immunodeficiency virus (HIV), cytomegalovirus (CMV), or bacterial infection. Exogenous causes include those associated with bladder catheters, endotracheal tubes, and intravenous catheters. All of these devices should be removed as soon as is feasible postoperatively. Infection surveillance should include intraoperative cultures of the bladder and kidney, pre- and postoperative chest radiographs, and a repeat urine culture before removal of the bladder catheter and as indicated by symptoms.

In an attempt to reduce the incidence of infection during the immediate postoperative period, most transplant protocols employ prophylactic antimicrobials. A second-generation cephalosporin with antistaphylococcal activity is frequently administered during the first 48 hours. Trimethoprim-sulfamethoxazole is occasionally used to prevent *Pneumocystis carinii* and UTIs. Antiviral agents may also be used. Acyclovir is often given to patients who have a history of herpes simplex infections. Acyclovir or ganciclovir and anti-CMV immunoglobulin preparations are used to reduce the incidence of CMV disease, particularly in CMV-seronegative patients who are receiving organs from CMV-positive donors. Oral and vaginal nystatin or clotrimazole is frequently given as prophylaxis against *Candida* species.

Immunosuppressive Therapy

Transplant immunosuppressive protocols vary widely among transplant centers. Currently employed regimens include cyclosporine with high- or low-dose prednisone, triple therapy (cyclosporine, azathioprine, prednisone), and conventional therapy (azathioprine, prednisone) with or without induction with antilymphocyte globulin, or quadruple therapy (induction antilymphocyte globulin followed by maintenance cyclosporine, azathioprine, and prednisone). Tacrolimus (FK506) is currently under study as an alternative to cyclosporine or as rescue therapy in patients failing or intolerant to cyclosporine-based immunosuppressive regimens. Its mechanism of action is similar to that of cyclosporine. Currently available monoclonal antibody therapy directed at the pan-T cell receptor CD3 (T3), OKT3, is effective in the treatment of acute rejection.

Glucocorticoids. Glucocorticoids have significant immunosuppressive, anti-inflammatory, and lymphocytolytic effects. The major glucocorticoids used in transplantation are prednisone, prednisolone, and methylprednisolone. The large number and frequent occurrence of side effects are well known and will not be recounted here.

Azathioprine. Azathioprine is an analogue of 6-mercaptopurine that functions as an antimetabolite to inhibit purine nucleotide synthesis. The major side effect is myelotoxicity, especially leukopenia and thrombocytopenia. Macrocytic anemia may also be seen. Less common side effects include intrahepatic cholestasis and acute pancreatitis. Interstitial pulmonary fibrosis and bladder carcinoma rarely occur.

Cyclosporine. Cyclosporine blocks an early stage of T lymphocyte activation and inhibits interleukin-2 release from activated helper T cells while sparing suppressor T lymphocytes. Unfortunately, it also has a wide range of side effects.

- **Renal,** including renal insufficiency, hyperuricemia, hyperkalemia, hypomagnesemia, type IV renal tubular acidosis, interstitial fibrosis, glomerular capillary thrombosis.
- **Vascular,** including hypertension, arteriolar hyalinosis, vasoconstriction, renal artery thrombosis, hemolytic-uremic syndrome.
- **GI,** including hepatotoxicity, cholestasis, cholelithiasis, pancreatitis.
- **Neurologic,** including tremors, paresthesias, seizures, encephalopathy.
- **Oncogenic,** including lymphomas, Kaposi's sarcoma.
- **Infectious,** including bacterial, viral, fungal infections.
- **Metabolic,** including diabetes, hypercholesterolemia, mammary hyperplasia.
- **Musculoskeletal,** including gout.
- **Other,** including hypertrichosis, gingival hyperplasia, acne, mild anemia, thrombocytopenia, leukopenia.

Cyclosporine use is complicated by tremendous individual variation in pharmacokinetics. It also has many drug interactions, including those that:

- **Increase cyclosporine levels,** such as antibiotics (erythromycin, norfloxacin, imipenem, doxycycline, aminoglycosides); antifungals (ketoconazole, fluconazole); antihypertensives (diltiazem, verapamil, nicardipine) acetazolamide; steroids; cimetidine; metoclopramide; colchicine.

- **Decrease cyclosporine levels,** such as antibiotics (rifampin, nafcillin, trimethoprim-sulfamethoxazole, isoniazid); anticonvulsants (phenytoin, phenobarbital, carbamazepine).
- **Potentiate cyclosporine nephrotoxicity,** such as nonsteroidal anti-inflammatory drugs; amphotericin B; antibiotics (aminoglycosides, trimethoprim-sulfamethoxazole); antivirals (ganciclovir, acyclovir); ranitidine; cimetidine.

A common and serious cyclosporine-associated complication is nephrotoxicity. This complication has led to the elimination of cyclosporine from the immediate or late post-transplant immunosuppressive regimen of many protocols. The nephrotoxicity of cyclosporine may be reversible or irreversible. Reversible nephrotoxicity is related to afferent arterial vasoconstriction, which reverses with a decrease in dose and may be lessened with the use of calcium channel blocking agents. Irreversible vasculopathy is caused by afferent arteriole occlusion and characterized by histologic findings of interstitial fibrosis and tubular atrophy.

OKT3. Within minutes of administration of OKT3, the circulating T lymphocyte count decreases. This effect is sustained by daily administration during the course of OKT3 therapy (10–14 days), and it reverses more than 90% of acute rejection episodes in the first 3 months after transplant, including those that are steroid resistant. Administration of OKT3 (especially the first two doses) is commonly associated with an influenza-like syndrome characterized by fever and chills as well as other symptoms reminiscent of leaky capillary syndrome. Severe pulmonary edema can develop in volume-expanded patients. Intravenous methylprednisolone before and hydrocortisone after OKT3 administration can mitigate these adverse effects.

Antilymphocyte Globulin. Polyclonal antibody directed against lymphocytes or thymocytes is used both as prophylaxis (induction) and as antirejection therapy. However, lack of standardization of potency and purity, earlier sensitization, and toxic and anaphylactic reactions make these preparations more difficult to use.

Transplant Rejection

Better histocompatibility matching and immunosuppressive protocols have led to improved long-term graft survival. Although with increasing time after transplantation the risk of rejection decreases as a result of both host (tolerance) and graft factors (adaptation), rejection remains an ever-present concern in nonidentical transplants. Difficulty arises, however, when rejection must be distinguished from other causes of worsening graft function, particularly in the immediate post-transplant period.

Hyperacute rejection occurs at the time of surgery. Within minutes of revascularization, preformed antibodies in the recipient initiate a dramatic destruction of the graft. This process is complete within hours. No therapy is possible. Fortunately, this form of rejection is rare with modern pretransplant crossmatching.

Acute rejection typically occurs within the first few months after transplant, but may also occur after the first year, particularly in patients who are noncompliant with their immunosuppressive regimen or after an abrupt change in immunosuppressive protocols. Typical signs include fever, graft swelling and tenderness, oliguria, hypertension, ileus, and lymphocyturia. Typical symptoms include graft and abdominal pain, nausea, and malaise. However, acute rejection, especially beyond the first post-transplant month, can occur in the absence of these classic signs and symptoms. Both antibody- and cell-mediated acute rejection responds to treatment. Successful therapy depends on rapid diagnosis and treatment. The differential diagnosis of acute rejection includes hypovolemia, acute tubular necrosis, vascular complications, urologic complications, lymphocele, cyclosporine toxicity, UTI, and recurrent glomerulopathy. The diagnosis rests on urinalysis, assessment of renal blood flow, and evaluation of the perinephric bed. Percutaneous renal biopsy is performed when less invasive methods do not establish the diagnosis.

Chronic rejection occurs after the sixth post-transplant month. It is characterized by steady deterioration of graft function that is unresponsive to antirejection therapy. As with acute rejection, other potentially reversible causes of renal failure must be excluded. In addition to those listed above, nonsteroidal anti-inflammatory drugs, angiotensin-converting enzyme inhibitors, and radiocontrast agents are common causes.

Other Long-Term Complications

Hypertension is the most common long-term complication, occurring in approximately 50% of renal transplant recipients. It may be caused by allograft dysfunction, renin production by the native kidneys, or transplant renal artery stenosis, as well as by medications (cyclosporine, corticosteroids). This complication, combined with hyperlipidemia, contributes to the development of arteriosclerotic vascular disease. Cerebrovascular and coronary artery disease are major causes of morbidity and mortality, especially in diabetic patients. Transplant recipients are at increased risk for the development of venous thromboembolic complications as well.

GI complications occur in approximately 40% of transplant recipients, and include peptic ulcer disease, colorectal bleeding and perforation, pancreatitis, and liver disease. Liver disease may be the result of infectious causes (viral hepatitis) or medications (azathioprine, methyldopa, isoniazid). Late urologic complications include vesicoureteral reflux and ureteral obstruction caused by scarring or rejection. Recurrence of the original renal disease in the allograft may occur, and can result in graft loss. Bone disease (osteoporosis, osteonecrosis), myopathy, and cataracts are common, disabling complications of chronic steroid use.

Post-transplant diabetes mellitus (in previously nondiabetic patients) is probably multifactorial in etiology, not solely the result of steroids. Another common metabolic derangement is hyperuricemia, occurring in 30–50% of patients who receive azathioprine and 50–90% of patients who receive cyclosporine. Clinical gout is rare in the former group, but occurs in approximately 10% of the latter group.

All forms of immunosuppression used in transplantation have been associated with an increased incidence of malignancy. The incidence increases over time. Epithelial carcinomas and lymphoma (especially non–Hodgkin's) are the most common.

Suggested Readings

Chan GL, Gruber SA, Skjei KL, et al. Principles of immunosuppression. *Crit Care Clin* 1990;6:841–892.

Excellent review of mechanisms and clinical use of cyclosporine, azathioprine, corticosteroids, antilymphocyte globulin, and OKT3 (356 references).

Dunn DL. Problems related to immunosuppression: Infection and malignancy occurring after solid organ transplantation. *Crit Care Clin* 1990;6:955–977.

Extensively discusses spectrum of infections to which the immunosuppressed transplant patient is susceptible.

Fabrega AJ, Lopez-Boado M, Gonzalez S. Problems in the long-term renal allograft recipient. *Crit Care Clin* 1990;6:979–1005.

Frey DJ, Matas AJ. Renal transplantation. *Crit Care Clin* 1990;6:899–910.

Reviews operative procedure, perioperative care, and survival statistics for renal transplantation.

Rao KV. Mechanism, pathophysiology, diagnosis, and management of renal transplant rejection. *Med Clin North Am* 1990;74:1039–1057.

Yoshimura N, Oka T. Medical and surgical complications of renal transplantation: Diagnosis and management. *Med Clin North Am* 1990; 74:1025–1037.

Covers operative, infectious, GI, orthopedic, oncologic, and other complications related to renal transplantation.

CHAPTER 58

Drug Dosing in Renal Insufficiency

(See Chapter 111)

Michael J. Ruffing and James A. Kruse

Many drugs that are commonly used in the management of critically ill patients require dosing modification if there is renal impairment (Table 58–1). Such modifications are usually based on the patient's creatinine clearance (Cl_{Cr}), a marker of renal function that closely parallels glomerular filtration rate (GFR). One formula that is commonly used for estimating Cl_{Cr} at the bedside is:

$$Cl_{Cr} = \frac{(140 - \text{age}) \times \text{IBW}}{72 \times Cr_s}$$

where Cr_s represents serum creatinine concentration (mg/dL), IBW represents ideal body weight (kg), and age is expressed in years. This equation is used for male patients; for use in female patients, the result is multiplied by 0.85. IBW can be determined with the following formulas:

$$\text{Male: IBW} = 50 + (2.3 \times \text{height in inches} > 5 \text{ feet})$$

$$\text{Female: IBW} = 45.5 + (2.3 \times \text{height in inches} > 5 \text{ feet})$$

The above formula for Cl_{Cr} is most accurate in patients with stable renal function and a GFR rate greater than 30 mL/min. Overestimation of renal function may occur in patients with acute renal deterioration because changes in Cr_s are generally delayed. Overestimation of GFR may also occur in patients with decreased creatinine production (e.g., malnutrition, hepatic insufficiency, muscular dystrophy) or lower GFRs, where tubular secretion plays a more significant role (e.g., glomerular disease). If Cr_s is less than 1.0 mg/dL, some clinicians substitute 1.0 mg/dL to account for the decrease in creatinine production common in ICU patients. Underestimation of GFR from Cl_{Cr} may occur if there is increased creatinine load (e.g., rhabdomyolysis), inhibition of creatinine secretion (e.g., trimethoprim, cimetidine), or interference with the creatinine assay. Interference can occur when the Jaffe assay method is employed because this colorimetric reaction cross-reacts with serum ketones (e.g., in diabetic ketoacidosis), ascorbic acid, barbiturates, and cefoxitin. The most accurate determination of Cl_{Cr} is obtained from a timed urine collection ($\geq$ 4 hours) and the following formula:

$$Cl_{Cr} = \frac{Cr_U \times V}{Cr_S \times t}$$

where Cl_{Cr} is expressed in milliliters per minute, Cr_U represents urine creatinine concentration (mg/dL), V is the volume of urine (mL), Cr_S is serum creatinine (mg/dL), and t is the collection time (minutes). Ideally, the serum creatinine level should be obtained during the midpoint of the urine-collection interval.

Besides affecting excretion, renal dysfunction has potential effects related to drug dosing. In patients with end-stage renal disease, drug absorption may be impaired secondary to gut edema or concomitant antacid administration. Severe renal insufficiency also affects protein binding. This effect is caused by decreased albumin levels, alterations in binding sites, and drug metabolites and endogenous substances that compete for binding. Many drugs, such as phenytoin, may increase the unbound to bound drug ratio, with the actual amount of unbound (active) drug remaining constant. The metabolism of certain drugs may be decreased because of diminished hepatic and renal microsomal enzyme activity. Some drugs are eliminated through hemodialysis, particularly those with high water solubility, low protein binding, low volume of distribution, and molecular weight less than 500 da. Supplemental doses may therefore be required after dialysis.

Aminoglycosides and vancomycin require careful initial dosing selection based on the level of renal function (Table 58–2). Subsequent dosing modifications are commonly required in patients with renal impairment, and are based on pharmacokinetic monitoring. Steady-state pre- (C_{pre}) and postdose (C_{post}) serum levels should be obtained. Estimates of the actual maximum (C_{max}) and minimum (C_{min}) plasma concentrations of aminoglycosides can then be calculated with the following equations:

$$K = \frac{-\ln\ (C_{post}/C_{pre})}{t_2 - t_1}$$

$$C_{max} = \frac{C_{post}}{e^{-K \times t}}$$

$$C_{min} = C_{pre} \times e^{-K \times t}$$

$$V = \frac{R \times (1 - e^{-K \times t'})}{K \times [C_{max} - (C_{min} \times e^{-K \times t'})]}$$

where K is the elimination constant (hr^{-1}); C_{post} is the measured postdose serum concentration (μg/mL); C_{pre} is the measured predose serum concentration (μg/mL); t_2 is the

Text continued on page 379

TABLE 58–1

DOSING SUGGESTIONS (% OF NORMAL) AND EFFECTS OF HEMODIALYSIS FOR DRUGS COMMONLY USED IN THE ICU SETTING (also see Table 111–1 in the main text)

Drug	Dose			Hemodialysis
	$Cl_{Cr} > 50$	Cl_{Cr} 10–50	$Cl_{Cr} < 10$	(% removed)
Acetaminophen	NC	75	50	0–50
Amikacin	(pharmacokinetic monitoring)			50–100
Amphotericin B	NC	NC	75	NS
Ampicillin	NC	50	25	25–50
Aspirin	NC	75	Avoid	50–100
Atracurium	NC	NC	NC	?
Aztreonam	NC	50	25	25–50
Bretylium	NC	25–50	Avoid	25–75
Cefazolin	NC	75	50	25–50
Cefoperazone	NC	NC	NC	< 25
Cefotaxime	NC	NC	50	25–50
Cefotetan	NC	50–75	25–50	25–50
Cefoxitin	NC	NC	50	25–50
Ceftazidime	NC	50	25	50–100
Ceftizoxime	NC	50	25	25–50

Ceftriaxone	NC	NC	NC	NS
Cefuroxime	NC	50	10	25–75
Cimetidine	NC	75	50	< 25
Ciprofloxacin	NC	50	25	< 25
Clindamycin	NC	NC	NC	NS
Clonidine	NC	NC	50–75	NS
Co-trimoxazole	NC	75	50	5–50
Digoxin	NC	25–75	10–25	NS
Enalapril	NC	75	50	25–75
Erythromycin	NC	NC	50–75	NS
Ethambutol	NC	75	50	< 50
Famotidine	NC	50	25	NS
Fluconazole	NC	50	25	25–50
Furosemide	NC	NC	NC	NS
Gentamicin	(pharmacokinetic monitoring)			50–100
Haloperidol	NC	NC	NC	NS
Hydralazine	NC	NC	50	NS
Imipenem	NC	50	25	25–50
Insulin	NC	75	50	NS
Isoniazid	NC	NC	75	50–100
Labetalol	NC	NC	NC	NS
Lidocaine	NC	NC	NC	NS
Lorazepam	NC	NC	50	NS

Table continued on following page

TABLE 58–1 *Continued*

DOSING SUGGESTIONS (% OF NORMAL) AND EFFECTS OF HEMODIALYSIS FOR DRUGS COMMONLY USED IN THE ICU SETTING (also see Table 111–1 in the main text)

Drug	Dose			Hemodialysis
	$Cl_{Cr} > 50$	Cl_{Cr} 10–50	$Cl_{Cr} < 10$	(% removed)
Meperidine	NC	NC	50–75	NS
Metoprolol	NC	NC	NC	?
Metronidazole	NC	75	50	50–100
Mezlocillin	NC	NC	50	< 50
Midazolam	NC	NC	75	?
Morphine	NC	NC	50–75	NS
Nafcillin	NC	NC	NC	NS
Nitroprusside	NC	NC	NC	Thiocyanate dialyzed
Pancuronium	NC	NC	Avoid	?
Penicillin G	NC	75	50	< 50
Pentamidine	NC	75	50	NS

Pentobarbital	NC	NC	NC	< 25
Phenobarbital	NC	NC	50–75	25–50
Phenytoin	NC	NC	NC	NS
Piperacillin	NC	75	50	25–50
Procainamide	NC	50–75	10–25	< 50
Quinidine	NC	NC	NC	< 25
Ranitidine	NC	75	50	< 25
Rifampin	NC	NC	NC	NS
Theophylline	NC	NC	NC	25–100
Ticarcillin	NC	50	25	25–50
Tobramycin	(pharmacokinetic monitoring)			50–100
Vancomycin	(pharmacokinetic monitoring)			NS
Vecuronium	NC	NC	NC	?
Verapamil	NC	NC	NC	NS
Warfarin	NC	NC	NC	NS

NC = no change; NS = no significant amount; ? = unknown.

TABLE 58–2

INITIAL DOSING GUIDELINES FOR AMINOGLYCOSIDES AND VANCOMYCIN

Drug	Dose (mg/kg)	Dosing interval (hours) based on Cl_{Cr}				
		A	*B*	*C*	*D*	*E*
Gentamicin/tobramycin	2–3	8	12	24	24–72	
	1–1.5					After HD
Amikacin	6–10	8	12	24	24–72	
	3–5					After HD
Vancomycin	15–20	8	12	24–48	48–120	120–200

Cl_{Cr} = creatinine clearance (A > 120 mL/min; B = 50–120 mL/min; C = 20–49 mL/min; D < 20 mL/min; E = end-stage renal disease); HD = hemodialysis.

time of C_{pre} after the previous infusion (hr); t_1 is the time of C_{post} after infusion (hr); t is the time between infusion and C_{post} or C_{pre} (hr); C_{max} is the maximum plasma concentration, i.e., immediately after infusion (μg/mL); C_{min} is the minimum plasma concentration, i.e., just before infusion (μg/mL); V is the volume of distribution (L); and t′ is the infusion time (hr). After the above variables are calculated, dosing adjustments can be made with the following formulas:

$$T = \frac{-1}{K} \times \ln \frac{C_{min*}}{C_{max*}} + t'$$

$$R = K \times V \times C_{max*} \times \frac{(1 - e^{-K \times T*})}{(1 - e^{-K \times t'*})}$$

$$C_{min} = C_{max*} \times e^{-K \times (T - t')}$$

$$MD = R \times t'$$

where T is the dosing interval (hr); * represents a desired value; R is the rate of infusion (mg/hr); and MD is the maintenance dose (mg). These calculations assume steady-state, one-compartment pharmacokinetics. Although vancomycin more closely resembles a two- or three-compartment model, a clinically acceptable adjustment of dosage can be achieved with the above formulas. C_{max} and C_{min} should be targeted as follows:

Gentamicin/tobramycin:
$C_{min} < 2$ μg/mL, $C_{max} = 4$ to 12 μg/mL,

Amikacin:
$C_{min} < 5$ μg/mL, $C_{max} = 20$ to 30 μg/mL,

Vancomycin:
$C_{min} = 5$ to 15 μg/mL, $C_{max} = 25$ to 40 μg/mL.

If C_{min} is high, the interval is extended. If C_{max} is high or low, the dose is adjusted. The target C_{max} is dependent on the source and severity of the infection.

Suggested Readings

Bennett W. Guide to drug dosage in renal failure. *Clin Pharmacokinet* 1988;15:326–354.

General review that contains a comprehensive list of commonly used drugs that includes the half-life, effects of dialysis, and dosing for patients with renal insufficiency.

Cockcroft DW, Gault HM. Prediction of creatinine clearance from serum creatinine. *Nephron* 1976;16:31–41.

Describes derivation of formula used for estimating creatinine clearance.

Gambertoglio J. Drug use in renal disease. In: Knoben JE, Anderson PO, eds. *Handbook of clinical drug data,* 7th ed. Hamilton, IL: Drug Intelligence Publications, Inc., 1993:161–194.

General review of drug dosing in renal failure. Includes table of drugs with corresponding percentage removed from the body through hemodialysis, peritoneal dialysis, and hemoperfusion.

Keller F, Offermann F, Lode H. Supplementary dose after hemodialysis. *Nephron* 1982;30:220–227.

Describes methods for calculating supplemental drug doses after hemodialysis. Includes list of drugs with percentage removed by hemodialysis and suggested supplemental doses.

Sawchuk RJ, Zaske DE, Cipolle RJ, et al. Kinetic model for gentamicin dosing with the use of individual patient parameters. *Clin Pharmacol Ther* 1977;21:362–369.

Assesses use of a one-compartment first-order elimination pharmacokinetic model to predict peak (C_{max}) *and nadir* (C_{min}) *serum levels.*

Metabolic Disorders

CHAPTER 59

Alcoholic Ketoacidosis

(See Chapters 62 and 106)

Cristina E. Cuevas-Korensky
and James A. Kruse

Alcoholic ketoacidosis is a syndrome that occurs in chronic, excessive alcohol users who have undergone prolonged fasting, usually after a drinking binge. The syndrome is characterized by:

- High anion gap metabolic acidosis.
- Ketonemia.
- Ketonuria.
- Low, normal, or slightly elevated serum glucose levels.

Etiology

Ethanol is irritating to the gastric mucosa, and when ingested in large quantities, may lead to gastritis, with nausea, vomiting, and epigastric pain. If they are severe enough, these symptoms may lead to abstinence from food and water. Ethanol inhibits gluconeogenesis, and promotes ketone and lactate production. If prolonged fasting takes place after ethanol ingestion, hepatic glycogen stores will be depleted, resulting in hypoglycemia, with release of epinephrine, cortisol, and growth hormone. This condition leads to hypoinsulinemia, which is responsible for increased lipolysis and an overabundance of free fatty acids presented to the liver for ketone production. In addition, oxidation of ketones by peripheral tissues is decreased. The result is ketonemia and ketonuria, ketone-induced osmotic diuresis with intravascular volume depletion, dehydration, and electrolyte loss.

Clinical Features

Patients frequently have the following signs and symptoms:

- Nausea, vomiting, or epigastric pain.
- History of recent heavy ethanol intake followed by anorexia or inability to eat or drink because of vomiting.
- Tachypnea (Kussmaul breathing).
- Tachyardia.
- Orthostatic changes in blood pressure and heart rate.
- Dry mucosa, decreased skin turgor, and other signs of dehydration.

Patients with severe intravascular volume depletion may have hypotension, oliguria, and mental obtundation. Hypothermia is not uncommon. Laboratory findings show increased anion gap metabolic acidosis, usually with normal or low serum glucose levels. Serum glucose level may be mildly increased in some patients. Serum and urine ketones will usually be detected by standard clinical tests that use the nitroprusside-based colorimetric assay. However, the degree of ketonemia and ketonuria may be substantially underestimated because β-hydroxybutyrate, the most abundant ketone body in this syndrome, is not detected by the nitroprusside test. Serum lactate levels are often somewhat elevated, but rarely exceed 5 mmol/L. Serum urea nitrogen and creatinine concentrations may be elevated; potassium and phosphorus levels may be low. The degree of acidemia can range from mild to severe. There is often concomitant metabolic alkalosis because of vomiting. In some cases, the alkalosis is more severe than the acidosis, resulting in an elevated blood pH despite the underlying ketoacidosis. Because this syndrome evolves as ethanol levels are decreasing, patients frequently have low or undetectable blood alcohol concentrations.

Differential Diagnosis

The diagnosis is made by recognizing the typical presentation and laboratory findings, which show high anion gap metabolic acidosis, ketonemia, ketonuria, and no significant hyperglycemia. It is important to differentiate this syndrome from other causes of high anion gap metabolic acidosis that require prompt recognition, such as salicylate overdose, ethylene glycol or methanol intoxication, diabetic ketoacidosis, and lactic acidosis as a result of circulatory shock or other causes. A serum and urine drug screen and serum osmolality determination should be obtained in all patients, and the osmole gap should be calculated (see Chapter 94 in this book). If lactate levels do not normalize with adequate hydration and dextrose administration, other causes of lactic acidosis should be sought.

Treatment

The treatment goal is to restore intravascular volume, replace total body water and electrolyte deficits, and provide dextrose. In patients with hypotension or evidence of end-organ hypoperfusion, such as decreased urine output, the initial IV solution should consist of 5% dextrose in normal saline, initially administered at a high infusion rate (e.g., 1 L/hr). To avoid precipitating Wernicke's encephalopathy, thiamine (100 mg IV) should be given before dextrose is administered. To guide fluid resuscitation and prevent precipitating congestive heart failure, pulmonary artery catheterization may be considered in patients with documented or suspected left ventricular dysfunction. Once blood pressure and urine output have been restored, the IV solution may be changed to 5% dextrose in 0.45% saline and the infusion rate decreased (e.g., to 200 mL/hr). IV fluid infusion should continue until the anion gap has normalized and other signs and symptoms of dehydration are no longer present.

Serum electrolyte levels should be monitored every 4 to 6 hours, and potassium should be replaced as needed. Special attention should be paid to the serum level of phosphorus. Even though serum phosphorus levels may initially be normal, patients with alcoholic ketoacidosis tend to be severely depleted of total body phosphorus. Intracellular oxidative phosphorylation, previously depressed for lack of substrate, resumes at an accelerated rate, with rapid phosphorus use once dextrose is given. Parenteral phosphorus supplementation should be initiated to maintain serum levels greater than 2.5 mmol/L. Insulin administration is not required unless diabetes is suspected. A normally functioning pancreas will increase insulin production adequately in response to dextrose administration. Bicarbonate administration is usually unnecessary in alcoholic ketoacidosis.

Because most of these patients have a history of chronic alcohol intake, alcohol withdrawal may occur. This condition should be anticipated and treated accordingly.

Prognosis

These patients usually recover without sequelae. The acidosis usually resolves within 12 to 24 hours after appropriate therapy is instituted. If patients are appropriately treated with dextrose, thiamine, IV fluids, and electrolytes, mortality and morbidity rates are related to concomitant underlying illness (e.g., pancreatitis, GI hemorrhage, or alcohol withdrawal) rather than to the ketoacidosis.

Suggested Readings

Adams SL, Matthews JJ, Flaherty JJ. Alcoholic ketoacidosis. *Ann Emerg Med* 1987;16:90–97.

Case report of alcoholic ketoacidosis followed by excellent discussion of clinical and laboratory findings of this disease as well as its treatment (83 references).

Dillon ES, Dyer WW, Smelo LS. Ketone acidosis in nondiabetic adults. *Med Clin North Am* 1940;24:1813–1822.

First description of alcoholic ketoacidosis.

Halperin ML, Hammeke M, Josse RG, et al. Metabolic acidosis in the alcoholic: A pathophysiological approach. *Metabolism* 1983;32:308–315.

Reviews pathophysiology of alcoholic ketoacidosis.

Miller PD, Heinig RE, Waterhouse C. Treatment of alcoholic ketoacidosis: The role of dextrose and phosphorus. *Arch Intern Med* 1978;138:67–72.

Compares saline versus dextrose solutions in treatment of alcoholic ketoacidosis and discusses physiologic importance of phosphorus administration.

Platia EV, Hsu TH. Hypoglycemic coma with ketoacidosis in nondiabetic alcoholics. *West J Med* 1979;131:270–276.

Clinical report of five patients with alcoholic ketoacidosis who were in a hypoglycemic coma. Contains an excellent discussion of the mechanism of ketosis in this syndrome and the clinical presentation, laboratory findings, treatment, and outcome.

CHAPTER 60

Diabetic Ketoacidosis and Hyperosmolar Syndrome

(See Chapter 106)

James A. Kruse and Michael A. Geheb

Diabetic ketoacidosis (DKA) and hyperglycemic, nonketotic dehydration (hyperosmolar) syndrome can be considered poles of a spectrum of life-threatening metabolic derangements that can occur because of lack of insulin. This lack of insulin results in impaired glucose utilization, increased glucose production, increased ketogenesis, and shifts in the distribution of water and electrolytes between the intracellular and extracellular space, mediated by the hypertonic (hyperglycemic) state. The major consequences of these disturbances are hyperglycemia, hyperosmolality and hypertonicity, metabolic acidosis, electrolyte disturbances, and glycosuria. Glycosuria results in osmotic diuresis that leads to dehydration and potentially to hypovolemic circulatory shock. In DKA, the major metabolic abnormality is metabolic acidosis as a result of excessive production of β-hydroxybutyric and acetoacetic acid. In hyperosmolar syndrome, ketoacid production is increased slightly or not at all, but extreme hyperglycemia occurs and leads to a significant increase in serum osmolality and tonicity, with resultant CNS dehydration that leads to adverse CNS consequences.

Diabetic Ketoacidosis

DKA can occur in patients with insulin-dependent diabetes, or it may occur as the first manifestation of diabetes. In either case, a specific precipitating factor can often be identified as triggering the episode of DKA. Among the most frequent precipitating factors are infection, noncompliance with long-term insulin therapy, trauma, acute myocardial infarction, and acute cerebrovascular events. However, in about half of cases, no precipitating cause can be found.

Clinical Findings. The symptoms and physical signs of DKA may be categorized as:

- **Constitutional,** such as weakness, malaise, myalgias, polydipsia and polyuria.
- **GI,** such as nausea, vomiting, anorexia, abdominal pain, and ileus.
- **Neurologic,** such as lethargy, headache, and delerium.
- **Respiratory,** such as hyperpnea (Kussmaul breathing), tachypnea, and odor of acetone on the breath.
- **Cardiovascular,** such as tachycardia, orthostatic hypotension, or frank circulatory shock.

The typical range of fluid deficit in DKA is 3.5–7 L. The chief clinical tools for assessing the degree of volume depletion and hypovolemia are assessment of heart rate, blood pressure (including postural changes), jugular venous distension, mucous membranes, and skin turgor. In most conditions, urine output is a valuable indicator of fluid status; however, the osmotic diuresis present in DKA may result in apparently adequate urine output despite severe dehydration.

Laboratory findings include:

- **Hyperglycemia** (serum glucose level typically ranges from 400–800 mg/dL), with associated hyperosmolality and glucosuria.
- **Electrolyte derangements,** such as hyperkalemia (typical before treatment is initiated), hypokalemia (typical after initiation of treatment), hyponatremia or hypernatremia, hypomagnesemia, and hypophosphatemia.
- **Metabolic acidosis,** usually in association with an elevated anion gap.
- **Ketonemia** and ketonuria.
- **Increased serum creatinine** level, which can be caused by underlying diabetic nephropathy, but can also be a spurious response to the presence of excessive β-hydroxybutyrate. The latter can interfere with some laboratory assays for creatinine.
- **Miscellaneous** laboratory abnormalities, which may include elevations in serum urea nitrogen, lipid, amylase, lipase, creatine phosphokinase, and transaminase levels.

Serum sodium level decreases in proportion to the degree of hyperglycemia, even if there is no derangement in total body water balance. Assuming that the baseline serum glucose level is 100 mg/dL, the expected decrease in serum sodium level (ΔNa_s, mmol/L) can be estimated from the measured serum glucose concentration (glucose$_s$, mg/dL) as:

$$\Delta Na_s = 0.016 \times (Glucose_s - 100)$$

The resulting hyponatremia is real, not artifactual, but it requires no special treatment other than the treatment of DKA. The utility of the formula is in detecting and quantifying concomitant derangements in total body free-water balance while the patient is hyperglycemic. In addition to this effect of glucose on sodium, spurious hyponatremia can occur if there is severe hyperlipidemia.

Nonanion gap metabolic acidosis usually evolves during the treatment phase of DKA. Rarely, a patient can have a significant degree of DKA and yet a nonanion gap acidosis at the time of presentation. This situation occurs chiefly in patients who have normal renal function and maintain a state of near-normal hydration, despite the glycosuria-induced osmotic diuresis.

Treatment. In addition to close monitoring of vital signs, routine laboratory studies (complete blood count, multiphasic serum chemistry panel, etc.) and, in severe cases, continuous ECG monitoring, the following measures constitute standard therapy:

- **IV fluid replacement** with normal saline. A typical regimen begins with rapid administration of 1 or 2 L, followed by 1 L/hr for 1 hour, then 500 mL/hr for 2 hours, then 200–400 mL/hr until dehydration is corrected. Maintenance IV fluid is then administered at 200–300 mL/hr, adjusted to ongoing losses, until DKA is resolved. Once hypovolemia is corrected, hypotonic saline is used if the serum sodium level exceeds 140 mmol/L.
- **Insulin administration** is initiated with 0.1–0.2 units/kg regular human insulin by IV injection, and a continuous infusion is initiated at 0.1 units/kg/hr. The infusion is titrated, ideally to achieve a decrease in serum glucose level of 75–100 mg/dL/hr. The insulin infusion is further slowed as the serum glucose level declines with therapy. The infusion should not be discontinued until there is evidence that the ketoacidosis has largely abated, e.g., near-normalization of pH, serum anion gap, acetone level, or CO_2 content.
- **Serial laboratory monitoring** while the patient is receiving IV insulin should include serum or blood glucose determinations every 1–2 hours, serum electrolyte testing every 2–6 hours and, in some cases, serial arterial blood gas measurements.
- **Potassium administration** is initiated (typically at 5–20 mmol/hr, occasionally at higher rates) in patients who are not hyperkalemic. Although many patients have

normal or elevated serum potassium levels on admission, essentially all have a deficit in total body potassium. Patients with hypokalemia are severely potassium depleted. Titration of further potassium administration is guided by serial serum assay findings and the level of renal function.

- **Bicarbonate administration** is generally unnecessary, even in severe DKA. Nevertheless, some clinicians administer sodium bicarbonate (e.g., 50 mmol) if blood pH is less than approximately 7.0 to maintain pH in the range of 7.0–7.2. If bicarbonate therapy is to be used, it is advisable to begin potassium administration first because alkali administration will lower serum potassium level. Normalization or overcorrection of pH should be avoided.
- **Phosphorus administration** is necessary in patients who have hypophosphatema. Routine supplementation of phosphorus in nonhypophosphatemic patients is commonly used, but has not been shown to affect the outcome. If used, it can be administered as potassium phosphate, 15 mmol of which contains 22 mmol potassium.
- **Dextrose administration** worsens hyperglycemia, so dextrose is not given initially. However, once insulin therapy decreases the serum glucose concentration to less than 250–300 mg/dL, a dextrose-containing saline solution is used and the insulin infusion is continued at a low rate. The goal of dextrose infusion is to maintain the serum glucose level within this range, allowing further insulin administration to reverse the ketoacidosis.

Because gastric atony and GI symptoms are common, patients are given nothing by mouth. Nasogastric suction may be necessary for patients with protracted vomiting. Central venous pressure measurement may be helpful in determining fluid requirements. Most patients do not require pulmonary artery catheterization, but this intervention may be helpful in unstable patients who do not respond to initial fluid resuscitation, in the elderly, and in patients with severe sepsis or underlying heart disease. Fluid intake and output should be accurately monitored and recorded.

A thorough search is made for any precipitating cause of DKA. Cultures of blood, urine and, when indicated, other body fluids are routine, particularly in patients with fever, leukocytosis, or other signs of possible infection. Urinalysis, a chest radiograph, and one or more 12-lead ECG readings are recommended as a routine screen for precipitating disorders.

In uncomplicated cases, hyperglycemia is typically controlled within the first 8 hours; however, the ketoacidosis persists for an additional 8 to 24 hours or longer. After both hyperglycemia and ketoacidosis are controlled, IV insulin is replaced by subcutaneous administration dosed on a sliding scale according to serum or blood glucose levels determined every 4 or 6 hours.

Complications of Therapy. Life-threatening hypokalemia can develop after treatment is begun, even in patients who are not initially hypokalemic. Severe hypoglycemia can occur, particularly during IV insulin administration. Circulatory shock can develop as a result of inadequate fluid loading in the face of ongoing urinary losses. On the other hand, fluid overload and pulmonary edema can occur because of excessive fluid administration, especially in patients with underlying cardiac or renal disease. Other complications include cardiac dysrhythmias, myocardial infarction, cerebral edema, and vascular thrombosis.

Hyperosmolar Syndrome

Three important manifestations differentiate this syndrome from DKA: extreme hyperglycemia, lack of severe ketoacidosis, and severe depression of the sensorium. Extreme hyperglycemia is responsible for severe hypertonic hyperosmolality that leads to intracellular dehydration. The disorder can occur in patients with either type I or type II, diabetes; in approximately half of cases, hyperosmolar nonketotic syndrome is the first manifestation of diabetes. Mild degrees of ketosis or ketoacidosis are not uncommon in hyperosmolar syndrome. In fact, hyperosmolar syndrome and DKA can coexist.

Clinical Findings. The degree of dehydration and hypovolemia can be profound, with fluid deficits sometimes exceeding 7 L. Dehydration of the brain results in alterations of consciousness that range from disorientation to deep coma, and may include seizures and focal neurologic deficits. The serum glucose level is frequently greater than 1000 mg/dL and sometimes greater than 2000 mg/dL. The severity of CNS manifestations is proportional to the severity of hypertonicity. Serum osmolality can be measured or calculated, but tonicity can only be calculated. The calculations are obtained from simultaneously drawn measurements of serum sodium (Na_s), glucose ($glucose_s$), and urea nitrogen (UN_s):

$$\text{Serum osmolality} = (2 \times Na_s) + (Glucose_s/18) + (UN_s/2.8)$$

$$\text{Serum tonicity} = (2 \times Na_s) + (Glucose_s/18)$$

where osmolality is expressed in milliosmoles per kilogram water, sodium level is expressed in millimoles per liter, and glucose and urea nitrogen levels are expressed in milligrams per deciliter. Neurologic signs generally occur clinically when serum tonicity values exceed 320 mOsm/L.

Precipitating factors include the same factors that precipitate DKA. Among these are cerebrovascular accidents, meningitis, and other neurologic catastrophes. Any of these conditions may be obscured by or confused with the neurologic effects of the hypertonic state. A number of drugs (e.g., corticosteroids, β-adrenergic receptor antagonists, calcium channel blocking drugs, thiazides, and phenytoin) may also be precipitating factors.

Treatment of hyperosmolar syndrome is similar to that of DKA. These patients are characteristically more severely dehydrated than patients with DKA. Correction of hypovolemia takes priority over correction of hypertonicity. Therefore, despite the hypertonic state, the initial fluid of choice is normal saline. Once adequate intravascular volume is restored and the patient is hemodynamically stable, the IV fluid is changed to hypotonic saline. Administering IV insulin without concomitant fluid resuscitation can precipitate or worsen circulatory shock by causing an osmotic shift of fluid from the extracellular space to the intracellular space. Therefore, fluid administration should be started immediately, before insulin therapy is initiated.

Suggested Readings

Basu A, Close CF, Jenkins D, et al. Persisting mortality in diabetic ketoacidosis. *Diabetic Med* 1993;10:282–284.

Of 929 episodes of diabetic ketoacidosis over a 21-year period, mortality rate was 3.9%. It did not change significantly from first half of the period to second half.

Kaminska ES, Pourmotabbed G. Spurious laboratory values in diabetic ketoacidosis and hyperlipidemia. *Am J Emerg Med* 1993;11:77–80.

Case report and discussion of artifactual laboratory results that can occur in diabetic ketoacidosis, including pseudonormoglycemia and pseudonormonatremia.

Malone ML, Klos SE, Gennis VM, et al. Frequent hypoglycemic episodes in the treatment of patients with diabetic ketoacidosis. *Arch Intern Med* 1992;152:2472–2477.

Of 220 patients admitted for diabetic ketoacidosis, 30% had hypoglycemia (serum glucose level <49 mg/dL) at some point during first 2 weeks of hospitalization. Patients with fever, renal disease, or hepatic disease, and those receiving nothing by mouth are at increased risk for this complication.

Wachtel TJ, Tetu-Mouradjian LM, Goldman DL, et al. Hyperosmolarity and acidosis in diabetes mellitus. *J Gen Intern Med* 1991;6:495–502.

Retrospective study of 613 cases. Diabetic ketoacidosis alone occurred in 22% of patients, hyperosmolar nonketotic syndrome occurred alone in 45%, and 33% had features that overlapped the two syndromes. Although both syndromes occurred in young and old adults, the mean age of the pure hyperosmolar group was 63 years versus 33 years for those with pure diabetic ketoacidosis.

Zonszein J, Baylor P. Diabetic ketoacidosis with alkalemia: A review. *West J Med* 1988;149:217–219.

Case report and review of published cases of diabetic ketoacidosis with frank alkalemia. The mechanism is concomitant metabolic alkalosis, most often caused by vomiting.

CHAPTER 61

Hypoglycemia

(See Chapters 62 and 106)

Cristina E. Cuevas-Korensky

Hypoglycemia is characterized by a decrease in the blood glucose concentration to levels insufficient to meet central nervous system (CNS) glucose requirements. This situation results in impairment of CNS function and release of counter-regulatory hormones.

Etiology

Fasting glucose levels are maintained within a range of approximately 90–100 mg/dL by strict hormonal regulation. Insulin is secreted in response to increased glucose levels. It lowers the blood sugar level by facilitating its diffusion into cells. Growth hormone, cortisol, epinephrine, and glucagon are released in response to decreased glucose levels. Growth hormone and cortisol raise glucose levels by promoting gluconeogenesis, whereas glucagon and epinephrine do the same by promoting glycogen breakdown and inhibiting insulin release. Conditions in which glucose requirements increase, glucose production decreases, or hormonal regulation is altered lead to hypoglycemia. These include:

- **Hyperinsulinemia,** such as insulinoma, insulin overdose, abrupt discontinuation of total parenteral nutrition, autoimmune hypoglycemia, nonislet cell tumors (secretion of insulin-like growth factors, e.g., mesenchymal and GI tumors, adrenocortical carcinoma, hepatoma, lymphoma, leukemia), drugs (sulfonylurea, pentamidine, quinidine, quinine, ritodrine, disopyramide).
- **Deficiency of counter-regulatory hormones,** such as hypopituitarism, adrenal insufficiency, deficiency of glucagon or catecholamines.
- **Increased glucose use,** such as pregnancy, excessive exercise, nonislet cell tumors.
- **Inadequate glucose production,** such as severe hepatic disease, congestive heart failure, ethanol ingestion, drugs (β-adrenergic blocking agents, salicylates), toxic plant ingestion (akee fruit, *Amanita* species), sepsis, congenital disorders (glycogen storage disease, impaired hepatic gluconeogenesis, nonketotic hypoglycemia of childhood).

- **Miscellaneous** causes such as renal failure, malaria, reactive or postprandial hypoglycemia, malnutrition.

Clinical Features

Signs and symptoms are related to sympathetic hyperactivity and CNS dysfunction. They may include diaphoresis, tachycardia, tremulousness, slurred speech, agitation, bizarre behavior, seizures, and coma. If treatment is delayed, severe hypoglycemia can result in a persistent vegetative state or death.

Diagnosis

Low serum glucose levels (generally < 50 mg/dL), symptoms of hypoglycemia, and relief of symptoms with glucose administration constitute Whipple's triad, which is diagnostic of clinical hypoglycemia. Definitive treatment of hypoglycemia requires determination of the etiology. A serum and urine drug screen should be obtained, and C peptide, proinsulin, and insulin levels should be measured concomitantly with glucose levels. Testing for the presence of anti-insulin and anti-insulin–receptor antibodies may be necessary if the etiology is obscure (see Table 106–8 in the main text).

Treatment

If hypoglycemia is suspected, or if a patient has a coma of unknown etiology, 50 mL 50% dextrose in water should be infused as soon as IV access is established. If the patient is awake, oral carbohydrate, such as orange juice with sugar, may be given as an alternative. If possible, blood should be drawn before glucose administration. However, it is not necessary to delay treatment if the blood sample cannot be immediately obtained or while awaiting the test result. When a diabetic patient has hypoglycemia because of an overdose of short- or intermediate-acting insulin, no further treatment may be needed. If the hypoglycemia is the result of surreptitious insulin administration, overdose with long-acting insulin, sulfonylurea agents, or is secondary to an insulinoma, an infusion of 5 or 10% dextrose may be needed for several hours or days, or until the underlying condition is resolved. In all cases, blood glucose level should be monitored every 1 to 4 hours by fingerstick or conventional serum testing, and the dextrose infusion should be adjusted to maintain blood sugar levels greater than 100 mg/dL. In some cases of insulinoma, the dextrose infusion may be supplemented with agents that inhibit insulin secretion, such as diazoxide, which may be given at a dose of 300 mg IV in 1L 5% dextrose in water at 100 mL/hr. Because diazoxide is a potent antihypertensive, hypotension precludes its use. When the etiology of refractory hypoglycemia cannot be determined, 100 mg hydrocortisone or 1 mg glucagon may be added per liter of dextrose-containing IV fluid as an empiric adjunct to glycemic control.

Suggested Readings

Bauman VA, Yalow RS. Hyperinsulinemic hypoglycemia: Differential diagnosis by determination of the species of circulating insulin. *JAMA* 1984;252:2730–2734.

Reports 14 cases of hyperinsulinemic hypoglycemia and discusses how to differentiate between hyperinsulinemia secondary to insulinomas and hyperinsulinemia caused by the administration of either exogenous insulin or insulin secretagogues.

Cryer PE, Gerich JE. Glucose counterregulation, hypoglycemia and intensive insulin therapy in diabetes mellitus. *N Engl J Med* 1985; 313:232–241.

Discusses glucose hormonal regulation and pathophysiology behind altered glucose homeostasis found in certain patients with type I diabetes at risk for hypoglycemia when tight blood sugar control is attempted with intensive insulin regimen (151 references).

Field JB. Hypoglycemia: Definition, clinical presentations, classification, and laboratory tests. *Endocrinol Metab Clin North Am* 1989;18:27–43.

This issue is devoted to hypoglycemia and contains excellent reviews on carbohydrate regulation and clinical presentation, laboratory findings, and many causes of hypoglycemia.

Waskin H, Stehr-Green JK, Helmick CG, et al. Risk factors for hyperglycemia associated with pentamidine therapy for *Pneumocystis* pneumonia. *JAMA* 1988;345–347.

Retrospective investigation of the association between pentamidine treatment for Pneumocystis carinii *pneumonia and development of hypoglycemia.*

White BJ, Warrell DA, Chanthavanich P, et al. Severe hypoglycemia and hyperinsulinemia in falciparum malaria. *N Engl J Med* 1983;309:61–66.

Studies incidence of hypoglycemia in patients with falciparum malaria. Discusses pathogenesis of hypoglycemia associated with malaria as well as with quinine used to treat it.

CHAPTER 62

Diabetes Insipidus

(See Chapter 100)

Michael J. Freeland

Diabetes insipidus (DI) is a disorder characterized by clinically euvolemic hypernatremia in association with polyuria and dilute urine. It may be caused by impaired release of antidiuretic hormone (ADH), or vasopressin, from the posterior pituitary gland, referred to as central DI, or renal resistance to ADH, referred to as nephrogenic DI. DI is not usually associated with clinically significant hypernatremia because thirst allows water balance to be maintained. However, severely ill patients with DI often cannot express or act on thirst, and severe hypernatremia and dehydration can develop. Because the causes of DI are conditions that frequently require ICU care, an awareness of its etiologies and means of diagnosis is essential.

Clinical Manifestations

Polyuria (commonly defined as urine output > 3 L/day or 30 mL/kg/day) or polydipsia is usually the first manifestation of DI to attract the attention of the patient or clinician. If free-water intake is inadequate to keep up with renal or extrarenal losses, significant hypernatremia may develop. The clinical manifestations of hypernatremia are reviewed in Chapter 51. Obviously, the multiple underlying causes of central or nephrogenic DI (see below) can result in signs and symptoms that are not attributable to DI or the associated hypernatremia.

Differential Diagnosis

Evaluation of the polyuric patient should begin with establishing whether the polyuria reflects water or solute (i.e., osmotic) diuresis and whether diuresis is appropriate or inappropriate. Urine osmolality (Osm_u) less than 250 mOsm/kg H_2O is indicative of water diuresis, whereas Osm_u greater than 300 mOsm/kg H_2O indicates solute diuresis. Water diuresis may be an appropriate response to a free-water load (e.g., because of primary polydipsia), or may be inappropriate, reflecting an inability to produce concentrated urine (i.e., because of DI). Solute, or osmotic, diuresis may be an appropriate response to saline loading or excretion of retained sodium and fluid after the release of bilateral urinary tract obstruction. Inappropriate solute diuresis may be caused by osmotic diuresis that accompanies hyperglycemia or occurs in response to high-protein feedings that result in increased urea production. Sodium-wasting nephropathy is a less common cause.

Measurement of serum sodium concentration (Na_s) may be helpful in the evaluation of water diuresis. Water-loaded patients tend to have a low–normal Na_s (135–138 mmol/L), whereas hospitalized patients with DI tend to have a Na_s in the high–normal range (143–145 mmol/L) because of their limited ability to access free water as a consequence of intercurrent illness. Because of their inability to act on thirst, critically ill patients with DI can have severe hypernatremia.

Central DI may result from a number of disorders that disrupt the osmoreceptors, hypothalamic nuclei, or hypophyseal tract, and thus impair ADH secretion from the posterior lobe of the pituitary gland.

- **Idiopathic** causes, which account for approximately 30% of cases.
- **Neurosurgery,** e.g., for craniopharyngioma, transphenoidal surgery.
- **Head trauma.**
- **Hypoxic or ischemic encephalopathy,** e.g., postcardiopulmonary arrest, circulatory shock, Sheehan's syndrome.
- **Neoplastic,** either primary (e.g., craniopharyngioma, pinealoma) or metastatic (e.g., breast or lung cancer).
- **Miscellaneous,** e.g., histiocytosis X, sarcoidosis, anorexia nervosa, cerebral aneurysm, encephalitis, meningitis.

Three distinct patterns of DI follow neurosurgery or head trauma. The most common is manifested by the acute onset of polyuria, typically within 24 hours, with resolution within 3 to 5 days, or occasionally longer. The second most common cause is permanent DI. The least common is the triphasic response manifested by an initial polyuric phase lasting 4 to 5 days, followed by an antidiuretic phase lasting from days 6 to 11 and then, finally, permanent DI. The first phase is believed to be caused by inhibition of ADH release as a consequence of hypothalamic dysfunction. The second phase is believed to reflect slow release of stored ADH from the degenerating posterior pituitary. The third phase is believed to reflect depletion of pituitary stores.

Nephrogenic DI may be congenital or acquired. Diminished ADH responsiveness may be caused by reduced ADH action on the collecting tubule or reduction of the corticomedullary osmotic gradient. An unusual form of acquired nephrogenic DI in women during the second half of pregnancy has been attributed to increased circulating levels of vasopressinase (probably released from the placenta) and rapid degradation of ADH. The major causes of acquired nephrogenic DI in adults are lithium toxicity, hypercalcemia, and hypokalemia. The causes of nephrogenic DI according to the probable mechanism of action can be summarized as follows:

- **Reduced ADH action on the collecting tubule** as a result of congenital causes, hypercalcemia, hypokalemia, certain drugs (e.g., lithium, demecocycline, amphotericin B), Sjögren's syndrome, amyloidosis, renal failure.
- **Reduction of the corticomedullary osmotic gradient** as a result of osmotic diuresis (e.g., glucose, mannitol, urea) loop diuretics, protein malnutrition, renal failure (especially chronic tubulointerstitial disease).

- **Increased peripheral degradation of ADH** as a result of pregnancy.
- **Unknown mechanisms,** including methoxyflurane, ifosfamide, propoxyphene.

Diagnostic Confirmation. After the presence of inappropriate water diuresis has been established, the patient's response to exogenous ADH (vasopressin) usually discriminates between central and nephrogenic DI. In stable, noncritically ill patients, vasopressin is usually administered as part of a dehydration test aimed at producing hypernatremia, assessing the adequacy of endogenous ADH secretion or action and, finally, determining the response to exogenous ADH. Water-deprivation testing is usually deferred in ICU patients because of the attendant risks of inducing hypovolemia in unstable patients. Additionally, some of these patients are already hypernatremic and hypovolemic secondary to DI and inability to act on their thirst.

When it can be safely carried out, the aim of water restriction is to increase serum osmolality (Osm_s) to greater than 295 mOsm/kg H_2O (or $Na_s > 145$ mmol/L). Normally, this intervention results in maximal stimulation of ADH release and maximally concentrated urine (osm_u 800–1400 mOsm/kg H_2O). At this point, the administration of exogenous ADH does not normally induce a further increase in osm_u. If a patient is already hypernatremic and has dilute urine, the diagnosis of DI is established. Water deprivation is not necessary and, in fact, is dangerous before the administration of vasopressin. However, patients with partial central or nephrogenic DI may produce urine with osm_u greater than 300 mOsm/kg H_2O, may not be polyuric if solute excretion is normal, and commonly have clearly normal Na_s if they have been provided adequate free water.

Although a number of variations of the test have been described, water intake is usually restricted until the patient loses 3–5% of body weight (determined hourly along with urine volume) or until two or three consecutive hourly urine samples show osm_u values that differ by less than 10% or by less than 30 mOsm/kg H_2O after the patient has lost at least 2% of body weight. Better discrimination is achieved if dehydration is continued until osm_s is greater than 295 mOsm/kg H_2O or Na_s is greater than 145 mmol/L (determined every 2 hours), but caution must be exercised to avoid excessive volume depletion. After osm_u plateaus or osm_s or Na_s reaches the previously stated end points, exogenous ADH is administered and a urine sample is collected for a final osm_u determination 1 hour later. At this point, the test is terminated. The test should be terminated at any point at which weight loss exceeds 5%. Patients with complete DI usually maintain osm_u less than

250 mOsm/kg H_2O. Primary polydipsia is excluded if osm_u remains less than 300 mOsm/kg H_2O.

Differentiation between central and nephrogenic DI rests on the response to exogenous ADH. Aqueous vasopressin (5 units) or desamino-D-arginine vasopressin (desmopressin, 1 μg) may be administered subcutaneously, or the latter may be administered by nasal insufflation (10 μg). Expected findings in normal subjects, compulsive water drinkers (i.e., primary polydipsia), and patients with DI are summarized in Table 62–1. Measurement of plasma ADH (i.e., vasopressin) levels is expensive, not widely available, and usually not necessary with severe, or complete, forms of DI. However, the indirect measure of ADH function provided by the standard dehydration and ADH administration test may not reliably distinguish between primary polydipsia and partial defects of ADH secretion or action. Direct measurement of plasma ADH, along with simultaneous determinations of osm_s and osm_u during the dehydration test, then becomes necessary.

Treatment

Patients with DI must be provided adequate free water. Treatment of hypernatremia by water replacement is discussed in Chapter 51. For central DI, the treatment of choice is administration of exogenous ADH. Aqueous vasopressin 5–10 units subcutaneously is useful for the acute management of central DI, but it is too short acting for long-term therapy, requiring dosing every 4 to 6 hours. Vasopressin tannate in oil (2–5 units IM) requires administration only every 1 to 2 days but for the most part, this agent has been supplanted by desmopressin (10–20 μg intranasally or 1–4 μg subcutaneously) once or twice daily. Desmopressin does not lead to antivasopressin antibody production with long-term use, as do other ADH preparations.

Partial central DI may also be treated with agents that simulate ADH secretion or potentiate its action. Chlorpropamide, 125–250 mg PO once or twice daily, enhances the action of ADH. Higher doses (up to 1250 mg/day) can increase antidiuresis, but carry increased risk of hypoglycemia. Carbamezapine, 100–300 mg PO twice daily, also potentiates ADH action, and may increase its secretion as well. However, hepatic and bone marrow toxicities limit its routine use. Clofibrate, 500 mg PO three to four times daily, is the agent more commonly used to increase ADH secretion, but it is associated with GI disturbances and cholelithiasis.

Thiazide diuretics at conventional doses, and usually in combination with amiloride, can substantially reduce urine output in patients with partial central or nephrogenic DI. Thiazide-induced volume depletion enhances

TABLE 62–1

INTERPRETATION OF DIAGNOSTIC FINDINGS AFTER WATER DEPRIVATION AND VASOPRESSIN ADMINISTRATION TESTING

	Osm_u with water deprivation (mOsm/kg H_2O)	Plasma ADH after dehydration (pg/mL)	% increase in Osm_u with exogenous ADH
Normal	> 800	> 2	< 5
Complete central DI	< 300	Undetectable	> 50
Partial central DI	300–800	< 1.5	> 10
Nephrogenic DI	< 300–500	> 5	0
Primary polydipsia	> 500	< 5	< 5

Osm_u = urine osmolality; ADH = antidiuretic hormone; DI = diabetes insipidus.

proximal sodium chloride and water reabsorption, and can lead to an increase in medullary interstitial osmolality, which further promotes water reabsorption. Amiloride alone is the treatment of choice for nephrogenic DI attributable to lithium because it blocks lithium absorption through sodium channels in the collecting tubule. However, induced volume depletion can secondarily increase proximal reabsorption of lithium and potentiate its toxicity. Loop diuretics should not be used in the treatment of DI because they further impair urine-concentrating ability. Nonsteroidal anti-inflammatory drugs may ameliorate polyuria of lithium toxicity or congenital nephrogenic DI.

In addition to pharmacotherapy, a low-sodium and moderately protein-restricted diet decreases urine output by reducing the rate of solute excretion and obligate water loss.

Suggested Readings

Blevins LS, Wand GS. Diabetes insipidus. *Crit Care Med* 1992;20:69–79.
Reviews pathophysiology, diagnosis, and treatment of syndromes of diabetes insipidus, with emphasis on likely situations in ICU.

Buonocare CM, Robinson AG. The diagnosis and management of diabetes insipidus during medical emergencies. *Endocrinol Metab Clin North Am* 1993;2:411–423.

Richardson DW, Robinson AG. Desmopressin. *Ann Intern Med* 1985;103:228–239.
Extensive review of desmopressin, its pharmacology, and its clinical use in many disease states, including diabetes insipidus (165 references).

Robertson GL. Differential diagnosis of polyuria. *Ann Rev Med* 1988;39:425–442.
Discusses diagnostic approach to diabetes insipidus that begins with routine clinical observations and progresses, as needed, to more sophisticated methods of laboratory analysis.

Hematology/ Oncology

CHAPTER 63

Bone Marrow Failure

(See Chapter 116)

Robert I. Parker

Bone marrow failure refers to disorders characterized by decreased or absent production of blood cell elements. This condition may be congenital or acquired, and it may be limited to a single cellular element or may affect cells of multiple lineages. Deficiencies of specific stem cell growth factors may result in deficient blood cell production. The clearest example is the anemia of chronic renal failure, in which the red cell growth factor erythropoietin is deficient. Occasionally, deficiency of a normal dietary nutrient may result in decreased production of a particular cellular element. This situation is most commonly noted in severe iron deficiency, but may also be seen with vitamin B_{12} or folate deficiency. Nutritional deficiencies of trace metals and severe calorie deprivation can also result in hypocellular marrow and pancytopenia. In the case of nutrient or calorie deficiency, replacement of the missing nutrient or improvement in calorie intake will be curative.

Because of the relative life spans of the cellular elements, decreased blood cell production on an acute basis is more likely to cause either granulocytopenia or thrombocytopenia rather than acute anemia. In the acutely ill patient, it is rarely possible on the first evaluation to definitively distinguish between decreased production and increased destruction as the cause of thrombocytopenia or granulocytopenia. The presence of rapidly falling hemoglobin not explained by phlebotomy or bleeding is indicative of increased red cell destruction. In most cases, the presence of anemia and reticulocytopenia indicates deficient red blood cell production. The definitive diagnostic test for bone marrow failure is bone marrow aspiration and biopsy. However, this study rarely needs to be performed on an emergent basis.

Complications of Bone Marrow Failure

Red Cell Aplasia or Hypoplasia

- Insidious onset of anemia; hemoglobin level decreases by approximately 1 g/wk.
- Oxygen delivery is adequate in stable patients to a hemoglobin value of 7 g/dL.

- Signs and symptoms include pallor, tachycardia, faintness, fatigue, angina pectoris, congestive heart failure.
- Treatment includes transfusion of packed red blood cells and careful monitoring for signs of circulatory overload.

Granulocytopenia

- Defined as an absolute granulocyte count $< 500\ mm^{-3}$.
- Patients are at increased risk of bacterial infection.
- Fever in the neutropenic patient should be treated empirically with broad-spectrum antibiotics, including coverage for *Pseudomonas* species. Antibiotics should be continued for the duration of neutropenia. If fever persists beyond 48–72 hours, the antibiotic spectrum should be broadened to include anaerobic coverage. If fever persists for 1 week with negative culture findings, antifungal therapy may be added.
- Regular surveillance cultures (e.g., blood, throat, urine) may be useful. Gut decontamination may be performed.
- Granulocyte colony-stimulating factor may be beneficial if granulocytopenia is a consequence of chemotherapy.

Thrombocytopenia

- Increased risk of traumatic and spontaneous bleeding.
- Risk of bleeding is moderate at platelet levels of 10,000–20,000 mm^{-3} and significant at 5000–10,000 mm^{-3}.
- Platelet size is sometimes helpful in distinguishing between decreased production and increased destruction as the cause of thrombocytopenia; younger platelets tend to be larger than older ones.
- Platelet transfusions should be given prophylactically if the platelet count is $< 10{,}000\ mm^{-3}$. Platelets are transfused at any level of thrombocytopenia if there is active bleeding. For invasive procedures, the platelet level should be $> 50{,}000\ mm^{-3}$.
- Patients may become sensitized with repeated platelet transfusions. Single-donor platelets or HLA-matched platelets may yield a better response.
- Transfusion with leukocyte-depleted or irradiated platelet units can minimize or delay alloimmunization in patients expected to receive repeated transfusions.

Treatment of Acquired Aplastic Anemia

Supportive measures include red blood cell transfusion, platelet transfusion, and administration of antibiotics for neutropenic fever, as outlined above. Bone marrow transplant is the definitive treatment, but an HLA-matched donor is required. Immunosuppressive regimens are generally effective in 30–50% of patients. Common regimens include antithymocyte globulin (may cause serum sickness or anaphylaxis), cyclosporine (see Chapter 57 in this book), and corticosteroids.

Suggested Readings

Doncy K, Pepe M, Storb R, et al. Immunosuppressive therapy of aplastic anemia: Results of a prospective, randomized trial of antithymocyte globulin (ATG), methylprednisolone and oxymetholone to ATG, very high-dose methylprednisolone and oxymetholone. *Blood* 1992;79:2566–2571.

This article and the next describe two large series of patients treated with aggressive immunosuppression. Response rates were between 30 and 50%.

Gluckman E, Esperou-Bourdeau H, Baruchel A, et al. Multicenter randomized study comparing cyclosporin-A alone and with antithymocyte globulin with prednisone for treatment of severe aplastic anemia. *Blood* 1992;79:2540–2546.

Pizzo PA. Management of fever in patients with cancer and treatment-induced neutropenia. *N Engl J Med* 1993;328:1323–1332.

Reviews infectious risks and management of febrile, neutropenic patients.

Robinson BE, Quesenbery PJ. Hematopoietic growth factors: Overview and clinical applications. *Am J Med Sci* 1990;300:163,237,311.

Excellent review of the rapidly expanding group of therapeutic molecules.

CHAPTER 64

Hemolysis

(See Chapter 118)

Robert I. Parker

Hemolysis is the abnormal destruction of red blood cells, resulting in decreased red cell survival and liberation of hemoglobin (Hb). Hemolysis may occur in intravascular or extravascular sites, may be the result of an acquired problem or an intrinsic red cell abnormality, may result from activation of the immune system, or may be mechanical. It is characterized clinically by the following findings:

- Anemia with no obvious blood loss.
- Elevated reticulocyte count (RC), corrected for the degree of anemia:

$$\text{Corrected RC} = \frac{\text{Observed Hb}}{\text{Expected Hb}} \times \text{Observed RC.}$$

  A corrected RC $\geq 3\%$ is consistent with hemolysis.

- Acute onset of pallor, fatigue, jaundice, or dark urine.

- Elevated serum indirect bilirubin level.
- Elevated serum lactate dehydrogenase (LDH) level.
- Reduced haptoglobin level (< 50 mg/dL).
- Characteristic red cell morphologic findings on peripheral blood smear. For example, microspherocytes suggest hereditary spherocytosis or immune hemolytic anemia, target cells suggest thalassemia or liver disease, and schistocytes or helmet cells are the hallmark of mechanical hemolysis.

Intravascular hemolysis is associated with free hemoglobin in the plasma and with hemoglobinuria. The absence of red cells on a fresh urine specimen in the presence of positive hemoglobin findings by dipstick testing is presumptive of hemoglobinuria, although it can also represent myoglobinuria from rhabdomyolysis. It occurs in mechanical hemolysis (e.g., from prosthetic heart valves), complement-fixing immune hemolysis, paroxysmal nocturnal hemoglobinuria, paroxysmal cold hemoglobinuria, glucose-6-phosphate dehydrogenase (G6PD) deficiency, and clostridial sepsis. Immune hemolytic anemia should be evaluated by direct antiglobulin test (direct Coombs test) and antibody screen (indirect Coombs test).

Extravascular hemolysis occurs within the spleen. It is associated with hypersplenism, autoimmune hemolysis, hemoglobinopathies, hemolysis with liver disease, hereditary spherocytosis, and delayed transfusion reactions.

Immune Hemolytic Anemia

Autoimmune Hemolytic Anemia

Warm Antibody Autoimmune Hemolytic Anemia. Antibodies interact with red blood cells at body temperature, leading to hemolysis. Microspherocytes are seen on the peripheral smear. The direct Coombs test results are positive for IgG, complement C3, or both; the indirect Coombs test results are positive in approximately half of cases. Treatment modalities include:

- **Corticosteroids:** prednisone 1–5 mg/kg/day.
- **Splenectomy** if steroid therapy is not effective.
- **Immunosuppressive drugs** (cyclophosphamide, chlorambucil, or cyclosporine) if splenectomy is ineffective or is not medically advisable.
- **Plasmapheresis** with plasma exchange may transiently improve hemolysis in emergency situations.

IV immunoglobulin is not an effective therapy for autoimmune hemolytic anemia. The goal of treatment is to produce a stable, but not necessarily normal, hemoglobin level to provide adequate oxygen delivery. Transfusions should be given with caution because they can be associated with increased hemolysis. Repeated small increments should be used, using the least incompatible blood available and monitoring for evidence of further hemolysis. Hydration and efforts to maintain good urine output should be initiated to minimize the risk of hemoglobin-induced nephrotoxicity.

Cold agglutinin syndrome is caused by immunoglobulin M antibodies that cause red cell agglutination below body temperature. Clinically significant hemolysis is uncommon unless the agglutinin reacts at least up to 30°C. There can be clinical evidence of hemolytic anemia, a negative Coombs test result for immunoglobulin G, and a positive test result for C3 and immunoglobulin M. It is most commonly caused by *Mycoplasma pneumoniae* infection, but may also be caused by infectious mononucleosis. Treatment is primarily supportive, avoiding cold conditions. Plasmapheresis may decrease the immunoglobulin M titer in emergency situations. Transfusions should be given with care, in small volumes, with an in-line blood warmer.

Paroxysmal cold hemoglobinuria occurs as acute attacks of shaking chills, fever, malaise, and abdominal and back pain, followed by hemoglobinuria. These symptoms usually occur after cold exposure. Treatment is supportive care and avoiding cold exposure. Patients are transfused with care, in small increments, with blood warmers.

Drug-induced hemolytic anemia can occur with α-methyldopa, quinine, quinidine, penicillins and cephalosporins. Mechanisms of drug-induced hemolysis include:

- Production of antidrug antibody that cross-reacts with cell membrane antigens.
- Production of antibody to drug bound to cell membrane (e.g., penicillin).
- Drug bound to plasma protein serves as antigen; antigen complex binds to the cell and is attacked by antibody (e.g., quinine and quinidine).
- Immune system is altered to produce true autoantibody (α-methyldopa).

Treatment consists of discontinuing the offending drug and providing supportive care. Corticosteroids may be necessary in some cases.

Immune Hemolytic Anemia Caused by Alloantibodies. Significant hemolysis may occur on the basis of transfused alloantibodies on exposure to plasma containing a high-titer of alloantibody directed against the patient's red cell antigens. The purpose of a crossmatch is to ensure that the transfused red cells are compatible with the patient, i.e., the patient does not have antibodies that would hemolyze the transfused blood. Platelet concentrates and fresh-frozen plasma are routinely transfused across ABO blood types. Consequently, platelets or plasma from a donor that contain a high titer of an anti-B (or anti-A) alloantibody transfused into a patient with type B (or type A) red cells may result in significant hemolysis of the patient's red cells. Rarely, the degree of hemolysis may be life threatening. Management is the same as for any acute hemolytic event. It is critical to stop the infusion of the blood product as soon as the problem is suspected and to maintain a high urine output with IV fluids and, if necessary, diuretics.

Major Transfusion Reactions

Acute hemolytic events can occur during transfusion. They are generally the result of the transfusion of ABO-incompatible blood. Major transfusion events are rare, with an incidence of 1 per 10,000–20,000 transfusions. Manifestations include fever, chills, hypotension, back pain, and hemoglobinuria. Management should include the following:

- Discontinuing the blood product infusion.
- Providing vigorous IV hydration to maintain blood pressure and urine flow.
- Administering antipyretics.
- Monitoring urine for hemoglobin.
- Sending the remaining blood product, along with a specimen of the patient's blood, to the blood bank for testing.

Disseminated intravascular coagulation (DIC) is uncommon, but may occur as a result of red cell stroma activating the coagulation system. It is usually self-limited. In severe cases, fresh-frozen plasma, platelet concentrates, and cryoprecipitate may be used. The use of heparin in this setting is controversial.

Delayed transfusion reactions occur 3–21 days after transfusion and are usually the result of an anamnestic immune response. In most cases, the patient has had previous sensitization to a red cell antigen as a result of pregnancy or previous transfusion, but the titer of this antibody is below the limits of detection. On rechallenge with red cells expressing this antigen, the patient's immune system responds with the production of significant amounts of antibody, with consequent hemolysis of the transfused cells. Unless records document previous red cell sensitization, delayed transfusion reactions are usually unavoidable. The degree of hemolysis with delayed transfusion reactions is generally mild.

Symptoms include low-grade fever and jaundice; chills and pallor are less common. Renal failure and DIC are rare. Laboratory studies will show positive direct and indirect Coombs test results, low haptoglobin level, elevated LDH level, and possibly hemoglobinuria. Identification of the antibody, showing its specificity for a transfused red cell antigen and not an intrinsic patient antigen, is necessary to differentiate between delayed transfusion reaction and autoimmune hemolytic anemia.

Miscellaneous Causes of Acquired Hemolytic Anemia

Paroxysmal nocturnal hemoglobinuria (PNH) is an uncommon disease in which hemolysis occurs as a result of increased sensitivity of red blood cells to complement. Complement is activated through the alternate pathway. Hemolysis generally occurs at night as a result of complement activation induced by the mild respiratory acidosis that occurs during sleep. Hemoglobinuria is noted in the first voided urine of the morning. More typically, patients have iron deficiency anemia of unexplained etiology.

Hemolytic crises can occur with acute illnesses or trauma. PNH should be suspected in any critically ill patient who has intravascular hemolysis and negative Coombs test results. Hemoglobin-induced nephropathy may be the presenting finding. There is an increased incidence of spontaneous thrombosis. Results of the Ham test and sucrose lysis test are positive; the former has greater specificity.

Corticosteroids (prednisone 1 mg/kg/day) may ameliorate the severity of hemolytic crisis. Transfusions are generally well tolerated, although transfusion of small amounts of activated complement contained within the donor plasma may precipitate a hemolytic crisis. Transfusion of saline-washed red cells will minimize this possibility. Thromboses should be treated aggressively by full anticoagulation with heparin followed by warfarin administration.

Hemolytic Anemia Resulting from Infection. Acute hemolysis has been associated with both bacterial (clostridial) and parasitic (malaria, babesiosis) infections. Mild transient hemolytic anemia has also been documented in association with bacteremia caused by infection with pneumococcus, *Staphylococcus* species, and *Escherichia coli.*

Toxin-induced hemolytic anemia has occurred with bites from the brown recluse spider, bee stings, elevated plasma copper levels (as seen in Wilson's disease), and exposure to heavy metals from environmental or industrial sources.

Hemolysis Associated with Acquired Defects of Red Blood Cell Membranes. Extensive burns and liver disease have been associated with an acquired hemolytic process caused by an alteration in red cell membranes. In both conditions, the treatment is supportive, providing replacement of red blood cells.

Hereditary Hemolytic Anemia

Hereditary spherocytosis (HS) is an intrinsic abnormality of the red cell membrane that results in episodic jaundice, splenomegaly, and mild to moderate anemia. It can be diagnosed by performing an osmotic fragility test. Splenectomy is indicated for patients who have critical splenomegaly or chronic severe anemia. Less severe forms of HS can be managed with episodic transfusion therapy. Patients are at increased risk of cholelithiasis. Abdominal pain in a patient with HS or any chronic hemolytic disorder must be evaluated for this possibility.

Aplastic crisis may develop after infection with parvovirus B19. Transfusion is the treatment of choice for this complication.

Deficiency of glucose-6-phosphate dehydrogenase results in red cells that are more susceptible to oxidant stress. The disorder is inherited as an X-linked recessive trait, and it is seen in all ethnic groups. Patients may experience acute hemolytic episodes in response to infections or on exposure to certain drugs, including the antimalarials, sulfonamides, and antipyretics that contain acetyl groups (e.g., acetylsalicylic acid and acetylphenetidine). Some patients exhibit sensitivity to fava beans. In severe cases, signs of intravascular hemolysis and vascular instability may be evident with fever, back pain, hemoglobinuria, and hypotension.

The diagnosis of G6PD deficiency or other red cell metabolic defects should be suspected in any patient who has an acute episode of nonimmune, nonmicroangiopathic hemolytic anemia, and especially in men. The diagnosis is made by the finding of a low steady-state red cell G6PD level, measured when the RC is normal. Because reticulocytes contain a higher level of the enzyme than older red cells, the presence of a significant elevation in RC may produce a falsely normal G6PD.

Specific therapy for G6PD deficiency is usually unnecessary because the hemolysis is generally self-limited. Occasionally, patients may require transfusion. Emphasis should be placed on the prevention of hemolytic episodes, minimizing exposure to drugs known to initiate hemolytic events.

Other red cell enzyme defects include pyruvate kinase deficiency and deficiencies of enzymes of the glycolytic pathway.

Unstable hemoglobins precipitate within the red cell, resulting in extravascular hemolysis on incubation of the cells within the splenic sinusoids. Hemolysis is exacerbated by infection and by drugs that induce oxidant stress on red blood cells. The precipitated hemoglobin is evident microscopically as Heinz bodies. Folate supplementation should be given. Splenectomy may benefit patients with severe disease, but it is not generally curative.

Sickle Cell Disease

This hemoglobinopathy leads to chronic anemia that is primarily hemolytic. A variety of acute sickle cell crises can occur:

- **Pain crisis** usually involves bone pain (caused by bone infarction or osteomyelitis, especially with *Salmonella* species) or abdominal pain (caused by splenic sequestration, mesenteric or hepatic vaso-occlusion, cholelithiasis, or an acute surgical abdomen).
- **Acute chest syndrome,** with chest pain and significant hypoxemia, is frequently accompanied by an infectious process with lobar consolidation (e.g., pneumococcus).
- **Priapism.**
- **Stroke.**
- **Aplastic crisis,** with acute, severe anemia and reticulocytopenia is generally secondary to parvovirus B19.
- **Hyperhemolytic crisis** (i.e., acute severe anemia accompanied by significant jaundice).

Management includes:

- **IV hydration** at 1.5–2 times maintenance levels. All patients with sickle cell crisis are dehydrated. Alkalinization may be considered to shift the oxyhemoglobin saturation curve to the left.
- **Analgesia.** Morphine sulfate is preferred over meperidine because of the risk of seizures with the latter agent.
- **Supplemental oxygen.** Intermittent administration is preferable. If continuous flow is necessary, the patient should be weaned gradually to avoid sudden bone marrow stimulation, with resultant production of sickle cells.
- **Packed red blood cell transfusion** is used for crises that are resistant to standard management.
- **Indications for exchange transfusion** include stroke, priapism or acute chest syndrome resistant to standard transfusion, and recurrent or resistant splenic sequestration crisis (seen in hemoglobin SC disease).

Suggested Readings

Embury SH, Garcia JF, Mohandas N, et al. Effects of oxygen inhalation on endogenous erythropoietin kinetics, erythropoiesis, and properties of blood cells in sickle cell anemia. *N Engl J Med* 1984;311:291–295.

Excellent study showing risks of continuous flow oxygen in patients with sickle cell anemia.

Engelfriet CP, Overbeeke MA, von dem Borne AE. Autoimmune hemolytic anemia. *Semin Hematol* 1992;29:3–12.
Good, broad review of types of autoimmune hemolysis with pharmacologic and transfusion therapies discussed.
Packman CH, Leddy JP. Drug-related immunologic injury of erythrocytes. In: Williams WJ, Beutler E, Ersiev AJ, et al., eds. *Hematology,* 4th ed. New York: McGraw-Hill, 1990, pp. 681–687.
Good, brief review including list of drugs most commonly associated with drug-induced hemolysis.
Pollack CV Jr. Emergencies in sickle cell disease. *Emerg Med Clin North Am* 1993;11:365–378.
Good, brief overview of assessment and management from an emergency care perspective.
Salama A, Mueller-Eckhardt C. Immune-mediated blood cell dyscrasias related to drugs. *Semin Hematol* 1992;29:54–63.
Overview of drug-induced hemolysis as well as thrombocytopenia and neutropenia.
Wayne AS, Kery SV, Nathan DG. Transfusion management of sickle cell disease. *Blood* 1993;81:1109–1123.
Comprehensive review of transfusion therapy in sickle cell disease with an extensive bibliography (194 references).

CHAPTER 65

Coagulation Disorders

(See Chapters 119 and 139)

Robert I. Parker

Disseminated Intravascular Coagulation

Disseminated intravascular coagulation (DIC) is a clinicopathologic syndrome characterized by microvascular thrombosis with resultant consumption of clotting factors and platelets. In its early stages, DIC may be primarily a thrombotic entity, although it more often occurs as diffuse bleeding. Sepsis, penetrating head injuries, and disorders associated with tissue necrosis (e.g., crush injuries, burns, ischemia) are strongly associated with the development of DIC. Other conditions associated with DIC include liver disease and disseminated carcinoma. Acute promyelocytic leukemia may occur with DIC, or DIC may occur on initiation of chemotherapy.

Diagnosis. DIC should be suspected by the clinical setting and confirmed by laboratory testing. In the earliest stages, prothrombin time (PT), partial thromboplastin time (PTT), platelet count, and fibrinogen level may be normal. As the microvascular thrombosis proceeds and clotting factors are consumed, platelet count and fibrinogen level decrease (typically by at least 50% from their baseline values), PT and PTT increase, and fibrin(ogen) degradation product (FDP) levels increase.

Treatment. The primary therapy for DIC is treatment of the underlying disease. The following supportive measures may be helpful, particularly in patients who are actively bleeding and have no clinical evidence of thrombotic complications:

- **Platelet transfusions** may be necessary to maintain the platelet count above 40,000–50,000 mm^{-3} in patients with active bleeding.
- **Cryoprecipitate** may be administered to maintain fibrinogen levels above 100 mg/dL.
- **Fresh-frozen plasma** (FFP) is given to replace deficient clotting factors and correct PT and PTT.

The use of heparin to treat DIC is controversial. The rationale is to prevent microvascular thrombosis and subsequent consumption of platelets and clotting factors. Although shown to be of some value in certain chronic forms of DIC, such as that associated with promyelocytic leukemia or prostate carcinoma, it is of unproven efficacy in acute forms of DIC. If used, the dose should be lower than normally used for systemic anticoagulation (e.g., 25 units/kg initially, followed by continuous IV infusion of 5–10 units/kg/hour; or, alternatively, with intermittent IV injection of 20–50 units/kg every 4–6 hours). The dose is titrated to the clinical response and to the response of the platelet count and fibrinogen level, rather than to a specific PTT value.

Antifibrinolytic agents (aminocaproic acid and tranexamic acid) are contraindicated in the absence of systemic anticoagulation because they can precipitate catastrophic thrombosis.

Liver Disease

Liver disease and hepatic insufficiency are common causes of abnormal hemostasis and bleeding in ICU patients.

Diagnosis. Abnormal coagulation study results or overt bleeding occurs in approximately 15% of patients with clinical or laboratory evidence of hepatic dysfunction. Both PT and PTT may be prolonged, but PT is more sensitive to hepatic dysfunction because of the short half-life of Factor VII. FDP levels may be mildly elevated because of an impairment in their clearance by the liver. Patients with liver disease and splenomegaly may be thrombocytopenic as a result of splenic sequestration of platelets. In contrast to DIC, however, patients with hepatic dysfunction will usually maintain fibrinogen levels unless there is severe hepatic failure. The absence of a microangiopathic hemolytic process is also helpful in differentiating DIC from bleeding diatheses caused by liver disease.

Treatment. Prophylactic treatment is generally not indicated. PT of as much as 4 seconds above the upper limit of normal rarely results in clinical bleeding. Patients who are to undergo invasive procedures or who are in the immediate postoperative period may benefit from prophylactic treatment to maintain hemostasis. In this setting, FFP or platelets may be indicated to maintain the PT below 15 to 16 seconds and the platelet count greater than 50,000 mm^{-3}. It is unusual to be able to normalize PT with intermittent FFP infusions, and it is generally not necessary.

Patients with active bleeding should be aggressively transfused with FFP and platelets. Because of the short half-life of Factor VII (6 hours), effective control of bleeding often requires the transfusion of 2–4 units of FFP every 6–8 hours until bleeding is controlled. Vitamin K should also empirically be administered to these patients, but in critically ill patients, the response to vitamin K, if it occurs at all, frequently takes longer than 12 to 24 hours.

Vitamin K Deficiency

Vitamin K deficiency can develop in the critically ill patient because of poor nutrition, increased turnover of Factor VII, and the use of broad-spectrum antibiotics or drugs that may be competitive inhibitors of vitamin K activity.

Diagnosis. Laboratory findings in patients with vitamin K deficiency include prolonged PT, normal fibrinogen level, normal platelet count, and normal Factor V level. Prolongation of PTT can occur as a late finding in severe cases.

Treatment. Vitamin K is available in both parenteral and oral preparations, although it is erratically absorbed by the oral route. The IM route of administration should be avoided when it is used to treat coagulopathy. There is a small, but finite risk of anaphylaxis when vitamin K_1 (phytonadione) is given IV. This risk can be minimized by administering it as an infusion over 30 to 45 minutes. The safest route is subcutaneous. In critically ill patients, it is reasonable to give vitamin K once daily for 3 consecutive days. If correction has not occurred after this treatment, further administration is unlikely to be beneficial.

Actively bleeding patients with vitamin K deficiency should be treated with FFP to restore hemostasis immediately. To increase Factor VII to hemostatic levels (i.e., 30–60%), administration of 4 to 6 units of FFP is frequently required over a relatively short period.

Massive Transfusion Syndrome

Banked blood is deficient in the labile clotting factors, particularly Factors V and VIII, and platelets. In addition, plasma washout occurs, resulting in depletion of clotting factors and platelets. Transfusion of large amounts of stored blood without transfusion of FFP or platelets may result in massive transfusion syndrome. This condition is generally seen in the setting of acute hemorrhage or coronary artery bypass surgery when large amounts of banked blood are used.

Diagnosis. This syndrome can mimic DIC. There is prolongation of PT and PTT, low fibrinogen level, low platelet count, and diffuse bleeding. It is differentiated from DIC by the clinical setting and by the absence of significant elevations of FDP levels.

Treatment is centered on replacing clotting factors and platelets through the transfusion of FFP, cryoprecipitate and, if necessary, platelets. For patients who are at high risk, prophylactic treatment has been recommended with 1 unit of FFP and 4 units of platelets for every 5 units of packed red blood cells transfused.

Anticoagulant Overdose

Heparin. In patients who are treated with heparin and become overanticoagulated, PTT and thrombin time are elevated beyond the normal range, but PT, platelet count, and fibrinogen level are usually normal. In severe cases, PT may be elevated. Serious bleeding associated with heparin can be rapidly reversed by protamine sulfate. As a general rule, 1 mg protamine will neutralize approximately 100 units of heparin. The required dose of protamine can be calculated from the number of units of active heparin remaining in the patient's system, determined from the original heparin dose and the half-life of the drug. Unfortunately, the half-life of heparin is nonlinear and variable. For a bolus of 100 units/kg, the half-life is roughly 1 hour; for bolus doses of 400 and 800 units/kg, the half-lives are approximately 2.5 and 5 hours, respectively. When protamine sulfate is used, the drug should be given by slow IV injection over 8 to 10 minutes. Single doses should not exceed 50 mg, and no more than 100 mg should be given as a cumulative dose. The major side effects of protamine are hypotension and anaphylactoid reactions.

Warfarin and related drugs competitively inhibit the effect of vitamin K on Factors II, VII, IX, and X by interfering with vitamin K metabolism. When overanticoagulation with warfarin produces clinically significant bleeding, immediate reversal with FFP is indicated. In addition to its use as a therapeutic anticoagulant, warfarin is the active agent in some rodenticides, and cases of human poisoning have been reported. Certain related anticoagulant rodenticides (e.g., brodifacoum) have similar effects, but can result in a prolonged state of anticoagulation, lasting for weeks or even months after a single ingestion.

Warfarin necrosis is a syndrome that occurs during the early stages of anticoagulation with warfarin. This disorder is seen as a consequence of microvascular thrombosis in patients with protein C deficiency. It generally occurs when large doses (e.g., > 15 mg) of warfarin are given as a bolus in the absence of heparin anticoagulation. The treatment is heparin anticoagulation or FFP to replace the protein C. The long-term treatment of patients with protein C deficiency is balanced anticoagulation with warfarin.

Primary Fibrinolysis

Primary fibrinolysis results from activation of the fibrinolytic system that is not in response to the generation of thrombin. This situation is seen most often in disseminated malignancy, particularly prostate carcinoma. Some snake venoms produce a primary fibrinolytic syndrome.

This syndrome must be suspected on the basis of clinical setting. Diagnostic confirmation is based on the following findings:

- Clinical bleeding; prolonged PT, PTT, and thrombin time; and decreased fibrinogen level. The platelet count may or may not be decreased.
- FDP levels will be elevated, although early on, the D-dimer assay result may be negative.
- The euglobulin clot lysis time is shortened.

Heparin therapy is not indicated for primary fibrinolysis. The preferred treatment is an antifibrinolytic agent (e.g., aminocaprioic acid or tranexamic acid).

Platelet Disorders

Thrombocytopenia can result from increased platelet destruction, decreased platelet production, or abnormal distribution (e.g., splenic sequestration).

Platelet Destruction. Increased destruction can occur by immune mechanisms (e.g., idiopathic, drug-related, or infection-related causes) or by mechanical destruction (e.g., prosthetic cardiac valves or microangiopathic processes, such as DIC, thrombotic thrombocytopenic purpura (TTP), or hemolytic uremic syndrome).

Heparin-Induced Thrombocytopenia. Heparin is frequently used in the ICU as therapy for thrombosis or as an adjunct to maintain the patency of central venous and arterial catheters. Its use is associated with two types of thrombocytopenia:

- **Nonimmune,** or type 1, heparin-induced thrombocytopenia results from the direct binding of heparin to the platelet surface. It occurs in most patients who receive

full-dose heparin. The associated thrombocytopenia is modest and generally transient.
- **Immune-mediated,** or type 2, heparin-induced thrombocytopenia occurs in fewer than 5% of patients, but is severe. The thrombocytopenia generally occurs on reexposure to heparin or after 7 days of continuous heparin therapy, and it is progressive. It may also be accompanied by microvascular thromboses because of the lodging of heparin aggregates in the microvasculature. This syndrome can be precipitated by exposure to minute amounts of heparin, including those used in vascular catheter flushes.

Treatment is removal of all exposure to heparin. Platelet transfusions are contraindicated as long as heparin is present because it may precipitate significant thrombosis.

Decreased Platelet Production

- Marrow suppression can occur in response to chemotherapy, viral illness, certain drugs (thiazides, alcohol, cimetidine), or the replacement of marrow with tumor or fibrosis.
- The diagnosis is suggested by the clinical setting. Other cellular elements are frequently involved.
- For bleeding patients or in those considered to be at significant risk for spontaneous or procedure-related bleeding, the treatment of choice is platelet transfusion. In general, spontaneous bleeding is unusual with platelet counts greater than 10,000–20,000 mm^{-3}.

Qualitative Platelet Disorders. Many drugs used in the ICU setting inhibit platelet function. Frequent offenders include:

- **Aspirin,** which irreversibly acetylates the active site for cyclooxygenase and impairs cyclooxygenase-mediated platelet activation for the life of the platelet. Platelets survive in the circulation approximately 8–10 days; measurable platelet inhibition can be seen for as long as 5 days after ingestion of a single 325-mg tablet of aspirin. Aspirin should be avoided in thrombocytopenic patients.
- **Nonsteroidal anti-inflammatory drugs** competitively inhibit platelet function, especially at high doses, but the effects are gone once the drug has been cleared from the circulation. If possible, these drugs should be avoided in patients with thrombocytopenia.

Uremia produces a state of acquired platelet dysfunction, presumably because of the accumulation of toxins that would otherwise be cleared by the kidney. Patients with uremia may experience significant bleeding, even with a normal platelet count. Dialysis generally results in improved platelet function. However, when dialysis is not possible, hemostasis can be improved in the uremic patient through the use of desmopressin, cryoprecipitate, or conjugated estrogens.

- **Desmopressin** has immediate effects that last for 6–8 hours. The dose is 0.3 μg/kg (maximum dose, 20 μg) infused over 20–30 minutes. Repeat doses may be given once or twice over a 24-hour period. Myocardial infarction has been anecdotally associated with its use in elderly patients and those with significant coronary artery disease.
- **Cryoprecipitate** may improve the bleeding in uremia, although frequently there is a 24-hour lag period from the transfusion of cryoprecipitate to the clinical benefit. The dose of cryoprecipitate is up to 1 unit for every 10 lb body weight, with repeated dosing at 12 hours and then every 24 hours, as needed.
- **Conjugated estrogens** are useful in some patients with uremia. Improvement in platelet function generally occurs within 3–7 days and lasts for as long as a week after cessation of estrogen therapy. Usual doses and preparations of estrogen used have been 50 mg/day estrogen, 2.5–5 mg/day norethynodrel, and 0.075–0.1 mg/day mestranol.

Anemia. Patients with significant anemia have prolonged bleeding times. This finding can be considered physiologic as a result of decreased interaction between circulating platelets and the vascular endothelial surface. Bleeding time is predictably prolonged with hematocrit values less than 30% and significantly prolonged with hematocrit values less than 20%. A straightforward intervention to improve hemostasis in anemic patients is the use of red cell transfusions. Maintaining the hematocrit level above 30% maximizes platelet interaction with vascular surfaces.

Suggested Readings

Bell WR. The pathophysiology of disseminated intramuscular coagulation. *Semin Hematol* 1994;31(suppl 1):19–25.

Concise review of current thought regarding disseminated intramuscular coagulation syndrome.

Bell WR. Heparin-associated thrombocytopenia and thrombosis. *J Lab Clin Med* 1988;111:600–605.

Bolan CD, Alving BM. Pharmacologic agents in the management of bleeding disorders. *Transfusion* 1990;30:541–551.

Good review of non–blood product therapies.

Bovill EG. Laboratory diagnosis of disseminated intramuscular coagulation. *Semin Hematol* 1994;31(suppl 1):35–41.

Understandable review with clear recommendations for basic evaluation of the patient with suspected disseminated intramuscular coagulation.

Edmunds HL, Salzman EW. Hemostatic problems, transfusion therapy, and cardiopulmonary bypass in surgical patients. In: Colman RW,

Hirsch J, Marder VJ, et al., eds. *Hemostasis and thrombosis: Basic principles and clinical practice,* 3rd ed. Philadelphia: JB Lippincott, 1994, pp 956–968.
Concise and comprehensive review of massive transfusion syndrome and other bleeding problems associated with cardiopulmonary bypass.
Joist JH. Hemostatic abnormalities in liver disease. In: Colman RW, Hirsch J, Marder VJ, et al., eds. *Hemostasis and thrombosis: Basic principles and clinical practice,* 3rd ed. Philadelphia: JB Lippincott, 1994, pp 906–920.
Comprehensive review of the myriad hemostatic abnormalities associated with liver disease. Includes short section on therapy and liver transplantation.
Warkentin TE, Kelton JG. Heparin-induced thrombocytopenia. *Annu Rev Med* 1990;40:31–44.
Comprehensive discussion of the problem, whereas Bell's review (listed above) provides a concise discussion of clinically relevant issues.

CHAPTER 66

Microangiopathic Hemolytic Anemia

(See Chapter 118)

Robert I. Parker

Microangiopathic hemolytic anemia is mechanical fragmentation of red blood cells in the microvasculature. It most commonly occurs in areas of fibrin deposition within the vascular space. It is frequently associated with thrombocytopenia because platelets are also trapped in the fibrin mesh. The degree of thrombocytopenia is often severe enough to produce clinical bleeding. A microangiopathic hemolytic process should be suspected in any patient with anemia and fragmented red blood cells on peripheral blood smear. Microangiopathic hemolytic anemia can be associated with autoimmune vasculitis, chemotherapy, vascular malformations (e.g., cavernous hemangioma producing Kasabach-Merritt syndrome), prosthetic cardiac valves, or infections. Thrombotic thrombocytopenic purpura (TTP), hemolytic-uremic syndrome (HUS), and disseminated intravascular coagulation (DIC) are three well-described entities in which a microvascular hemolytic process is a central component. For a discussion of DIC, see Chapter 65 in this book.

Thrombotic Thrombocytopenic Purpura

The primary pathophysiologic process in TTP is the formation of microvascular fibrin thrombi, which can involve virtually any organ. The classic presentation of TTP is the triad of:

- **Hemolytic anemia,** which is generally moderate. Results of tests for immune markers of hemolysis are negative. The serum haptoglobin level is low, and there may be free hemoglobin in the serum and urine.
- **Thrombocytopenia** that is severe, with the platelet count often in the range of 20,000 mm^{-3}.
- **Neurologic manifestations,** which range from headache to gross behavioral and sensorimotor dysfunction, to seizures, stupor, and coma.

Renal involvement and fever may also be present. Microvascular fibrin thrombi seen on tissue biopsy in the appropriate clinical setting are thought to be diagnostic.

Treatment. Improved recognition of TTP and response to therapy has dramatically improved survival rates, which are now greater than 80%. Plasmapheresis with plasma exchange is the treatment of choice. If plasmapheresis is not available, aggressive treatment with fresh-frozen plasma (20 mL/kg/day) should be initiated. In some patients with TTP, platelet transfusions accelerate the disease; therefore, platelet transfusion should be reserved for use in emergency situations, such as intracranial bleeding. Methylprednisolone may be of benefit. Treatment can be monitored by following the platelet count, with an increase indicating successful therapy. Platelet counts should be monitored weekly until they are stable for at least 1 month. The presence of unusually large von Willebrand factor multimers in plasma between episodes of TTP may serve as a marker to identify patients who are at risk for chronic relapsing TTP.

Hemolytic-Uremic Syndrome

HUS and TTP have many clinical similarities. The primary difference between them is the major end-organ affected. In TTP, the CNS is the major organ affected, whereas in HUS, the kidneys are primarily involved.

Clinical Presentation. HUS is generally seen in children younger than 10 years, but it may occur in older patients. It is usually preceded by an acute gastroenteritis syndrome, and it has been linked to infection with toxin-producing *Escherichia coli* O157:H7. Patients typically are acutely ill, with pallor, vomiting, irritability, and some evidence of renal failure. Neurologic symptoms, such as seizures or altered consciousness, may occur, but are much less common than in TTP. Irritability is common. The degree of anemia frequently parallels the severity of the renal failure, whereas the degree of thrombocytopenia does not.

Urinalysis shows proteinuria, hematuria, and casts. Anuric or oliguric renal failure is common. Although serum fibrin degradation product levels are frequently elevated, convincing evidence for DIC is usually absent.

Treatment consists of supportive care, focusing on the management of renal failure. Short-term dialysis may be necessary. Full recovery is the rule. Plasmapheresis with plasma exchange is not indicated on a routine basis, but may be considered in patients with severe disease. Early onset of anuria, a white blood cell count of greater than 20,000 mm^{-3} at presentation, and anuria lasting more than 14 days are all indicators of poor prognosis, with an increased risk for residual renal failure.

Chemotherapy-Induced Hemolytic-Uremic Syndrome

A syndrome characterized by microangiopathic hemolytic anemia, thrombocytopenia, and renal failure has been reported in patients receiving cancer chemotherapy with mitomycin C, bleomycin, or cisplatin. Chemotherapy-related HUS generally occurs approximately 1 year after cancer chemotherapy, and is not associated with the presence of residual tumor. The mortality rate for this syndrome is high, approaching 70%.

Treatment. Aggressive management is indicated because these patients are usually free of their underlying malignancy. Supportive therapy should be directed toward control of hypertension, pulmonary edema, and renal failure.

- Dialysis is often required.
- Corticosteroids appear to be ineffective.
- Patients may benefit from plasmapheresis with plasma exchange.
- Transfusions with red blood cells should be used carefully because they frequently cause exacerbation of the syndrome.

Other Disorders Associated with Microangiopathic Hemolytic Anemia

- Widespread carcinomatosis.
- Preeclampsia.
- Abnormal cardiac structures, especially aortic valve disease.

Suggested Readings

Lesesne JB, Rothschild N, Erickson B, et al. Cancer-associated hemolytic uremic syndrome: Analysis of 85 cases from a national registry. *J Clin Oncol* 1989;7:781–789.

Reviews cases, outcome, and prognosis from national database.

Bell WR, Brain HG, Ness PM, et al. Improved survival in thrombotic

thrombocytopenic purpura: Hemolytic uremic syndrome. Clinical experience in 108 patients. *N Engl J Med* 1991;325:398–403.
Large, single institution experience showing improved survival with prednisone and plasma exchange versus prednisone alone. Editorial on pages 426–427 of the issue.

Kwaan HC. Miscellaneous secondary thrombotic microangiopathy. *Semin Hematol* 1987;24:141–147.
Excellent brief review with good list of references.

Rock GA, Shumak KH, Buskard NA, et al. Comparison of plasma exchange with plasma infusion in the treatment of thrombotic thrombocytopenic purpura. *N Engl J Med* 1991;325:393–397.
Strong study showing increased efficacy of plasma exchange versus simple plasma infusion. Includes brief, but good, review of other treatment options.

Stewart CL, Tina LU. Hemolytic uremic syndrome. *Pediatr Rev* 1993;14:218–224.

CHAPTER 67

Blood Product Use

(See Chapter 119)

Robert I. Parker

Critically ill patients frequently require multiple blood products to maintain their oxygen-carrying capacity, intravascular volume, and hemostatic effectiveness. In most cases, the blood product used is packed red blood cells (PRBCs). The indications for blood product use have changed over the years with the increasing awareness of the risks of transfusion therapy and the development of alternate modalities.

Red Blood Cell Transfusion

The increase in oxygen-carrying capacity results in increased oxygen delivery to the tissues. Oxygen delivery to the tissues is usually maintained at near-normal levels down to a hemoglobin of approximately 7 g/dL, assuming a normal cardiac rsponse to anemia. However, the optimal level in a critically ill patient may be about 10 g/dL.

- **PRBCs** are the component of choice in patients who are anemic. The volume of PRBCs (mL) to be transfused can be calculated from the patient's estimated blood volume (mL) and hemoglobin (Hb) level (g/dL) by the formula:

$$\frac{(\text{Target Hb} - \text{Observed Hb}) \times \text{Blood volume}}{20}$$

PRBCs leak potassium progressively during storage. Patients who cannot tolerate a potassium load should be transfused with washed, saline-suspended PRBCs.

- **Whole blood** transfusions may be given to patients who require replacement of both red cells and plasma volume. In most circumstances, this replacement can be accomplished effectively by the transfusion of both PRBCs and fresh-frozen plasma (FFP).
- **Washed red blood cells** should be used when transfusion of plasma proteins included with the red cells is potentially detrimental to the patient, as in immunoglobulin A-deficient patients, who are at risk for anaphylaxis on exposure to even the small amounts of immunoglobulin present in the residual plasma of a packed cell unit.
- **Irradiated blood products** may be used during transfusion to patients who are immunoincompetent because of underlying disease or therapy to prevent the transfusion of immunocompetent cells and the development of graft-versus-host disease (GVHD).

Platelet Transfusion Therapy

Normal surgical hemostasis can usually be maintained at platelet counts greater than 40,000 to 50,000 mm^{-3}. A threshold platelet count of 20,000 mm^{-3} has been used as the point at which patients undergoing cancer chemotherapy should be prophylactically transfused with platelets. Spontaneous bleeding rarely occurs at a level above 10,000 mm^{-3}. More aggressive use of platelet transfusions may be indicated in patients with underlying coagulopathy (such as uremia or hemophilia), uncontrolled hypertension, peptic ulcer disease, or intracranial abnormalities. Patients with thrombocytopenia should not receive IM injections. Medications that inhibit platelet function should be avoided.

A unit of platelets is that derived from the donation of a unit of whole blood or its equivalent. A single unit of platelets will raise the platelet count by 5,000 to 10,000 mm^{-3} in a normal 70-kg person. A typical platelet transfusion consists of 1 unit/10 kg body weight. Because critically ill patients may have an element of increased platelet consumption contributing to their thrombocytopenia, determination of peak platelet increments after transfusion should be obtained within 1 hour of transfusion. Patients who are expected to receive multiple platelet transfusions over a prolonged period should receive single-donor or HLA-matched platelet packs to minimize the risk of alloimmunization.

Fresh-Frozen Plasma

A unit of fresh-frozen plasma (FFP) has a volume of 200 or 250 mL, and contains all of the plasma coagulation factors and inhibitors. FFP is the product of choice in patients suspected of having a clotting factor deficiency. Specific indications include:

- Coagulopathy caused by congenital or acquired factor deficiency and detected by abnormal coagulation study results (prothrombin time > 18 seconds, activated partial thromboplastin time >55 seconds, or coagulation factor activity assay < 25%).
- Treatment of bleeding or prophylaxis during surgery or invasive procedures in patients with coagulopathy.
- Massive blood transfusion, i.e, more than one circulating blood volume transfused over several hours, with abnormal coagulation study results or clinical bleeding.
- Rapid reversal of warfarin-induced anticoagulation.
- Miscellaneous indications, including treatment of protein C or S deficiency, thrombotic thrombocytopenic purpura, and hemolytic-uremic syndrome.

Limitations of FFP therapy are related to volume; multiple units are often needed to cause a significant increase in the level of a deficient clotting protein. FFP is not recommended for use merely as a volume expander.

Cryoprecipitate

Cryoprecipitate is prepared from plasma. It contains high concentrations of fibrinogen, Factor VIII, and von Willebrand factor. It is indicated in bleeding patients with isolated deficiencies of any of these three factors. It has also been beneficial in the treatment of patients with uremic bleeding. The usual dose of cryoprecipitate is up to 1 unit/5 kg body weight.

White Blood Cell Transfusions

White blood cell transfusion is used to treat septic newborns, patients with chronic granulomatous disease, and patients with neutropenia caused by cancer chemotherapy who also have established fungal infections. Because of their short intravascular half-life, these transfusions are generally required every 8–12 hours in adults. Pulmonary leukoagglutinin reactions with noncardiogenic pulmonary edema have been documented in patients receiving granulocyte transfusion.

Adverse Effects of Transfusion

Febrile reactions are common and usually clinically insignificant. Hemolytic reactions can occur (see Chapter 64 in this book). Other adverse effects include leukocyte febrile reactions, plasma protein febrile reactions, urticaria, anaphylactic reactions (caused by reactions to plasma proteins, such as immunoglobulin A), noncardiogenic pulmonary edema (believed to result from leukoagglutination within the pulmonary vasculature), infection, and immune sensitization of blood cells. GVHD, which is rare, is usually fatal, and results from the transfusion of lymphocytes to an immunoincompetent host (e.g., patients with acquired immune deficiency syndrome and patients undergoing chemotherapy). GVHD can be prevented by the irradiation of all cellular blood products. Transmission of viral disease is a small, but significant, possibility with any transfusion.

Suggested Readings

Beutler E. Platelet transfusions: The 20,000 trigger. *Blood* 1993;81:1411–1413.

Good review of development and rationale for prophylactic platelet transfusion practices.

Fresh-Frozen Plasma, Cryoprecipitate, and Platelets Administration Practice Guidelines Development Task Force of the College of American Pathologists. Practice parameter for the use of fresh-frozen plasma, cryoprecipitate, and platelets. *JAMA* 1994;271:777–781.

Lane TA, Anderson KC, Goodnough LT, et al. Leukocyte reduction in blood component therapy. *Ann Intern Med* 1992;117:151–162.

Strong, retrospective review indicating benefits of leukocyte depletion and identifying those patients most likely to benefit from this procedure.

Nacht A. The use of blood products in shock. *Crit Care Clin* 1992;8:255–291.

(141 references.)

Office of Medical Applications of Research, National Institutes of Health. Platelet transfusion therapy. *JAMA* 1987;257:1777–1780.

Excellent, short review of clinically relevant points developed by consensus conference. Full document is available through NIH.

Spitzer TR. Transfusion-induced graft-vs-host disease. In: Burakoff SJ, Deeg HS, Ferrara J, Atkinson K, eds. *Graft-vs-host disease: Immunology, pathophysiology, and treatment.* New York: Marcel Dekker, 1990, pp 539–555.

Excellent, comprehensive review of topic, with clear recommendations regarding those patients believed to be at risk for transfusion-induced graft-versus-host disease.

CHAPTER 68

Oncologic Emergencies

(See Chapter 120)

Herold Duroseau

Acute metabolic or anatomic complications from neoplastic disease often necessitate admission to the ICU.

Superior Vena Cava Syndrome

There is obstruction of blood flow through the superior vena cava (SVC) as a result of external compression, invasion, thrombosis, or stenosis. Malignancy is the most common cause. Benign causes are less frequent, and include mediastinitis or thrombosis caused by indwelling catheters.

Diagnosis

- **Symptoms** include dyspnea, facial swelling, cough, arm and trunk swelling, chest pain, dysphagia, headache, dizziness, hoarseness, and syncope.
- **Physical findings** include facial edema with plethora, neck vein distension, cyanosis, arm edema, and dilation of veins on the chest and abdominal wall.
- **Chest radiograph** may show widening of the mediastinum, a lung mass, or pleural effusion.
- **Computed tomography** of the chest using contrast infusion helps to define the anatomy.
- **Diagnostic procedures** that aid in defining the underlying etiology include sputum cytology, thoracentesis, lymph node biopsy, bronchoscopy, and mediastinoscopy.

Treatment

- **General measures** include elevation of the head of the bed, oxygen administration, and administration of diuretics, with careful monitoring of fluid balance and cardiac function. Steroids may be helpful in reducing inflammation and edema.
- **Surgery** in the form of bypass grafting between the innominate or jugular vein on the left and the right atrial appendage is not generally used.
- **Chemotherapy** is the treatment of choice when the cause is small cell lung cancer or malignant lymphoma.
- **Radiation therapy** is effective for chemoresistant malignancies.

- **Anticoagulants,** thrombolytics, or angioplasty may be useful in some cases.

Airway Obstruction

Obstruction of the airway most commonly occurs in patients with bronchogenic carcinoma. Obstruction can be complete or partial. Symptoms include dyspnea, cough, and hemoptysis. Partial obstruction can be successfully treated with laser therapy, providing immediate relief of symptoms. Complete obstruction is more difficult to treat. Laser therapy along the linear axis of the trachea and bronchus is the initial therapy, providing temporary relief. The use of corticosteroids may help to prevent airway edema, which can exacerbate the obstruction.

Leptomeningeal Disease

Leptomeningeal carcinomatosis occurs in 5–8% of patients with solid tumors, most commonly lung or breast cancer. The leptomeninges may be involved in leukemia, lymphoma, melanoma, or gastric cancer.

Clinical manifestations include headache, alteration of sensorium, nausea, diplopia, weakness, and paresthesias. Physical findings include cranial nerve palsy, sensory loss, motor weakness, or signs of cerebral dysfunction.

Diagnosis is made by lumbar puncture and cerebrospinal fluid (CSF) analysis. There should be no evidence of a mass lesion or midline shift before the lumbar puncture is performed. Characteristic CSF findings are intracranial hypertension, elevated protein level, and low glucose concentration.

Treatment is directed toward the neoplastic etiology. For CNS leukemia, neuroaxis radiation and systemic and intrathecal therapy with methotrexate and cytosine arabinoside often lead to complete resolution. Some solid tumors respond to intrathecal chemotherapy.

Spinal Cord Compression

This compression can be caused by tumor of the cord itself or, more commonly, by an expanding paraspinal mass. The most common causes are breast, lung, and prostate cancer; myeloma; and lymphoma. The most frequent location is in the thoracic vertebrae.

Clinical manifestations include back pain, weakness, and sensory, motor, or autonomic deficits.

Diagnosis. Prompt and immediate evaluation is crucial. A neurologic examination is performed to assess the deficit. Myelography is the diagnostic test of choice. CT and MRI may be helpful.

Treatment. Once compression is documented, corticosteroids (dexamethasone) should be initiated immediately. Radiation therapy is used as soon as possible in a patient with a known primary tumor and other evidence of metastatic disease. Neurosurgical consultation should be obtained for possible decompression laminectomy if the symptoms progress despite radiation therapy and steroids or if the tumor is radioresistant.

Prognosis is directly related to the level of disability.

Urologic Complications

Hemorrhagic cystitis usually occurs in patients who have received high-dose cyclophosphamide. It may be preventable by aggressive hydration during therapy, bladder catheterization, and irrigation. Mesna (mercaptoethanesulfonate) given during and after chemotherapy prevents cystitis.

Obstructive uropathy is seen with lymphomas; carcinoma of the cervix, ovary, prostate, or colon; or primary ureteral, bladder, or urethral tumors. Obstruction may be secondary to radiation or surgery. Management consists of placement of an in-dwelling bladder catheter. If the obstruction is not relieved, suprapubic bladder catheterization or percutaneous nephrostomy is recommended.

Uric acid nephropathy may result from underlying neoplastic disease or, more often, its treatment. It usually develops after the initiation of treatment for leukemia or lymphoma. Aggressive hydration, including alkalinization with sodium bicarbonate, and administration of allopurinol before therapy are recommended.

Other Oncologic Emergencies

Other emergencies that can be caused by underlying malignancy include massive hemoptysis, pericardial tamponade, intracranial hypertension, status epilepticus, hypercalcemia, hypoglycemia, and severe hyponatremia caused by the syndrome of inappropriate antidiuretic hormone release (see respective chapters in this book and the main text).

Suggested Readings

Arrambide K, Toto RD. Tumor lysis syndrome. *Semin Nephrol* 1993; 13: 273–280.

Current review of acute tumor lysis syndrome: diagnosis, etiology, and management.

Chang AY-C, Kuebler JP, Pandya KJ, et al. Pulmonary toxicity induced by mitomycin C is highly responsive to glucocorticoids. *Cancer* 1986;57:2285–2290.

Study of five cases of biopsy-proven pulmonary toxicity caused by administration of mitomycin C, vincristine, and cisplatin in 64 patients. All responded dramatically well to high-dose glucocorticoids.

Fleming DR, Doukas MA. Acute tumor lysis syndrome in hematologic malignancies. *Leuk Lymphoma* 1992;8:315–318.
Brief review of risk factors and preventive and therapeutic measures; useful, short algorithm is presented.
Morris JC, Holland JF. Oncologic emergencies. In: Holland JF, Frei III E, Bast RC Jr, et al., eds. *Cancer medicine,* 3rd ed. Philadelphia: Lea and Febiger, 1993, pp 2442–2465.
Comprehensive review.
Warrell RP Jr. Clinical trials of gallium nitrate in patients with cancer-related hypercalcemia. *Semin Oncol* 1991;18:26–31.
Brief review of experience with gallium nitrate versus calcitonin or bisphosphonates in treatment of malignancy hypercalcemia. In general, gallium nitrate is more effective than standard- (low-) dose diphosphonates or calcitonin in controlling hypercalcemia.

CHAPTER 69

Complications of Therapy of Neoplastic Disease

(See Chapter 121)

Herold Duroseau

The care of patients with neoplastic disorders poses many complications, including those caused by the malignancy itself and those resulting from its treatment.

Pancytopenia

The most common and predictable complication of cancer therapy is myelosuppression. The degree of treatment-related pancytopenia depends on:

- Intrinsic myelosuppressive activity of the drug.
- Concomitant or previous exposure to radiation therapy.
- Age and nutritional status of the patient.
- Extent of bone marrow reserve.

Neutropenia is defined as an absolute neutrophil count of less than 500 cells/mm^{-3}. Gram-negative bacilli (especially *Pseudomonas* species) and gram-positive cocci are the most common organisms identified in febrile, neutropenic patients. *Staphylococcus epidermidis* is a prominent pathogen in patients with an in-dwelling vascular device. Management of the febrile neutropenic patient requires:

- **History and physical examination,** with attention to the skin, vascular access devices, oropharyngeal mucosa, and perianal region.
- **Blood cultures,** obtained peripherally and from indwelling catheters, as well as cultures of other relevant body fluids.
- **Isolation,** with strict hand washing and neutropenic precautions.
- **Antibiotic treatment** with empiric broad-spectrum antibiotics that cover gram-negative bacilli (including *Pseudomonas* species) and gram-positive cocci.
- **Growth factors** that stimulate marrow recovery significantly reduce the duration of neutropenia as well as the number of days antibiotic therapy is needed.

Thrombocytopenia is defined as a platelet count of less than 150,000 mm^{-3}. It develops and resolves later than neutropenia that occurs after chemotherapy. The depth and duration of the platelet count nadir depend on:

- Type, dose, and intensity of chemotherapy agents.
- Previous radiation therapy.
- Presence of underlying fever and infection.
- Concomitant use of drugs that may depress platelet count, such as antibiotics, amphotericin, or heparin.
- Coexistent consumptive coagulopathy.
- Splenomegaly with hypersplenism and sequestration.

Clinical manifestations usually do not occur until the count decreases to less than 50,000 mm^{-3}. Ecchymosis and spontaneous petechiae develop with platelet counts less than 20,000 mm^{-3}. At this level, there is serious risk of spontaneous hemorrhage. Spontaneous intracranial bleeding can occur if the platelet count is less than 10,000 mm^{-3}.

Management consists of:

- Identification and correction of coexisting coagulopathies, bleeding precautions (such as prolonged pressure over needlesticks), and avoidance of potential platelet toxins and heparin.
- Platelet transfusions are necessary in actively bleeding patients to maintain a platelet count greater than 50,000 mm^{-3}.
- In nonbleeding patients with platelet counts less than 50,000 mm^{-3}, platelet transfusions just before invasive procedures or surgery.
- For patients with platelet counts less than 10,000 mm^{-3}, prophylactic platelet transfusions to avoid the small, but devastating, risks of spontaneous intracranial hemorrhage.

Anemia. In the assessment of anemia, it is important to exclude the possible coexistent etiology of anemia in the critically ill cancer patient.

Management depends on the clinical condition of the patient rather than on laboratory values. In general, a hemoglobin level of 9–10 g/dL is adequate. Transfusion of packed red blood cells is indicated for patients who require greater oxygen-carrying capacity to meet the demands of a febrile illness or cardiopulmonary compromise. With the use of recombinant erythropoietin, there may be a decreased requirement for transfusion.

Renal and Metabolic Abnormalities

Acute Urate Nephropathy and Acute Tumor Lysis Syndrome. Characterized by hyperuricemia, hyperphosphatemia, hyperkalemia, and hypocalcemia, along with progressive azotemia, these conditions occur during the first 3 to 5 days after initiation of chemotherapy. There is an abrupt release of large quantities of intracellular contents (uric acid, phosphorous, and potassium) into the blood as a result of rapid tumor cell lysis. These materials overwhelm the renal capacity and result in renal damage, culminating in acute renal failure.

Management

- **IV hydration** to decrease the concentration of solutes and prevent their precipitation. A typical regimen is 3 $L/m^2/day$.
- **Urine alkalinization** with IV $NaHCO_3$ to achieve urine $pH > 7$ facilitates the solubility of uric acid.
- **Allopurinol** is given before chemotherapy in a loading dose of 600–900 mg, followed by 100–300 mg/day.
- **Hemodialysis** may be indicated if the patient has progressive renal insufficiency, life-threatening metabolic abnormalities, or cardiac or pulmonary disease that contraindicates vigorous hydration.

Divalent Cation Wasting. Severe hypomagnesemia with mild to moderate hypocalcemia is associated with repeated cycles of platinum-containing compounds. Clinical manifestations include seizures and tetany. Patients who are receiving platinum should have periodic measurement of serum calcium and magnesium levels, with magnesium supplementation as necessary.

Nephrotoxicity of Antineoplastic Agents

- **Cisplatin** causes distal tubular necrosis; dilation of tubules, with relative sparing of glomeruli; and renal wasting of divalent cations. Factors predisposing patients to nephrotoxicity are higher doses and concurrent use of aminoglycosides. Toxicity can be minimized by prehydration and vigorous ongoing hydration, diuretics, and mannitol to induce osmotic diuresis.

- **Methotrexate** is nephrotoxic at intermediate and high doses. It is excreted primarily by the kidneys. In high concentrations, it may precipitate in the renal tubules, decreasing its elimination and causing further renal injury. Preventive measures include vigorous hydration, alkalinization with $NaHCO_3$ to maintain urine pH > 7, monitoring of serum creatinine and methotrexate levels, and leucovorin rescue 24 hours after infusion and continuing until the methotrexate level is $< 5 \times 10^{-8}$ mol/L.
- **Mitomycin** can cause a syndrome of microangiopathic hemolytic anemia, progressive renal insufficiency, and thrombocytopenia, which carries a high mortality rate (> 50%).
- **Radiation** involving the kidney almost always causes alterations in renal function. Radiation nephritis consists of progressive renal insufficiency, hypertension, and proteinuria, occurring from 6 months to many years after radiation.

Pulmonary Toxicity

Chronic Pneumonitis with Pulmonary Fibrosis. Bleomycin is the major agent. Clinical manifestations include insidious onset of progressive dyspnea, nonproductive cough, fatigue, and malaise. Physical examination shows tachypnea, fever, bibasilar crackles, and occasionally a pleural friction rub. Laboratory findings incude hypoxemia, hypocapnia, diffuse interstitial infiltrates on chest radiography, restrictive defect, and diminished carbon monoxide diffusion capacity on pulmonary function testing. The diagnosis is established by lung biopsy. Treatment is prompt withdrawal of the offending agent, corticosteroids (prednisone 1 mg/kg/day), and supportive care. Supplemental oxygen may exacerbate the pneumonitis, and should be kept at the lowest possible level.

Hypersensitivity pneumonitis is associated with bleomycin, methotrexate, and procarbazine. It is clinically characterized by subacute onset of dyspnea, nonproductive cough, fever, and occasionally rash. Lung biopsy shows marked eosinophilic infiltrate of the pulmonary parenchyma. Treatment is corticosteroids. The prognosis is better than that for chronic pneumonitis.

Noncardiogenic pulmonary edema is caused by cytosine arabinoside, methotrexate, cyclophosphamide, and biologic agents, such as interleukin-2 and colony-stimulating factors. Clinically, capillary leak syndrome is indistinguishable from other causes of noncardiogenic pulmonary edema.

Acute chest syndrome is caused by bleomycin and methotrexate. Pleuritic pain is common, and may be retrosternal, but a friction rub is rarely heard. Chest radiograph and ECG findings are normal. Management consists of analgesia for pain.

Radiation-Related Pulmonary Toxicity. Lung tissue is sensitive to radiation because of its high oxygen content and the local generation of toxic oxygen free radicals. Lung damage is dose related. Acute radiation pneumonitis occurs 2 to 3 months after initiation of therapy. Patients have dyspnea, hacking cough, and fever. The chest radiograph shows a reticular interstitial pattern, which may progress to consolidation and then to chronic radiation fibrosis. Most patients improve over a few months. Treatment with steroids should be initiated at the earliest signs of acute pneumonitis, with prednisone 1 mg/kg/day, and slowly tapered. Steroids should not be used if chronic changes are seen.

Cardiac Toxicity

Cardiac complications of cancer therapy can occur soon after treatment or many months to years later.

Anthracycline cardiotoxicity occurs acutely as ECG changes in as many as 40% of cases, most commonly with ST and T wave abnormalities occurring within hours of drug administration. This finding does not indicate drug discontinuation. Acute pericarditis-myocarditis syndrome rarely occurs. Myocardial dysfunction with intractable heart failure is seen with relatively low cumulative doses (60–180 mg/m^2). Chronic toxicity can also occur, and is treated with supportive care, digoxin, diuretics, and vasodilator therapy. The prognosis is more favorable with early detection and discontinuation of the drug.

5-Fluorouracil-induced ischemia is caused by inducing coronary spasm and is diagnosed by the occurrence of anginal symptoms minutes to hours after administration. The ischemia may be fatal. There is no dose–toxicity relationship, but preexisting heart disease is a risk factor. Ischemia may be prevented with calcium channel blockers.

Cyclophosphamide-induced myocardial necrosis occurs in the treatment of pre–bone marrow transplantation patients, who receive high doses of cyclophosphamide (120–270 mg/kg). Patients have impaired systolic function, pericardial effusion, and ECG abnormalities 5–16 days after initiation of therapy. The mortality rate is 10–20%. Treatment is supportive, with treatment of heart failure and, if necessary, pericardiocentesis.

Radiation-induced cardiac toxicity that results in pericarditis occurs in approximately 50% of patients undergoing radiation to the chest. It usually develops 6–24 months after therapy. Patients may have pericarditis or pericardial tamponade. Treatment is drainage of pericardial fluid. Myocardial ischemia and fibrosis may occur as a consequence of radiation-related coronary artery disease in young patients who have received more than 3,500 cGy to the mediastinum. Treatment is the same as for other ischemic syndromes.

GI and Hepatic Toxicity

GI Toxicity. Emesis begins within hours of chemotherapy and may last for days. Management can include combination treatment with metoclopramide 1 to 3 mg/kg IV, given 30 minutes before chemotherapy and repeated every 2 hours in combination with diphenhydramine 50 mg IV every 6 hours. Metoclopramide is contraindicated in pheochromocytoma. Ondansetron 0.15 mg/kg 30 minutes before chemotherapy and repeated 4 and 8 hours after treatment is highly effective in preventing emesis caused by highly emetogenic drugs. Dexamethasone may enhance the effect of ondansetron.

Mucositis. The degree of mucositis is related to the properties of the agent and to the overall condition of the patient. The clinical manifestations range from stomatitis, glossitis, esophagitis, or diarrhea to more severe damage that results in tissue ulceration and subsequent sepsis. Treatment includes giving the patient nothing by mouth if necessary, vigorous IV hydration, palliative mouth care with warm saline rinses, and dyclonine hydrochloride to relieve pain. Chlorhexidine gluconate rinse may reduce oral colonization with bacteria and fungus. Recovery often occurs in conjunction with white blood cell count recovery.

Hepatic Toxicity. Therapy with antineoplastic agents is associated with a vast spectrum of liver injury, ranging from elevation of liver enzyme levels to acute parenchymal necrosis to chronic fibrosis and cirrhosis. Almost all chemotherapeutic drugs can cause some degree of hepatotoxicity. The agents most often related to hepatotoxicity are methotrexate, 6-mercaptopurine, and cytarabine.

Veno-occlusive Disease. This syndrome occurs in bone marrow transplant patients and is characterized by hepatomegaly, jaundice, ascites, and right upper quadrant tenderness. The incidence varies with the pretransplant hepatic function, the preparative regimen, and the nature of the original neoplasm. It occurs more commonly in patients with leukemia than in those with solid tumors. Treatment is supportive, consisting of managing fluid levels carefully, maintaining intravascular volume while using spironolactone to control edema, and minimizing encephalopathy with protein restriction and lactulose.

Neurotoxicity

Acute and chronic encephalopathies as well as acute cerebellar syndromes are chemotherapy-induced neurotoxicities that may require ICU care.

Methotrexate Neurotoxicity

- **Arachnoiditis** is a self-limited process that occurs after intrathecal (IT) administration and resolves within a few days.
- **Paraplegia** (acute encephalomyelopathy) also results from IT therapy and resolves spontaneously.
- **Chronic encephalopathy,** ranging from mild intellectual impairment to debilitating necrotizing leukoencephalopathy, occurs several months after IT administration, high-dose systemic methotrexate or, more often, with either type of therapy after a course of cranial irradiation.
- **Risk factors** for methotrexate neurotoxicity include treatment at a young age, long-term prophylaxis therapy (in leukemia or lymphoma), and previous cranial irradiation.
- **Diagnosis** is presumptive. Electroencephalography, CT, or MRI may provide supportive information.
- **Treatment** is discontinuation of further methotrexate and supportive care. Complete recovery is rare.

Ifosfamide Encephalopathy. Clinical characteristics include abrupt onset of mental status changes, with confusion, irritability, personality changes, drowsiness, stupor, coma, cranial nerve palsies, seizures, or cerebellar dysfunction. The incidence is 15–20% of courses of therapy. Risk factors are impaired renal or hepatic function, a high cumulative dose of cisplatin, and rapid infusion of ifosfamide. Treatment is discontinuation of the agent and supportive care, including anticonvulsant therapy if necessary. Full recovery is typical.

Cytosine Arabinoside Neurotoxicity. Cerebellar dysfunction or acute encephalopathy may be seen with high-dose cytarabine. Risk factors include a high cumulative or individual dose, pre-existing renal or hepatic dysfunction, and antecedent neurologic disease. Recovery occurs in 80% of cases; full recovery may be followed with subsequent courses of cytarabine at lower doses. Treatment is supportive care.

Suggested Readings

Baker WT, Royer GL, Weiss RB. Cerebellar toxicity during cytarabine therapy associated with renal insufficiency. *Cancer Chemother Pharmacol* 1990;27:76–78.

Case report of evidence of renal insufficiency as major risk in development of cerebellar toxicity during cytarabine therapy.

Dafnis EK, Laski ME. Fluid and electrolyte abnormalities in the oncology patient. *Semin Nephrol* 1993;13:281–296.

Excellent comprehensive review pointing out major drugs implicated and treatment approaches.

Dangaurd G, Abildgaard U. Cisplatin nephrotoxicity. *Cancer Chemother Pharmacol* 1989;25:1–9.

Reviews pathophysiologic mechanism of cisplatin-induced nephrotoxicity and prophylactic means to reduce its toxicity.

Hughs WT, Armstrong D, Bodey GP, et al. Guidelines for the use of antimicrobial agents in neutropenic patients with unexplained fever. *J Infect Dis* 1990;161:381–396.

Excellent consensus report on recommendations for antibiotic therapy in febrile, neutropenic patients.

Pizzo PA. Management of fever in patients with cancer and treatment-induced neutropenia. *N Engl J Med* 1993;328:1323–1332.

Excellent review of development of empiric antimicrobial therapy for patients with chemotherapy-induced neutropenia, patients at risk, and likely infections and organisms. Includes discussion of use of growth factors.

Rolston KVI, Bodey GP. Infections in patietns with cancer. In: Sutton XL, Holland JF, Frei E III, et al., eds. *Cancer medicine,* 3rd ed. Philadelphia: Lea and Febiger, 1993, pp 2416–2441.

Comprehensive review of cancer therapy–related infections with up-to-date bibliography.

Sutton XL, Holland JF, Frei E III, et al., eds. *Cancer medicine,* 3rd ed. Philadelphia: Lea and Febiger, 1993, pp 2219–2415.

This section, entitled "Complications of cancer and its treatment," presents a comprehensive, although rather lengthy, review of the topic. It is organized by organ-specific toxicities and includes excellent reveiw on cancer pain management.

Twohig KJ, Matthay RA. Pulmonary effects of cytotoxic agents other than bleomycin. *Clin Chest Med* 1990;11:31–54.

Infectious Diseases

CHAPTER 70

Sepsis Syndrome

(See Chapters 22–27)

Robert A. Balk

Sepsis has traditionally been viewed as the systemic inflammatory process that develops in response to an infection. In the past, confusion has centered around the terminology used to describe patients with this systemic response. Recently, the difficulties with nomenclature have been highlighted because of attempts to identify septic patients at an early stage with predominantly clinical criteria. This approach facilitates the use of various investigational therapies and treatment approaches. The many clinical studies directed at this critically ill population of patients have underscored the need for consensus regarding the terminology used to describe the septic patient.

Definitions

In the past, bacteremia and sepsis were often considered similar, if not identical, phenomena. Some early definitions of sepsis required the presence of hypotension. With an ever-increasing number of septic patients and clinical trials that required early intervention with investigative therapies, it became necessary to develop clinical criteria to identify the septic patient. Waiting 24–48 hours for the results of blood cultures to confirm sepsis was impractical. Any delay might represent an unacceptable alternative in view of the results of experimental animal studies indicating that the earlier the intervention, the more beneficial the response. It thus became necessary to develop clinical criteria that could identify the critically ill septic patient who would be likely to benefit from new therapies.

To this end, the concept of sepsis syndrome was developed. This clinical definition allows for early identification of septic patients and allows for early institution of therapy, whether conventional or investigational. This definition was subsequently evaluated in the control group of a large clinical trial studying the efficacy of early high-dose methylprednisolone in the treatment of sepsis. Forty-five percent of the patients were bacteremic. Patients meeting this definition were relatively similar despite their blood culture status. The only significant difference between the bacteremic and nonbacteremic groups was a higher incidence of circulatory shock with bacteremia. The overall mortality rate was 26%. The major determinant of mortality was the presence of adverse sequelae, such as shock or adult respiratory distress syndrome (ARDS).

The lack of any positive microbiologic culture result in approximately 25% of the sepsis syndrome population has created concern and confusion over the proper use of terminology. In an attempt to resolve some of the confusion, a consensus conference was held by the American College of Chest Physicians and the Society of Critical Care Medicine, with representation from critical care physicians, surgeons, infectious disease specialists, cardiologists, pulmonologists, and others. Their recommendations for terminology regarding sepsis and other causes of systemic inflammatory response are listed in Table 70–1.

Epidemiology of Sepsis

Recent reports have claimed an alarming increase in the frequency of sepsis. The exact incidence has been difficult to determine because of the lack of uniform definitions; however, a survey based on discharge diagnoses of bacteremia showed a 139% increase over the last 10 years. Recent estimates of the annual number of episodes of sepsis in the United States have reached as high as 300,000 to 500,000.

TABLE 70–1

AMERICAN COLLEGE OF CHEST PHYSICIANS/ SOCIETY OF CRITICAL CARE MEDICINE CONSENSUS CONFERENCE COMMITTEE DEFINITIONS

Bacteremia	Presence of viable bacteria in the blood
Hypotension (due to sepsis)	A systolic blood pressure of < 90 mm Hg or a reduction of > 40 mm Hg from baseline in the absence of other causes of hypotension
Infection	Microbial phenomenon characterized by an inflammatory response to the presence of microorganisms or the invasion of normally sterile host tissue by those organisms
Multiple organ dysfunction syndrome	Presence of altered organ function in an acutely ill patient such that homeostasis cannot be maintained without intervention

TABLE 70–1 *Continued*

AMERICAN COLLEGE OF CHEST PHYSICIANS/ SOCIETY OF CRITICAL CARE MEDICINE CONSENSUS CONFERENCE COMMITTEE DEFINITIONS

Sepsis	Systemic inflammatory response to infection (see below)
Septic shock	Sepsis with hypotension, despite adequate fluid resuscitation, along with the presence of perfusion abnormalities that may include, but are not limited to, lactic acidosis, oliguria, or an acute alteration in mental status. Patients who are receiving inotropic or vasopressor agents may not be hypotensive at the time that perfusion abnormalities are measured
Severe sepsis	Sepsis associated with organ dysfunction, hypoperfusion, or hypotension. Hypoperfusion and perfusion abnormalities may include, but are not limited to, lactic acidosis, oliguria, or an acute alteration in mental status
Systemic inflammatory response syndrome	Systemic inflammatory response to a variety of severe clinical insults. The response is manifested by two or more of the following conditions: Temperature > 38°C or < 36°C Heart rate > 90 beats/min Respiratory rate > 20 breaths/min or Pa_{CO_2} < 32 torr White blood cell count > 12,000 cells/mm^3, < 4000 cells/mm^3, or > 10% immature (band) forms

Pa_{CO_2} = arterial carbon dioxide tension.

(ACCP/SCCM Consensus Conference Committee. American College of Chest Physicians/Society of Critical Care Medicine Consensus Conference: Definitions for sepsis and organ failure and guidelines for the use of innovative therapies in sepsis. *Crit Care Med* 1992;20:864–874 with permission of Williams & Wilkins.)

Possible causes of the increased prevalence of sepsis include:

- Increased recognition.
- Increased elderly population.
- Expanded use of invasive procedures.
- Greater use of immunosuppressive agents.
- Increased numbers of immunosuppressed patients.
- Increased numbers of patients with chronic diseases.
- Aggressive management of malignant conditions.
- Increased use of transplantation.

Clinical Features

The clinical manifestations of sepsis are varied, and may involve almost any organ system. It is important to recognize the wide range of clinical presentations of septic processes and to be particularly attuned to this potential diagnosis in the setting of known or presumed infection. The most common clinical manifestations of sepsis include fever, tachycardia, tachypnea, leukocytosis with a leftward shift, and alterations in mental status. It is important to remember that sepsis is a syndrome and that none of these clinical manifestations is by itself pathognomonic of the diagnosis. Some common clinical manifestations of sepsis are listed below.

Temperature Abnormalities in Sepsis

- Fever (more common than hypothermia; inability to increase the temperature to > 99.6°F is a poor prognostic sign).
- Hypothermia (most common in the extremes of age and in patients with chronic debilitated or immunosuppressed conditions).

Pulmonary Manifestations

- Tachypnea, hyperventilation, and hypoxemia are common manifestations.
- ARDS (develops in 5%–40% of septic patients; see Chapters 23, 26, 27, and 73 in the main text).

Cardiovascular Manifestations

- Tachycardia (an early clinical manifestation).
- Typical hemodynamic profile (see Table 70–2).
- Biventricular myocardial depression (reversible and associated with decreased ejection fraction) or frank circulatory shock.

GI and Hepatic Manifestations

- Risk of stress-related GI bleeding.
- Hepatic dysfunction is frequent.
- Patients at risk for translocation of intestinal bacteria and toxins.

TABLE 70–2

HEMODYNAMIC ALTERATIONS IN SEPTIC SHOCK

	Early Septic Shock	Late Shock	Refractory Shock
Blood pressure	↓	↓	↓
Heart rate	↑	↑	↑
Systemic vascular resistance	↓↓	↓	Nl
Cardiac output	↑↑	↑	Nl or ↓
Volume responsiveness	+	±	−

Nl = normal; + = responsive; − = unresponsive; arrows denote relative magnitude and direction of change from normal.

Renal Manifestations

- Renal dysfunction (oliguria and acute tubular necrosis may develop in the absence of hypotension).
- Antibiotic-induced nephrotoxicity.

Hematologic Manifestations

- Leukocytosis with a leftward shift is the most common manifestation.
- Neutropenia (usually transient and occurring early in the course; underlying neutropenia is a risk factor for gram-negative infection).
- Thrombocytopenia (with or without disseminated intravascular coagulation).
- Prolonged prothrombin time or partial thromboplastin time.
- Increased fibrin(ogen) split products and D-dimer levels.
- Decreased fibrinogen, Factor V, Factor VIII, and antithrombin III levels.

Neurologic Manifestations

- Mental status changes are common.
- Confusion, disorientation, lethargy, obtundation, agitation, coma, seizures, polyneuropathy of critical illness.

Metabolic and Endocrine Manifestations

- Hypermetabolism. Sepsis is a catabolic state.
- Hyperglycemia, glucose intolerance, relative insulin resistance (seen in as many as 40% of septic patients).
- Elevated levels of stress hormones.
- Lactic acidosis.

Adverse Sequelae of Sepsis

The mortality rate for sepsis is directly related to the adverse sequelae that complicate the clinical course. These include the development of septic shock, acute lung injury (ARDS), and multiple organ dysfunction or failure. Most studies of septic patients have used an operational definition of shock (usually systolic blood pressure < 90 mm Hg, mean pressure < 70 mm Hg, or a drop in systolic pressure > 40 mm Hg, in the absence of antihypertensive therapy) and have found that approximately 40% of sepsis is complicated by the development of shock at some point in the course.

The timing of the onset of shock has prognostic significance. In a large multicenter study, shock at presentation had a 28% mortality rate, whereas shock that developed later during the course of sepsis had a 43% mortality rate. Patients who never had shock had a 13% mortality rate.

Most reports show higher mortality rates for septic shock, in the range of 50%.

The development of multiple organ failure is also associated with increased mortality rates. Some studies demonstrated higher morbidity and mortality rates when selected organs, such as the liver or CNS, are involved. Other studies emphasized that the duration of organ system failure is a critical determinant of prognosis. The more organ systems that fail and the longer the duration of failure, the higher the mortality rate.

Prognosis

The overall mortality rate associated with sepsis is highly variable, and is dependent on multiple factors. Among these factors are the underlying health status of the patient, the development of adverse sequelae of sepsis, the specific causative microorganisms, and the extent of involvement at the time of diagnosis.

The key to improved survival is prompt recognition of sepsis and early institution of appropriate therapy (see Chapter 71 in this book). It is also important to perform appropriate cultures to help to direct therapy. Future therapy may involve the use of specific agents to modify or direct the inflammatory response of the host.

Suggested Readings

ACCP/SCCM Consensus Conference Committee. American College of Chest Physicians/Society of Critical Care Medicine Consensus Conference: Definitions for sepsis and organ failure and guidelines for the use of innovative therapies in sepsis. *Crit Care Med* 1992; 20:864–874.

Publication of definitions and guidelines concerning sepsis, septic shock, and organ dysfunction. Also contains discussion of scoring systems and the role they play in assessing the severity of illness in this group of patients. Guidelines are given to direct the use of experimental and innovative new therapies in treatment of septic patients.

Bone RC. Gram-negative sepsis: Background, clinical features, and intervention. *Chest* 1991;100:802–808.

Excellent review of pathophysiology and clinical features of gram-negative sepsis. Brief discussion of newer treatments directed at endotoxin and gram-negative sepsis.

Bone RC, Fisher CJ Jr, Clemmer TP, et al. Sepsis syndrome: A valid clinical entity. *Crit Care Med* 1989;17:389–393.

One of the initial descriptions of sepsis syndrome. Supports the concept that there is no major difference between patients with and without bacteremia.

Harris RL, Musher DM, Bloom K, et al. Manifestations of sepsis. *Arch Intern Med* 1987;147:1895–1906.

Excellent review of common clinical manifestations of sepsis and pathophysiology of these manifestations.

Mizock B. Septic shock: A metabolic perspective. *Arch Intern Med* 1984;144:579–585.

Excellent, comprehensive review of metabolic disturbances that occur during sepsis. Reviews specific organ-related disturbances as well as global response.

Snell RJ, Parrillo JE. Cardiovascular dysfunction in septic shock. *Chest* 1991;99:1000–1009.
Reviews complex cardiovascular changes seen in septic patients and probable mechanisms behind dysfunction.

CHAPTER 71

Essentials of the Standard Management of Septic Shock

(See Chapters 25–28)

Robert A. Balk

Chapter 70 in this book describes the various clinical manifestations in the patient with sepsis. This chapter describes the standard conventional approach to sepsis and septic shock (Table 71–1). Further discussion of the rationale behind the suggested approaches and a review of new therapies on the horizon can be found in the sepsis section (Chapters 25–28) of the main text and in the Suggested Readings at the end of this chapter.

Diagnostic Studies

When sepsis is suspected, it is imperative that there be a directed history and physical examination. The initial level of detail is dictated by the gravity of the clinical condition. If the patient is hemodynamically unstable or is oxygenating poorly, initial resuscitative efforts must be promptly instituted (see following). Appropriate laboratory and radiologic tests should also be performed, directed by the historical features of the illness and guided by the findings on physical examination. Appropriate microbiologic cultures are obtained, typically including blood cultures from at least two sites. Areas of abscess or loculated purulent fluid collections should be appropriately drained, with samples sent for culture and susceptibility testing.

Antimicrobial Therapy

The early initiation of appropriate antibiotic therapy, as determined by eventual culture and susceptibility testing results, is associated with a decreased incidence of shock and improved survival rates in patients with bacteremia. Because culture and susceptibility results are typically unavailable for the first 24 to 48 hours, selection of initial antimicrobial therapy often must be empiric, taking into account:

- Patient's historical and physical examination features.
- Typical clinical presentations.
- Patient's underlying health status and immunocompetence.
- Severity of the patient's current illness.
- Institution-specific pathogen and antibiotic susceptibility patterns.
- Results of gram stains.

The importance of tailoring initial empiric therapy according to the above information is underscored by the fact that blood culture findings are negative in many patients with clinically defined sepsis syndrome. The initial antibiotic regimen is usually broad spectrum, directed at both gram-positive and gram-negative organisms. Specific modification of the antibiotic regimen based on suspected organisms or complicating underlying processes should also be considered. In the immunocompromised patient, opportunistic as well as common pathogens should be considered. Neutropenic patients are at increased risk of gram-negative infection, and many clinicians provide coverage with two antibiotics of different classes against gram-negative organisms.

When the clinical situation suggests that *Pseudomonas* species, *Legionella* species, or methicillin-resistant *Staphylococcus* species are involved, it is important to select antibiotic therapy that is effective against these organisms. After the culture and susceptibility results are available, the initial antibiotic regimen can be modified as necessary. Lack of positive culture results does not necessarily indicate that antibiotics are not warranted.

Provision of Intensive Care

The patient with severe sepsis and septic shock is critically ill and requires the expertise and intensity of care that is provided by an ICU staffed with experienced personnel who are trained to care for the complex needs of these patients. The high nurse-to-patient ratio allows frequent patient assessments. Studies have shown improved survival rates in patients with septic shock when an on-site critical care physician team cared for the patients as compared with retrospective control subjects. The ICU environment is designed to provide intensive monitoring, including invasive (e.g., pulmonary artery catheters and arterial lines) and noninvasive (e.g., continuous cardiac rhythm and

TABLE 71–1

THERAPY FOR SEVERE SEPSIS AND SEPTIC SHOCK

Diagnostic studies	History, physical examination, laboratory and radiologic tests, microbiologic smears and cultures
Empiric antimicrobial therapy	Initial antibiotic selection is based on patient's historical and clinical features, patient's severity of illness, susceptibility patterns of the institution
Specific antimicrobial therapy	Based on culture and susceptibility results
Drainage of closed-space infections	If indicated
Fluid resuscitation and hemodynamic support	Appropriate use of fluid loading, inotropic and vasoactive agents
Ensuring adequate oxygenation and oxygen delivery	Supplemental oxygen to ensure Sa_{O_2} > 0.90, mechanical ventilatory support as needed, blood transfusion for significant anemia
Provision of intensive supportive care	Critical care unit admission; use of noninvasive monitors (pulse oximeter, noninvasive blood pressure, continuous ECG monitoring); use of invasive hemodynamic monitors (pulmonary

	artery catheter, arterial catheter, mixed venous oxygen saturation, etc.), as indicated; correction of electrolyte and other metabolic abnormalities
Nutritional support	Enteral nutritional support may prevent translocation of intestinal bacteria and toxins
Prevention of complications	Stress-related GI bleeding prophylaxis (cytoprotective agents, H_2-receptor blocking agents, enteral nutrition); prophylaxis against venous thrombosis (minidose subcutaneous heparin, lower-extremity pneumatic compression devices)
Investigational therapies	Nonsteroidal anti-inflammatory agents, antiendotoxin monoclonal antibodies, antitumor necrosis factor monoclonal antibodies, interleukin-1 receptor antagonist, bradykinin antagonist, platelet-activating factor antagonist, immunoglobulins, antithrombin III (all currently considered investigational)

SaO_2 = arterial oxygen percent saturation.

pulse oximetry) monitoring. The availability of intensive monitoring often guides the treatment decisions related to vasoactive pharmacotherapy and oxygen delivery.

Fluid Resuscitation and Hemodynamic Support

Appropriate antibiotics are the cornerstone of improved overall survival rates; however, early mortality often is related to cardiovascular collapse. Unless contraindicated, the initial resuscitative efforts in the hypotensive patient should focus on fluid therapy (see Chapter 3 in this book). Critically ill patients with septic shock often require invasive hemodynamic monitoring to assist with their management. Assessment of pulmonary artery occlusion (wedge) pressure, cardiac output, systemic vascular resistance, and mixed venous oxygen saturation may aid in the diagnosis and etiology of shock, and also may guide the choice of therapy and gauge the response to therapy. Initial fluid resuscitation is directed at achieving a mean arterial blood pressure greater than 60 mm Hg or a systolic blood pressure greater than 90 mm Hg. Care is taken to avoid elevating the pulmonary artery wedge pressure to more than approximately 18 mm Hg. If adequate fluid resuscitation does not sufficiently increase the blood pressure, then inotropic or vasopressor therapy should be instituted.

Dopamine is probably the most commonly used vasopressor agent. The dose is titrated upward until the desired effect is obtained. When higher doses of dopamine are administered, usually more than 15–20 μg/kg/min, many recommend gradual reduction of the dose to renal perfusion levels (usually 2–3 μg/kg/min) and maintenance of blood pressure by an agent such as norepinephrine. The latter intervention is less likely to cause tachycardia than dopamine. Low doses of dopamine are used to increase perfusion of the kidneys and splanchnic bed during vasopressor therapy. Additional supportive therapy includes treatment of electrolyte abnormalities and other metabolic disturbances.

Respiratory Support and Oxygen Delivery

There is general agreement that supplemental oxygen is necessary for the patient with hypoxemia. However, there is controversy regarding the timing of intubation and ventilatory support in the patient with septic shock. Some argue for early intervention to reduce the workload placed on the diaphragm and muscles of respiration and to increase the percentage of cardiac output available to fuel vital organs. Others point out the negative aspects of endotracheal intubation, such as the inability to cough effectively, the loss of protective airway reflexes, and the propensity for mishaps in patients receiving mechanical ventilatory support.

An equally controversial issue is the level of tissue oxygen delivery to achieve. Several studies have suggested that there is a critical threshold of oxygen delivery below which there is supply dependency for oxygen use. Other studies have questioned this finding, and contend that it is a representation of the methods used to measure oxygen delivery and oxygen use. Systemic oxygen delivery is the product of arterial blood oxygen content and cardiac output. Therefore, it is influenced by hemoglobin concentration as well as oxygen saturation and cardiac output. Blood transfusions can be an important means of increasing oxygen delivery in anemic patients. A number of studies have tested the hypothesis that increased oxygen delivery is associated with increased patient survival. This topic remains controversial, and the goal is to achieve adequate oxygen delivery, not necessarily supranormal tissue oxygen delivery.

Nutritional Support and Prevention of Complications

Patients with severe sepsis and septic shock are at risk for complications of critical illness. These complications include stress-related GI bleeding, deep venous thrombosis, pulmonary embolism, multiple organ system dysfunction or failure, and malnutrition. Prophylactic measures to prevent stress-related GI bleeding, deep venous thrombosis, and pulmonary embolism should be implemented unless there are specific contraindications. H_2-blocking agents and sucralfate appear to have prophylactic efficacy, and probably do not increase the incidence of nosocomial pneumonia. In addition to providing nutritional support, enteral feeding may be an effective method of stress ulcer prophylaxis. Subcutaneous heparin and pneumatic compression boots have been effective methods of prophylaxis against venous thrombosis.

Recent studies have supported a potential benefit of the early institution of enteral nutritional support of the critically ill patient in an attempt to prevent the translocation of bacteria and toxins from the intestinal lumen to the bloodstream. Malnutrition and intestinal ischemia promote this translocation. Early enteral feeding may help to preserve the integrity of the intestinal mucosal barrier. Definitive studies are needed to confirm this potential benefit.

Investigational Approaches

Current therapy that employs new technology, improved antibiotics with expanded spectrums of coverage, and aggressive monitoring has not significantly improved survival rates in patients with severe sepsis and septic shock. A number of experimental or innovative approaches to the management of septic patients has been proposed (see Chapter 28 in the main text and the suggested readings at the end of this chapter). Animal investigations have suggested a potential therapeutic role for the early administration of high-dose corticosteroid therapy. However, several large prospective, placebo-controlled, multicenter trials have clearly shown that no significant benefit is offered by the use of large doses of corticosteroids in patients with severe sepsis and septic shock. In fact, there may even be a detrimental effect in some subpopulations of these patients. Naloxone, an endorphin antagonist, was found to lack efficacy in human sepsis. Current studies are underway to evaluate other anti-inflammatory agents and a variety of immune modulators and specific inhibitors of the potential mediators of the inflammatory response that is characteristic of sepsis (see Table 71–1).

Suggested Readings

Alexander JW. Nutrition and translocation. *J Parenter Enteral Nutr* 1990;14(5 suppl):170S–174S.

Excellent review of mechanisms and ramifications of intestinal translocation and its potential relationship to production of sepsis and organ system failure.

Bone RC. A critical evaluation of new agents for the treatment of sepsis. *JAMA* 1991;266:1686–1691.

Excellent review that contrasts antiendotoxin and other innovative therapies used in treatment of severe sepsis and septic shock.

Bone RC, Fisher CJ Jr, Clemmer TP, et al. A controlled clinical trial of high-dose methylprednisolone in the treatment of severe sepsis and septic shock. *N Engl J Med* 1987;317:653–658.

One of several large, multicenter, placebo-controlled, prospective trials that showed a lack of beneficial effect of high-dose steroids in patients with sepsis and septic shock. In subgroup of patients with elevated serum creatinine levels, there was actually an increase in mortality rate with high-dose steroid administration.

Luce JM. Pathogenesis and management of septic shock. *Chest* 1987; 91:883–888.

Concise review of basic pathophysiology of septic shock and approach to standard therapy.

Martin LF, Booth FVM, Karlstadt RG, et al. Continuous intravenous cimetidine decreases stress-related upper gastrointestinal hemorrhage without promoting pneumonia. *Crit Care Med* 1993;21:19–30.

Trial that evaluated the use of continuous infusion of H_2-blocking agents in prevention of stress-related upper GI bleeding. Continuous infusion of cimetidine decreased the incidence of GI hemorrhage without increasing the incidence of nosocomial pneumonia.

Meadows D, Edwards JD, Wilkins RG, et al. Reversal of intractable septic shock with norepinephrine therapy. *Crit Care Med* 1988;16:663–670.

Studies use of norepinephrine in patients with septic shock who were unresponsive to dopamine and dobutamine treatments.

Parker MM, McCarthy KE, Ognibene FP, et al. Right ventricular dysfunction and dilatation, similar to left ventricular changes, characterize the cardiac depression of septic shock in humans. *Chest* 1990; 97:126–131.

Excellent study of the myocardial depression seen in some patients with severe sepsis. Includes in-depth description of parameters that reflect this dysfunction and implications of the abnormality.

St. John RC, Dorinsky PM. Immunologic therapy for ARDS, septic shock, and multiple-organ failure. *Chest* 1993;103:932–943.
Excellent review of innovative therapies for treatment of septic shock and adult respiratory distress syndrome.

CHAPTER 72

Gram-Positive Bacterial Sepsis

(See Chapter 31)

David Tompkins

Staphylococci

Staphylococci are gram-positive cocci that have characteristic microscopic morphologic features, occurring primarily in clusters, but also as single organisms, pairs, or sometimes short chains. There are three clinically important species of staphylococci: *Staphylococcus aureus, S. saprophyticus* (a cause of acute cystitis in young women), and *S. epidermidis.*

S. aureus is the most virulent of the staphylococci. It is the second leading cause of nosocomial bacteremia, and overall it accounts for 10–40% of nosocomial infections. Two patterns of disease are caused by *S. aureus:* infections with tissue invasion and destruction, and toxin-mediated disease.

Invasive Staphylococcal Disease. The initial infections may be localized to the skin and subcutaneous tissues, and can rapidly lead to tissue destruction and abscess formation. Progressive infection may lead to bacteremia, seeding of the endovascular tree, endocarditis, metastatic abscess formation in various organs (brain, kidney, liver, muscle), sepsis, and death.

In patients with blood cultures that grow *S. aureus,* it is crucial, but often difficult, to determine whether endocarditis is present. The most reliable evidence for infection of a heart valve or vessel is continuous bacteremia in which several blood culture results are positive over time. The rate of endocarditis is less than 5% in patients with a recognized primary site of infection caused by *S. aureus.* Conversely, in patients with a clinically occult source of bacteremia, particularly community-acquired bacteremia, the risk of endocarditis and secondary bacterial seeding is much higher, 60% and 90%, respectively.

Diagnostic evaluation should include gram stain and culture of any purulent material and cultures of normally sterile body fluids, such as blood (3–4 sets at timed intervals) and urine. Echocardiography, ideally a transesophageal study, should be considered in patients without an identifiable focus of infection or with stigmata of endocarditis.

Treatment includes eradication of the source of infection by removal of any infected foreign body, when feasible, or drainage of abscess collections. Most strains of *S. aureus* produce β-lactamase and require therapy with a penicillinase-resistant penicillin, such as semisynthetic penicillins or cephalosporins. Certain strains of *S. aureus* are resistant to all β-lactam antibiotics (methicillin-resistant *S. aureus*), including semisynthetic penicillins, cephalosporins, and imipenem-cilastatin. Such strains are increasing in frequency in certain areas and patient populations (e.g., IV drug abusers, nursing home residents). When methicillin resistance is suspected on clinical grounds or documented by microbial susceptibility results, vancomycin should be used.

The duration of antibiotic treatment is generally at least 2 weeks; however, patients with endocarditis from metastatic seeding require a more extended course of 4 weeks or more. Criteria for short-course therapy are:

- No valvular heart lesions and no other obvious sites of infection other than the bloodstream, a removable catheter, or the primary site.
- Immunocompetence.
- Obvious and easily managed primary infection source.
- Prompt response to initial therapy.
- Causative *S. aureus* organism that is fully susceptible to the antibiotics chosen.
- No evidence of metastatic infection complications during the 14-day period of therapy.

Toxin-mediated staphylococcal disease is the result of a variety of toxins produced by *S. aureus*. Staphylococcal food poisoning is a self-limited disease that is caused by ingestion of a preformed toxin. Localized infections with toxin production and cutaneous manifestations are staphylococcal scalded skin syndrome and toxic shock syndrome.

Staphylococcal scalded skin syndrome primarily occurs in infants. It results from the production of an exfoliative toxin in the setting of a cutaneous *S. aureus* infection. The characteristic rash begins with perioral erythema that, over several days, spreads to the entire body before desquamating. Therapy is supportive, and consists primarily of prevention of dehydration and secondary infection.

Toxic shock syndrome is a multisystem illness characterized by rapid onset of high fever, rash, hypotension, and multiple organ system failure. It commonly affects young, otherwise healthy patients who have often trivial infections with toxin-producing (TSST-1 or related exotoxin) strains of *S. aureus.* Since the removal of superabsorbent tampons from the market, the incidence of nonmenstrual toxic shock syndrome (postsurgical, influenza-associated, postpartum toxic shock syndrome) exceeds that of the menstrual type. Diagnostic criteria include:

- Temperature > 38.9°C.
- Systolic blood pressure < 90 mm Hg.
- Rash with subsequent desquamation, especially on palms and soles.
- Involvement of more than three organ systems:
  - **GI:** Vomiting or profuse diarrhea.
  - **Muscular:** Severe myalgias or greater than fivefold increase in creatine phosphokinase level.
  - **Mucous membranes** (vagina, conjunctivae, or pharynx): frank hyperemia.
  - **Renal:** Serum urea nitrogen or creatinine level at least twice the upper limit of normal, with pyuria in the absence of urinary tract infection.
  - **Liver (hepatitis):** Serum bilirubin and transaminase levels at least twice the upper limit of normal.
  - **Blood:** Thrombocytopenia < $100{,}000/mm^{-3}$.
  - **CNS:** Disorientation without focal neurologic signs.

The differential diagnosis includes Rocky Mountain spotted fever, leptospirosis, and measles. Treatment includes:

- **Antibiotic treatment** with an antistaphylococcal antimicrobial agent.
- **Removal of foci** of infection, including removal of foreign bodies and drainage of infected sites.
- **Methylprednisolone** for severe cases (no controlled studies).
- **IV immune globulin.** Almost all patients have an absent or low-titer antibody to TSST-1 early in the course of disease, and high levels of antibody are found in commercial immune globulin preparations.
- **Management of complications,** which include hypovolemia, hypotension, myocardial dysfunction, adult respiratory distress syndrome, cerebral edema, disseminated intravascular coagulation, acute renal insufficiency, and fluid and electrolyte abnormalities.

Coagulase-negative staphylococci (*S. epidermidis*) are the most commonly reported causes of nosocomial bacteremia. Risk factors for bacteremia include the presence of a foreign body (e.g., intravascular catheter, prosthetic joint, prosthetic heart valve), neutropenia, antibiotic therapy, chronic peritoneal dialysis, and the neonatal period. *S. epidermidis* is a component of normal skin flora, and it may contaminate blood culture specimens. The clinical presentation of *S. epidermidis* bacteremia may be relatively subtle, with low-grade fever and no evidence of systemic toxicity. Features suggestive of true bacteremia include:

- Growth in multiple sets of blood cultures.
- Growth in both aerobic and anaerobic bottles.
- Identical antibiotic susceptibility pattern of organisms from several sets of cultures.
- When available, identification of identical species of staphylococci.

Patients who are not septic or febrile, have no risk factors for the acquisition of the organism, and have only a single positive blood culture finding may be observed without therapy while the results of follow-up blood cultures are awaited.

Therapy for true infections includes removal of the infected foreign body (if possible) and administration of antibiotics. β-Lactam antibiotic resistance is so common that vancomycin is the empiric therapy of choice. For susceptible strains, a semisynthetic penicillin (e.g., nafcillin) or cephalosporin is effective. The duration of therapy for bacteremic infection in a patient with a removable focus is generally 14 days. Therapy for prosthetic valve endocarditis is discussed elsewhere (see Chapter 80 in this book).

Enterococci

Two species account for most clinical infections: *Enterococcus faecalis* is responsible for 85% of infections, and *E. faecium* is responsible for the remaining 15%. Enterococci are components of the normal flora of various body sites (bowel, vagina, urethra, and occasionally oral cavity).

Enterococcal bacteremia, which originates from extracardiac sites (e.g., gut, urinary tract, or genital tract), may be associated with endocarditis. Clinically, enterococcal endocarditis can have a subacute presentation, with low-grade fever, malaise, fatigue, and weight loss, or a more acute presentation, with high fever and evidence of valve dysfunction.

Nosocomial enterococcal bacteremia is usually associated with an identifiable focus of infection, is often polymicrobial, and is less frequently a cause of endocarditis than enterococcal infections acquired outside of the hospital. Sources of nosocomial bacteremia include intra-abdominal infections, surgical wounds, burns, decubitus ulcers, vascular catheters, and the genitourinary and biliary tracts.

An important consideration in the treatment of enterococcal infections is the relative resistance of these bacteria to antibiotics. Cell wall–active agents, such as the penicillins, carbapenems, and vancomycin are only bacteriostatic (cephalosporins are not active). Because of this relative resistance, infections that are ideally treated with bactericidal agents, such as endocarditis, should be treated with a synergistic combination of a cell wall–active agent (penicillin, ampicillin, or vancomycin, if penicillin allergic) and an aminoglycoside. The recent increase in enterococcal resistance to penicillin, vancomycin, and aminoglycosides necessitates susceptibility testing of all clinically significant isolates. If high-level aminoglycoside resistance (> 500 μg/mL) is found, single-agent therapy for endocarditis with penicillin or vancomycin is effective if prolonged (6–8 weeks).

Streptococci

Group A streptococci (e.g., *S. pyogenes*) are classically a cause of pediatric pharyngitis, but may also be a pathogen in adults. In addition to pharyngitis, group A streptococci can cause soft tissue infections and bacteremia. Bacteremia is more common in patients with underlying disease (e.g., chronic renal failure, alcoholism, IV drug abuse, diabetes, connective tissue disease, or malignancy). The source is usually a skin or soft tissue infection, and clinical presentation is abrupt, with fever, rigors, GI symptoms, and mental status changes. Circulatory shock develops in as many as 40% of cases. Group A streptococcal infection can also cause a syndrome similar to staphylococcal toxic shock syndrome, with sepsis, shock, diffuse erythroderma, and multiple organ system failure. See Table 72–1 for treatment.

Group B streptococci (*S. agalactia*) are a component of GI and genitourinary tract flora that can result in several disease syndromes:

- **Neonatal sepsis** is frequently the result of intrapartum transmission of the bacteria from mother to infant.
- **Postpartum infection** is the most common infection in adults. It presents as endometritis, usually developing within 48 hours of delivery. Women with cesarian sections are at the greatest risk.
- **Bacteremia** in adults is seen primarily among elderly patients with an underlying disease (e.g., diabetes, malignancy, renal failure). Despite a subacute presentation, the mortality rate is high (approximately 70%).

See Table 72–1 for treatment.

Group C streptococci are a relatively rare cause of bacteremia. The classic occurrence is a community-acquired

TABLE 72–1

ANTIBACTERIAL THERAPY FOR GRAM-POSITIVE BACTERIA

Infecting Organism	Drug of Choice	Alternate Drug Choice
S. aureus, penicillinase-producing organisms	Penicillinase-resistant penicillin (nafcillin)	Cephalosporins (cephalothin, cefotaxime), vancomycin, clindamycin, ampicillin-sulfbactam, ticarcillin-clavulanate, imipenem-cilastatin
Methacillin-resistant staphylococci	Vancomycin	Trimethaprim-sulfamethoxazole; fluoroquinolone (ofloxacin, ciprofloxacin)
S. epidermidis	Vancomycin	Trimethaprim-sulfamethoxazole; fluoroquinolone (ofloxacin ciprofloxacin)
Enterococcus species	Penicillin G, ampicillin with gentamicin or amikacin	Vancomycin with gentamicin or amikacin

High-level gentamicin resistance	Penicillin G, ampicillin, or vancomycin	
S. pyogenes Groups A, C, and G	Penicillin	Macrolide, cephalosporin, vancomycin, clindamycin
Streptococcus, group B	Penicillin, ampicillin	Macrolide, cephalosporin, vancomycin
Streptococcus, viridans group	Penicillin, ampicillin	Cephalosporin, vancomycin
S. pneumoniae	Penicillin*	Vancomycin, cephalosporin, macrolide
Rhodococcus equi	Vancomycin, erythromycin, aminoglycoside, chloramphenicol	
Corynebacterium group JK	Vancomycin	
L. monocytogenes	Ampicillin or penicillin with or without gentamicin	Trimethoprim-sulfamethoxazole

*Penicillin-resistant pneumococci must be treated with cephalosporin or vancomycin (see text).

infection in a patient with serious underlying disease (e.g., malignancy, diabetes, chronic liver and renal disease). *S. equisimilis* and *S. zooepidemicus* are the primary causes of infections in humans. Infection is frequently related to animal exposure, with entry through the skin, upper respiratory tract, or GI tract. Presentation is usually acute, with fever, chills, and prostration. Endocarditis is seen in 30% of cases. The mortality rate is greater than 25% (33% with endocarditis).

Nonenterococcal group D streptococci (e.g., *S. bovis, S. equinus*) are normal components of the gut flora. They are relatively uncommon causes of bacteremia. *S. bovis* bacteremia is a marker of GI abnormality, particularly colon carcinoma.

Group G streptococci are normal flora of the gut, vagina, pharynx, and skin. An unusual cause of bacteremia, Group G streptococci cause endocarditis, meningitis, pneumonia, arthritis, pharyngitis, and soft tissue infections. When bacteremia occurs, the source is the skin in 70–80% of cases. Most patients have an underlying disease (e.g., alcoholism, diabetes, malignancy) or are taking steroids. The rate of endocarditis may be as high as 47%.

With in vitro testing, most strains are susceptible to penicillin, but reports of in vitro tolerance to the bactericidal activity of penicillins have led to the suggestion that severe infections (e.g., endocarditis) be treated with a penicillin and aminoglycoside combination.

S. pneumoniae is a frequent cause of community-acquired pneumonia and bacterial meningitis as well as osteomyelitis, sinusitis, endocarditis, septic arthritis, and spontaneous bacterial peritonitis. In addition to advanced age, risk factors include asplenia, sickle cell anemia, congenital agammaglobulinemia, hematologic malignancies (e.g., multiple myeloma, acute and chronic lymphocytic leukemia) and human immunodeficiency virus infection.

Penicillin has historically been the treatment of choice, but moderate to high-level penicillin resistance is seen with variable frequency. Therefore, all clinically significant pneumococcal isolates should have susceptibility testing performed. Treatment for penicillin-sensitive strains (minimal inhibitory concentration [MIC] < 0.6 μg/mL) is:

- **Uncomplicated pneumonia:** 300,000–600,000 units procaine penicillin IM every 12 hours.
- **Complicated pneumonia** (e.g., hypotension, empyema): 5–10 million units aqueous crystalline penicillin daily.
- **Meningitis, endocarditis, septic arthritis:** 18–20 million units aqueous crystalline penicillin daily.

For penicillin-resistant strains (MIC > 2.0 μg/mL), vancomycin is used, and for intermediate strains (MIC 1–2 μg/mL), cefotaxime, ceftriaxone, or vancomycin is used.

Corynebacterium Group JK

This bacterium is a cause of sepsis in patients with underlying neoplasm, neutropenia, prolonged hospitalization, antibiotic use, central venous lines, and cardiac surgery. In addition to bacteremia, this organism can cause endocarditis, pneumonia, and infection of prosthetic material. For treatment, see Table 72–1.

Listeria monocytogenes

This gram-positive aerobic bacillus causes infections in several distinct settings. Risk groups include peripartum women, neonates, and immunosuppressed patients (primarily deficient in cell-mediated immunity, such as those with leukemia or lymphoma, transplant recipients, or those undergoing corticosteroid therapy). Food-borne outbreaks occur, especially with dairy products, in immunocompetent hosts. Clinical syndromes include bacteremia with sepsis and meningoencephalitis, which may complicate bacteremia. The signs and symptoms of meningitis may be subtle; therefore some suggest lumbar puncture of all patients with bacteremia. For treatment, see Table 72–1.

Suggested Readings

Ahmed AJ, Kruse JA, Haupt MT, et al. Hemodynamic responses to Gram-positive versus Gram-negative sepsis in critically ill patients with and without circulatory shock. *Crit Care Med* 1991;19:1520–1525.

Study showing no difference between hemodynamic responses to gram-positive and gram-negative sepsis.

Kain KC, Schulzer M, Chow AW. Clinical spectrum of nonmenstrual toxic shock syndrome (TSS): Comparison with menstrual TSS by multivariate discriminant analysis. *Clin Infect Dis* 1993;16:100–106.

Authors contrast clinical and laboratory features of 24 patients with nonmenstrual toxic shock syndrome and 21 patients with menstrual toxic shock syndrome.

Klugman KP, Koornhof HJ. Drug resistance patterns and serogroups or serotypes of pneumococcal isolates from cerebrospinal fluid or blood, 1979–1986. *J Infect Dis* 1988;158:956–964.

Murray BE. The life and times of the enterococcus. *Clin Microbiol Rev* 1990;3:46–65.

Reviews microbiology, mechanisms of antibiotic resistance, spectrum of diseases, and treatment of enterococcal infections.

Stevens DL. Invasive group A *Streptococcus* infections. *Clin Infect Dis* 1992;14:2–11.

Comprehensive review of severe group A streptococcal *infections, including streptococcal toxic shock syndrome.*

CHAPTER 73

Gram-Negative Bacterial Infections

(See Sections 3 and 4)

Victor Jimenez

Infections caused by gram-negative organisms are associated with significant morbidity and mortality rates in the ICU setting. The frequency of isolation of gram-negative organisms ranges from 60–80% of all bacterial isolates in these settings.

Etiologic Agents

Gram-Negative Bacteria of Respiratory Origin. *Haemophilus influenzae* and *Moraxella catarrhalis* are significant causes of community-acquired pneumonia. They are also found as part of the normal respiratory flora of elderly patients.

Enteric Gram-Negative Aerobes. *Escherichia coli, Proteus* species, and *Klebsiella* species constitute part of the normal intestinal flora and commonly cause urinary tract infections. They also colonize the respiratory tract of hospitalized patients and are a frequent cause of nosocomial pneumonia.

Nonenteric Gram-Negative Aerobes. *Pseudomonas* species, *Acinetobacter* species, *Serratia* species, and *Aeromonas* species are not usually part of the normal flora, but develop as a result of exposure of the patient to the hospital environment. These organisms may become resistant to multiple antibiotics, can be spread from one patient to another through hospital personnel, and may contaminate equipment such as mechanical ventilators.

Gram-Negative Anaerobes. *Bacteroides* species and *Fusobacterium* species are part of the normal respiratory and intestinal flora. They are typically found along with aerobic organisms in polymicrobial infections, such as aspiration pneumonia, intra-abdominal infections, or infected decubitus ulcers.

Gram-Negative Cocci. *Neisseria gonorrhoeae* infection may be complicated by disseminated gonococcal sepsis. *N. meningitidis* causes meningococcal meningitis.

Identification and Culture

Gram stain of a pertinent body fluid can be helpful in:

- Providing a rapid preliminary identification of a gram-negative infection.

- Helping to differentiate infection from colonization by the presence or absence of white blood cells (WBCs).
- Demonstrating whether the infection is polymicrobial by the presence of multiple types of bacteria.

The finding of previously identified organisms from an infected site may assist in the assessment of possible pathogens. Overnight culture results can provide initial identification of likely organisms involved.

Risk Factors for Gram-Negative Bacterial Infection

Drugs. This category includes the use of antacids and H_2-receptor antagonists that reduce gastric acidity and thereby predispose to bacterial colonization of gastric contents. In addition, the use of broad-spectrum antibiotics can select out resistant gram-negative organisms.

Malnutrition is a frequent finding in critically ill patients. It may lead to depression of immune defenses.

Comorbidity caused by underlying disease, such as diabetes mellitus, pulmonary disease, malignancy, burns, or human immunodeficiency virus infection, increases the risk of gram-negative infection.

Medical devices, such as endotracheal and nasogastric tubes, mechanical ventilation, urinary catheterization, and intravascular catheters, invade the body's natural barriers and predispose to gram-negative and other types of infection.

Colonization Versus Infection

Gram-negative colonization at multiple sites is common in ICU patients and usually precedes active infection. The distinction between colonization and infection is important to determine the need for treatment.

Colonization is the presence of microorganisms in tissues, but without overt clinical manifestations of an inflammatory reaction (i.e., absence of WBCs in the involved body fluid).

Infection is the growth of microorganisms in tissues, with subsequent clinical expression of disease or associated inflammatory reaction (presence of WBCs).

Diagnosis and Specific Risk Factors

The diagnosis of a gram-negative infection is based on the isolation of the organism from the specific site of infection.

Surgical wound infection is the presence of inflammation or drainage at a surgical incision within 30 days after surgery. It may be superficial (incisional), deep (involving soft tissues), or complicated by abscess formation. Ultrasonography or CT may be useful in identifying deep abscesses. Risk factors include prolonged surgical procedures, surgery in contaminated sites, or devitalized tissues. Staphylococci are a more common cause than are gram-negative organisms. Intra-abdominal abscesses are often polymicrobial.

Urinary tract infection usually results in the growth of more than 10^5 colony-forming units/mL from fresh clean-catch or catheter-obtained urine specimen. Risk factors include advanced age, female sex, diabetes, renal dysfunction, and indwelling catheter use. Gram-negative enteric bacteria are the most common etiologic agents.

Pneumonia and Tracheobronchitis. Pneumonia occurs clinically as a new infiltrate on chest radiography, consistent physical findings, and purulent tracheobronchial secretions. Tracheobronchitis is the presence of purulent secretions in the absence of a lung infiltrate. Mechanical ventilation, nasogastric tube use, and an impaired gag reflex are major risk factors. Common pathogens are *H. influenzae, M. catarrhalis,* enteric aerobes, gram-negative anaerobes, and nonenteric aerobes.

Catheter-associated bacteremia occurs as fever and leukocytosis, with or without local signs of inflammation at the site of catheterization. A bacterial pathogen may be isolated from peripheral blood cultures and from the catheter tip or from blood culture samples obtained through the catheter. Duration of catheterization is a major risk factor. Common etiologic agents are staphylococci, enteric organisms, and *Pseudomonas aeruginosa.*

Gram-negative meningitis is diagnosed by isolation of a gram-negative pathogen from cerebrospinal fluid (CSF) in association with meningeal signs and CSF pleocytosis. Risk factors include head trauma, neurosurgery, and severe neutropenia. Enteric organisms and *Pseudomonas* species are common etiologic agents.

Disseminated Neisserial Infections. Fulminant meningococcemia is characterized by the rapid progression of sepsis, purpura, and disseminated intravascular coagulation, with meningococcus (or its antigen) detected in blood, skin, or CSF. Disseminated gonococcal infection (DGI) is characterized by polyarthritis and multiple pustular lesions, with gonococcus organisms isolated from the blood, synovial fluid, skin, or genitals. Children and young adults are more susceptible to meningococci; young menstruating women are more prone to DGI.

Nosocomial sinusitis is diagnosed by the finding of purulent sinus drainage, consistent findings by computed tomography, and isolation of a bacterial pathogen from the paranasal sinus. Risk factors include nasotracheal or nasogastric intubation for more than 6 days. These infections are usually polymicrobial, often occurring with *Pseudomonas* species and enteric gram-negative organisms.

Infections in ischemic areas can lead to cellulitis, with soft tissue swelling, erythema, and warmth. Necrotizing cellulitis or fasciitis is accompanied by necrosis of the subcutaneous tissue, fascia, or overlying skin. Foul odor is suggestive of the diagnosis. Patients with diabetes and compromised arterial vascular supply may have lesions after minor trauma. These infections are often polymicrobial, and include anaerobes.

Antimicrobial Treatment

Prompt elimination of the cause of the infection is important whenever possible (e.g., drainage of an abscess, removal of an intravascular catheter that is the nidus of infection). Empiric antimicrobial treatment should be initiated immediately, pending results of the cultures. Typical initial regimens for the following gram-negative organisms (with alternatives in parentheses) are:

- ***Acinetobacter calcoaceticus:*** imipenem (piperacillin plus aminoglycoside, trimethoprim-sulfamethoxazole [TMP-SMX]).
- ***Aeromonas hydrophila:*** TMP-SMX (imipenem, fluoroquinolones).
- ***Bacteroides fragilis:*** metronidazole (cefoxitin, ticarcillin-clavulanate, ampicillin-sulbactam, imipenem, clindamycin).
- **Enteric gram-negative bacteria** (such as *E. coli, Klebsiella* species, *Proteus* species): third-generation cephalosporin (piperacillin, aminoglycosides, TMP-SMX, fluoroquinolones).
- ***Enterobacter aerogenes:*** imipenem (piperacillin plus aminoglycoside, aztreonam, fluoroquinolones).
- ***H. influenzae:*** third-generation cephalosporin (TMP-SMX, chloramphenicol, fluoroquinolones).
- ***N. gonorrhoeae*** (causing DGI): ceftriaxone (cefotaxime, ceftizoxime, spectinomycin).
- ***N. meningitidis:*** penicillin G (chloramphenicol).
- ***P. aeruginosa:*** ceftazidime (piperacillin plus aminoglycoside, aztreonam, imipenem, fluoroquinolones).
- ***Pseudomonas cepacia:*** TMP-SMX (chloramphenicol, fluoroquinolones).
- ***Xanthomonas maltophilia:*** TMP-SMX (ceftazidime, fluoroquinolones).

Local susceptibility patterns may vary, and must be considered.

Infection Control

- **Hand washing** before and after each patient contact is the single most important factor in infection control.

- **Patient isolation** is necessary for highly antibiotic-resistant organisms.
- **Barrier precautions** can be used for selected high-risk patients.

Suggested Readings

Bion JF, Badger I, Crosby HA, et al. Selective decontamination of the digestive tract reduces gram-negative pulmonary complications, but not systemic endotoxemia in patients undergoing elective liver transplantation. *Crit Care Med* 1994;22:40–49.

One of many recent reports on the use of selective gut decontamination. Authors conclude that failure of this intervention to enhance survival in some studies may be related to its inability to eliminate endotoxemia.

Calandra T, Cometta A. Antibiotic therapy for gram-negative bacteremia. *Infect Dis Clin North Am* 1991;5:817–834.

Review that includes a discussion of the management of neutropenic patients. Authors summarize data on single-agent versus combination therapy.

Caplan ES. Role of immunomodulator therapy in sepsis. *Am J Surg* 1993;165(2A suppl):20S–25S.

Reviews results from clinical trials examining use of monoclonal antiendotoxin antibody therapy.

King JW, White MC, Todd JR, et al. Alterations in the microbial flora and in the incidence of bacteremia at a university hospital after adoption of amikacin as the sole formulary aminoglycoside. *Clin Infect Dis* 1992;14:908–915.

Report of prospective study of aminoglycoside resistance and bacteremia after institution of amikacin as the sole formulary aminoglycoside. Incidence of aminoglycoside resistance and bacteremia decreased significantly.

Meyer KS, Urban C, Eagan JA, et al. Nosocomial outbreak of *Klebsiella* infection resistant to late-generation cephalosporins. *Ann Intern Med* 1993;119:353–358.

Report of more than 400 ceftazidime-resistant isolates of Klebsiella pneumoniae *recovered in 19-month period. Incidence of colonization and infection was reduced with a decrease in ceftazidime use and with use of barrier precautions.*

Verhoef J. Prevention of infection by gram-negative microorganisms. *Infect Dis Clin North Am* 1991;5:835–846.

Reviews host defenses to gram-negative infections, the epidemiology, and prevention, including selective gut decontamination.

CHAPTER 74

Viral Infections

(See Chapter 30)

Margaret M. Parker

Viral Respiratory Infections

Influenza virus infection causes both epidemic and pandemic respiratory tract infections. Four patterns of pulmonary disease are seen with influenza:

- Influenza with signs of lower respiratory tract disease, but no pneumonia on chest radiograph (bronchiolitis).
- Influenza complicated by secondary bacterial pneumonia.
- Primary influenza pneumonia, most commonly seen in patients with heart disease.
- Combined influenza and bacterial pneumonia.

The clinical manifestations of primary influenza pneumonia classically involve a prodrome of fever, chills, sore throat, dry cough, and myalgias followed by respiratory distress with tachypnea, cyanosis, and rales on chest examination. Aerosolized ribavirin shortens the duration of fever and decreases viral shedding.

Cytomegalovirus (CMV). Primary infection in immunocompetent hosts is usually a mild, mononucleosis-like illness. This illness is followed by lifelong latent infection that may reactivate if host immunity is compromised. CMV frequently causes life-threatening infection in profoundly immunocompromised patients, especially those with acquired immune deficiency syndrome (AIDS) and recipients of bone marrow transplants. Solid organ transplant recipients are also at risk for severe CMV disease.

CMV pneumonia is the most life-threatening manifestation of CMV disease. It is characterized by fever, cyanosis, nonproductive cough, dyspnea, hypoxemia, and bilateral interstitial infiltrates. In bone marrow transplant patients, it occurs 1–3 months after transplant, and carries an 85% mortality rate. Risk factors for the development of CMV pneumonia include graft-versus-host disease, CMV seropositivity before transplant, and the presence of viremia.

- **Diagnosis** of CMV infection is made by the finding of intranuclear viral inclusions (owl's eyes) on cytopathology, most commonly from lung tissue. Viral cultures may be useful to monitor the response to therapy and to distinguish CMV infection from other viral infections, especially herpes simplex virus.
- **Treatment** is ganciclovir, 5 mg/kg every 12 hours for 14–21 days. CMV immune globulin, in combination with gancyclovir, has been shown in some studies to be of benefit. Foscarnet is active in some CMV disease, particularly retinopathy, but it has no demonstrated benefit in CMV pneumonia.

Varicella zoster virus (VZV) infection is common in childhood, causing chickenpox, a highly contagious disease spread by aerosolized droplets. Patients are contagious 2 days before and at least 5 days after the onset of the rash. The incubation period is 11–20 days. The clinical illness is characterized by a prodrome of fever, chills, myalgias, and arthralgias, followed by the eruption of skin lesions. Acute infection is followed by lifelong latent infection that may reactivate, particularly with advancing age or immunosuppression.

Zoster (shingles) is reactivation of VZV harbored in the dorsal root ganglia. The patient has a painful vescicular eruption in a single dermatome. The skin lesions are contagious.

Pulmonary involvement with VZV is the most common cause of mortality from the virus. It is much more common in adults than in children; smokers have a higher risk than nonsmokers. The mortality rate for VZV pneumonitis is 10% in normal adults and as high as 30% in pregnant women. Pulmonary involvement occurs within 72 hours of the onset of the rash. Patients have a dry cough, dyspnea, and hypoxia. There are usually few physical findings other than the rash. The chest radiograph is characterized by diffuse interstitial or nodular infiltrates. Results of a Tzanck smear of sputum may be positive.

Immunocompromised hosts may have progressive varicella infection, with new lesions forming for more than a week, high spiking fevers (> 40°C), and visceral organ involvement. The mortality rate is 20%. The risk of reactivation of zoster is increased in immunocompromised patients, and dissemination may occur.

Acyclovir is active against VZV, although less so than against herpes simplex virus (HSV). Immunocompromised patients should receive 10 mg/kg IV every 8 hours. The dose must be adjusted in patients with renal failure. Respiratory isolation is necessary. Exposed susceptible individuals also require respiratory isolation from 10 days after the first day of exposure to 21 days after the last day of exposure.

Viral Infections of the CNS

Viral meningitis usually occurs as a subacute process, with symptoms of fever, headache, stiff neck, and photophobia evolving over 24 to 48 hours. Most commonly, it is caused by enteroviruses. It occurs more often in the summer months. The diagnosis is made by the finding of moderate cerebrospinal fluid (CSF) pleocytosis (usually < 1000 white blood cells mm^{-3}). CSF glucose and protein levels are usually normal.

- **Enterovirus** infections are spread by fecal–oral transmission, usually in the summer months. The incubation period is 4 to 8 days. Patients with enteroviral meningitis may have abdominal pain or may have a rash that mimics that of meningococcal meningitis. The illness usually resolves spontaneously over 5 to 7 days.
- **Poliovirus** causes a painful flaccid paralysis with associated aseptic meningitis. The incidence is low since the institution of widespread immunization. The risk of

disease from the vaccination is 3 per 1,000,000 vaccinations. The virus is excreted in the stool for as long as 1 month after administration of the live oral vaccine.

- **Coxsackieviruses** cause widespread muscle inflammation. Serogroup B also affects the myocardium, pericardium, CNS, and pancreas. Coxsackie A7 occasionally causes an aseptic meningitis with paralysis, mimicking poliomyelitis.
- **Mumps virus** is spread by airborne droplets, with an incubation period of 14–21 days. Patients are infectious 2 days before and 4 days after the onset of symptoms of meningitis. Parotitis is present in two-thirds of cases. The absence of parotitis makes the diagnosis difficult. Adults have symptoms of meningitis more commonly than do children; they may also have associated encephalitis. The disease resolves spontaneously in 5 to 7 days; it is rarely fatal.
- **Lymphocytic choriomeningitis virus** is an infrequent cause of viral meningitis, but may cause marked CSF pleocytosis and hypoglycorrhachia. A lymphocytic predominance of CSF white blood cells helps to differentiate this illness from bacterial meningitis.
- **Human immunodeficiency virus** (HIV) infection, in the acute phase, may include aseptic meningitis, CSF white blood cell count of 5 to 12, with a lymphocyte predominance, and CSF protein level of 40–60 mg/dL. Infection with the virus may cause these CSF abnormalities, with no symptoms of meningitis.

Encephalitis may be caused by a diverse group of arboviruses, which are spread by arthropod vectors. The symptoms are fever, chills, headache, nausea, and vomiting, followed within 2 days by confusion and somnolence, sometimes with progression to coma or seizures. The diagnosis is made by serologic confirmation of viral infection in a compatible clinical setting. The virus may be cultured from brain tissue after death, but is not present in CSF. Common arboviruses include the California subgroup, eastern equine encephalitis virus, western equine encephalitis virus, Venezuelan equine encephalitis virus, and St. Louis encephalitis virus.

Therapy for encephalitis caused by these viruses is supportive, and may include mechanical ventilation, careful monitoring of fluid balance, and control of intracranial pressure.

HSV is the most common cause of severe sporadic encephalitis in the United States. The illness is typically subacute, with symptoms evolving over a period of hours to days. Patients have headache, fever, and progressive obtundation. They may have focal cortical signs, such as localized weakness, seizures, dysphasia, or personality changes.

The definitive diagnosis of HSV encephalitis is made by brain biopsy. The use of this invasive technique is controversial because of the potential morbidity of the procedure and the relative safety of empiric treatment. The diagnosis is supported by focal abnormalities on electroencephalogram or computed tomography, typically showing hypodensity in the temporal lobe, and CSF pleocytosis greater than 5 cells mm^{-3}. A polymerase chain reaction is under investigation as a technique for rapid identification of HSV in the CSF, but it is not widely available.

The treatment for HSV encephalitis is acyclovir 10 mg/kg IV every 8 hours for 10 days. Early therapy is the most effective. The dose must be adjusted in patients with renal failure.

Measles Virus. Measles is increasing in incidence in young adults, especially those vaccinated before 1980. The illness is defined by fever, a rash lasting at least 3 days, and cough, conjunctivitis, or coryza. The acute illness may be followed by subacute sclerosing panencephalitis, with progressive cognitive and motor dysfunction.

Rabies Virus. In the United States, there is approximately one case per year of human rabies. After a bite by an infected animal, there is a 30- to 90-day incubation period. This incubation period may be prolonged for several years in some patients. The risk of clinical rabies after a bite is 5–15%. The symptoms of the prodrome include fever, headache, malaise, fatigue, anorexia, abdominal pain, nausea, vomiting, and occasionally upper respiratory symptoms. The prodrome is followed by hydrophobia, with painful laryngopharyngeal contractions leading to choking or aspiration. Seizures may develop. There is a high mortality rate.

The diagnosis of rabies may be made by histopathologic examination, isolation of the virus, or serologic studies. Postexposure use of human rabies immunoglobulin and human diploid cell vaccine can prevent the development of clinical disease in patients who have been bitten.

Viral Hepatitis

The clinical presentation of hepatitis A, B, C, and delta viruses is similar. After a variable incubation period, the patient has malaise, anorexia, nausea, vomiting, and abdominal pain, followed by jaundice. The mortality rate for type A is 0.5% and that for type B is 2%. On physical examination, the patients are usually afebrile; there is jaundice and occasionally spider angiomata. On laboratory studies, there is an eight- to 10-fold increase in transaminase levels. The bilirubin level is increased, with both direct and indirect bilirubin values elevated. An increased prothrombin time suggests severe hepatic dysfunction and is a poor prognostic indicator in acute hepatitis.

Differential Diagnosis of Acute and Chronic Hepatitis

- **Other viruses,** including Epstein-Barr virus, CMV, HSV, VZV, rubella, rubeola, mumps, and yellow fever.
- **Bacterial infection,** including pneumococcal pneumonia, leptospirosis, syphilis, and *Brucella* species.
- **Drugs,** e.g., isoniazid, rifampin, acetaminophen, and anticonvulsants.
- **Hepatotoxins,** such as carbon tetrachloride, beryllium, and vinyl chloride.
- **Miscellaneous causes,** such as circulatory shock, right heart failure, Wilson's disease, hemochromatosis, and α_1-antitrypsin deficiency.

Treatment is primarily supportive, with maintenance of nutrition, careful fluid and electrolyte balance, management of coagulopathy and bleeding, monitoring for hypoglycemia, and management of encephalopathy (see Chapter 48 in this book). Caution should be used with drugs that are hepatotoxic or undergo hepatic metabolism.

Hepatitis A is highly contagious and is transmitted by the fecal–oral route. It is usually spread through contaminated food or drink. It is also common among children in day care centers and among persons with many sexual partners. The diagnosis is made by the presence of anti-hepatitis A virus antibodies in the appropriate clinical setting. Immunoglobulin G anti-hepatitis A virus confers lifelong immunity from recurrent infection.

Hepatitis B risk factors include IV drug abuse, blood transfusion (especially in hemophiliacs), hemodialysis, multiple sexual partners, and accidental needlesticks. Ninety-two percent of patients have self-limited clinical illness, 1% have fulminant hepatitis, and 7% have chronic hepatitis B (chronic persistent hepatitis, chronic active hepatitis, or cirrhosis). Treatment with interferon α-2b can produce an improvement in transaminase levels in patients with chronic hepatitis B. Immunization with three serial injections in the deltoid is 90% successful; immunization in the gluteal region is less successful. Treatment with hepatitis immune globulin is indicated after percutaneous or mucosal exposure to blood infected with hepatitis B surface antigen or sexual exposure to a person infected with this virus.

Hepatitis C risk factors are the same as those for hepatitis B. The disease is clinically the same, although usually somewhat milder than hepatitis B. Hepatitis C tends to cause a chronic increase in transaminase levels.

Hepatitis delta is an incomplete ribonucleic acid virus that requires the presence of hepatitis B surface antigen for replication. It may be found as acute delta infection in a patient with chronic B, acute delta infection with acute B infection, or chronic delta infection with chronic B infection. The illness is similar to hepatitis B, with a high tendency for chronic active hepatitis or cirrhosis in patients with chronic hepatitis B and hepatitis delta infection.

Viral Hemorrhagic Fever

Viral hemorrhagic fever is a triad of fever, renal dysfunction, and hemorrhagic manifestations that occurs endemically in Europe and Asia.

Dengue Hemorrhagic Fever. In southeast Asia, dengue is a frequent cause of hospitalization and death in children. In the United States, the disease is usually imported, although it has been transmitted in the southeastern United States by a mosquito vector closely related to the Asian vector. Treatment is supportive care.

Korean Hemorrhagic Fever. Also known as hemorrhagic fever with renal syndrome, this illness has five phases: febrile, shock, oliguric, polyuric, and convalescent. Laboratory studies show an increased hematocrit value (from hemoconcentration), thrombocytopenia, and proteinuria. There is not frank hemorrhage, but patients may have intracranial hemorrhage that may be fatal. The mortality rate is approximately 5%. The disease is caused by the Hantaan virus, and is carried and spread by a rodent vector.

Ribavirin is active against the Hantaan virus. Supportive care, with careful fluid management and dialysis if needed, is important as well. Ribavirin is given as an initial load of 33 mg/kg (IV or PO), then 16 mg/kg every 6 hours for 4 days, followed by 8 mg/kg every 8 hours for 3 days.

Hantavirus. This new disease was identified in an outbreak in New Mexico in 1993. The virus is closely related to that causing Korean hemorrhagic fever. The disease is carried by a rodent vector, and is characterized by fever and chills, followed by respiratory distress, severe hypoxemia, and pulmonary edema as well as myocardial dysfunction. Initial symptoms of nausea, vomiting, diarrhea, or abdominal pain, followed by respiratory symptoms in 1–2 days, are common. The major cause of death is cardiogenic shock. Treatment is aggressive supportive care; the mortality rate once respiratory failure has occurred is high.

Congo-Crimean Hemorrhagic Fever. This tick-borne disease occurs during the summer months in the Middle East. Nosocomial spread to health care workers can occur, and it appears to have a higher mortality rate than tick-borne disease. Universal precautions should be observed. The clinical manifestations are headache, fever, rigors, myalgias, sore throat, abdominal pain, and petechial rash, with laboratory abnormalities suggestive of disseminated intravascular coagulation. Laboratory abnormalities that are associated with a poor prognosis are white blood cell count greater than 10,000 mm^{-3}, platelet count less than 20,000 mm^{-3}, hepatic transaminase levels greater than 200 units/L, activated partial thromboplastin time greater than 60 seconds, and fibrinogen level less than 110 mg/dL.

The use of immune sera for treatment is controversial and not currently recommended. A trial of ribavirin is warranted in high-risk patients because this agent is highly active in vitro. An IV loading dose of 2 g should be given, followed by 1 g IV every 8 hours for 4 days. Postexposure prophylaxis with ribavirin is effective, with 400 mg PO every 6 hours for 1 day, then 400 mg PO every 8 hours for 6 days.

Lassa Fever. The vector is a rat for this disease, which is endemic to western Africa. Secondary spread (human to human) through body fluids has occurred; universal precautions are advised. Ribavirin may be effective when used before day 7 of illness.

Yellow Fever. This mosquito-borne disease is endemic to South America and Africa. The incubation period of 3–6 days is followed by the onset of fever, chills, headache, and then myalgias, flushing, hemorrhagic manifestations, and jaundice. There is no specific therapy; supportive care is important.

Antiviral Agents

Acyclovir is highly effective against HSV, less so against CMV. The dose for HSV encephalitis is 10 mg/kg IV every 8 hours. Side effects include azotemia, phlebitis, GI irritation, and confusion. High-dose acyclovir (4000 mg/day) may ameliorate HSV in normal hosts.

Vidarabine is effective in HSV encephalitis and neonatal herpes. The toxicity includes dose-dependent GI and CNS toxicity, some myelosuppression, hepatotoxicity, and nephrotoxicity. The toxicity limits the usefulness of this drug.

Ganciclovir has greater activity against CMV than does acyclovir. The dose is 5 mg/kg every 12 hours. The dose must be reduced in patients with renal failure. The major side effect is neutropenia.

Ribavirin has been used in an aerosolized form with some efficacy in infants with respiratory syncitial virus. It is also effective against some strains of influenza and parainfluenza and for some viruses causing hemorrhagic fever. Toxicity includes reversible anemia and thrombocytosis. Aerosolized ribavirin may cause conjunctival irritation in health care workers.

Foscarnet is effective for CMV retinitis in patients with AIDS. It may also be effective in mucocutaneous HSV lesions that are resistant to acyclovir in patients with AIDS.

Suggested Readings

Balfour HH Jr. Management of cytomegalovirus disease with antiviral drugs. *Rev Infect Dis* 1990;12:S849–S860.
Reviews treatment of different cytomegalovirus clinical syndromes, including retinitis, GI disease, and pneumonia, as well as prophylactic therapy for transplant patients.

Haake DA, Zakowski PC, Haake DL, et al. Early treatment with acyclovir for varicella pneumonia in otherwise healthy adults: Retrospective controlled study and review. *Rev Infect Dis* 1990;12:788–798.
Thirty-eight previously normal adults hospitalized with varicella pneumonia were reviewed retrospectively. The 11 patients who received acyclovir early appeared to have more rapid clinical improvement compared with those who did not have early acyclovir.

Perrillo RP, Schiff ER, Davis GL, et al. A randomized, controlled trial of interferon alpha-2b alone and after prednisone withdrawal for the treatment of chronic hepatitis B. *N Engl J Med* 1990;323:295–301.
Randomized controlled trial compared interferon α-2b versus prednisone withdrawal followed by interferon in patients with chronic hepatitis B. Describes biochemical, histologic, and virologic improvements after 5 million units daily of interferon. In one-third of the patients, transaminase levels returned to normal.

Wallace MR, Bowler WA, Murray NB, et al. Treatment of adult varicella with oral acyclovir: A randomized, placebo-controlled trial. *Ann Intern Med* 1992;117:358–363.
One hundred forty-eight adults hospitalized for varicella were randomized to receive either oral acyclovir or placebo. Early therapy with acyclovir decreased the duration of illness compared with the placebo group.

CHAPTER 75

Tuberculosis and Other Mycobacterial Infections

(See Chapter 32)

Roy T. Steigbigel

Myrobacterium tuberculosis causes more deaths throughout the world than any other single microorganism. The incidence of tuberculosis (TB) in the United States increased each year from 1985 to 1993, when the surge in incidence began to abate. The causes for the increase include homelessness; transmission in clinics, hospitals, substance-abuse treatment centers, and prisons; immigration from areas where TB is endemic; and human immunodeficiency virus (HIV) infection.

Pulmonary Tuberculosis

The initial site of *Mycobacterium tuberculosis* infection is almost always the lung. Even with resolution of the primary infection, there may be spread of tubercle bacilli to other sites in the body, with the potential for reactivation there as well as in the lung. In the immunocompetent person, primary TB most often occurs in the anterior segment of the upper lobes or right middle lobe, whereas reactivation of pulmonary TB commonly affects the upper lobes. In the immunodeficient patient, such as the patient with acquired immune deficiency syndrome (AIDS), any lobe can be involved in either primary or reactivative disease.

The clinical presentation of pulmonary TB can range from the entirely asymptomatic person, who may develop a positive reaction to the purified protein derivative (PPD) skin test, to the ill patient with fever, diaphoresis, weight loss, productive cough, hemoptysis, and extensive infiltrates evident on chest radiograph. Patients with advanced HIV infection are more likely to be asymptomatic on presentation with TB.

Diagnosis. Pulmonary TB should be suspected in the patient with a positive skin test finding and an infiltrate shown on chest radiograph for which another cause cannot be found. Finding more than 10 mm of induration 48–72 hours after intradermal injection of 5 tuberculin units of PPD constitutes a positive test result, and this result will be present in most immunocompetent people with active or latent TB. In the elderly and in patients with HIV infection, 5 mm of induration may indicate a positive reaction.

The finding of tubercle bacilli by smear or culture is vital for diagnosis, and culture is important for drug susceptibility testing, which should be routinely performed because of the increasing incidence of resistant organisms. The best sample is usually expectorated sputum. The likelihood of finding organisms depends on the extent of disease, the adequacy of sample collection and specimen processing, and the expertise of the laboratory. Concentrating the specimens increases the chance of a positive result, as does repeating the collection as many as three times. In infected individuals, one-third of specimens that have negative smear findings can still yield a positive culture result. If the patient does not have a spontaneous cough, aerosol-induced sputum production is useful and more efficient than gastric aspirates. A bronchoalveolar lavage specimen or postlavage coughed specimen may also be useful.

A problem associated with the initial diagnosis of pulmonary TB in patients with HIV infection or chronic lung disease is the frequent presence of nontuberculous acid-fast organisms in the sputum. The diagnosis cannot be made until the organism is growing in culture and can then be speciated; this procedure is most rapidly performed with a nucleic acid probe. Other laboratory findings that may be present in patients with pulmonary tuberculosis include anemia, mild leukocytosis and neutrophilia, and hyponatremia caused by unregulated antidiuretic hormone release.

Tuberculous Pleuritis

The pleural space can be involved during the primary infection or, less frequently, with reactivation of latent infection. Tuberculous pleuritis can have a sudden onset. Systemic symptoms include night sweats, chills, dyspnea, weakness, weight loss, and chest pain. A large proportion of pleural space infections are accompanied by effusions. The fluid is often copious at first, and gradually ceases by 6 to 8 weeks. It is an exudate with a predominance of lymphocytes, often more than 80%. The pleural fluid glucose concentration is highly variable.

The chest radiograph usually does not show a parenchymal infiltrate. The tuberculin skin test result is usually positive. The diagnosis is made by the finding of tubercle bacilli from pleural fluid or pleural biopsy specimen. The sputum finding is usually negative in the absence of active pulmonary TB. The most sensitive method of diagnosis is pleural biopsy.

Extrapulmonary Tuberculosis

TB may involve many organs besides the lungs. The symptoms are related to the site of involvement and may be insidious. Fever is not universally present. In most cases, the PPD result is positive. Diagnosis is made by histologic examination and culture of the involved tissue or body fluid. The following TB syndromes can be seen:

- Tuberculous pericarditis.
- TB of the lymph nodes (e.g., scrofula).
- Renal TB.
- Genital TB.
- TB of bones and joints (predilection for involvement of spine and weight-bearing joints).
- Peritoneal TB.
- Tuberculous enteritis.

CNS Tuberculosis. Meningitis resulting from TB causes symptoms of meningitis, usually ranging from hours to weeks, most commonly several days. Cranial nerve palsies, particularly of the ocular nerves, should raise the suspicion of TB. Examination of the cerebrospinal fluid (CSF) is the single most useful procedure. The cell count is most often 100–500 mm^{-3}, with a predominance of mononuclear cells, but up to one-third will have a predominance of polymorphonuclear leukocytes on the initial study. The protein level is usually 100 to 500 mg/dL, and the glucose level is less than 45 mg/dL. Often, the initial examination shows an abnormality in only one or two values. Acid-fast bacilli may be seen in the concentrated CSF, but most commonly they are not seen on the initial sample. The result of CSF culture is positive in 50% to 90% of patients. The sensitivity is dependent on the volume of CSF: at least 10–15 mL should be sent for analysis. Treatment should not await confirmation of diagnosis, but should be initiated when there is suspicion of TB meningitis. Earlier treatment is associated with better outcome.

Intracranial tuberculomas occur as space-occupying lesions. Symptoms include headache, vomiting, visual changes, and seizures. CT with contrast or MRI shows the mass. Biopsy should be performed for histologic examination, staining, and culture.

Disseminated Tuberculosis

Disseminated mycobacterial disease has become more common with the HIV pandemic. Most is caused by *M. avium-intracellulare* complex (MAI), but disseminated *M. tuberculosis* has also been increasing in incidence. The symptoms are usually not specific, and include weakness, anorexia, fatigue, weight loss, and fever. Cough is less common, and hemoptysis is infrequent. The duration of symptoms before diagnosis is variable. Most patients do not have a history of tuberculosis. Predisposing factors other than HIV infection include alcoholism, pregnancy, neoplastic disease, injected drug use, and cerebrovascular disease.

Diagnosis. The PPD result is less often positive in disseminated tuberculosis than in other forms. The white blood cell count is normal in two-thirds of cases, with an increase in early forms present in one-fifth to one-half. Pancytopenia, granulocytopenia, and leukemoid reactions are infrequent, but important, clues to the diagnosis. Consumptive coagulopathy may be present.

The chest radiograph shows the classic miliary pattern in approximately two-thirds of patients on initial presentation, with the development of this pattern within weeks in many others. Sputum culture grows *M. tuberculosis* in one-half to two-thirds of patients. CSF should be examined because signs of meningeal infection may be overshadowed by other manifestations of illness. The most sensitive means of making the diagnosis is by biopsy of bone marrow or liver, even when liver function test results are normal.

Nontuberculous Mycobacterial Infection

Infection caused by MAI is the most common mycobacterial infection in the United States because of the AIDS epidemic. Patients with HIV infection and a CD4 lymphocyte count less than 100 mm^{-3} are prone to disseminated MAI infection. This infection may be partially prevented by prophylaxis with rifabutin. MAI bacteremia is often a reflection of infection at multiple sites, including the lymph nodes, liver, spleen, bone marrow, and colon. Symptoms include fever, weight loss, and diarrhea. Physical examination may show lymphadenopathy and hepatosplenomegaly. The diagnosis is usually easily made by culture of blood. Other studies that can show infection are bone marrow, liver, or colon biopsies.

Treatment

The most important principle in the treatment of *M. tuberculosis* infection is ensuring patient compliance with medication over the prescribed treatment period. The treatment regimens are the same for all sites, except that therapy is longer for infections involving the CNS. The drugs used for initial treatment are based on the likelihood that the patient has resistant organisms (e.g., patients who have been previously treated or those who reside in areas in which there is a high incidence of resistance). Typical daily dosing of commonly used drugs (and the most common, potentially serious side effects) are:

- **Isoniazid:** 5 mg/kg PO or IM (hepatic toxicity).
- **Rifampin:** 10 mg/kg PO (hepatic toxicity, flu-like syndrome).
- **Pyrazinamide:** 15–30 mg/kg PO (hepatic toxicity, hyperuricemia).
- **Ethambutol:** 15–25 mg/kg PO to a maximum of 2.5 g (optic neuritis).
- **Streptomycin:** 15 mg/kg IM (auditory, vestibular, and renal toxicity).

The regimen chosen is based on the results of susceptibility testing, which should be performed on all isolates. Pyridoxine (10–50 mg/day) is given prophylactically to patients who receive isoniazid and have malnutrition, alcoholism, diabetes, pregnancy, peripheral neuropathy, seizures, or renal failure.

Initial empiric treatment and treatment of immunocompetent patients with susceptible organisms is a combination of isoniazid and rifampin for 6 months, plus pyrazinamide for the first 2 months.

Treatment of possibly resistant organisms should be initiated with a combination of at least four drugs: isoniazid, rifampin, pyrizinamide, and either ethambutol or streptomycin. If full drug susceptibility is documented, treatment can be completed with the regimen listed above for susceptible organisms.

For patients with HIV infection or with disseminated or CNS TB, treatment should be continued for at least 9 months, assuring treatment for 6 months after culture results become negative. Some recommend therapy with pyrazinamide throughout the treatment period.

Treatment for multiply-resistant organisms is attempted with at least three drugs to which the organism is susceptible. Treatment is continued for 12 to 24 months. This approach may require the use of drugs such as capreomycin (15 mg/kg IM daily), cycloserine (250–500 mg PO twice daily), ethionamide (250–500 mg PO twice daily), ciprofloxacin (500–750 mg PO twice daily), or ofloxacin (400 mg every 12 hours or 800 mg PO daily), para-aminosalicylic acid (4–6 g PO twice daily), or clofazimine (100–200 mg PO daily). When there is suspicion of multiply-resistant organisms, the initial treatment is begun with five to seven drugs, until susceptibilities have been determined.

Prophylactic treatment is recommended for patients whose skin test result has converted, those who are immunocompromised, and those who are in close contact with patients with active pulmonary TB. Isoniazid given for 6 to 9 months at 300 mg PO daily is standard prophylaxis; for patients with HIV infection, it is given for at least 12 months. If the exposure is to a person infected with organisms that are resistant to isoniazid, some recommend treatment with rifampin, with or without ethambutol, for 1 year.

Treatment of *M. avium-intracellulare* Complex. There is evidence that treatment of MAI infection in patients with AIDS prolongs life and improves the quality of life. The optimal treatment regimen is not clearly defined, but should include a macrolide antibiotic such as clarithromycin. A suggested regimen is: clarithromycin (500 mg PO twice daily), ethambutol (15 mg/kg PO daily), and a third drug, such as rifampin (600 mg PO daily). Therapy should continue for the duration of the patient's life. Patients who have CD4 lymphocyte counts of less than 100 mm^{-3} may benefit from prophylaxis with rifabutin 300 mg PO daily.

Suggested Readings

Chin DP, Reingold AL, Stone EN, et al. The impact of MAC bacteremia and its treatment on survival of AIDS patients: A prospective study. *J Infect Dis* 1994;170:578–584.

Indicates that treatment of disseminated Mycobacterium avium *complex infection is effective in prolonging lives.*

Goble M, Iseman MD, Madsen LA, et al. Treatment of 171 patients with pulmonary tuberculosis resistant to isoniazid and rifampin. *N Engl J Med* 1993;328:527–532.

Reviews difficulties of curing drug-resistant tuberculosis and analysis of outcome with various regimens.

Horsburgh CR Jr. *Mycobacterium avium* complex infection in the acquired immunodeficiency syndrome. *N Engl J Med* 1991;325:1332–1338.

Reviews clinical manifestations of M. avium-intracellulare *complex infection.*

Masur H, the Public Health Service Task Force on Prophylaxis for Therapy of MAC. Recommendations on prophylaxis and therapy for disseminated MAC disease in patients infected with HIV. *N Engl J Med* 1993;329:898–904.

Van Scoy RE, Wilkowske CJ. Antituberculous agents. *Mayo Clin Proc* 1992;67:179–187.

Reviews drugs used to treat tuberculosis, their dosing and side effects, and recommendations for monitoring to detect adverse effects.

CHAPTER 76

Candida and Other Fungal Infections

(See Chapters 33 and 34)

Jack Fuhrer

The ICU, where vascular catheters, tracheal intubation, invasive monitoring devices, and antibiotics are used extensively, is a high-risk area for certain fungal infections, particularly *Candida* species. In addition, immunocompromised patients become infected with fungi and may require ICU care. Fungal infections are also prevalent in burn units.

Candida Infections

There has been a significant increase in the number of nosocomial *Candida* infections in recent years. In some medical centers, *Candida* is among the more frequent bloodstream isolates. High-risk patients include patients who have undergone transplantation, neutropenic patients, seriously ill postoperative patients, and patients with severe burns. In addition to resulting in significant morbidity and mortality rates, these infections often prolong hospitalization. There are numerous species of *Candida;* the most common isolated from patients with invasive candidiasis are *C. albicans, C. tropicalis,* and *Torulopsis glabrata.*

Candidemia and Disseminated Candidiasis. The signs and symptoms of candidemia or disseminated candidiasis can be variable and indistinguishable from bacterial sepsis. The longer the duration of fungemia, the greater the chance of metastatic spread to other organs. On the other hand, catheter-related candidemia may resolve without sequelae on removal of the catheter. Nonetheless, the management of candidemia includes the removal of possible foci of infection as well as the administration of amphotericin B in the immunocompromised patient and the septic-appearing patient. Amphotericin B in doses of 0.3–0.5 mg/kg daily for a total dose of 1–2 g is generally recommended, depending on the severity of infection and the immune status of the patient. Combination therapy with 5-flucytosine could be considered, although data showing improved outcome are scant. Azole (i.e., ketoconazole, fluconazole, or itraconazole) therapy, with and without amphotericin B, remains controversial, and thus is not recommended. Afebrile immunocompetent patients may be able to be managed with foci removal alone, although some advocate low-dose amphotericin B administration.

Other Sites of *Candida* Infection. Because fungemia can result in hematogenous seeding of various organs, the practitioner must be alert to the following possibilities:

- **Skin** involvement usually produces firm, pink to red, raised nodules. There may be associated muscle involvement. The diagnosis is made by biopsy identification of *Candida* organisms in the dermis.
- **Eye:** Endophthalmitis is associated with multiple organ involvement, and is usually unilateral. Some patients have acute visual symptoms, whereas others are asymptomatic. On examination, fundi show fluffy white infiltrates representing microabscesses. Some recommend routine ophthalmologic evaluation in candidemic patients.
- **GI tract:** Esophagitis is a common manifestation in immunosuppressed patients, such as those with leukemia and acquired immune deficiency syndrome (AIDS). Patients usually have dysphagia or odynophagia. The diagnosis can be made by upper endoscopy with biopsy, a barium swallow result showing a cobblestone pattern, or presumptively after a therapeutic response to systemic antifungal therapy.
- **CNS** involvement includes meningitis, diffuse cerebritis, mycotic aneurysms, parenchymal hemorrhage, and fungus ball formation. Because of the variability of clinical and cerebrospinal fluid (CSF) findings, the diagnosis is often delayed or mistaken for a cerebrovascular accident.
- **Heart:** Endocarditis should be considered in the presence of persistent fungemia or emboli to large vessels. Vegetations tend to be left-sided, large, and more commonly found on prosthetic valves.
- **Lungs:** Although *Candida* species are commonly cultured from sputum and bronchial secretions, pulmonary involvement is unusual. It occurs as a result of hematogenous spread in severely neutropenic leukemic patients. The diagnosis is made by biopsy evidence of invasive infection.

- **Catheter-related candidemia** is a common problem that may resolve with catheter removal alone or in combination with low-dose amphotericin B administration. The threshold for removal of such catheters should be low in patients with persistent or relapsing candidemia despite medical therapy.

Other Fungal Infections

The focus is on the more common fungi, with particular emphasis on disease presentations in the immunosuppressed patient.

Aspergillosis is caused by inhalation of ubiquitous *Aspergillus* spores or inoculation of traumatized skin. Disease presentation is variable, and differs by host. Some patients have hypersensitivity to *Aspergillus* antigens; this condition can lead to episodic bronchial obstruction and eventually to steroid-dependent asthma. In patients with cavitary lung disease, colonization by *Aspergillus* that proliferate can lead to a fungus ball or to aspergilloma formation. In its most severe form, aspergilloma can lead to massive hemoptysis requiring surgical excision. Invasive aspergillosis is typically seen in immunosuppressed patients (those with hematologic malignancies, organ transplant recipients, patients with AIDS, recipients of corticosteroids or cytotoxic agents). This form causes invasion of blood vessels, resulting in thromboembolic phenomena and infarction of surrounding tissue. Less common manifestations of aspergillosis include rhinocerebral aspergillosis (similar to rhinocerebral mucormycosis), ocular aspergillosis, endocarditis, and invasion of the CNS. The diagnosis is made by serologic studies, sputum cultures, and elevated immunoglobulin E levels in bronchopulmonary aspergillosis; by serologic studies and chest radiograph in aspergillomas; and by culture and histopathologic identification in invasive aspergillosis. Similarly, treatment varies by presentation: amphotericin B or itraconazole for invasive disease; surgical resection for hemoptysis-producing aspergillomas; surgical debridement plus amphotericin B or itraconazole for rhinocerebral infection, CNS infection, and endocarditis.

Mucormycosis. The responsible agents are found in soil and in decaying organic matter. Disease is acquired through inhalation or inoculation of traumatized skin. Patients with diabetic ketoacidosis and patients with hematologic malignancies are most likely to have fulminant infection. Rhinocerebral mucormycosis, with its characteristic thrombosis and hemorrhagic infarction, may lead to a black necrotic eschar involving the nasal mucosa or the hard palate. Spread into the orbit can result in proptosis, impairment of the extraocular muscles, and diplopia. Direct invasion into the brain can result in significant neurologic dysfunction.

Pulmonary mucormycosis similarly occurs with thrombosis and infarction of blood vessels. Patients may report pleuritic chest pain; the chest radiograph typically shows a necrotizing nodular pneumonia. Occasionally, wedge-shaped densities, pleural effusions, and fungus balls have been described. Unlike rhinocerebral mucormycosis, which is more common in diabetic patients, pulmonary infection is more common in patients with hematologic malignancies.

Other organ involvement has been described, including the GI tract, skin, CNS (primary), spleen, kidney, pancreas, and heart. Diagnosis is made by the histopathologic finding of broad, nonseptate thick-walled hyphae that branch at right angles, invading blood vessels and causing thrombosis, hemorrhage, and infarction. Therapy consists of high-dose amphotericin B and aggressive surgical debridement where appropriate.

Cryptococcosis. Patients with cell-mediated immune defects (e.g., human immunodeficiency virus infection, Hodgkin's disease, sarcoidosis) are prone to dissemination, often after initial subclinical pneumonia. Dissemination to the CNS with resultant meningitis is the most common presentation. Severe pneumonitis; dissemination to the skin, muscle, and bone marrow; and endocarditis have also been described. Diagnosis can be made by the finding of cryptococcal antigen in the serum or CSF, a positive CSF India ink preparation finding, blood culture growth of *Cryptococcus neoformans,* or histological evidence of involved tissues.

Therapy is administration of amphotericin B (0.7–1.0 mg/kg/day), with or without 5-flucytosine. The total recommended dose varies by host. Patients with AIDS require long-term therapy to prevent relapses. Maintenance therapy is fluconazole 200 mg/day after an initial course of amphotericin B.

Histoplasmosis, Blastomycosis, and Coccidiomycosis are dimorphic fungi endemic to certain geographic areas. They most often cause asymptomatic or mildly symptomatic pulmonary infection. Coccidiomycosis observed in residents of the southwestern United States and South and Central America can result in meningitis, pneumonia, and disseminated infection. Histoplasmosis is observed in patients who have lived in southeastern and central parts of the United States and in some temperate and tropical zones throughout the world. It can result in chronic pulmonary infection or a progressive disseminated form involving the oral mucosa, adrenal glands, bone marrow, and cardiac valves. Patients with AIDS are more prone to severe forms of histoplasma and coccidioides infection. Blastomycosis is endemic to the states surrounding the Mississippi River and, although described in immunosuppressed patients, occurs most frequently in normal hosts.

ICU practitioners should be alert to the possibility of adult respiratory distress syndrome associated with blastomycosis. Therapy for these infections includes administration of amphotericin B initially, with possible oral azole therapy thereafter.

Suggested Readings

Bradsher RW. Systemic fungal infections: Diagnosis and treatment. I. Blastomycosis. *Infect Dis Clin North Am* 1988;2:877–898.
(116 references.)

Bross J, Talbot GH, Maislin G, et al. Risk factors for nosocomial candidemia: A case-control study in adults without leukemia. *Am J Med* 1989;87:614–620.
Defines seven major risk factors for nosocomial candidemia: presence of a central venous or bladder catheter, use of two or more antibiotics, azotemia, transfer from another hospital, diarrhea, and candiduria.

Sugar AM. Empiric treatment of fungal infections in the neutropenic host: Review of the literature and guidelines for use. *Arch Intern* 1990;150:2258–2264.
Author recommends early consideration of empiric antifungal therapy in the febrile neutropenic patient who has not defervesced after a course of broad-spectrum antibiotics.

Terrell CL, Hughes CE. Antifungal agents used for deep-seated mycotic infections. *Mayo Clin Proc* 1992;67:69–91.
Comprehensive, practical review of available and investigational antifungal drugs (227 references).

Wheat LJ. Systemic fungal infections: Diagnosis and treatment. I. Histoplasmosis. *Infect Dis Clin North Am* 1988;2:841–859.
(95 references.)

Zuger A, Louie E, Holzman RS, et al. Cryptococcal disease in patients with the acquired immune deficiency syndrome: Diagnostic features and outcome of treatment. *Ann Intern Med* 1986;104:234–240.
In this study of 396 patients with acquired immune deficiency syndrome, 34 had cryptococcal infections, most commonly with brain or meningeal involvement.

CHAPTER 77

Pneumonia

(See Chapter 39)

David Tompkins

Pneumonia is a frequent problem in ICU patients. By some estimates, approximately one-fifth of patients have pneumonia either on arrival or during their ICU stay. In patients receiving mechanical ventilation, there is a direct correlation between the duration of mechanical ventilation and the incidence of pneumonia. The mortality rate of patients in the ICU with pneumonia is significantly higher than that in patients without pneumonia.

Diagnosis

The pathogens responsible for pneumonia vary based on the patient's risk factors, the geographic location, and the type of institution, as well as whether the infection is community or nosocomially acquired. A variety of noninfectious processes (e.g., congestive heart failure, atelectasis, adult respiratory distress syndrome) produce fever, leukocytosis, purulent respiratory secretions, and radiographic infiltrates that mimic pneumonia. The following guidelines are helpful in determining whether the patient has pneumonia as well as its possible etiology:

History. Specific pathogens are seen with increased frequency in particular settings:

- **Chronic lung disease:** *Streptococcus pneumoniae* and *Haemophilus influenzae.*
- **Cystic fibrosis:** *Pseudomonas* species and *Staphylococcus aureus.*
- **When influenza is prevalent:** *S. aureus, S. pneumoniae,* group A *Streptococcus,* and *H. influenzae.*
- **Patients already hospitalized** or residing in long-term care facilities are more likely to have oropharyngeal colonization with enteric gram-negative bacilli, *Pseudomonas* species, and *S. aureus.*
- **AIDS:** *Pneumocystis carinii,* cytomegalovirus, and mycobacteria.

Chest Radiography. The presence of a pulmonary infiltrate supports the diagnosis of pneumonia, but may be nonspecific. Persistent or progressive infiltrates are consistent with a bacterial etiology, particularly if there is lobar consolidation and a large pleural effusion. Necrotizing pneumonia with cavitation suggests infection with *S. aureus* or gram-negative bacilli (including *Pseudomonas* species), or aspiration pneumonia. Diffuse infiltrates suggest *P. carinii, Legionella* species, or viral infection.

Blood Tests. White blood cell (WBC) count elevation, especially with a shift to band and other immature forms, suggests bacterial infection. However, in the elderly and in immunocompromised patients, the WBC count may be normal or low, even with overwhelming infections. Blood cultures should be obtained in all patients with suspected bacterial pneumonia; findings are positive in 10% to 30% of cases. Serologic studies are useful in the diagnosis of *Legionella, Mycoplasma, Chlamydia,* and *Coxiella burnetti* infections.

Sputum Analysis. Microscopic examination of respiratory secretions should include a gram stain to detect WBCs

(≥ 20 WBC/low-power field) and suspected bacterial organisms. If clinically indicated, a potassium hydroxide preparation is used for fungal elements, Ziehl-Nielsen stain for acid-fast bacilli, silver methenamine stain for *P. carinii,* and direct fluorescent antibody staining for *Legionella* species. In addition to bacterial culture, viral, mycobacterial, and fungal cultures are indicated in certain settings. In community-acquired pneumonia, good-quality (see below) expectorated sputum is a useful guide for making the diagnosis and for initial antibiotic selection. However, in nosocomial pneumonia, noninvasive sampling of respiratory secretions is less reliable because of increased colonization of the respiratory tract with potential pathogens and because of upper airway inflammation, particularly in endotracheally intubated patients. In patients who have possible pneumonia in the ICU setting, other diagnostic strategies can be useful to guide antibiotic selection.

Expectorated Sputum

- **Advantage.** Noninvasive; provides a sample of respiratory secretions for immediate evaluation.
- **Disadvantage.** Contamination with oropharyngeal flora limits the reliability of culture results.
- **Guidelines.** Sputum samples containing ≥ 25 neutrophils and ≤10 epithelial cells/low-power field (100×) contain minimal oropharyngeal contamination. Specimens with more epithelial cells and fewer neutrophils may be misleading and should be discarded.

Transtracheal Aspiration

- **Advantage.** Reduced oropharyngeal contamination.
- **Disadvantage.** Requires a cooperative patient with a palpable cricothyroid membrane, adequate oxygenation reserve, normal clotting function, and a skilled operator. Cannot be performed in patients who are endotracheally intubated.

Percutaneous Needle Aspiration

- **Advantage.** Minimal risk of contamination.
- **Disadvantage.** Limited to peripheral lesions, requires a skilled operator, patient cannot be intubated. There is a 10% risk of pneumothorax or hemorrhage.

Transbronchial Biopsy

- **Advantage.** Directed sampling.
- **Disadvantage.** Limited sampling; risk of pneumothorax.

Bronchoalveolar Lavage

- **Advantage.** Low complication rate; samples a large segment of lung; useful for the diagnosis of *P. carinii* and cytomegalovirus infection in patients with human immunodeficiency virus infection; rapid results (by gram stain).

- **Disadvantage.** High rate of contamination limits the validity of routine bacterial cultures.

Protected Specimen Brush

- **Advantage.** Low-risk of contamination; sensitive. Quantitative cultures improve the diagnostic accuracy of this technique (>10^3 colony-forming units/mL often used as a cutoff point for defining infection).
- **Disadvantage.** Limited availability of equipment and quantitative cultures.

Open-Lung Biopsy

- **Advantage.** No risk of contamination; accurate; considered the criterion standard for the diagnosis of nosocomial pneumonia.
- **Disadvantage.** Requires thoracotomy; 10% complication rate. Therefore, generally reserved for patients in whom less invasive diagnostic procedures have been unsuccessful in establishing the diagnosis.

Etiologic Agents

Mycoplasma pneumoniae may be the most frequent cause of community-acquired pneumonia, followed by *S. pneumoniae* and then *S. aureus* (occurring after influenza or by hematogenous seeding). Gram-negative organisms are relatively infrequent, except for *H. influenzae* and *Moraxella catarrhalis,* which are common pathogens in patients with underlying lung disease. Gram-negative bacilli, particularly *Pseudomonas aeruginosa,* assume increasing importance as pathogens in nosocomial pneumonia. Because there may be distinct flora with unique antibiotic susceptibility patterns in a specific hospital or a particular area of a hospital (e.g., the ICU), knowledge of the prevalent organisms in each particular geographic area is important for empiric antibiotic selection. Certain pathogens, for example, *Legionella* species, may show regional variation in incidence. Table 77-1 lists frequently identified pathogens in community-acquired and nosocomial pneumonias.

Complications of Pneumonia

Empyema. When a parapneumonic effusion is noted, thoracentesis is usually necessary to exclude pleural space infection unless the volume of fluid is small (< 1 cm on lateral decubitus radiograph), the patient is doing well, and the radiographic picture is improving. Chest tube drainage is indicated when thoracentesis shows:

TABLE 77-1

COMMON PATHOGENS CAUSING PNEUMONIA

Community-acquired Pneumonia
Mycoplasma pneumoniae
Streptococcus pneumoniae
Staphylococcus aureus
Haemophilus influenzae
Legionella species
Rarely, aerobic gram-negative bacilli
Nosocomial Pneumonia
Enterobacteriaceae
Proteus mirabilis
Escherichia coli
Serratia marcescens
Klebsiella pneumoniae
Pseudomonas aeruginosa
S. aureus
H. influenzae
S. pneumoniae

- Grossly purulent drainage.
- Visible organisms on gram stain.
- Pleural fluid pH < 7.0.
- Glucose level < 40 mg/dL.
- Lactic dehydrogenase level > 1000 units/L.

Purulent pericarditis should be considered in patients who have persistent fever or leukocytosis despite appropriate antibiotic therapy, an enlarged cardiac silhouette shown by radiography, atrial dysrhythmias, chest pain, or clinical signs of cardiac tamponade. Risk factors include pneumonia with pleural evolvement (empyema), thoracic surgery, and infection with certain pathogens (*S. aureus, S. pneumoniae,* group A *Streptococcus,* and gram-negative bacilli). Echocardiography can confirm the presence of fluid in the pericardium. Surgical drainage, in conjunction with appropriate antibiotics, is indicated in most patients.

Meningitis can complicate pneumonia, particularly with *S. pneumoniae* infection. Lumbar puncture should be considered in patients with pneumonia and altered mental status or coma.

Treatment

Supportive Measures. Supplemental oxygen should be administered if hypoxemia is documented. Clearance of respiratory secretions can be improved by control of pleuritic chest pain (analgesics and pulmonary toilet measures). Nasogastric suction may be needed if gastric dilatation or ileus complicates pneumonia. Severe respiratory distress, refractory hypoxemia, and respiratory failure may necessitate endotracheal intubation and mechanical ventilation.

Antimicrobial Therapy. Initial antibiotic selection is based on information gathered from the history, physical examination, results of gram stain of respiratory secretions, and antibiotic susceptibility patterns of the specific hospital. Therapy can be amended once culture and susceptibility data are available. Typical empiric antibiotic regimens and alternatives for common pathogens include:

- ***S. pneumoniae:*** penicillin G (erythromycin).
- ***H. influenzae:*** second-generation cephalosporin (e.g., cefuroxime or cefamandole) or third-generation cephalosporin (e.g., ceftizoxime or ceftriaxone) (ampicillin, if β-lactamase negative).
- ***Legionella* species:** erythromycin, with or without rifampin.
- ***S. aureus:*** if methicillin sensitive, nafcillin (first-generation cephalosporin, imipenem-cilastatin, or vancomycin); if methicillin resistant, vancomycin.
- ***K. pneumoniae:*** third-generation cephalosporin, with or without an aminoglycoside (aztreonam or imipenem-cilastatin).
- ***P. aeruginosa:*** aminoglycoside (tobramycin or amikacin) plus either an antipseudomonal penicillin (piperacillin) or ceftazidime (aztreonam, imipenem-cilastatin).
- ***Serratia marcescens:*** third-generation cephalosporin plus aminoglycoside (aztreonam, imipenem-cilastatin).
- ***P. carinii:*** trimethoprim-sulfamethoxazole, with or without corticosteroids (pentamidine).

Suggested Readings

Craven DE, Steger KA. Nosocomial pneumonia in the intubated patient: New concepts of pathogenesis and prevention. *Infect Dis Clin North Am* 1989;3:843–866.

Comprehensive review of epidemiology and pathogenesis of microbial spread, colonization, and infection of intubated patients (103 references).

Gleeson K, Reynolds HY. Pneumonia in the intensive care unit setting. *J Intensive Care Med* 1992;7:24–35.

Nosocomial pneumonia develops in approximately 20% of ICU patients. The mortality rate approaches 70% (88 references).

Kollef MH. Ventilator-associated pneumonia: A multivariate analysis. *JAMA* 1993;270:1965–1970.

Of 277 consecutive ICU patients who received mechanical ventilation longer than 24 hours, ventilator-associated pneumonia occurred in 43. Identified risk factors include age older than 60 years, degree of organ system failure, previous antibiotic use, and supine head position during the first 24 hours of mechanical ventilation.

Mayhall CG. New techniques for the accurate diagnosis of nosocomial pneumonia. *Infect Dis Clin Pract* 1994;3:56–61.

Concise review of epidemiology and pathogenesis of nosocomial pneumonia, difficulties in establishing accurate etiologic diagnosis, and performance of various diagnostic techniques.

Montecalvo MA, Steger KA, Farber HW, et al. Nutritional outcome and pneumonia in critical care patients randomized to gastric versus jejunal tube feedings. *Crit Care Med* 1992;20:1377–1387.
Of 38 patients studied, half were randomized to gastric tube feedings and half to feedings delivered by an endoscopically placed jejunal tube. The latter group had a lower rate of pneumonia, but the difference was not statistically significant.
Niederman MS, Craven DE, Fein AM, et al. Pneumonia in the critically ill hospitalized patient. *Chest* 1990;97:170–181.
Case report and interesting discussion (88 references).
Ruiz-Santana S, Garcia-Jimenez A, Esteban A, et al. ICU pneumonias: A multi-institutional study. *Crit Care Med* 1987;15:930–936.
Comparison of microbial etiologies of community and nosocomial pneumonias in patients requiring care in the ICU.

CHAPTER 78

Sinusitis and Other Serious Upper Respiratory Tract Infections

(See Chapter 38)

David Tompkins

Sinusitis

Sinusitis is an uncommon cause of admission to the ICU, but it frequently develops as an unrecognized infection in the ICU patient. Nosocomial sinusitis is directly related to use of nasotracheal and nasogastric tubes, which cause irritation and edema of the nasal mucosa and secondary obstruction of the sinus ostia. Additional risk factors include nasal packing, craniofacial injuries, corticosteroid therapy, diabetes mellitus, prolonged mechanical ventilation, and broad-spectrum antibiotic use.

Pathogens. Community-acquired acute bacterial sinusitis is most commonly associated with *Streptococcus pneumoniae* and *Haemophilus influenzae* infection. Nosocomial sinusitis is usually polymicrobial. The more frequently isolated pathogens include *Staphylococcus aureus,* the enterobacteriaceae, *Pseudomonas* species, and anaerobes.

Clinical Features. Symptoms associated with community-acquired sinusitis, such as headache, facial pain, nasal congestion, and discharge, are less frequent in nosocomial sinusitis. Fever is more common in nosocomial sinusitis, and may be the only clue.

Diagnosis. Sinusitis should be considered in all ICU patients with cryptogenic fever, particularly if there is a foreign body in the nasal passage. Evidence of an air–fluid level, mucosal thickening, and opacification, shown by sinus radiographs or CT, supports the diagnosis of purulent sinusitis. Sinus puncture, for both drainage and culture, can be helpful in some circumstances to guide antibiotic therapy for nosocomial sinusitis.

Treatment. Removal of all nasal tubes and application of vasoconstricting agents (e.g., oxymetazoline spray) will decrease mucosal swelling and improve sinus drainage. Initial empiric antibiotics should target staphylococci, gram-negative bacteria, and anaerobes. Further antibiotic decisions can be guided by culture and susceptibility data from sinus cultures, if available. Surgical drainage may be needed if the infection persists despite the above measures.

Complications of Nosocomial Sinusitis. In addition to sepsis, sinus infection may be complicated by local extension to surrounding bone, the orbits, and the CNS. Osteomyelitis is most frequently seen with frontal sinus infection. Orbital complications can be divided into five stages of progressively serious involvement:

- **Inflammatory edema,** with nontender swelling of the eyelids. Therapy is antibiotics.
- **Orbital cellulitis,** with fever, lid edema, erythema, pain and, with progressive infection, proptosis. Therapy is antibiotics.
- **Subperiosteal abscess** is usually associated with frontal or ethmoid sinus infection, with downward or lateral displacement of the globe. Therapy is surgical drainage in conjunction with antibiotics.
- **Orbital abscess,** which can lead to ophthalmoplegia and progressive loss of vision. Therapy is surgical drainage in conjunction with antibiotics.
- **Cavernous sinus thrombosis,** with headache, nausea, vomiting, fever, chills, and change in mental status. On examination, there is venous congestion, with chemosis, proptosis, and purplish discoloration of the eyelids. Compression of cranial nerves III, IV, and VI results in ophthalmoplegia which, if bilateral, is diagnostic of cavernous sinus thrombosis. Therapy is surgical drainage in conjunction with antibiotics.

Epiglottitis

Epiglottitis is inflammation and edema of the supraglottic structures (epiglottis, arytenoid cartilages, aryepiglottic folds, and false vocal folds). The potential for rapid progression from the onset of symptoms to the abrupt development of airway obstruction must be recognized and managed as a medical emergency.

Pathogens. A variety of bacteria have been implicated, including *H. influenzae,* other *Haemophilus* species, *Klebsiella pneumoniae,* pneumococcus, other streptococci, and staphylococci.

Clinical Features. Patients with epiglottis can have fever, sore throat, dysphagia and hoarseness, stridor, drooling, and progressive respiratory distress.

Diagnosis is confirmed by direct visualization with a laryngoscope or bronchoscope that shows erythema and edema of the supraglottic area. These procedures may precipitate airway closure; therefore, they should be performed in a setting in which an artificial airway can be established if needed. Lateral soft tissue radiographs of the neck may show generalized swelling or enlargement of the epiglottis (thumb sign). Cultures of the supraglottic area and blood should be obtained to guide antibiotic therapy.

Treatment. Maintenance of airway patency is the primary concern. The risk of airway obstruction is greatest early in the course; therefore, patients should be observed closely in an ICU for the first 24 to 48 hours. Markers of high risk for airway obstruction include subjective respiratory distress, stridor on examination, and positive blood culture findings. If the patient is not prophylactically intubated, equipment and personnel to perform this procedure quickly should be available. The endotracheal tube can be removed after inflammation and swelling subside (usually in 36–48 hr). IV antibiotics targeting *H. influenzae,* other gram-negative organisms, and staphylococci (such as some second- or third-generation cephalosporins or ampicillin-clavulanate) should be used. High-dose corticosteroids may be useful in reducing edema.

Oropharyngeal Space Infection

Oropharyngeal space infections are usually the result of extension of dental, tonsillar, or pharyngeal infections. Infection of the submandibular, lateral pharyngeal, or retropharyngeal–prevertebral space is potentially life threatening, either by leading to mechanical airway occlusion or extending infection to vital areas. Infections in these areas can dissect into and along tissue planes to involve the mediastinum and carotid sheath, with secondary hemorrhage or septic phlebitis.

Submandibular Space Infection. Submandibular space infections (Ludwig's angina) result from an initial odontogenic infection (mandibular molars) in most cases. Other risk factors include mandibular fracture and laceration, foreign bodies, or tumors of the floor of the mouth. Infection of the submandibular space classically causes a woody cellulitis with elevation of the tongue that can lead to asphyxiation. Less commonly, the infection can extend to the lateral pharyngeal space, retropharyngeal area, and mediastinum. Trismus is unusual unless there is lateral pharyngeal space involvement.

Lateral Pharyngeal Space Infection. The source of lateral pharyngeal space infection is usually an initial infection of the peritonsillar space, pharynx, teeth, or parotids. Clinically, patients have fever, trismus, lateral neck swelling, a bulging pharyngeal wall, and dysphagia. Complications include suppurative jugular venous thrombosis and carotid artery erosion and rupture.

Retropharyngeal Space Infection. The retropharyngeal area is composed of three potential spaces: the retropharyngeal space, the prevertebral space, and the intermediate *danger space,* so called because of its free communication with the posterior mediastinum. The retropharyngeal space has a rich lymphatic system that drains the nasopharynx, middle ear, and paranasal sinuses. Initial infection of these structures, with lymphatic spread and lymph node suppuration, is a frequent cause of retropharyngeal space infection. Esophageal trauma, for example, from endoscopy, nasogastric tube passage, or traumatic intubation, is the usual cause of retropharyngeal space infection. Prevertebral space infection usually arises from cervical spine infection. Infection of the danger space arises most commonly from contiguous spread of retropharyngeal or prevertebral space infections.

Manifestations include fever, sore throat, neck stiffness, dysphagia, and dyspnea. A pharyngeal mass is often visible. Severe respiratory distress, particularly if associated with chest pain, suggests extension to the mediastinum. Complications of retropharyngeal space infection include meningitis, mediastinitis, pneumonia, empyema, and purulent pericarditis.

Pathogens

Oropharyngeal space infections result from extension of dental, tonsillar, or pharyngeal infection. The bacteria responsible are often components of normal oral flora that become pathogenic when mucosal barriers are breached. These infections are usually polymicrobial, with a mixture of aerobic (primary streptococci) and anaerobic organisms (*Peptostreptococcus* species, *Fusobacterium* species, *Bacteroides* species, and *Actinomycetes* species), with anaerobes predominating. *Eikenella corrodens* is an important pathogen in this setting and is clindamycin resistant. Staphylococci and aerobic gram-negative bacilli are rare causes of deep neck infections, except in the setting of cervical osteomyelitis, extension from salivary gland infection, or external penetrating trauma.

Diagnosis

In addition to the clinical symptoms and physical findings, computed tomography scanning is useful for both confirming the diagnosis and showing which spaces are involved. For retropharyngeal infections, the diagnosis can be supported by lateral neck radiographs showing prevertebral soft tissue widening ($>$ 7 mm at the C2 level and $>$ 22 mm at the C6 level), loss of cervical lordosis, or evidence of vertebral osteomyelitis.

Purulent collections should be drained by needle aspiration, ideally using an extraoral route to limit contamination by normal flora. Aspirated pus should undergo gram stain and culture, both aerobically and anaerobically.

Therapy

There are three components to the treatment of deep neck infections:

- **Airway control:** Artificial airway control is not universally needed, but close observation in an ICU is necessary, with frequent evaluation of respiratory status. Rapidly progressive cellulitis and swelling, dyspnea, and stridor are indications for intubation.
- **Antibiotic therapy:** Penicillin had been the drug of choice for deep neck infections, although clinical failures associated with β-lactamase-producing *Bacteroides* species have been reported. High-dose IV penicillin G (12–20 million units/day) is frequently used as initial therapy. In critically ill patients or those with progressive disease, metronidazole can be added. Penicillin-allergic patients may be treated with erythromycin or cephalosporin with metronidazole. Agents that are active against staphylococci and gram-negative bacilli are usually not indicated, except if these organisms are identified on culture or in the setting of prevertebral space infection secondary to cervical osteomyelitis.
- **Surgical intervention** is reserved for cases in which crepitus, fluctuance, or purulent collections are identified, or when antibiotic therapy is unsuccessful. Ultrasonography and computed tomography scanning of the neck can aid in the identification of collections before surgical drainage.

Suggested Readings

Blomquist IK, Bayer AS. Life threatening deep fascial space infections of the head and neck. *Infect Dis Clin North Am* 1988;2:237–264.
Concise, well-referenced review of anatomy, pathogenesis, and clinical features of deep oropharyngeal infections.

Holzapfel L, Chevret S, Madinier G, et al. Influence of long-term oro- or nasotracheal intubation on nosocomial maxillary sinusitis and

pneumonia: Results of a prospective, randomized, clinical trial. *Crit Care Med* 1993;21:1132–1138.
In this study of 300 patients randomized to receive either oro- or nasotracheal intubation, there was a nonsignificant trend in favor of the oral route with respect to the rate of nosocomial sinusitis and pneumonia.
Mayo-Smith I. Fatal respiratory arrest in adult epiglottitis in the intensive care unit: Implications for airway management. *Chest* 1993; 104:964–965.
Case report of an adult with acute epiglottitis, review of literature on epiglottitis in adults, and suggestions for management.

CHAPTER 79

Bacterial Meningitis

(See Chapter 36)

Peter R. Mariuz

Bacterial meningitis is a medical emergency. Despite the advent of potent antimicrobials, it remains an important cause of morbidity and mortality.

Epidemiology and Etiology

Bacteremia is the source of most cases of bacterial meningitis. The overall annual attack rate is approximately 3 cases per 100,000 population in the United States. *Haemophilus influenzae, Neisseria meningitidis,* and *Streptococcus pneumoniae* cause more than 80% of all cases. Mortality rates were higher (e.g., approximately 84% with *Pseudomonas aeruginosa*) before the advent of potent newer β-lactam antimicrobials.

Streptococci. *S. pneumoniae* accounts for approximately 13% of cases and is the most common pathogen among adults older than 30 years. It is associated with high mortality (as high as 27%) and morbidity rates (neurologic sequelae in 30–50% of survivors). It is often associated with distant foci of infection, such as pneumonia, sinusitis, otitis media, and endocarditis. Risk factors include asplenic state, multiple myeloma, hypogammaglobulinemia, alcoholism, and skull fractures with cerebrospinal fluid (CSF) leak. There is an increasing incidence of pneumococci resistant to penicillin.

S. agalactiae (group B *Streptococcus*) is a frequent cause of meningitis and sepsis in neonates. It occurs rarely in postpartum women and other adults, and it is associated with a high mortality rate (22%) and a high rate of neurologic complications.

Neisseria. *N. meningitis* is isolated from 20% of patients with bacterial meningitis. It is most often seen in children and young adults, and carries a mortality rate of 10%. It can occur in epidemics (serogroups A and C), whereas type B strains are isolated most frequently in sporadic cases. Type Y strains may be associated with pneumonia. A risk factor is deficiency of one of the terminal complement components (C5–C9) so that the membrane attack complex (C5b–C9) cannot be formed and lysis of organisms entering the bloodstream does not occur.

Staphylococci. *Staphylococcus epidermidis* is the most common cause of meningitis associated with CSF shunts, accounting for 75% of cases. *S. aureus* is associated with neurosurgical procedures, penetrating head trauma, CSF shunts, and endocarditis. Other predisposing factors include diabetes mellitus, alcoholism, hemodialysis, IV drug abuse, and malignancies.

Haemophilus. *H. influenzae* type B has been a common cause of meningitis, occurring primarily in young children. The incidence has decreased significantly in the United States with widespread use of the conjugate vaccine. The overall mortality rate is 6%, whereas residual hearing deficits occur in at least 10% of patients. Risk factors other than age include sinusitis, epiglottitis, pneumonia, otitis media, diabetes mellitus, alcoholism, asplenia, hypogammaglobulinemia, and anatomic defects (e.g., skull fractures and dermal sinus tracts).

Listeria. *Listeria monocytogenes* represents 2% of cases, and has a high mortality rate (29%). Infection is most likely in neonates and the elderly, and in patients with alcoholism, cancer, organ transplants, and other immunocompromised states. Thirty percent of adults and approximately 50% of children and young adults have no apparent underlying risk factors. It has been associated with food-borne outbreaks (e.g., contaminated coleslaw, milk, cheese).

Gram-Negative Bacilli. *Escherichia coli* causes 30–50% of cases in infants younger than 2 months. *Klebsiella* species, *E. coli,* and *P. aeruginosa* are associated with head trauma, neurosurgical procedures, advanced age, immunosuppression and, rarely, bacteremia. Mortality rates were higher (approximately 85% with *P. aeruginosa*) before the advent of potent newer β-lactam antimicrobials.

Clinical Presentation

- Fever, headache, meningismus, and signs of cerebral dysfunction, including confusion, delirium, or a decreasing level of consciousness ranging from lethargy to coma.

- Seizures are present in one-third of patients.
- Kernig's or Brudzinski's signs are elicited in only half of cases.
- Focal cerebral signs (e.g., visual field defects, dysphasia, hemiparesis) suggest a parameningeal focus of infection. Cranial nerve palsies (particularly nerves III, IV, and VI) suggest basilar meningitis that is often associated with mycobacterial or fungal etiology.
- With disease progression, signs of increased intracranial pressure may develop and are associated with a poor prognosis.
- In the elderly, a change in mental status should not be ascribed to other causes until bacterial meningitis is considered.
- The onset of meningitis varies from fulminant, occurring over a period of 24 hours (25%), to acute, occurring over 1 to 7 days, sometimes after respiratory symptoms occur.
- Recurrent bacterial meningitis is associated with CSF leaks (otorrhea and rhinorrhea) that complicate basilar skull fractures.

Diagnosis

The diagnosis rests on the results of lumbar puncture (LP). The opening pressure is elevated in most cases, usually 20 to 30 cm H_2O. The CSF fluid may appear cloudy or turbid if the white blood cell (WBC) count is greater than 200 mm^{-3}, and it shows a predominance of neutrophils. Ten percent of patients have a lymphocytic predominance that suggests a viral etiology. A low CSF WBC count indicates a poor prognosis. Low CSF glucose concentration (< 40 mg/dL if not hyperglycemic) is found in 60% of cases. CSF protein level is elevated (100–500 mg/dL) in most cases.

Gram stain of a centrifuged CSF specimen permits rapid and accurate identification of causative organisms in 60–90% of cases. CSF culture findings are usually positive in bacterial meningitis if the patient has not received antimicrobial therapy. Blood cultures are positive in 40–60% of patients with *H. influenzae, N. meningitidis,* and *S. pneumoniae.* Counterimmunoelectrophoresis and latex agglutination tests of CSF for detection of bacterial antigens are rapid diagnostic indicators that are particularly useful in partially treated patients. These tests can detect antigens in the CSF when meningitis is caused by meningococci, *H. influenzae* type B, group B streptococci, pneumococci, and *E. coli* K1.

The most feared complication after lumbar puncture is tonsillar herniation from increased intracranial pressure (ICP). If increased ICP is suspected (e.g., related to the presence of an intracranial mass lesion), antibiotic therapy should be initiated and computed tomography scan with contrast of the head performed before the LP is performed.

Differential Diagnosis

- **Viral meningitis:** Pathogens include enteroviruses (coxsackie A, B serotypes, echoviruses, and polioviruses), lymphocytic choriomeningitis virus (often associated with exposure to rodents, including pet hamsters), herpesviruses, and human immunodeficiency virus. Measles, mumps, Epstein-Barr virus, cytomegalovirus, and adenovirus infections can be complicated by meningitis. The onset is usually more insidious and the progression slower than with bacterial meningitis. Patients often report severe headache, but are otherwise alert and awake. Stupor, obtundation, and coma are unusual.
- **Spirochetes:** Acute syphilitic meningitis is a well-known, although rare, manifestation of neurosyphilis. Serologic tests on both CSF and serum establish the diagnosis. *Borrellia burgdorferi* may cause meningitis during the secondary stage of Lyme disease. Bell's palsy frequently develops in these patients.
- **Mycobacteria:** Tuberculous meningitis usually occurs subacutely or chronically. Cranial nerve palsies are common. Early in the course, CSF neutrophilic pleocytosis may be present, but typical CSF findings are increased protein levels, hypoglycorrhachia, and lymphocytic pleocytosis. Results of CSF smears for acid-fast bacilli are usually negative. Results of CSF cultures, although positive in most cases, are not rapidly available. A positive tuberculin skin test result, an abnormal chest radiograph, and evidence of infection at other sites support the diagnosis.
- **Fungi:** *Cryptococcus neoformans* typically causes subacute, chronic meningitis in immunocompromised patients (e.g., those with acquired immune deficiency syndrome, lymphoma, organ transplantation, or prolonged steroid use). CSF studies may be indistinguishable from those of tuberculous meningitis, but India ink stains (positive results in 50–60% of cases), CSF cryptococcal polysaccharide antigen (positive results in > 90% of cases), and culture establish the diagnosis.
- ***Rickettsia:*** Rocky Mountain spotted fever (caused by *Rickettsia rickettsii*) can cause fever, headache, and altered mental status. The macular rash, first involving wrists and ankles, then spreading centrally without mucous membrane involvement, is characteristic and helps to establish the diagnosis.
- **Noninfectious disorders** include neoplasia, cerebral vasculitis, granulomatous angiitis, sarcoidosis, and chemical meningitis (e.g., caused by the use of indo-

methacin, trimethoprim-sulfamethoxazole, radiocontrast agents, or anesthetics).

Treatment

Antimicrobial Therapy. Emergent antimicrobial therapy should be initiated and is based on age and underlying disease status, gram stain results, and other rapidly available diagnostic information.

- **Neonates and infants** younger than 3 months old: The most likely organisms are *E. coli, S. agalactiae,* or *Listeria monocytogenes. H. influenzae* and *S. pneumoniae* must also be considered in infants. The empiric therapy of choice is ampicillin plus a third-generation cephalosporin (i.e., cefotaxime or ceftriaxone).
- **Children 3 months to 18 years old:** *H. influenzae* has been the most frequent pathogen in children 3 months to 18 years old. Pneumococci and meningococci are also prevalent. Empiric therapy with a third-generation cephalosporin that crosses the blood–brain barrier is indicated. Vancomycin is the drug of choice for highly resistant strains of pneumococci.
- **Adults 18 to 50 years old:** Most cases are caused by *S. pneumoniae.* Penicillin G or ampicillin should be used, and a third-generation cephalosporin should be added if *H. influenzae* is suspected (risk factors include sinusitis, otitis media, epiglottitis, pneumonia, head trauma with CSF leak, diabetes mellitus, alcoholism, splenectomy, and immunodeficiency) or if there is a high incidence of penicillin-resistant pneumococci in the area.
- **Adults 50 years and older:** Pneumococci and meningococci are possible causes, as are *L. monocytogenes* and gram-negative bacilli. Ampicillin combined with a third-generation cephalosporin is indicated.

In documented *L. monocytogenes* infection, an aminoglycoside should be added. In postneurosurgical patients with CSF shunts or foreign bodies, meningitis is usually caused by staphylococci (*S. epidermidis* or *S. aureus*), diphtheroides, and gram-negative bacilli (including *P. aeruginosa*). A combination of vancomycin and ceftazidime is indicated pending culture results.

The optimal duration of therapy for bacterial meningitis has not been established in standardized prospective studies. However, treatment for 10 to 14 days is recommended for most cases of nonmeningococcal meningitis, and treatment for 3 weeks is recommended for gram-negative meningitis. Seven days of therapy appears to be adequate for meningococcal infection.

Monitoring Response to Therapy. Response to therapy is assessed by evaluation of temperature and neurologic signs and symptoms. Repeat examination of CSF is not routinely necessary in an adult who is responding well to antibiotic therapy. Indications for considering a repeat LP include:

- Uncertain initial diagnosis.
- New or progressive signs and symptoms.
- Inadequate or atypical clinical response.
- Documentation of early CSF sterilization (after 24–48 hours of therapy) with unusual organisms (e.g., gram-negative bacilli, *Listeria* species, fungi, mycobacteria, or resistant organisms).
- Intrathecal or intraventricular therapy.

Adjuvant Therapy. The high morbidity and mortality rates associated with bacterial meningitis despite the advent of potent antibiotics have led to the development of adjunctive treatment strategies based on the pathogenesis of this disease.

- **Corticosteroids** (e.g., dexamethasone) decreased hearing loss as a sequela meningitis in children with *H. influenzae* type B infection in one study, and decreased the case fatality rate and overall neurologic sequelae in children and adults with pneumococcal meningitis in another study. However, controversy exists regarding the routine use of corticosteroids in all cases of bacterial meningitis. A dose of 0.15 mg/kg IV every 6 hours for the first 4 days of therapy has been used, beginning immediately before the first dose of antibiotics.
- **Reduction of ICP** in patients with signs of increased ICP (e.g., altered level of consciousness; dilated, poorly reactive, or nonreactive pupils; and ocular movement disorders). Increased ICP can preclude assessment of worsening neurologic function, and patients may benefit from the insertion of an ICP monitoring device. Pressures greater than 20 mm Hg should be treated (see Chapter 39 in this book).
- **Treatment of seizures** must be initiated promptly to avoid status epilepticus and further brain injury. A short-acting agent (diazepam or lorazepam) should be initiated, followed immediately by a long-acting agent (phenytoin).

Suggested Readings

Dougherty JM, Roth RM. Cerebral spinal fluid. *Emerg Clin North Am* 1986;4:281–297.

Comprehensive review of cerebrospinal fluid analysis, including physiology of its production and technique of its sampling.

Girgis NI, Farid Z, Mikhail IA, et al. Dexamethasone treatment for bacterial meningitis in children and adults. *Pediatr Infect Dis J* 1989;8:848–851.

Nonplacebo controlled trial of the efficacy of dexamethasone as adjunctive therapy for S. pneumoniae *meningitis in children and adults.*

Lebel MH, Freij BJ, Syrogiannopoulos GA, et al. Dexamethasone therapy

for bacterial meningitis: Results of two double-blind, placebo-controlled trials. *N Engl J Med* 1988;319:964–971.
Controlled study of efficacy of adjunctive therapy with dexamethasone in infants and children with bacterial meningitis.
Quagliarello V, Scheld WM. Bacterial meningitis. *N Engl J Med* 1992; 327:864–872.
Excellent review of current understanding of pathogenesis and pathophysiology of bacterial meningitis and possible therapeutic implications.
Roos KL, Scheld WM. The management of fulminant meningitis in the intensive care unit. *Infect Dis Clin North Am* 1989;3:137–154.
Concise, clinically oriented review of the management of bacterial meningitis in the ICU. Includes informative discussion of treatment modalities of increased intracranial pressure.
Tunkel AR, Wispelwey B, Scheld M. Bacterial meningitis: Recent advances in pathophysiology and treatment. *Ann Intern Med* 1990; 112:610–623.

CHAPTER 80

Endocarditis

(See Chapters 40 and 48)

Roy T. Steigbigel

Infectious endocarditis (IE) has substantial morbidity and mortality rates. The diagnosis may be obvious, with acute symptoms, or subtle, with nonspecific symptoms of fatigue, weight loss, and low-grade fever. In both instances, rapid institution of appropriate therapy will likely result in a better outcome.

The older classification system based on presentation (i.e., acute, subacute, or chronic) has been largely replaced by systems based on the etiologic agent (e.g., *Staphylococcus aureus*), the type of valve involved (e.g., prosthetic vs. native valve), or the portal of entry (e.g., IV drug abuse). This classification allows for better descriptions of the presentation, clinical course, and diagnostic and therapeutic options.

Epidemiology

Although the incidence of rheumatic fever and valvulitis has declined, improved medical and surgical therapy has allowed for longer survival of people at increased risk for IE. These people include patients with congenital heart defects, degenerative heart disease (e.g., calcified mitral annulus, aortic valve calcification, or mitral valve prolapse, especially with associated mitral insufficiency), and prosthetic heart valves. Invasive devices, such as central venous catheters, also contribute to the increasing incidence of IE. The use of injected drugs remains a major predisposing factor for repetitive episodes of IE. Other predisposing factors include dental procedures (approximately 15%) and genitourinary or gynecologic surgical procedures.

IE is likely to occur when there is bacteremia in the setting of abnormal blood flow in the heart, so that eddy currents are generated. Bacteria settle on the low-pressure side of flow through a valve or defect in the septum where there is a gradient from high to low pressure. Hence, IE is often associated with mitral insufficiency (high pressure from the left ventricle to low pressure in the left atrium), with organisms infecting the atrial side of damaged mitral leaflets. IE is rarely seen in pure mitral stenosis because the pressure gradient from the left atrium to the left ventricle is not sufficient to lead to the conditions that are necessary for IE. Similarly, IE is associated with ventricular, not atrial, septal defects. The valves most commonly affected in non–IV drug users are, in order of prevalence, the aortic, mitral, and tricuspid valves.

In addition to host factors, some organisms are more likely to adhere to endothelium and cause IE, so that among the non–group A, B, and G streptococci (sometimes called viridans streptococci), *Streptococcus sanguis* and *S. mutans* cause a high proportion of cases of IE.

Clinical Manifestations

The classic presentation of IE, with fever, heart murmur, skin lesions, and splenomegaly, is easily recognized. However, more subtle presentations are more common, and have the potential for delay in diagnosis. The range of symptoms and signs is extensive, and they are related to events such as embolization within the heart and to other organs, destruction of the heart valve, and host immune response to the infection. Common symptoms are anorexia, weight loss, nonspecific GI symptoms, malaise, myalgia, and arthralgias.

Fever is present in 90–95% of patients with IE. Fever may not develop in the elderly, in those with renal failure or severe congestive heart failure, or in patients partially treated with antimicrobial drugs. A heart murmur is heard in 85–95% of cases, and is suggestive of IE when it is a new regurgitant murmur. Peripheral signs include petechiae in 20–30% of cases, Osler's nodes (small, tender nodules most often seen on the fingers or toe pads) or Roth spots (retinal hemorrhages) in approximately 5% and, rarely, Janeway lesions (nontender hemorrhagic areas on the palms or soles) or clubbing of the fingers or toes. These peripheral manifestations are more common in patients with IE of longer duration. Splenomegaly is present in 25–45% of cases, with a higher incidence in patients with a more prolonged course.

Major embolic events occur in approximately one-fourth of patients and may be the only manifestation of IE at presentation, especially when the IE is caused by fungi or *Haemophilus* species. Emboli from within the heart can result in myocardial infarction or myocarditis. Emboli to a renal artery may result in renal dysfunction or parenchymal infection, whereas immune complex deposition may cause glomerulonephritis. Emboli to the CNS can result in focal neurologic deficits, seizures, transient ischemic attacks, meningitis, encephalitis, visual impairment, and severe headache. CNS emboli can also lead to the formation of mycotic aneurysms. Other consequences of emboli include arthritis, osteomyelitis, diskitis, and pyomyositis.

Laboratory Evaluation

IE causes bacteremia that is relatively continuous; therefore, blood cultures are almost always positive in patients who have not been partially treated. A major indicator that bacteremia is caused by IE is that almost all blood cultures drawn over a period of many hours grow the same organism. Ninety-five to 98% of patients who have not received antimicrobial drugs will have an organism isolated from at least one of the first two sets of blood cultures when at least 10 mL of blood is drawn. Therefore, it is usually not necessary to perform more than three sets of blood cultures before empiric antimicrobial therapy is considered. Patients with right-sided endocarditis may have fewer positive cultures because the organism can be filtered out in the lung.

If there is suspicion of fastidious organisms (e.g., nutritionally deficient streptococci, *Rickettsia* species, or *Brucella* species) or fungi, additional sets should be drawn and the laboratory should be notified to ensure that the culture media used will support the growth of nutritionally deficient organisms. Patients who have recently received antibiotics should have blood cultures drawn daily for 5 to 7 days, after the last dose of antimicrobials.

Hematologic abnormalities in IE are common, but not specific. They include normocytic, normochromic anemia, with low serum iron and transferrin levels and, less frequently, leukocytosis, thrombocytopenia, or leukopenia. Leukopenia is usually associated with splenomegaly. The erythrocyte sedimentation rate is almost always elevated. With more prolonged IE, patients often have positive findings for rheumatoid factor or circulating immune complexes, or decreased levels of some complement proteins (especially C3 and C4). Some studies have shown a correlation between the rate of decline of immune complex levels and the clinical course, with prolonged higher levels associated with more complications.

Echocardiography

Two-dimensional transthoracic echocardiography can detect vegetations as small as approximately 2 mm. Transesophageal echocardiography is even more sensitive, especially for right-sided lesions, and may be able to detect a vegetation as small as 1 mm. Echocardiography can also provide information about the degree of valvular destruction, and can identify valve ring abscesses. It is also useful in assessing the need for valve replacement surgery. The size of a vegetation alone does not directly correlate with the likelihood of embolization, although a large vegetation (≥ 10 mm) is more likely to embolize, as are those caused by fungi and some *Haemophilus* species. Patients with IE involving a prosthetic valve should undergo cineradiography to detect valve dehiscence.

Etiologic Agents

Native Valve

- **Streptococci** account for 60–80% of infections. Viridans streptococci (*S. mutans, S. sanguis, S. mitis,* and others) occur in 40–50% of cases, Group D streptococci occur in 10–15%, and *S. bovis* occur in approximately 5%. These organisms are usually penicillin sensitive. There is an association between *S. bovis* bacteremia and GI malignancy, especially of the colon. Enterococci account for approximately 10% of cases, and are generally resistant to the killing action of all β-lactam antibiotics.
- **Staphylococci** occur in approximately 20% of cases. *S. aureus* are usually sensitive to semisynthetic penicillins (e.g., nafcillin or methicillin), but there is increasing incidence of methicillin-resistant *S. aureus.* The latter organisms are susceptible to vancomycin.
- **Gram-negative organisms** account for approximately 10% of cases. These include Enterobacteriaceae, *Pseudomonas* species, and slow-growing, fastidious gram-negative bacteria (the HACEK group: *Haemophilus* species, *Actinobacillus actinomycetemcomitans, Cardiobacterium hominis, Eikenella corrodens,* and *Kingella kingae*).
- **Miscellaneous organisms** include pneumococci, gonococci, and fungi.

Prosthetic valve endocarditis is defined as early (≤ 60 days after valve insertion) or late (> 60 days) because the predisposing factors and causative agents differ. Common early pathogens include *S. epidermidis* and *S. aureus.* Less common during this period are gram-negative bacilli, streptococci, enterococci, and fungi. The etiology of late infections is similar to that of native valve endocarditis.

IE in IV drug abusers is more often right-sided and is usually caused by *S. aureus* or *Pseudomonas aeruginosa.* It is commonly associated with septic pulmonary emboli that may persist for weeks, even when the patient is receiving appropriate antibiotics.

Complications

Cardiac Complications

- **Valvular dysfunction** results from the destruction of leaflets or of supporting structures, and causes valvular insufficiency or, rarely, obstruction because of large vegetations, especially if the etiology is fungal.
- **Myocardial abscesses** are most often associated with more virulent organisms (e.g., *S. aureus*). They are usually paravalvular and occur as conduction disturbances or mural perforation.
- **Myocardial infarction** is caused by embolic occlusion, thrombosis, or mycotic aneurysm.
- **Myocarditis** is probably caused by vasculitis.
- **Pericarditis** is usually associated with *S. aureus* infection. It occurs by extension or bacteremic spread.

CNS Complications

- **Intracranial mycotic aneurysms** usually occur at bifurcation points in branches of the middle cerebral artery. Signs and symptoms are variable, and include headache, focal neurologic deficits, seizures, and meningismus. The diagnosis is made by computed tomography or magnetic resonance imaging, with and without contrast. Hemorrhage or infarction can be further evaluated with angiography. Because two-thirds of mycotic aneurysms rupture, with a mortality rate of 30–80%, many recommend repair. However, approximately one-third disappear with medical management alone. Some recommend clipping for single peripheral cerebral aneurysms that have bled or those that are asymptomatic but easily accessible. Others should be followed by serial angiography and repaired if enlargement occurs. The role of antihypertensive therapy or antifibrinolytic agents is not defined.
- **Brainstem syndromes** are caused by emboli. They cause nausea, vomiting, singultus, and dyskinesia.
- **Meningitis** may be caused by leakage of mycotic aneurysms, infarction from emboli, brain abscess, thrombosis, vasculitis, or bacteremia.
- **Cranial nerve palsies** may result from emboli, and can involve cranial nerve III, IV, or VI.

- **Psychiatric disturbances** result from vasculitis or anatomic abnormalites.
- **Alteration in consciousness** may have multiple causes, including metabolic abnormalities and hypoxia.
- **Seizures** may be focal, caused by infarction, or generalized and associated with mycotic aneurysms, abscess, meningitis, hypoxia, or high-dose penicillin therapy in patients with renal failure.
- **Peripheral neuropathy** occurs rarely, and may be caused by immune injury.
- **Stroke** is usually the result of emboli or mycotic aneurysm.
- **Subarachnoid hemorrhage** is usually caused by leakage of a mycotic aneurysm.
- **Visual disturbances** may be caused by cranial nerve dysfunction, embolus to the central retinal artery, or endophthalmitis.

Miscellaneous Complications

- **Emboli** occur in approximately 30% of cases, and can be nonseptic or septic. Metastatic abscesses can occur in any organ, and are more common with virulent bacteria, such as *S. aureus.* Large emboli are seen with fungal IE.
- **Glomerulonephritis** can be focal (caused by emboli) or diffuse (secondary to immune complex deposition or infarction from renal artery emboli).
- **Vasculitis** can involve the CNS, renal glomerulus, myocardium, or skin. It is caused by immune complex deposition onto the endothelium, with activation of the complement cascade and localization of inflammatory cells.
- **Mycotic aneurysms** occur in 2–10% of patients with IE, and are multiple in 25%. They usually occur in abnormal vessels, such as an atherosclerotic abdominal aorta. They are often caused by less virulent bacteria.

Treatment

Streptococci. Aqueous penicillin G, 10–20 million units IV daily for 4 weeks, with or without an aminoglycoside during the first 2 weeks, is the basic regimen. Inclusion of an aminoglyside is suggested for those with a complicated course (e.g., heart failure or metastatic foci of infection), prosthetic heart valves, or relatively resistant organisms. Vancomycin 15 mg/kg IV every 12 hours for 4 weeks is recommended for patients who are allergic to penicillin.

Enterococci. Aqueous penicillin G, 20 million units daily IV accompanied by an aminoglycoside to which the organism does not show high-level resistance, is given for 4 weeks. Penicillin-resistant enterococci should be treated with vancomycin. Some enterococci are resistant to both penicillin and vancomycin, but may be sensitive to teicoplanin, which is available on a compassionate basis from Marion Merrell

Dow. If the organism is also resistant to teicoplanin, surgical replacement of the valve may be required.

S. aureus infection is treated with nafcillin 2 g every 4 hours IV for 4 to 6 weeks. Patients with a complicated course or metastatic infection should also receive rifampin (600 mg PO daily) or an aminoglycoside. Vancomycin is used for patients who are allergic to penicillin or to treat infections with methicillin-resistant *S. aureus.*

Other organisms are treated on the basis of the results of susceptibility testing. Fungal endocarditis has a poor prognosis, and may require valve replacement.

Suggested Readings

Bayer AS. Infective endocarditis. *Clin Infect Dis* 1993;17:313–322.

Reviews changes in responsible organisms, diagnostic criteria (including utility of echocardiography), and treatment regimens.

Dajani AS, Bisno AL, Chung KJ, et al. Prevention of bacterial endocarditis: Recommendations by the American Heart Association. *JAMA* 1990;264:2919–2922.

Authoritative indications for prophylaxis and suggested regimens.

Durack DT, Lukes AS, Bright DK, et al. New criteria for diagnosis of infective endocarditis: Utilization of specific echocardiographic findings. *Am J Med* 1994;96:200–210.

Useful criteria for patients with suspected infective endocarditis, but no obvious evidence. Defined two major criteria (blood culture and echocardiographic findings) and six minor criteria.

Hecht SR, Berger M. Right-sided endocarditis in intravenous drug users: Prognostic features in 102 episodes. *Ann Intern Med* 1992; 117:560–566.

Study involving 121 IV drug users with right-sided endocarditis showing that vegetation size may be an important predictor of outcome and that vegetations larger than 2 cm are associated with increased mortality rates.

Shively BK. Transesophageal echocardiography in endocarditis. *Cardiol Clin* 1993;11:437–446.

Review concluding that a technically adequate study with negative findings almost always means a low probability of endocarditis (57 references).

Tucker KJ, Johnson JA, Ong T, et al. Medical management of prosthetic aortic valve endocarditis and aortic root abscess. *Am Heart J* 1993;125:1195–1197.

CHAPTER 81

Urosepsis

(See Chapter 44)

Peter R. Mariuz

Nosocomial Urinary Tract Infections

Nosocomial infections of the urinary tract are the most common infections that occur in hospitals, accounting for 35% to 45% of all hospital-acquired infections. Catheter-associated bacteriuria is the most common source of nosocomial gram-negative bacteremia. Most of these infections are associated with bladder catheterization or other urologic instrumentation.

- Bacteriuria occurs in 10–30% of catheterized patients.
- The per-day risk of bacteriuria is 3–10%.
- Bacteriuria develops in 50% of patients catheterized for more than 7–10 days.

Patient-related risk factors include advanced age, female sex, diabetes mellitus, and the presence of renal dysfunction. Catheter-related risk factors include the duration of catheterization, errors in catheter care, and meatal colonization.

Etiology

Microorganisms enter the urinary tract from colonic flora, from the hands of health care personnel, and from contaminated urinometers or measuring containers. The colonic flora is composed of native organisms plus organisms acquired from the hospital environment. More than 80% of nosocomial urinary tract infections (UTIs) are caused by aerobic gram-negative rods. *Escherichia coli* is the most frequently isolated organism. Other commonly isolated gram-negative pathogens include *Pseudomonas aeruginosa, Klebsiella pneumoniae, Proteus mirabilis, Enterobacter* species, and *Serratia* species. Among the gram-positive organisms, Group D streptococci (*Enterococcus faecalis* and *E. faecium*) and staphylococci (especially *Staphylococcus saprophyticus*) account for periurethral infections. These include urethritis, urethral fistulas, epididymitis, prostatitis, and scrotal or prostatic abscesses. Fournier gangrene is a form of necrotizing fasciitis associated with diabetes mellitus, at first involving the scrotum and then rapidly spreading to the genitalia, perineum, and abdominal wall. Immediate surgical evaluation, debridement, and broad-spectrum antibiotics are necessary.

Diagnosis

A definitive diagnosis is dependent on culture of urine that is freshly voided or collected from the catheter. Organism concentrations of $\geq 10^5$ colony-forming units/mL urine are most likely to represent true bacteriuria if the sample is properly collected. Lower concentrations ($\leq 10^3$) also may reflect true bacteriuria, particularly when associated with pyuria. Catheter-tip cultures play no role in the diagnosis of UTI.

Treatment

Symptomatic Catheter-Associated Bacteriuria. After cultures of blood and urine have been obtained, treatment can be initiated with parenteral antibiotics at initial doses adequate to treat bacteremia. The dose may be reduced if there is no evidence of bacteremia. The antibiotics should be selected based on urine gram stain results and knowledge of organisms that are common to the specific hospital. Concomitant infections outside the urinary tract, catheter obstruction and, especially among men, periurethral infections, should also be noted. Cure is unlikely unless the indwelling catheter is removed. Initial therapy should be designed to treat the likely organism, including *Pseudomonas* species. Antipseudomonal third-generation cephalosporin (ceftazidime), ticarcillin-clavulanate, antipseudomonal penicillins (piperacillin, mezlocillin), aminoglycosides, monobactams (aztreonam), fluoroquinolones (ciprofloxacin, ofloxacin), and imipenem are all useful as initial therapy. Therapy should be adjusted after culture results are available to permit the use of antimicrobials with the narrowest spectrum of activity, lowest cost, and least toxicity. The optimal length of treatment is not known, but treatment for 5 to 7 days results in a high rate of cure. Prostatitis may require treatment for as long as 4 weeks. Prostatic involvement is common in catheterized male patients with UTI. The only antimicrobials that reach significant levels in the prostate and have activity against UTI pathogens are trimethoprim and the quinolones.

Asymptomatic Catheter-Associated Bacteriuria. Treatment should not be initiated unless the patient is at risk for sepsis (e.g., advanced age, underlying disease, diabetes, or pregnancy).

Asymptomatic Bacteriuria and Catheter Removal. In women with bacteriuria that persists 48 hours after catheter removal, particularly those 65 years and older, treatment should be considered.

Uncomplicated Cystitis in Nonpregnant Patients. Single-dose therapy with trimethoprim-sulfamethoxazole (TMP-SMX; 2–3 double-strength tablets) is usually effective, although a 3-day regimen results in fewer relapses than the single-dose regimen.

Acute, Uncomplicated Pyelonephritis Requiring Hospitalization (e.g., in the setting of pregnancy, diabetes, dehydration, vomiting, or a severely ill-appearing patient). Third-generation antipseudomonal cephalosporins, ticarcillin-clavulanate, antipseudomonal penicillins, aminoglycosides, or fluoroquinolones can be used.

Acute, Complicated Pyelonephritis (e.g., catheter-related pyelonephritis or that associated with obstruction, reflux, renal transplant, azotemia, diabetes, or structural or neurologic genitourinary abnormalities). Treatment is the same as for symptomatic catheter-associated bacteriuria. The duration of therapy is 14 days. Renal abscess should be suspected when fever persists beyond 48–72 hours despite appropriate treatment.

Prostatitis. Effective antibiotics include fluoroquinolones (ciprofloxacin, ofloxacin) and TMP-SMX for 4 weeks.

Prevention of Catheter-Associated Bacteriuria

If patients can be managed without a catheter or other urine-collection devices, the incidence of bacteriuria and its complications are minimized. If this type of management is not possible, collection devices other than indwelling catheters may be associated with a lower incidence of bacteriuria. Two principles are universally recommended for the prevention of bacteriuria: (1) maintaining a closed catheter system and (2) minimizing the duration of catheterization.

The closed drainage system should be considered a sterile site, and aseptic precautions should be observed when any portion of the system is manipulated. Urine specimens should be collected without opening the catheter–collection tube junction. The system should be opened only at the bag drainage tube. Continuous downhill gravity drainage should be maintained.

Techniques that are ineffective for the prevention of bacteriuria include:

- Antibacterials placed at the catheter–urethra interface.
- Silver-coated catheter.
- Irrigation of the collection system with antibacterial agents or saline.
- Devices to ensure a discontinuous column of urine in the catheter-collection tube.
- Systemic antibiotic prophylaxis.

Suggested Readings

Boscia JA, Kobasa WD, Knight RA, et al. Epidemiology of bacteriuria in an elderly ambulatory population. *Am J Med* 1986;80:208–214.
Demonstrates transient nature of asymptomatic bacteriuria and shows that attempts to eradicate asymptomatic bacteriuria are unsuccessful and unwarranted.
Garibaldi RA, Burke JP, Dickman ML, et al. Factors predisposing to bacteriuria during indwelling urethral catheterization. *N Engl J Med* 1974;291:215–219.
Discusses risk factors for bacteriuria as well as modes of prevention.
Hirsh DD, Fainstein V, Musher DM. Do condom catheter collecting systems cause urinary tract infections? *JAMA* 1979;242:340–341.
Discusses risk of urinary tract infection with this type of catheter use.
Stamm WE. Catheter-associated urinary tract infections: Epidemiology, pathogenesis and prevention. *Am J Med* 1991;91(suppl 3B):65S–71S.
Stamm WE, Hooton TM. Management of urinary tract infections in adults. *N Engl J Med* 1993;329:1328–1334.
In-depth review of management of specific groups of adult patients with urinary tract infections.
Warren JW. Catheter-associated urinary tract infections. *Infect Dis Clin North Am* 1987;1:823–854.
Excellent review of nosocomial urinary tract infections.

CHAPTER 82

Gastrointestinal and Intra-Abdominal Infections

(See Chapters 41 and 42)

Jennifer A. Schranz

Secondary Peritonitis

Primary or spontaneous bacterial peritonitis is reviewed in Chapter 44 in this book. Secondary peritonitis may be localized or related to diffuse abdominal infection. The distinction is necessary to determine the appropriate therapy. Localized infection is amenable to therapy such as resection or percutaneous drainage. Diffuse suppurative infections are more complex, often requiring peritoneal debridement, lavage, or repeated explorations.

Microbiology. Polymicrobial infection results from endogenous bacteria that colonize the visceral mucosa. Aerobes and anaerobes are frequently isolated and include *Escherichia coli, Klebsiella* species, and *Enterobacter* species, enterococci, and *Bacteroides* species. Antibiotic-resistant strains, such as *Pseudomonas aeruginosa, Serratia marcescens, Acinetobacter* species, and *Xanthomonas* species are frequently isolated in the nosocomial setting.

Clinical Presentation. Symptoms include abdominal pain, anorexia, nausea, vomiting, fever, and chills. On physical examination, there may be tachycardia, a hyperresonant abdomen with decreased or absent bowel sounds, rebound pain, and involuntary guarding.

Prognostic indicators of survival in secondary peritonitis are:

- **Age** of the patient.
- **Duration** of peritoneal contamination.
- **Contamination** with foreign materials, such as bile, pancreatic secretions, or barium.
- **Specific pathogens** involved, their virulence, and the inoculum size.
- **Underlying disease,** i.e., the primary intra-abdominal process.
- **Comorbidity,** i.e., severity of illness, concomitant diseases, organ system failure.

Laboratory findings include leukocytosis (typically, the peripheral white blood cell [WBC] count is 17,000–25,000 mm^{-3}), with a predominance of neutrophils, hemoconcentration, elevated serum urea nitrogen level, and acidosis. If the infection is close to the genitourinary system, there may be pyuria and hematuria. Abdominal radiography may show ileus, multiple air–fluid levels, widening between bowel loops, gas within the bowel wall, obliteration of the psoas shadow, or fat lines and free air if there has been perforation of a viscus.

Treatment initially includes fluid replacement, decompression of gastric contents, surgical intervention to correct the underlying disease process, empiric broad-spectrum antibiotics, and institution of an alternate form of nutrition. Therapeutic goals in secondary peritonitis include:

- Control of bacteremia.
- Treatment of metastatic foci of infection.
- Reduction of suppurative complications (abscess formation).
- Prevention of local spread of existing infection.

Both monotherapy and combination antibiotic regimens have been used successfully, for example:

- Metronidazole plus either a third-generation cephalosporin or an aminoglycoside.
- Metronidazole plus ampicillin plus an aminoglycoside.
- Cephalosporin monotherapy (e.g., cefoxitin or cefotetan for pelvic infections and appendicitis).

- Broad-spectrum penicillin plus a β-lactamase inhibitor (e.g., ticarcillin-clavulanic acid or piperacillin-tazobactam).
- Imipenem-cilastatin.

An aminoglycoside should be included in the regimen when there is isolation of resistant gram-negative bacilli. In established intra-abdominal infection, 7 to 10 days of therapy is usually sufficient. However, a longer duration may be required if leukocytosis or fever persists. One-third of afebrile patients with persistent leukocytosis have infection. If the patient remains febrile, the likelihood of intra-abdominal infection is 80%.

Peritoneal Dialysis-Associated Peritonitis

Nearly one-half of patients receiving chronic ambulatory peritoneal dialysis (CAPD) have peritonitis during the first 6 months of treatment. This rate increases to 60–70% by 12 months. Recurrent peritonitis occurs in one-fourth of patients with CAPD. Skin contamination is the leading cause of infection. Coagulase-negative staphylococci, *Staphylococcus aureus,* streptococci, and diphtheroids are the pathogens in approximately 70% of cases. Enterobacteriaceae such as *E. coli, Klebsiella* species, *Enterobacter* species, *Proteus* species, *Pseudomonas* species, and fungi are responsible for the remainder of cases.

Patients report abdominal pain (70%), nausea and vomiting (30%), fever (15%), and diarrhea (10%). Dialysate should be sent for culture, cell count, and differential. Fluid analysis usually shows > 100 WBC mm^{-3}, with a predominance of granulocytes. Gram stain results are positive in as many as one-half of patients. Peritonitis occurs with negative culture findings in 5–10% of patients.

Treatment consists of IV vancomycin or intraperitoneal third-generation cephalosporin or aminoglycoside for 10 days to 3 weeks. Longer duration may be necessary in infections with *P. aeruginosa, Candida albicans,* or *S. aureus.* Fungal peritonitis usually requires removal of the peritoneal catheter and administration of IV amphotericin B for 10 to 14 days. The mortality rate is low, with most patients defervescing within 1 to 4 days of treatment.

Appendicitis

Appendicitis usually begins as midepigastric pain localizing to the right lower quadrant. Persistent obstruction of the appendiceal lumen leads to gangrene and eventual rupture. Either a diffuse peritonitis or a local inflammatory mass will develop. Treatment consists of surgery and administration of antimicrobials as described above.

Diverticulitis

Diverticulitis is common in older patients, and usually is located in the sigmoid and descending colon. Symptoms include right lower quadrant pain, diarrhea, fever, and hematochezia. Complications include confined perforation that remains localized, pericolic abscess, fistula formation, and free perforation with generalized peritonitis. Nonoperative therapy with antibiotics covering colonic flora is preferred for uncomplicated cases.

Acute Cholecystitis

Complications include gangrenous or emphysematous cholecystitis, empyema, pericholecystic abscess, cholangitis, liver abscess, bacteremia, and peritonitis. The risk of infectious complications increases with longer duration and severity of symptoms, in elderly or jaundiced patients, and when there is obstruction of the common bile duct.

Pelvic Inflammatory Disease

Pelvic inflammatory disease (PID) can result in bilateral lower abdominal pain, adnexal tenderness, cervical tenderness, vaginal discharge, abnormal vaginal bleeding, dysuria, or dyspareunia. Pathogens such as *Neisseria gonorrhoeae, Chlamydia trachomatis, Mycoplasma hominis,* and *Ureaplasma urealyticum* are recovered in one-half of cases. Other organisms include enteric gram-negative bacilli and anaerobes. Patients with gonococcal etiology may have septic arthritis, septic emboli, tubo-ovarian abscess, or perihepatitis (Fitz-Hugh-Curtis syndrome). Antibiotic coverage may include IV cefoxitin or cefotetan, metronidazole plus a third-generation cephalosporin or aminoglycoside, and tetracycline. Any localized abscesses, regardless of its etiology, should be treated surgically or percutaneously.

Pseudomembranous Colitis

This disorder is caused by infection with *Clostridium difficile.* The organism has a wide clinical spectrum, including asymptomatic carriage, antibiotic-associated colitis without pseudomembranes, pseudomembranous colitis (PMC), and fulminant colitis with toxic megacolon. Although as many as 30% of hospitalized patients receiving antibiotics carry *C. difficile,* only 1% will have PMC. Previous antibiotic use, malignancy, uremia, burns, ICU stay, and colonic stasis are associated with increased risk of contracting PMC.

Patients can be asymptomatic, or may have crampy abdominal pain associated with fever and diffuse, watery diarrhea. Symptoms usually begin 3 to 9 days after antibiotics are initiated. In 20% of patients, symptoms may be delayed for as long as 6 weeks after antibiotics are discontinued. The rectosigmoid colon is the most common site of disease, with pseudomembranes visualized on endoscopy. However, in 10% of patients, the cecum or transverse colon is inflamed, resulting in fever and abdominal pain without pseudomembranes.

The diagnosis is made by identifying the causative toxin by immunoassay, finding evidence of a cytopathic effect in a cell monolayer, or performing culture for *C. difficile.* Stool leukocytes are present in 50% of cases. Endoscopy is the criterion standard for identifying pseudomembranes. Treatment options are described in Chapter 47 in this book.

Toxic Shock Syndrome

S. aureus strains that produce toxic shock syndrome toxin-1 (TSST-1) and other toxins are implicated in causing this syndrome. Initial symptoms include diarrhea, fever, and myalgias, followed by erythroderma, conjunctivitis, hypotension, and multiple organ system failure. Physical examination shows mucosal and vaginal erythema in TSS associated with menstruation. *S. aureus* can often be cultured from the vaginal discharge. Diagnostic criteria include fever, hypotension, rash followed by desquamation, and involvement of at least three organ systems. Management includes supportive care and aggressive fluid hydration. Antibiotics play little role in the immediate management because the syndrome is toxin mediated. Nonetheless, therapy should be instituted with a penicillinase-resistant penicillin (nafcillin) or vancomycin (if the patient is penicillin allergic) for a total of 10 to 14 days (see Chapter 72 in this book).

Acute Dysentery

Dysentery is the passage of frequent, small bowel movements accompanied by blood and mucus. Bacterial invasion of the bowel mucosa results in fecal leukocytes.

Shigellosis is caused by *Shigella* species. These organisms induce high fever, bloody diarrhea, abdominal pain, headache, malaise, and occasionally reactive arthritis or meningismus. Only small numbers of organisms need to be ingested; the incubation period is less than 72 hours. Bacteremia and dissemination are uncommon features, but severe cases may result in pseudomembranous colitis, hemolytic uremic syndrome, or a leukemoid reaction. Stool specimens should be sent for culture. Antibiotics shorten the course of illness and decrease the period of fecal excretion. Antibiotics of choice include trimethoprim-sulfamethoxazole, quinolones (norfloxacin, ciprofloxacin), third-generation cephalosporins and, less often, ampicillin or tetracycline. Antidiarrheal agents should be avoided.

Escherichia coli strains can mediate several forms of GI infection:

- Enteroinvasive *E. coli* produces a syndrome identical to acute shigellosis.
- Enterotoxigenic *E. coli* is the major cause of traveler's diarrhea and diarrhea in the third world.
- Enteropathogenic *E. coli* causes a form of chronic diarrhea.
- Enterohemorrhagic *E. coli* is associated with outbreaks of hemorrhagic colitis and, rarely, with hemolytic-uremic syndrome (*E. coli* O157:H7). Treatment is generally supportive because the infection is self-limited.

***Campylobacter* species** cause inflammatory colitis, with abdominal pain, fever, and bloody diarrhea. Bacteremia also can occur, and is seen in patients infected with human immunodeficiency virus (HIV). Treatment with macrolides (erythromycin or clarithromycin) or quinolones (ciprofloxacin) is effective.

Salmonellosis causes many clinical syndromes, depending on the *Salmonella* serotype. Patients can have fever, myalgias, headache, and diarrhea. When *S. typhi* is the pathogen, the patient may also have a maculopapular rash (rose spots), cervical lymphadenopathy, cough, dyspnea, and hepatosplenomegaly. Bacteremia can occur from any *Salmonella* serotype, but *S. typhimurium* is most frequently isolated in the United States. Localized *Salmonella* infection, such as meningitis, lung abscess, osteomyelitis, hepatic or splenic abscess, or soft-tissue abscess, occurs after bacteremia. A chronic carrier state can occur after *Salmonella* enterocolitis or enteric fever. Treatment options for *Salmonella* infection depend on the clinical syndrome. Treatment is not required in transient carriers or in patients with enterocolitis because a chronic carrier state may be enhanced by the use of antimicrobials. Antibiotic choices for *S. typhi* include third-generation cephalosporins, quinolones, chloramphenicol, and ampicillin (when susceptible).

Amebiasis. *Entamoeba histolytica* can cause an asymptomatic carrier state or amebic dysentery. Extra-intestinal amebiasis is more frequently associated with severe illness in patients who are malnourished, immunosuppressed (e.g., from chemotherapy or HIV infection), or pregnant. Treatment for invasive and symptomatic amebic colitis is metronidazole 750 mg three times daily for 5–10 days.

Suggested Readings

Bohnen JMA, Solomkin JS, Dellinger EP, et al. Guidelines for clinical care: Anti-infective agents for intra-abdominal infection: A surgical infection policy statement. *Arch Surg* 1992;127:83–89.

Developed by committee of the Surgical Infection Society, this report gives guidelines for antibiotic selection for intra-abdominal infections. Regimens that have limited activity against facultative and anaerobic gram-negative bacilli are not considered acceptable.

Kelly, CP, Lamont JT. *Clostridium difficile* colitis. *N Engl J Med* 1994;330:257–262.

Nichols RL, Smith JW. Wound and intra-abdominal infections: Microbiological considerations and approaches to treatment. *Clin Infect Dis* 1993;16(suppl 4):S266–S272.

Excellent review of microbiology and medical and surgical treatment.

Von Graevenitz A, Amsterdam D. Microbiological aspects of peritonitis associated with continuous ambulatory peritoneal dialysis. *Clin Microbiol Rev* 1992;S:36–48.

Good review of peritonitis in continuous ambulatory peritoneal dialysis patients. Discusses pathophysiology, diagnosis, and management.

Wilson SE. A critical analysis of recent innovations in the treatment of intra-abdominal infection. *Surg Gynecol Obstet* 1993;177(suppl):11–17.

Discusses newer surgical techniques for complex intra-abdominal infections. Discussion follows on pages 35–40.

CHAPTER 83

Infections in the Immunocompromised Host

(See Chapters 45, 46, and 49)

Jennifer A. Schranz

Infections in Solid Organ Transplant Recipients

Medical and surgical advances have led to a 1-year graft survival rate of 80–85% in most solid organ transplants. However, infection is expected in 75% of patients after transplantation, and it poses a significant threat to both patient survival and graft function. The duration, type, and temporal sequence of immunosuppressive therapy and the presence of neutropenia play an important role in the management of infection. The time after transplantation can be divided into three periods.

First Month. There are three categories of infection:

- **Pre-existing infections** (peritonitis, bacteremia, pneumonia), which must be treated before transplantation.
- **Infection from the allograft,** resulting in mycotic aneurysms and infected suture lines.
- **Postoperative infections,** e.g., wound, urine, pulmonary, and catheter-related, account for 90% of infections in this period.

The highest and lowest incidences of wound infections occur in liver and renal transplants, respectively. Common organisms include staphylococci and aerobic gram-negative bacilli.

1 to 6 Months. Viral infections, such as cytomegalovirus (CMV), Epstein-Barr virus (EBV), hepatitis B and C, and rarely human immunodeficiency virus (HIV) or protozoa (e.g., toxoplasmosis, leishmaniasis, malaria), predominate by 4 months. The combination of immunomodulating viruses and immunosuppression increases the risk of opportunistic infection, such as *Pneumocystis carinii* pneumonia (PCP).

- Chronic and recurrent urinary tract infections in renal transplant recipients may be secondary to anatomic abnormalities. Papovavirus infection occurs by 3 months, and is generally asymptomatic. CMV infection can result in fever, leukopenia, and allograft dysfunction, especially when a CMV-negative recipient receives a CMV-positive kidney.
- Bacterial mediastinitis occurs in heart transplant recipients in the first month. In addition to CMV, toxoplasmosis and nocardiosis may emerge as opportunistic pathogens.

6 Months and Longer. Three categories of infection occur in patients receiving maintenance immunosuppression.

- Chronic viral infections (10–15%), such as CMV chorioretinitis, EBV-induced lymphoproliferative disease, or hepatitis B- and C-associated liver disease.
- Community-acquired infections (e.g., influenza, parainfluenza, pneumococcal pneumonia, or urinary tract infection) in patients with functional allografts with no evidence of chronic viral infection.
- Opportunistic pathogens (e.g., *Aspergillus* species, *Nocardia* species, *P. carinii, Cryptococcus* species) in the setting of poor allograft function, chronic viral infection, and the use of immunosuppressive drugs.

Infectious Disease Syndromes

Fever of Unknown Origin. Noninfectious causes include adverse drug reactions, thromboembolism, and malignancy. Bacterial infections predominate in the first month. Frequent cultures of blood, urine, surgical wounds and, in some cases, cerebrospinal fluid, in addition to examination of catheter and wound sites, sinuses, and lungs, are important. Empiric broad-spectrum antimicrobial therapy is initiated in neutropenic or toxic-appearing patients according to the nosocomial flora of the institution. CMV infections cause two-thirds of febrile episodes 1–6 months after transplant. Because of toxicity associated with antifungal and antiviral drugs, documentation of viral or fungal infection is necessary unless the patient is acutely ill.

Pulmonary Infiltrates. Diagnostic clues include the rate of progression, degree of hypoxemia, and radiographic pattern.

- Acute onset (within 24 hours) of symptoms, with productive cough, dyspnea, fever, and pulmonary infiltrates usually indicates bacterial origin. A sputum gram stain shows organisms with many neutrophils. Noninfectious causes include pulmonary embolism, pulmonary edema, and hemorrhage.
- Subacute course (2–7 days) can be seen with viral or fungal infections or with PCP. Allogeneic bone marrow transplant recipients with chronic graft-versus-host disease (GVHD) and long-term survivors of heart–lung transplantation may have airflow obstruction as a result of bronchiolitis obliterans.
- Insidious course (>1 week) with nodular or diffuse infiltrates and a nonproductive cough is suggestive of an opportunistic infection (e.g., fungal, mycobacterial, nocardial, or PCP). Bronchoalveolar lavage (BAL) or open-lung biopsy is often required for diagnosis.

Hypoxemia is often worse in acute and subacute pneumonia and with PCP or CMV. Identification of the organism by sputum gram stain and culture, BAL, or open-lung biopsy is important. There is an association between BAL fluid neutrophil count of greater than 20% and bacterial pneumonia. Because CMV isolation by BAL is common, active disease must be distinguished from colonization. Open-lung biopsy should be performed early in rapidly evolving pulmonary syndromes:

CNS infections occur 1 to 6 months after transplantation in 5–10% of recipients. They occur as four distinct clinical syndromes:

- Acute meningitis with *Listeria monocytogenes.*
- Subacute and chronic meningitis caused by mycobacterial and fungal infections.
- Focal infection resulting in focal neurologic deficits caused by *Aspergillus fumigatus* (aspergilloma), *Toxoplasma gondii, Nocardia asteroides,* or *Mycobacterium tuberculosis* (tuberculoma).

TABLE 83–1

PROPHYLAXIS AGAINST CYTOMEGALOVIRUS INFECTION OR DISEASE ACCORDING TO ALLOGRAFT SITE

Donor	Recipient	Kidney	Liver	Lung	Heart
−	−	No	No	No	Yes
−	+	No	No	Yes	Yes
+	+	No	Yes	Yes	Yes
+	+	Yes	Yes	Yes	Yes

- Progressive dementia associated with papovavirus (JC virus).

CMV infections occur in two-thirds of transplant recipients within 6 months as shown by a serologic rise in CMV titer or isolation of CMV in urine, blood, or throat specimens. The infection rate is higher in CMV-positive recipients (85%) compared with CMV-negative recipients (53%) before transplantation. The allograft is the site of viral reactivation in the CMV-negative recipient who receives a CMV-positive organ, leading to numerous clinical syndromes such as pneumonitis or hepatitis in lung and liver allografts, respectively. There are three patterns of CMV reactivation.

- Primary CMV infection in which a CMV-negative recipient receives a CMV-positive allograft or blood product.
- Reactivation of CMV in positive recipients (estimated at 50–70%); 20% have symptomatic disease.
- Superinfection of a CMV-positive allograft in a CMV-positive recipient. CMV infection can be asymptomatic, or may have systemic manifestations such as fever, myalgias, and leukopenia. Other presentations include pneumonia, hepatitis, GI ulcerations, encephalitis, and transverse myelitis. CMV infection increases the risk of opportunistic infection and allograft rejection. Treatment of CMV disease with hyperimmune globulin (250 mg/kg IV on days 1, 3, 5, and 7) and ganciclovir (5 mg/kg IV every 12 hours for 14 days) is widely used, but is only proven to be effective in the bone marrow transplant population. Suggestions for CMV prophylaxis with high-dose oral acyclovir or ganciclovir and CMV hyperimmune globulin are given for the transplantation scenarios outlined in Table 83–1.

Infection in Bone Marrow Transplant Patients

These infections can be categorized into four clinical stages.

Pretransplant Stage. The risk of infection depends on chemotherapy exposure, degree and duration of neutropenia, previous infections, and disruption of mucosal barriers. When treated, infection in this period does not delay engraftment or alter success. Sixty percent of infections involve the skin, soft tissue, or urinary tract. Less common are sepsis (24%) and pneumonia (10%).

Pre-engraftment Period (Days 0–30). Previous total body irradiation increases the incidence of diarrhea, bacteremia, and reactivation of herpes zoster. Veno-occlusive disease of the liver occurs in 20–50% of patients, and can mimic bacterial and fungal infections.

- **Bacteremia** occurs in 15–50% of patients with staphylococci (*Staphylococcus aureus* and *S. epidermidis*) and *Corynebacterium* species infection. Most catheter-related infections (60–90%) respond to antibiotics.
- **Bacterial pneumonia** occurs in 35% of patients, with gram-negative bacilli (e.g., *Escherichia coli, Klebsiella* species) identified in 4–20% of cases.
- **Neutropenic typhilitis** has a mortality rate of 50–100%. Symptoms include nausea, vomiting, or abdominal pain. Radiographic features include bowel wall thickening, pneumatosis intestinalis, or a cecal mass. Urgent surgical resection and administration of broad-spectrum antibiotics covering enteric organisms are required.
- **Fungal infections** are common in the setting of prolonged neutropenia, steroid use, broad-spectrum antibiotic use, advanced age, and graft-versus-host disease (GVHD). *Candida* infection commonly occurs 2 weeks after transplant, with *C. albicans* the most common isolate and *C. tropicalis* occurring in 25% of cases. Prophylactic fluconazole decreases colonization and may reduce the incidence of invasive disease. Infection can be disseminated or localized to the GI or genitourinary tract. *Aspergillus* infection occurs in 4–20% of patients, with 1% risk per day after bone marrow transplantation and as great as 4% risk per day if neutropenia persists for more than 3 weeks.
- **Herpes simplex virus (HSV)** reactivation and clinical disease occur in 80% of seropositive patients. The maximal incidence is at 4 weeks after transplant. HSV-1 accounts for one-half of nonspecific oral lesions, with gingivostomatitis accounting for 85% of HSV-1 disease. Oropharyngeal infection is a risk factor for bacterial infection, HSV pneumonitis, and esophagitis. HSV-2 is less common, causing genital ulcer disease in 10–15% of patients.

Postengraftment Period (Days 30–100)

- **CMV infection,** defined by seroconversion or isolation, develops in as many as 50% of patients. It is fatal in 15–20%. Risk factors for CMV infection include being a

CMV-positive recipient or a CMV-negative recipient receiving unscreened blood products, advanced age, GVHD and total body irradiation. CMV pneumonitis occurs in 10–30% of allogeneic transplants, with a mortality rate approaching 80%. Open-lung biopsy is usually required for diagnosis, with positive BAL findings and CMV viremia indicating a population at risk. Treatment with CMV hyperimmune globulin and ganciclovir or foscarnet is required.

- **Viral pneumonia** can develop from adenovirus, influenza, parainfluenza, and respiratory syncytial virus.
- **Viral gastroenteritis** is caused by rotavirus and coxsackie virus. It has a mortality rate of as high as 50%.
- **Chronic disseminated candidiasis** (hepatosplenic candidiasis) develops in patients recovering from neutropenia. Symptoms include fever, abdominal pain, and elevated alkaline phosphatase level. Liver biopsy with culture and fungal stains is required for diagnosis. The treatment is amphotericin B.

Fourth Stage After Transplant (Days > 100). Viral infections, e.g., varicella zoster virus (VZV), occur in 40%, bacterial pulmonary infection in 33%, and fungal infections in 20% of recipients.

- **VZV infections** are usually caused by reactivation of latent virus. Risk factors for VZV infection include GVHD, previous diagnosis of lymphoma, and allogeneic transplantation. More than 85% of cases occur within the first year, with most occurring as localized herpes zoster. Herpes zoster can be prevented in recipients with a history of varicella infection with administration of parenteral acyclovir for 25–35 days followed by high-dose oral therapy for 6 months. Relapses are common once oral therapy is discontinued.
- **Bacterial upper respiratory tract infection** with encapsulated organisms commonly occurs in patients with chronic GVHD. Prophylaxis with biweekly trimethoprim-sulfamethoxazole (TMP-SMX) has been successful in preventing these infections.

Infections in Nonneutropenic Cancer Patients

Malignancy and its treatment results in many defects in host defenses, increasing susceptibility to infection.

Bacteremia in nongranulocytopenic patients is usually a consequence of malignant obstruction and is caused by gram-negative organisms. Relief of the obstruction along with 10 to 14 days of antibiotic therapy is required. *Streptococcus bovis* bacteremia is associated with carcinoma of the GI tract (especially the colon), and *Clostridium septicum* infection is associated with hematologic and intestinal malignancies.

Catheter-related infection is suggested when a catheter tip grows > 15 colony forming units/mL in the setting of bacteremia. The exit site and tunnel must be examined for tenderness, erythema, and purulent discharge. Cultures of the exit site and both peripheral and central venous catheter blood cultures are required. Vancomycin, which is effective against staphylococci, is usually initiated. An aminoglycoside or cephalosporin can be instituted in suspected gram-negative infections. Catheter removal is usually required in the setting of a tunnel infection, persistent bacteremia, or isolation of organisms such as *Acinetobacter* species, *Bacillus* species, or fungi.

Upper respiratory tract infections are common in cancer of the nasopharynx or maxillary sinus, and are often related to obstruction. Therapy includes relieving the obstruction and administering antibiotics effective against upper respiratory tract flora (e.g., ampicillin-clavulanic acid, cephalosporin, macrolide, or TMP-SMX). In chronic sinusitis, antibiotics effective against anaerobes and colonizing gram-negative bacilli are used. Treatment failures are usually secondary to persistent obstruction or fungal infection.

Pulmonary infiltrates in cancer patients can be categorized according to the temporal course and pattern of infiltrate. Bacterial pneumonia occurs acutely with focal infiltrates, fever, cough, and sputum production. Miliary tuberculosis, agents of atypical pneumonia (*Legionella pneumophila* and *Mycoplasma hominis*), PCP, and viral etiologies should be considered when diffuse infiltrates are present. Subacute focal infiltrates occur with fungi (e.g., *Cryptococcus* species), tuberculosis, or tumor recurrence. Subacute diffuse infiltrates are common with viral infections (VZV, CMV, adenovirus, or influenza), PCP, or noninfectious causes, such as radiation pneumonitis and lymphangitic carcinomatosis. PCP occurs with corticosteroid treatment, especially during tapering, chemotherapy, and thoracic radiotherapy. The clinical course is rapid, with fever, nonproductive cough, and bilateral interstitial or alveolar infiltrates. Patients should empirically be treated with TMP-SMX and erythromycin to cover atypical organisms until the etiology is determined.

Esophagitis is commonly seen in cancer patients with radiation- or chemotherapy-induced mucositis or strictures. *Candida* esophagitis sometimes responds to topical clotrimazole or nystatin, but usually requires oral ketoconazole, fluconazole, or low-dose parenteral amphotericin B. Esophageal biopsy to exclude CMV or HSV infection should be considered in resistant esophagitis.

Skin infections are common because cutaneous barriers are often breached in the critically ill patient. Skin breakdown caused by pressure or the effects of corticosteroids on skin integrity and ulcerated skin metastases are potential portals of entry. Perioral HSV caused by reactivated HSV-1 is common, and is effectively treated with acyclovir (200 mg PO 5 times daily). Localized VZV infections also occur. Aspiration or biopsy should be performed on skin lesions. Depending on the appearance of the specimens, they may be sent for viral, mycobacterial, and bacterial cultures, gram stain, Tzanck smear, potassium hydroxide preparation, or fungal fluorescent stains. For VZV, acyclovir (800 mg 5 times daily) is sufficient, but parenteral doses (10 mg/kg every 8 hours) should be used when there is associated disseminated disease. Acyclovir decreases the duration of symptoms, viral shedding, and the risk of dissemination.

CNS infection in the critically ill patient with cancer is often difficult to diagnose because of the use of narcotics and sedatives.

- Intraventricular shunt or Ommaya reservoir infection may cause headache, fever, persistent leukocytosis, meningismus, or a change in the level of consciousness. Cerebrospinal fluid (CSF) must be sent for gram stain and culture, determination of glucose and protein levels, and cell count with differential. Initial antimicrobial therapy includes vancomycin and ceftazidime or an aminoglycoside to provide coverage for staphylococci and gram-negative organisms. In patients who do not defervesce, removal of the device is required.
- Meningitis caused by *L. monocytogenes* usually has a subacute presentation, with low-grade fever, meningismus, CSF findings that include pleocytosis (usually with a predominance of neutrophils), gram-positive coccobacilli on gram stain, low glucose level, and elevated protein level. Treatment with ampicillin and an aminoglycoside is indicated.
- Cryptococcal meningitis is an indolent process that causes chronic headaches, low-grade fever, altered level of consciousness and, rarely, focal neurologic deficits. CSF studies show lymphocytic pleocytosis, elevated protein level, low glucose level, and cryptococcal antigen. Treatment with amphotericin B, with or without flucytosine, for 4–6 weeks is required.
- Viral encephalitis with HSV or VZV is associated with cognitive function or personality changes, seizures, low-grade fever, and CSF findings of mononuclear cells, reduced glucose level, and elevated protein level. VZV encephalitis is usually accompanied by cutaneous lesions. Electroencephalographic abnormalities in HSV encephalitis are localized to the temporal lobe. Treatment with parenteral acyclovir (10 mg/kg every 8 hours) is indicated.

Urinary tract infections are common with tumor obstruction or foreign bodies (e.g., urethral catheters, stents, nephrostomy tubes). Common organisms include *E. coli*, *Proteus* species, *Klebsiella* species, and *Enterococcus* species, as well as more resistant organisms, such as *Serratia* species, *Enterobacter* species, and *Pseudomonas* species. Relief of obstruction and antibiotics are required. Chronic suppressive antimicrobial therapy is indicated for infected foreign bodies. When *Candida* is isolated in a patient with a Foley catheter, the catheter should be removed and urine culture repeated. If the patient is at high risk of dissemination (e.g., diabetic, immunosuppressed) and the foreign body cannot be removed, fluconazole (200 mg daily for 3 days) or amphotericin B bladder irrigation can be given.

Infections in Neutropenic Patients

The frequency and severity of infection increase when the total granulocyte count decreases to less than 1000 mm^{-3}. The greatest risk of infection occurs with rapid declines and an absolute value of less than 250 mm^{-3}. Empiric antibiotics are initiated in febrile patients (temperature > 38.3°C) when the granulocyte count decreases to less than 750 mm^{-3}. The most common sites of infection are the alimentary tract, including the oropharynx, esophagus, and anorectal region; the respiratory tract, including the sinuses; and the skin, particularly at sites of vascular catheter insertion. The most common causes of infection are aerobic bacteria (staphylococci, *E. coli*, *Klebsiella* species, and *Enterobacter* species) arising from the host's endogenous flora and the hospital environment. Gram-positive bacteria, especially coagulase-negative staphylococci, have occurred with increasing frequency. In 80% of neutropenic patients, primary bacteremia results from endogenous microflora. Superinfection with fungi, especially *Candida* species, must be considered in patients who do not respond to antibacterial therapy.

Fever in the Neutropenic Patient. Fever may be the only sign of infection in the neutropenic patient. A detailed history, physical examination, and laboratory evaluation will show the source of infection in as many as 60% of febrile neutropenic patients. Routine tests should include complete blood count with differential, serum chemistry profile, urinalysis and culture, chest radiograph, two sets of blood cultures, and cultures from any accessible site suggestive of infection.

Empiric treatment with broad-spectrum antibiotics decreases the mortality rate, frequency of bacteremia, and incidence of clinically evident foci of infection. Historically, combination regimens were used to improve synergistic interaction and prevent the emergence of resistant organisms. Typical combination antimicrobial regimens for febrile neutropenic patients are:

- Ceftazidime plus an aminoglycoside (tobramycin, amikacin, or gentamicin).
- Antipseudomonal penicillin (e.g., piperacillin) plus an aminoglycoside.
- Two β-lactam antibiotics (e.g., piperacillin and ceftazidime).
- Aztreonam plus vancomycin.

No particular combination has clearly been shown to be superior. The choice should reflect the local resistance patterns in the hospital. Monotherapy is increasing in popularity because of the ease of administration, lower cost, and lower toxicity. Agents in use include ceftazidime and imipenem-cilastatin. After antibiotics are initiated, an endpoint (e.g., 48–72 hours) should be defined before the current regimen is modified. Patients may defervesce initially, but often fever recurs or a site of infection becomes obvious. In this setting, a list of antimicrobial modifications is given in Table 45–4 in the main text to guide therapy.

Patients who are persistently febrile after 4–7 days of antibiotic administration have a high risk of fungal infection. Empiric amphotericin B (0.5 mg/kg/day) may decrease the frequency and mortality rate of invasive fungal infections. Therapy should be continued until the neutropenia resolves. If fever continues, persistence or recrudescence of an infection is probable. More resistant fungi, including *Aspergillis fumigatus,* disseminated trichosporosis, or systemic fusariosis, must be considered. In this instance, the dose of amphotericin B is increased to 1–1.5 mg/kg/day. There is some evidence that itraconazole is useful for invasive aspergillosis.

Patients with unexplained fever while taking antibiotics can be divided into two categories. In low-risk patients, the granulocyte count recovers within 1 week of antibiotic administration. Generally, antibiotics should be given until the granulocyte count is greater than 500 mm^{-3}. In high-risk febrile patients, granulocytopenia occurs for more than 7 days. Some patients defervesce while taking broad-spectrum antibiotics. If antibiotics are discontinued on day 7, many patients experience fever recrudescence within 3 days, with organisms remaining sensitive to the original antibiotics. Therefore, antibiotic administration should be maintained for at least 14 days in this setting. If fever remains, antibiotics should be continued.

Suggested Readings

Armstrong D. Empiric therapy for the immunocompromised host. *Rev Infect Dis* 1991;13(suppl 9):S763–S769.

Reviews various empiric antimicrobial options for immunocompromised hosts.
Lee JW, Pizzo PA. Management of the cancer patient with fever and prolonged neutropenia. *Hematol Oncol Clin North Am* 1993;7:937–960.
Excellent review of antimicrobial management of infection in cancer patients.
Milliken ST, Powles RL. Antifungal prophylaxis in bone marrow transplantation. *Rev Infect Dis* 1990;12(suppl 3):S374–S379.
Discusses risk of fungal disease in bone marrow transplantation and use of antifungal prophylaxis.
Pauw BE, Derenski SC, Feld R, et al. Ceftazidime compared with piperacillin and tobramycin for the empiric treatment of fever in neutropenic patients with cancer. *Ann Intern Med* 1994;120:834–844.
Evaluation of monotherapy for febrile neutropenic patients.
Sable CA, Donowitz GR. Infections in bone marrow transplant recipients. *Clin Infect Dis* 1994;18:273–285.
Detailed review of infectious complications in bone marrow transplant patients.
Steinberg RI, Baugham RP, Dohn MN, et al. Utility of bronchoalveolar lavage in assessing pneumonia in immunosuppressed renal transplant recipients. *Am J Med* 1993;95:358–364.
Discusses bronchoalveolar lavage fluid analysis and the effect on antimicrobial management.
Walsh TJ, Lee JW, Roilides E, et al. Recent progress and current problems in management of invasive fungal infections in patients with neoplastic disease. *Curr Opin Oncol* 1992;4:647–655.
Discusses management of fungal infections in patients with malignancy.

CHAPTER 84

Human Immunodeficiency Virus Infection and Acquired Immune Deficiency Syndrome

(See Chapter 50)

Jack Fuhrer

Acquired immune deficiency syndrome (AIDS) is of pandemic proportions in the United States. Although it has primarily occurred in homosexual or bisexual men and IV drug users, it is becoming more prevalent through heterosexual transmission, particularly in women of child-bearing age, with a resultant growth in pediatric cases. It is characterized by profound immunodeficiency secondary to infection with the human immunodeficiency virus (HIV).

The spectrum of HIV infection ranges from the asymptomatic state to advanced disease manifested by opportunistic infections, aggressive malignancies, dementia, and severe wasting. Shortly after initial infection, many patients experience an acute mononucleosis-like illness known as acute retroviral syndrome. After this initial phase, most patients become asymptomatic, with the possible exception of having chronic lymphadenopathy. This phase of infection can last 7–10 years. The next phase, characterized by chronic fever, weight loss, malaise, and evidence of oral candidiasis, oral hairy leukoplakia, or shingles, has been referred to as symptomatic HIV infection (or AIDS-related complex). Eventually, full-blown AIDS develops.

Epidemiology

Transmission of HIV occurs by sexual contact with infected partners; direct exposure to contaminated blood, blood products, or tissues; and vertical transmission from infected mothers to their infants. Nonsexual transmission in the household and in the nonmedical workplace is unproven. The rate of transmission from an infected patient to a health care worker through accidental percutaneous needle exposure or mucocutaneous exposure to infected blood is estimated at 0.3%. The risk of transmitting HIV infection from an infected health care worker to a patient is estimated at between 1 in 42,000 and 1 in 420,000.

Clinical Syndromes

Respiratory. Respiratory insufficiency, generally secondary to pneumonia, is the most common reason for ICU treatment of the patient with AIDS. Whereas acute bacterial pneumonia occurs, the most common cause of pneumonia in patients with AIDS is *Pneumocystis carinii.*

***P. carinii* Pneumonia**

- **History:** subacute to chronic onset of fever; dry, hacking cough; progressive dyspnea; and atypical chest pain.
- **Physical examination:** few rales or clear lung fields.
- **Laboratory findings:** arterial blood gas studies may show respiratory alkalosis and hypoxemia; serum lactate dehydrogenase level is usually elevated.
- **Chest radiograph** typically shows bilateral diffuse infiltrates.
- **Diagnosis** is made from special stains of induced sputum (50–75% sensitivity), from bronchoalveolar lavage (BAL) fluid (> 90% sensitivity), or by open-lung biopsy (criterion standard).

- **Therapy** of choice is trimethaprim-sulfamethoxazole (TMP-SMX) 15–20 mg/kg (TMP portion) IV or PO in 3–4 divided doses for 2–3 weeks. Alternatives are pentamidine 4 mg/kg IV daily; trimethoprim 15–20 mg/kg in 3–4 divided doses PO plus dapsone 100 mg PO daily for mild to moderate disease; atovaquone 750 mg PO three times a day for mild to moderate disease; or trimetrexate 45 mg/m^2 IV daily plus leucovorin 20 mg/m^2 every 6 hours for moderate to severe disease in patients who cannot tolerate TMP-SMX or for whom this therapy is unsuccessful. Steroids (prednisone 40 mg PO twice daily, tapered over 3 weeks) are added for patients with abnormal oxygenation.

Cytomegalovirus Pneumonia

- **History and physical examination** are similar to those for *P. carinii* pneumonia (PCP); patients are likely to have extrapulmonary disease, particularly retinitis.
- **Laboratory findings:** arterial blood gas studies may show mild to severe hypoxemia.
- **Chest radiograph** is the same as for PCP.
- **Diagnosis** is empiric if the patient has evidence of extrapulmonary disease or biopsy evidence of cytomegalovirus (CMV) inclusions or CMV antigen.
- **Therapy** is ganciclovir 5 mg/kg IV twice daily for 2 to 3 weeks or foscarnet 60 mg/kg IV every 8 hours. Neither of these agents has proven efficacy for pneumonitis in patients with AIDS.

Tuberculosis

- **History** of subacute to chronic onset of fever, usually productive cough, weight loss.
- **Physical examination** may show evidence of consolidation.
- **Chest radiograph** can show a range of abnormalities, from upper lobe cavitary disease to reticulonodular infiltrates.
- **Diagnosis** is by detecting acid-fast bacilli on smears and culture of *Mycobacterium tuberculosis* from sputum, BAL fluid, or biopsy specimen. Positive acid-fast bacillus smear findings may be secondary to atypical mycobacteria, e.g., *M. avium* complex (MAC).
- **Therapy.** Because of the increasing number of cases of multidrug-resistant tuberculosis, a four-drug regimen is currently recommended, e.g., isoniazid 300 mg PO daily, rifampin 600 mg PO daily, pyrazinamide 25 mg/kg PO daily, and ethambutol 15–25 mg/kg PO daily. Addition of streptomycin may be advisable in some localities.

Bacterial Pneumonia

- **History** usually is of acute onset of fever with productive cough.
- **Physical examination** may show evidence of pulmonary consolidation.
- **Chest radiograph** typically shows infiltrates of bronchopneumonia.
- **Diagnosis** is by sputum gram stain and culture or by protected bronchial brush for culture.
- **Therapy** should be based on whether pneumonia is nosocomial versus community acquired and on sputum evaluation. If pneumonia is community acquired, coverage for *Streptococcus pneumoniae* and *Haemophilus influenzae* should be considered.

Fungal pneumonia may occur secondary to *Aspergillus* species, *Cryptococcus* species, *Coccidiomyces* species, *Histoplasma* species, *Blastomyces* species, and other fungi in patients with AIDS (see Chapter 76 in this book and Chapters 33 and 34 in the main text).

Cardiac. Most patients with AIDS are young, so coronary artery disease is not commonly encountered. However, cardiomyopathy in patients with AIDS is well described, and may be secondary to infection with an opportunistic pathogen (e.g., *Toxoplasma gondii* or MAC), infiltrating malignancy (e.g., lymphoma), HIV infection itself, or the immune response to HIV. In addition, there have been reports of drug-induced cardiomyopathy, e.g., zidovudine (AZT). Large pericardial effusions leading to pericardial tamponade have been observed. The approach to the management of these cardiac complications should be individualized and based on the overall functional status of the patient, the ability of the clinician to make a definitive diagnosis, and the ability to treat the underlying etiology.

GI. The most common GI complications in patients with AIDS are esophageal candidiasis and severe chronic diarrhea, but these rarely lead to ICU treatment.

Pancreatitis. In addition to alcohol-induced and gallstone-induced pancreatitis, a number of etiologies should be considered in patients with AIDS. These include drugs such as pentamidine, dideoxyinosine (DDI), and sulfa drugs; opportunistic infections such as CMV and MAC; malignancies such as lymphoma causing biliary obstruction; and severe hypertriglyceridemia. The approach to treating these patients should be geared to eliminating potential drug toxicities and determining a potentially treatable cause.

Perforated viscus can occur secondary to an opportunistic infection of the small bowel or colon or an infiltrating malignancy, e.g., lymphoma with possible obstruction. Colonic tuberculosis or CMV infection can result in a perforated viscus and acute abdomen. Treatment requires surgical intervention as well as treatment of the underlying cause.

GI Hemorrhage. In addition to peptic ulcer disease, patients with AIDS commonly have ulcerations secondary to opportunistic infections, such as CMV and herpes simplex virus. These infections usually lead to abdominal pain, but can result in GI bleeding. Although rarely a cause of symptoms, GI Kaposi's sarcoma (a highly vascular malignancy) occasionally leads to hemorrhage. Treatment is based on the etiology.

Renal dysfunction in AIDS is primarily caused by prerenal azotemia, drug-induced nephropathy (e.g., amphotericin B or foscarnet), and HIV-induced nephropathy. HIV-induced nephropathy usually causes focal segmental glomerulosclerosis; however, other potentially treatable nephropathies (e.g., minimal change disease) have been reported. The long-term benefit of chronic dialysis for patients with AIDS is in question, but deserves consideration.

Hematologic. Anemia, neutropenia, and thrombocytopenia, alone or in combination, are common in HIV-infected patients. Anemia is usually chronic or drug induced (e.g., a result of AZT use). Neutropenia can similarly be drug induced (e.g., AZT, ganciclovir, or TMP-SMX), but infection of the bone marrow (e.g., MAC) or infiltration of the bone marrow by malignancy (e.g., lymphoma) should be considered. Thrombocytopenia can occur secondary to drug toxicity (e.g., ganciclovir, TMP-SMX), secondary to an opportunistic infection (e.g., MAC), or secondary to peripheral destruction (e.g., idiopathic thrombocytopenic purpura) and defective megakaryocyte function. Therapy is based on the underlying etiology.

Neurologic. Although the neurologic complications of AIDS include dementia, progressive multifocal encephalopathy, and peripheral neuropathies, special attention to chronic meningoencephalitis and to CNS mass lesions will be addressed.

Chronic Meningitis

- **History** of headache and fever is common.
- **Physical examination** may show cranial nerve abnormalities; meningeal signs may be absent.
- **Differential diagnosis** includes cryptococcosis, tuberculosis, histoplasmosis, coccidiomycosis, and B cell lymphoma.
- **Laboratory tests** include cerebrospinal fluid analysis for glucose and protein, white blood cell count and differential, gram stain, acid-fast bacillus smear and culture, cryptococcal antigen, India ink stain, fungal culture, and cytology, and serum analysis for cryptococcal antigen, antibody to histoplasma, and coccidiomyces.
- **Therapy** is directed at the etiology. For cryptococcal

meningitis, amphotericin B with or without 5-fluorocytosine is given for at least 2 weeks, followed by fluconazole 200 mg PO daily. (See the chapters on fungal infections for other regimens.)

Tuberculous Meningitis. See the drug regimen above for tuberculosis pneumonia. Adjunctive steroids also may be used.

CNS Mass Lesion. Symptoms include focal neurologic deficit, seizure, and change in mental status.

- **History** may include headache, seizure, mental status changes, or focal neurologic deficits.
- **Differential diagnosis** includes *Toxoplasma gondii* and B cell lymphoma. Tuberculoma, cryptococcoma, and bacterial brain abscess are possibilities, but are much less common.
- **Imaging studies** should include either computed tomography or magnetic resonance scanning of the head.
- **Laboratory tests** include *Toxoplasma* serology, brain biopsy, cerebrospinal fluid analysis (if lumbar puncture is not contraindicated), as for meningitis.
- **Therapy:** Empiric treatment with sulfadiazine and pyrimethamine for toxoplasmosis should be instituted pending *Toxoplasma* serology. If the patient is *Toxoplasma* seropositive, pyrimethamine 200 mg PO is given as a loading dose, then 50–75 mg PO daily; sulfadiazine 6–8 g PO daily is given in 4 divided doses; and folinic acid 10 mg PO is given daily, or clindamycin 600 mg PO is given every 6 hours. Adjunctive steroids are considered. A clinical or neuroradiologic response should occur within 2 to 3 weeks; if there is no response or deterioration occurs, brain biopsy should be considered. If the patient is *Toxoplasma* seronegative, brain biopsy is considered, and therapy is based on the biopsy findings.

Endocrine. Both hypoglycemia and hyperglycemia are associated with previous pentamidine therapy for PCP. Severe hyperglycemia may require close monitoring as well as IV insulin. Lifelong insulin therapy may be required because pentamidine can permanently destroy islet cells. Recently, hyperglycemia has been attributed to megestrol used to stimulate weight gain in patients with AIDS. Patients with megestrol-induced hyperglycemia may have normalization of the blood glucose level after discontinuation of megestrol.

Suggested Readings

Acierno LJ. Cardiac complications of acquired immunodeficiency syndrome (AIDS): A review. *J Am Coll Cardiol* 1989;13:1144–1154. *(94 references.)*

Grinspoon SK, Bilezikian JP. HIV disease and the endocrine system. *N Engl J Med* 1992;327:1360–1365.

Meredith T, Acierno LJ. Pulmonary complications of acquired immunodeficiency syndrome. *Heart Lung* 1988;17:173–178.

Rao TK, Friedman EA, Nicastri AD. The types of renal disease in the acquired immunodeficiency syndrome. *N Engl J Med* 1987;316:1062–1068.

Of 750 hospital-treated patients with acquired immune deficiency syndrome, 10% needed evaluation for renal disorders. Authors discuss potential role of hemodialysis in patients with acquired immune deficiency syndrome and renal failure.

Rosen MJ, DePalo VA. Outcome of intensive care for patients with AIDS. *Crit Care Clin* 1993;9:107–114.

Adjunctive use of corticosteroids for treatment of P. carinii *pneumonia is probably a major factor resulting in improved survival of ICU patients with acquired immune deficiency syndrome.*

Wachter RM, Luce JM, Hopewell PC. Critical care of patients with AIDS. *JAMA* 1992;267:541–547.

From their review of literature, the authors conclude that the provision of critical care for P. carinii *pneumonia and respiratory failure specifically or acquired immune deficiency syndrome generally cannot be considered futile (105 references).*

Zon L, Groopman J. Hematologic manifestations of the human immunodeficiency virus. *Semin Hematol* 1988;25:208.

Poisoning and Overdose

CHAPTER 85

Antidepressant Drug Overdose

(See Chapter 146)

Michael J. Ruffing and James A. Kruse

Cyclic Antidepressants

(see Table 85–1)

Most cyclic antidepressants (CAs) inhibit the reuptake of biogenic amines (norepinephrine, serotonin, and dopamine); alter the responsiveness of adrenergic and serotonergic receptor sites; block muscarinic acetylcholine, histamine (H_1 and H_2), and α-adrenergic receptors; and exhibit quinidine-like effects. Other important pharmacologic points include the following:

- Absorption is usually rapid and complete, but bioavailability is low because of first-pass metabolism. Peak levels occur in 2 to 8 hours, but may be delayed by 12 hours or more in toxic ingestions.
- The volume of distribution (Vd) of CAs is large (10–50 L/kg), and there is substantial protein binding (85–95%).
- Metabolism is largely by microsomal enzymes in the liver, with excretion of glucuronide conjugates in the urine. A small fraction undergoes enterohepatic recirculation. The elimination half-life is variable (10–200 hr); at toxic levels, nonlinear kinetics have been shown.

Clinical Features. Manifestations of CA overdoses are usually apparent within a few hours after ingestion. Although there are differences in side-effect profiles, acute toxicity is generally similar among the various agents. Exceptions are the newer serotonergic CAs (fluoxetine, sertraline, and paroxetine), which are probably less toxic. Manifestations include:

- **Anticholinergic effects,** such as tachycardia, mydriasis, blurred vision, dry mouth, hyperpyrexia, dizziness, urinary retention, decreased GI motility, agitation, CNS excitation.
- **Cardiovascular effects,** such as hypotension, supraventricular tachycardia, quinidine-like effects, atrioventricular block, right bundle branch block, ventricular tachycardia, torsades de pointes, ventricular fibrilla-

TABLE 85-1

CYCLIC ANTIDEPRESSANTS AND MONOAMINE OXIDASE INHIBITORS AVAILABLE IN THE UNITED STATES

Cyclic antidepressants	
Unicyclic	Bupropion
Bicyclic	Fluoxetine
Tricyclic	Amitriptyline, desipramine, doxepin, imipramine, nortriptyline, protriptyline, trimipramine
Tetracyclic	Maprotiline
Dibenzoxazepine	Amoxapine
Triazolpyridine	Trazodone
Other structures	Paroxetine, sertraline
Monoamine oxidase inhibitors	
Hydrazine	Phenelzine
Nonhydrazine	Isocarboxazid, tranylcypromine

tion, idioventricular rhythms, electromechanical dissociation, asystole.

- **CNS toxicity,** such as mild sedation, confusion, agitation, delirium, hallucinations, myoclonic jerks, dystonic reactions, seizures, coma.
- **Pulmonary complications,** such as pulmonary edema, adult respiratory distress syndrome, or aspiration pneumonitis. These complications occur in one-third of serious intoxications.

Quinidine-like effects include ST and T wave changes, PR and QT interval prolongation, increased QRS duration, and right-axis deviation. Severe hypotension can often occur because of quinidine-like myocardial depression and α-adrenergic blockade. Transient hypertension can occur as a result of inhibition of norepinephrine uptake. Seizures are more common with amoxapine, maprotiline, and probably bupropion.

Treatment. IV access and cardiac monitoring should be established early. Administration of naloxone, thiamine, and dextrose should be routine for patients with altered consciousness. An adequate airway and, if necessary, ventilatory support, should be ensured. A 12-lead ECG, chest radiograph, arterial blood gas determinations, and serum electrolyte levels should be obtained. Because quantitative CA serum levels do not correlate well with toxicity, they are rarely necessary.

- Decontamination should be done by gastric lavage with a large (36–40 Fr) orogastric tube. Activated charcoal (1 g/kg; 50–100 g) with a cathartic (sorbitol, magnesium sulfate, or magnesium citrate) should be administered as soon as feasible. If bowel sounds are present, charcoal administration should be repeated with one-half this dose, without cathartic, every 2–4 hours for one or more additional doses. Ipecac should be avoided because CNS depression may develop and lead to aspiration.

- Sinus tachycardia requires no treatment unless it is symptomatic. Other supraventricular tachycardia may be treated by alkalinization with parenterally administered $NaHCO_3$ or hyperventilation, aiming for an arterial blood pH of 7.45–7.55. If necessary, vagal maneuvers, β-blocking agents, or calcium channel blocking agents may be used cautiously.
- Ventricular tachydysrhythmias should also be treated with alkalinization. Lidocaine and cardioversion are the initial treatments of choice, followed by overdrive pacing and bretylium. Class Ia, Ic, and III antiarrhythmics are generally contraindicated because they have quinidine-like effects. Phenytoin and β-blocking agents may be useful, but the potential negative inotropic and proarrhythmic effects preclude their routine use.
- Second-degree, Mobitz type II, and third-degree atrioventricular blocks should be managed with alkalinization and temporary pacing. Atropine is generally ineffective because the block is low in the atrioventricular node.
- Hypotension should be treated with volume expansion as well as alkalinization. If refractory, α-adrenergic agents such as norepinephrine, phenylephrine, or high-dose dopamine should be used and titrated to the response. Dobutamine and digoxin may improve severe myocardial depression, but hypotension and proarrhythmic effects limit their use to refractory cases.
- Seizures are generally short (< 2 minutes). Diazepam should be given, followed by phenobarbital. Phenytoin may be used, but it is ineffective in many cases, and has potential adverse effects.
- Physostigmine (0.5–2.0 mg IV) may reverse the anticholinergic effects of CNS depression and supraventricular dysrhythmias, but can cause cholinergic crisis, bradycardia, and seizures. Therefore, if physostigmine is used at all, it should be reserved for refractory cases.

Sinus tachycardia, QRS interval prolongation, and right-axis deviation are often harbingers of potentially serious complications, such as seizures and dysrhythmias. Acidosis increases the free fraction of CAs and enhances cardiovascular toxicity. Hyponatremia and hyperkalemia can worsen cardiac conduction, and therefore should be corrected. Patients without major symptoms (dysrhythmias; QRS >100 ms; seizures; decreased blood pressure, respiratory rate, or level of consciousness) who are improving clinically and have bowel sounds 6 hours after admission are unlikely to have serious toxicity and may not require

ICU admission. Hemodialysis and hemoperfusion remove only a minimal amount of the total body load.

Monoamine Oxidase Inhibitors

(see Table 85–1)

Monoamine oxidase inhibitors (MAOIs) irreversibly inhibit the degradation of the enzyme monoamine oxidase, resulting in the accumulation of intraneural catecholamines (norepinephrine, epinephrine, dopamine) and serotonin. These drugs are well absorbed, highly protein bound (> 90%), and metabolized by the liver. Signs and symptoms of overdose are delayed for 6–12 hours and manifest as a combination of sympathomimetic and sympatholytic actions. Peak effects occur in 24–48 hours.

Clinical Features

- Initially, stimulation of the autonomic nervous system occurs as agitation, tachycardia, hypertonicity, hyperreflexia, mydriasis, hyperpyrexia, nausea, diaphoresis, convulsions, altered mentation, and hypertension.
- CNS and cardiovascular depression may follow, leading to coma, hypotension, and cardiac arrest.
- Other complications include disseminated intravascular coagulation, intracerebral hemorrhage, acute renal failure, and pulmonary edema.

Treatment

- Initial management requires gut decontamination (gastric lavage and charcoal administration) and initiation of supportive care.
- Severe hypertension is best managed initially with nitroprusside or phentolamine (depending on the patient's status). Methyldopa and β-blocking agents are generally avoided.
- Hyperthermia may be managed with acetaminophen and external cooling. Dantrolene (2.5 mg/kg every 6 hours) may reverse malignant hyperthermia.
- Seizures and muscle rigidity can be treated with diazepam and phenytoin. Phenobarbital may be added for refractory seizures.
- Hypotension should be managed with fluid resuscitation and α-adrenergic agonists, such as norepinephrine.
- Forced acid diuresis, dialysis, and hemoperfusion offer little benefit.

The action of agents such as theophylline, caffeine, hypoglycemic agents, barbiturates, cocaine, codeine, meperidine, antihistamines, anticholinergics, alcohol, and phenothiazines may be enhanced when administered with MAOIs. All patients should be observed for symptoms for at least 24 hours after ingestion. Full recovery depends in part on the regeneration of monoamine oxidase, which may take several weeks. Agents with indirect-acting sympathomimetic actions (e.g., amphetamines, phenylpropanolamine, ephedrine), opiates, tyramine-rich diets (e.g., aged cheese, yeast, smoked or pickled meat and fish, red wine), and CAs (particularly fluoxetine) can enhance the toxicity of MAOIs, and should be avoided for at least 1–2 weeks after ingestion.

Suggested Readings

Boehnert M, Lovejoy F. Value of the QRS duration versus the serum drug level in predicting seizures and ventricular arrhythmias after an acute overdose of tricyclic antidepressants. *N Engl J Med* 1985; 313:474–479.

Callaham M. Epidemiology of fatal tricyclic antidepressant ingestion: Implications for management. *Ann Emerg Med* 1985;14:1–9.
Discusses signs and symptoms as well as a disposition algorithm.

Frommer D, Kulig K, Marx J, et al. Tricyclic antidepressant overdose: A review. *JAMA* 1987;257:521–526.

Krishel S, Jackimczyk K. Cyclic antidepressants, lithium, and neuroleptic agents: Pharmacology and toxicology. *Emerg Med Clin North Am* 1991;9:53–86.

Linden C, Rumack B, Strehlke C. Monoamine oxidase inhibitor overdose. *Ann Emerg Med* 1984;13:1137–1144.
Case report and review of the various stages and treatment of monoamine oxidase inhibitor overdose.

CHAPTER 86

Cocaine Intoxication

(See Chapter 146)

David B. Levy and James E. Cisek

Cocaine is widely abused, both in its crystalline form (cocaine hydrochloride) and in its solid alkaloid form (freebase or crack cocaine). It is a potent CNS stimulant and sympathomimetic agent with local anesthetic and vasoconstrictor effects. Its systemic adverse actions are similar to those of amphetamines.

Pharmacokinetics and Mechanism of Action

Cocaine is used illicitly by nasal insufflation (snorting), oral ingestion, or IV injection. In addition, the freebase form (but not the hydrochloride form) can be smoked.

Higher-peak blood levels are achieved by smoking than by nasal insufflation. It is rapidly and well absorbed from the nasal mucosa, in the GI tract, and through the alveoli when smoked. The onset of effect occurs within seconds to minutes.

Cocaine is rapidly hydrolyzed by plasma cholinesterase to ecgonine methyl ester and by nonenzymatic hydrolysis to benzoylecgonine. A small fraction is demethylated to norcocaine. The longer half-life of these metabolites allows detection by urine testing for 2 days or more after cocaine use. The local anesthetic effects of cocaine are mediated by blockade of fast sodium channels. Sympathomimetic effects occur through centrally mediated α- and β-adrenergic stimulation and through blockade of the reuptake of catecholamines. Street cocaine is often impure, containing cocaine substitutes or adulterants such as local anesthetics (e.g., lidocaine, tetracaine, benzocaine), sugars (e.g., lactose, mannitol), stimulants (e.g., phenylpropanolamine, caffeine, amphetamine, ephedrine), toxins (e.g., strychnine, quinine), inert substances (e.g., talc, cornstarch), and other substances (e.g., heroin, phencyclidine, flour, plaster of Paris, aspirin, acetaminophen).

Clinical Manifestations

CNS signs and symptoms include:

- Mental status changes, such as anxiety, restlessness, euphoria, delirium, hyperactivity, psychosis, syncope, and coma. True hallucinations are uncommon.
- Seizures, which are generally brief and self-limited.
- Subarachnoid and intracerebral hemorrhage.
- Miscellaneous effects, including headache, transient ischemic attacks, cerebral infarction, CNS vasculitis, and cerebral atrophy.

Cardiovascular effects are common. They include:

- Hypertension as a result of peripheral vasoconstriction.
- Tachydysrhythmias, e.g., sinus tachycardia and ventricular tachycardia.
- Myocardial ischemia and infarction, which may be caused by coronary vasospasm, increased myocardial oxygen demand, intimal smooth muscle proliferation, and premature coronary atherosclerosis.
- Depressed systolic function as a result of myocarditis, cardiomyopathy, or contraction band necrosis.
- Aortic dissection and rupture.
- Endocarditis and valvular heart disease, usually as a consequence of IV administration.

Other adverse effects include:

- Pulmonary effects, particularly respiratory distress caused by pulmonary edema, pulmonary hemorrhage, hypersensitivity pneumonitis, bronchiolitis obliterans, or barotrauma.

- GI effects, which may consist of mesenteric ischemia and infarction as well as bowel obstruction in "body packers" (see below).
- Obstetric complications, such as preterm labor, abruptio placentae, chorioamnionitis, spontaneous abortion, and stillbirth.
- Adverse prenatal effects, including teratogenesis, growth retardation, microcephaly, myelomeningocele, agenesis of the corpus callosum, and other congenital anomalies.
- Miscellaneous effects, including rhabdomyolysis, hyperthermia, disseminated intravascular coagulation, metabolic acidosis, renal failure, and hepatotoxicity.

Ongoing drug absorption can occur as a result of body packing, i.e., swallowing cocaine-filled packets to avoid detection during smuggling. Severe manifestations can occur if the packets rupture in the GI tract. Mechanisms of death in acute cocaine intoxication include hyperthermia, myocardial infarction, CNS hemorrhage, and status epilepticus (SE) leading to respiratory arrest and ventricular arrhythmias.

Treatment

Cocaine has no specific antagonist or antidote; therefore, supportive measures are the mainstays of therapy. Intractable seizures, hyperthermia, respiratory arrest, and tachydysrhythmias are the greatest dangers from cocaine intoxication. Close monitoring for toxic manifestations is imperative, including frequent monitoring of vital signs and continuous ECG monitoring in patients with severe intoxication. A 12-lead ECG reading should also be examined. IV access should be secured. Urine toxicologic assay is performed to confirm the presence of cocaine metabolites. Routine hematologic, coagulation, and serum chemistry studies, including analysis of serum creatine phosphokinase levels, should be performed. Arterial blood gas analysis, computed tomography of the brain, and other special diagnostic studies may be indicated in selected cases. Therapeutic priorities in unstable patients include:

- Ensuring a patent airway and adequate oxygenation and ventilation. Early endotracheal intubation and mechanical ventilation may be essential, particularly in patients with SE or incipient respiratory failure.
- Gastric evacuation is considered for cases of recent oral consumption; activated charcoal should be administered.
- Body packing may be confirmed by plain or contrast-

enhanced abdominal radiography. Specific treatment includes administration of activated charcoal and whole gut lavage. Endoscopic or surgical removal has been used, but its role remains controversial.

- Mild hypertension can sometimes be treated with benzodiazepines, but severe hypertension necessitates the use of antihypertensive drugs. Previously, β-adrenergic blocking agents, such as propranolol, have been recommended. However, they may potentiate cocaine-induced hypertension by blocking β_2-mediated vasodilation and allowing unopposed α-adrenergic stimulation.
- Myocardial ischemia and infarction should be treated in the standard way, although thrombolytic therapy may be contraindicated because of hypertension. β-Adrenergic blocking agents could potentiate cocaine-induced coronary vasospasm. However, labetolol, with its combined α- and β-adrenergic antagonist effects, may be useful.
- Supraventricular tachydysrhythmias may respond to benzodiazepines alone, although IV calcium channel blocking agents or labetolol can also be used if supportive measures do not control heart rate.
- Ventricular tachycardia may respond to intravenous labetolol or magnesium sulfate. Lidocaine has some effects that are similar to those of cocaine but can probably be safely used, especially if a patient is not severely hyperadrenergic.
- Hypotension is treated initially with isotonic fluid loading. If necessary, norepinephrine can be used if hypotension persists despite adequate volume loading.
- Seizures are managed with conventional anticonvulsant drug therapy (IV benzodiazepines followed by barbiturates or phenytoin).
- Hyperthermia may require external cooling measures or other methods of reducing body temperature.

Benzodiazepines may ameliorate several toxic manifestations, including seizures, hypertension, and tachycardia. They reduce mortality rates in animal models of cocaine intoxication.

Suggested Readings

Goldfrank LR, Hoffman RS. The cardiovascular effects of cocaine. *Ann Emerg Med* 1991;20:165–175.

Reviews pathophysiology of cardiovascular manifestations of cocaine intoxication (143 references).

Lange RA, Cigarro RG, Flores ED, et al. Potentiation of cocaine-induced coronary vasoconstriction by beta-adrenergic blockade. *Ann Intern Med* 1990;112:897–903.

Spivey WH, Euerle B. Neurologic complications of cocaine abuse. *Ann Emerg Med* 1990;19:1422–1428.

Reviews historical aspects, pharmacology (local anesthetic action and neurotransmitter activity), patterns of use, and neurologic complications (including

pre- and postnatal exposure). Briefly covers treatment of neurologic complications (81 references).
VanDette JM, Cornish LA. Medical complications of illicit cocaine use. *Clin Pharmacol* 1989;8:401–411.
Reviews chemistry, pharmacology, pharmacokinetics, and medical complications of illicit cocaine use (107 references).
Warner EA. Cocaine abuse. *Ann Intern Med* 1993;119:226–235.
General comprehensive review describing complications of cocaine use (144 references).

CHAPTER 87

Sedative, Hypnotic, and Opioid Drug Overdose

(See Chapter 146)

Michael T. Imperato

Sedative, hypnotic, and opioid drugs include:

- **Benzodiazepines,** e.g., alprazolam, chlordiazepoxide, clonazepam, clorazepate, diazepam, flurazepam, halazepam, lorazepam, midazolam, oxazepam, prazepam, temazepam, triazolam.
- **Barbiturates,** e.g., amobarbital, barbital, butabarbital, pentobarbital, phenobarbital, secobarbital.
- **Opiates and opioids,** e.g., codeine, diphenoxylate, fentanyl, heroin, hydrocodone, hydromorphone, levorphanol, meperidine, methadone, morphine, opium, oxycodone, oxymorphone, paregoric, pentazocine, propoxyphene, sufentanil.
- **Miscellaneous drugs,** e.g., chloral hydrate, ethchlorvynol, glutethimide, meprobamate, methaqualone, paraldehyde.

Ethanol can also be considered a sedative drug (see Chapter 62 in the main text and Chapter 93 in this book).

Clinical Manifestations

The effects of these drugs include sedation, sleep induction (hypnosis, narcosis), and generalized CNS depression. The most common symptom of overdose involving these agents is depressed mentation. In severe cases, the patient may be in a deep coma, and there may be associated respiratory or cardiovascular depression. Hypothermia can occur. Opiate and opioid narcotics can cause miosis. Noncardiogenic pulmonary edema has been described, particularly with opiates and ethchlorvynol. Metabolites of oral meperidine and propoxyphene may cause seizures and cardiac dysrhythmias, respectively.

Management of Acute Ingestions

Management involves the following steps:

- Ensuring a patent airway and adequate ventilation. Endotracheal intubation and mechanical ventilation may be required.
- Monitoring the patient closely (frequent assessment of vital signs, continuous ECG monitoring, etc.).
- Instituting supportive measures (general ICU care, supplemental oxygen, correction of electrolyte abnormalities, pharmacologic support of blood pressure, prophylaxis against venous thrombosis, etc.), as necessary.
- Considering IV administration of concentrated dextrose, thiamine, naloxone, and flumazenil in patients with depressed consciousness.
- Administering activated charcoal (1 g/kg) enterally every 4–6 hours for several doses. A cathartic (e.g., sorbitol or magnesium citrate) is given with the first dose only. Charcoal dosing is not repeated if there is evidence of decreased gut motility (e.g., absent bowel sounds or abdominal distension).
- Excluding other causes of sensorial depression or coma.
- Identifying coingestants (e.g., ethanol, tricyclic antidepressants, acetaminophen).
- Avoiding extracorporeal elimination (e.g., hemodialysis or hemoperfusion) of these agents because this intervention has little role in treatment.

Naloxone for Opiate and Opioid Overdose

- If respiratory depression is present, naloxone 2 mg IV push is administered. If IV access cannot be secured, naloxone can be given IM, subcutaneously, sublingually, or through an endotracheal tube.
- If the patient has a depressed sensorium, but respiration is not impaired, naloxone can be given in smaller doses, starting with 0.4 mg IV push. If there is no response or only a partial response, an additional 0.8 mg is administered.
- Establishment of an adequate airway and ventilation takes precedence over administration of naloxone.
- A positive response may include improvement in level of consciousness, pupillary dilation, increase in respira-

tory rate and depth, and increase in heart rate and blood pressure.

- Naloxone may precipitate acute withdrawal in an addict (e.g., diaphoresis, agitation, body aches, lacrimation, piloerection, nausea, vomiting, abdominal pain, diarrhea). A reasonable goal is to titrate the naloxone dose to reverse respiratory depression, yet minimize withdrawal effects.
- Because the half-life of IV naloxone is only 20–60 minutes, repeat doses may be required.
- Naloxone may be given by continuous IV infusion. This method of administration is especially useful in the treatment of longer-acting opioids, such as methadone or propoxyphene. The amount of naloxone required per hour is approximately two-thirds of the dose that was initially required to reverse respiratory depression. For example, if 2 mg IV was required initially, an infusion rate of 1.3 mg/hr can be initiated. The infusion can be maintained for 12 hours or more in the ICU. A dose of 10 mg naloxone in 250 mL normal saline at 25 mL/hr delivers a dose of 1 mg/hr.

Flumazenil for Benzodiazepine Overdose. Flumazenil is a relatively new agent that antagonizes the actions of benzodiazepines on the CNS. It acts as a competitive inhibitor at benzodiazepine receptor sites and is a specific antidote for this class of drugs. Flumazenil should be used with caution in the emergency department and ICU setting because:

- In patients with concurrent cyclic antidepressant poisoning, seizures may be precipitated by reversal of the anticonvulsive effects of the benzodiazepine.
- Withdrawal seizures may be precipitated in a patient with previously unrecognized benzodiazepine dependence.
- Benzodiazepine dependence can be established after only a few days of high-dose sedation as is sometimes used in ICU settings.

To treat suspected benzodiazepine overdose, 0.2 mg flumazenil is given by slow IV injection. If no response is seen after 30 seconds, an additional 0.3-mg dose can be given. Further doses of 0.5 mg can be given over a period of 30 seconds at 1-minute intervals, to a cumulative dose of 3 mg.

Withdrawal Reactions

Tolerance develops in chronic users of these drugs, i.e., higher doses are required to achieve a given level of effect. Cessation of drug use or marked dose reduction in a chronic user results in withdrawal symptoms, which may range from mild to life threatening. These withdrawal symptoms are similar to those that occur in chronic ethanol users, and are characterized by:

- A typical onset occurring 1–5 days after the last dose.
- Duration ranging from approximately 2 days to 2 weeks.
- Manifestations that, in mild cases, may include tachypnea, tachycardia, tremors, irritability, insomnia, and apprehension.
- Manifestations that, in severe cases, may include delirium, hyperthermia, seizures, psychosis, and death.

Many sedative-hypnotic drugs, including ethanol, are cross-reactive with one another. Withdrawal reactions can be prevented by prompt administration of another sedative-hypnotic agent (see Chapter 93 in this book). Benzodiazepines and phenobarbital are commonly used in the ICU setting for this purpose. Patients who have developed tolerance to sedative-hypnotic agents can be weaned off by progressive dose reduction over several days to weeks under close medical supervision. Withdrawal seizures can occur if blood levels of the sedative-hypnotic drug decrease too quickly. Seizures should be treated by administration of additional sedative-hypnotic doses. Phenytoin is frequently ineffective in controlling withdrawal seizures.

Suggested Readings

Augenstein WL, ed. Emergency aspects of drug abuse. *Emerg Med Clin North Am* 1990;8:467–730.

Issue contains 16 articles related to drug abuse and overdose, including reviews on cocaine, opioids, adulterants, substance withdrawal, and general topics in clinical toxicology.

Challoner KR, McCarron MM, Newton EJ. Pentazocine (Talwin®) intoxication: Report of 57 cases. *J Emerg Med* 1990;8:67–74.

Case series of patients who had overdoses of the opioid agonist-antagonist pentazocine. Mixed drug ingestions were common. One patient had opioid-induced noncardiogenic pulmonary edema, and one patient died.

Höjer J, Baehrendtz S, Gustafsson L. Benzodiazepine poisoning: Experience of 702 admissions to an intensive care unit during a 14 year period. *J Intern Med* 1989;226:117–122.

Of 702 patients who had benzodiazepine overdose, 144 ingested benzodiazepine alone, 200 ingested benzodiazepine combined with ethanol, and 358 ingested benzodiazepine combined with various other drugs. The mortality rate was low (5 patients), but 10% of patients had hypotension, aspiration pneumonia, pressure injuries, or other complications.

Merigian KS, Woodard M, Hedges JR, et al. Prospective evaluation of gastric emptying in the self-poisoned patient. *Am J Emerg Med* 1990;8:479–483.

Large-scale study comparing gastric emptying followed by activated charcoal administration with administration of activated charcoal alone. Supports management of selected patients with acute overdose without gastric evacuation.

Utecht MJ, Stone AF, McCarron MM. Heroin body packers. *J Emerg Med* 1993;11:33–40.

Describes 14 patients who smuggled between 2 and 112 packages containing heroin within their bodies by swallowing or rectal insertion, usually with the heroin wrapped in latex gloves or condoms. There were two complications: one case of bowel obstruction requiring laparotomy and one case of heroin intoxication with noncardiogenic pulmonary edema.

Winkler E, Almog S, Kriger D, et al. Use of flumazenil in the diagnosis and treatment of patients with coma of unknown etiology. *Crit Care Med* 1993;21:538–542.

Describes use of flumazenil in cases of coma, excluding metabolic, neurologic, or traumatic causes. Most patients responded to flumazenil. Concludes that flumazenil is safe and effective in diagnosis of benzodiazepine-induced coma.

Yell RP. Ethchlorvinol overdose. *Am J Emerg Med* 1990;8:246–250.

Thorough review of effects and treatment of ethchlorvinol intoxication.

CHAPTER 88

Salicylate Toxicity

(See Chapter 146)

James E. Cisek
and James A. Kruse

Salicylates are available in a variety of product formulations other than aspirin tablets. Many over-the-counter analgesic and other preparations are combinations of agents that may include aspirin (acetylsalicylic acid) or nonacetylated salicylic acid derivatives. For example, each milliliter of bismuth subsalicylate (Pepto-Bismol®) contains 8.8 mg salicylate. Methylsalicylate (oil of wintergreen) is the most potent salicylate formulation by strength. One teaspoon contains 7 g salicylate. It is well absorbed orally and across intact epidermis. Many external liniments (e.g., methylsalicylate [Ben-Gay®]) contain methylsalicylate. Concentrated topical salicylates used as keratolytic agents can also cause systemic toxicity if they are applied to a large area of skin.

Clinical toxicity from aspirin can occur after acute ingestion of 150 mg/kg. Mild to moderate reactions occur with ingestion of 150–300 mg/kg, and serious reactions occur with ingestion of more than 300 mg/kg. These guidelines do not apply to chronic intoxication, which may be more serious. Simple observation of the patient for the presence and severity of symptoms is useful in evaluating the severity of intoxication. When the time of ingestion is known, the Done nomogram (Figure 88–1) can often be used initially to assess the severity of acute intoxication. However, this

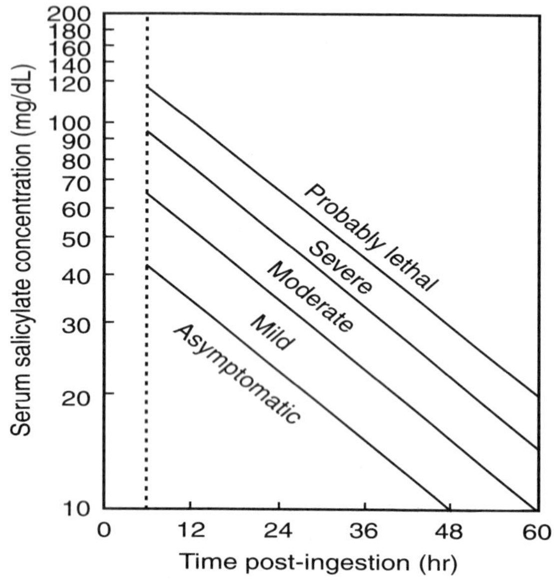

Figure 88–1. The Done nomogram for early assessment of clinical severity in salicylate intoxication. Serum levels obtained less than 6 hours after ingestion may not reflect the severity of the intoxication. (Redrawn from Done AK. Salicylate intoxication: Significance of measurement of salicylate in blood in cases of acute ingestion. *Pediatrics* 1960;26:800–807, with permission.)

nomogram may be invalid in mixed ingestions involving aspirin, in ingestions of enteric-coated preparations, and in cases of chronic overdosage.

Pharmacokinetics

Most salicylates are poorly absorbed in the stomach; absorption occurs best in the small bowel. Enteric-coated formulations may take 12–24 hours to reach maximal effect. Aspirin is rapidly deacetylated to salicylic acid, which is highly bound to albumin and has a volume of distribution of approximately 0.2 L/kg. Many drugs (e.g., coumarin) may compete for albumin binding sites, and certain disease states (e.g., cirrhosis, nephrosis) may be associated with low albumin levels or decreased protein binding. Any condition that increases the free fraction of plasma salicylate increases toxicity. Elimination kinetics change from first order to zero order within the therapeutic range. Small changes in dosage may therefore be associated with large changes in serum levels.

Alkaline urine traps salicylate anions in the renal tubule,

mitigating tubular reabsorption and promoting excretion. This activity is the basis for alkalinization therapy, which can be moderately effective at increasing renal salicylate clearance if renal function is normal.

Signs and Symptoms

Serum salicylate concentration greater than 30 mg/dL is usually associated with toxic manifestations. These may include:

- **Central nervous system:** tinnitus, decreased auditory acuity, tachypnea, irritability, delirium, hallucinations, coma, seizures, cerebral edema.
- **GI:** nausea, vomiting, epigastric pain, GI bleeding, and perforation. Nonacetylated formulations are associated with less GI and platelet toxicity.
- **Metabolic:** metabolic acidosis, hypokalemia, hypoglycemia, hypocalcemia, hyperpyrexia.
- **Hepatic:** hepatocellular necrosis, inhibition of synthesis of vitamin K–dependent clotting factors.
- **Renal:** impaired glomerular filtration, oliguria, interstitial nephritis, acute tubular necrosis.
- **Pulmonary:** respiratory alkalosis, noncardiogenic pulmonary edema. The risk of the latter is increased in smokers, patients with metabolic acidosis, and patients with chronic intoxication.
- **Hematologic:** hemorrhagic diathesis caused by impaired platelet function (persisting for the life span of the platelet), coagulopathy.

Treatment of Toxicity

General Principles

- Serum is obtained for quantitative salicylate assay, but initiation of treatment is not delayed pending the results. Vital signs are monitored frequently. Cardiac monitoring and early endotracheal intubation can be employed if necessary.
- Concentrated glucose solution is administered if there are any mental status abnormalities. Serum glucose concentration results are not reliable because the brain glucose level may be low despite normal serum glucose levels.
- Intravascular volume deficits are restored rapidly, and an attempt is made to achieve a urine output of > 1 mL/kg/hr.
- Gastric lavage should be performed after acute ingestions.
- Activated charcoal is administered at an initial dose of 1 g/kg. Subsequent dosing of activated charcoal (0.5

g/kg every 6 hours) may be used, but is probably of marginal value in further hastening elimination.

- IV sodium bicarbonate is administered to alkalinize the urine. Urine pH should be titrated to 7.5 or higher, if possible. Arterial blood pH level is monitored to avoid inducing significant alkalemia (i.e., arterial pH > 7.5). To prevent the development of severe hypokalemia, urinary alkalinization therapy requires a normal serum potassium level, careful monitoring of this electrolyte and, in most cases, potassium supplementation.
- Ionized calcium is monitored and supplemented as necessary. IV calcium should be administered if there is symptomatic hypocalcemia or associated hemodynamic instability.
- Enteric-coated preparations result in peak serum levels 12–24 hours after ingestion. All forms of salicylates have the potential for formation of concretions in the GI tract, with slow release and prolonged high serum levels. Therefore, serum salicylates concentration should be monitored serially until the level decreases.
- Oxygenation and respiratory function are monitored carefully because noncardiogenic pulmonary edema can occur and may be exacerbated by IV fluids and administration of sodium bicarbonate. Pulmonary artery catheterization may be necessary in some cases.
- Seizures can usually be controlled by rapidly correcting hypoglycemia, electrolyte, and acid–base disturbances; by treating hyperthermia; and by administering anticonvulsants (e.g., benzodiazepines, phenytoin, barbiturates).
- Patients are at risk for GI bleeding and should receive H_2-blocking agents or other prophylactic measures. Fresh-frozen plasma and vitamin K may be required to reverse coagulopathy.

Extracorporeal Elimination of Salicylates. Hemodialysis effectively increases the clearance of salicylate and improves fluid and electrolyte imbalances. Specific clinical indications include seizures, hemodynamic instability, pulmonary edema, intractable acidosis, and severe fluid and electrolyte imbalance. Serum salicylate concentration of 100 mg/dL or greater as a result of a single acute ingestion indicates the need for hemodialysis. Chronic intoxication is often associated with profound symptoms at relatively low serum levels. The use of hemodialysis for chronic intoxication is best guided by the above clinical parameters. Although charcoal hemoperfusion effectively removes salicylates from the blood, hemodialysis is preferred because it can also correct fluid, electrolyte, and acid–base abnormalities. Hemodialysis is continued until symptoms resolve and the serum salicylate level is less than 10 mg/dL.

Suggested Readings

Chapman BJ, Proudfoot AT. Adult salicylate poisoning: Deaths and outcome in patients with high plasma salicylate concentrations. *Quart J Med* 1989;72:699–707.

Descriptive review covering large number of salicylate-poisoned patients, with emphasis on clinical findings, treatment, and outcome.

Dugandzic RM, Tierney MG, Dickinson GE, et al. Evaluation of the validity of the Done nomogram in the management of acute salicylate intoxication. *Ann Emerg Med* 1989;8:1186–1190.

Reviews limitations of Done nomogram.

Raschke R, Arnold-Capell PA, Richeson R, et al. Refractory hypoglycemia secondary to topical salicylate intoxication. *Arch Intern Med* 1991;151:591–593.

Case report of patient with type II diabetes who had hypoglycemia as a result of salicylate intoxication from overuse of salicylate-containing topical cream. The hypoglycemia was severe and refractory to glucose supplementation.

Temple A. Acute and chronic effects of aspirin toxicity and their treatment. *Arch Intern Med* 1981;141:364–369.

Review of acute and chronic salicylate intoxication.

Thurston JH, Pollack PG, Warren SK, et al. Reduced brain glucose with normal plasma glucose level in salicylate poisoning. *J Clin Invest* 1970;49:2139–2145.

Describes animal model demonstrating occurrence of reduced brain glucose level despite normal plasma glucose level.

CHAPTER 89

Acetaminophen Poisoning

(See Chapter 146)

David B. Levy and James A. Kruse

Acetaminophen (also known as paracetamol) is a widely used drug found in many over-the-counter preparations, prescription analgesics, and cold remedies. It acts as an antipyretic and analgesic for mild to moderate pain. As a sole ingestant, serious toxicity is uncommon, but it can lead to serious morbidity and death. In overdoses involving coingested opioid substances (e.g., propoxyphene or codeine), the mild and nonspecific symptoms of acetaminophen toxicity may be masked by the more dramatic acute effects of the opioid, thus resulting in delayed recognition of toxicity and delayed initiation of antidotal treatment.

Toxicity

Acetaminophen is rapidly absorbed, reaching peak therapeutic levels in 30 minutes to 2 hours. It has a mean duration of effect of 4 hours. Delayed absorption can occur if it is taken with drugs that delay gastric emptying or, in massive overdoses, as a result of the formation of drug bezoars. Although the usual plasma half-life is approximately 2 hours, it may increase to 10 hours or more after an overdose. Approximately 5% of an ingested dose of acetaminophen is excreted unchanged by the kidneys. Most of the rest is metabolized to sulfate and glucuronide conjugates that are nontoxic and readily excreted by the kidney. The remainder is metabolized by the cytochrome P-450 mixed-function oxidase pathway in the liver to a putative, highly reactive intermediate compound known as *N*-acetyl-*p*-benzoquinone imine (NAPQI). This compound is a potent intracellular toxin, but normally it is promptly inactivated by conjugation to the sulfhydryl group of glutathione present within the hepatocytes. After an overdose, toxic quantities of acetaminophen are suddenly presented to the liver for metabolism, the sulfate and glucuronide conjugation enzymes become saturated, large amounts of NAPQI are produced, and glutathione stores become depleted. Additional glutathione cannot be synthesized rapidly enough to detoxify the high NAPQI load, and hepatic necrosis ensues. Renal damage may occur by the same mechanism. The degree of hepatic damage does not correlate well with the amount of drug ingested because of individual differences in metabolism. The risk of toxicity is increased if there is preexisting depletion of glutathione stores, as occurs in malnutrition or chronic alcoholism, or if there is preexisting increased cytochrome P-450 activity, as occurs with long-term use of drugs that induce these enzymes (e.g., phenobarbital, phenytoin, or ethanol). For these reasons, alcoholics are at higher risk of hepatic damage from acetaminophen. Toxicity sometimes occurs in these individuals, even at therapeutic doses.

In adults, some degree of toxicity is generally expected with an acute ingestion of more than 7.5 g. Fatalities typically involve ingestions of more than 13 g.

Clinical Manifestations

The clinical features of toxicity are reasonably uniform. They have been divided into four phases.

- **Phase 1** occurs from the time of ingestion to approximately 24 hours after ingestion. Symptoms and signs may include anorexia, nausea, vomiting, pallor, and diaphoresis. There may be no symptoms during this phase if acetaminophen is the sole ingestant, regardless of the dose. Alterations in sensorium suggest concomitant overdose with a narcotic or other sedating drug.
- **Phase 2** typically begins 24–48 hours after ingestion. It is characterized by the resolution of first-phase signs and symptoms. Right upper quadrant pain and tender-

ness can occur, but the patient may feel well during this phase. However, there is biochemical evidence of developing hepatic necrosis, i.e., increasing levels of serum transaminase and lactate dehydrogenase. In mild cases, these enzyme elevations resolve without further progression to the next phase.

- **Phase 3** typically begins 72–96 hours after ingestion. It is characterized by the development of the clinical entity known as fulminant hepatic failure. Serum transaminase activity increases to high levels (in some cases to > 20,000 IU/L), serum bilirubin level increases, and prothrombin time increases. Overt liver failure develops and may be accompanied by a variety of sequelae, such as hypoglycemia; coagulopathy; GI bleeding; hepatic encephalopathy or coma; cerebral edema; myocardial, pancreatic, or renal dysfunction; sepsis; and death. The duration and severity of this phase depends on the degree of hepatic necrosis and the severity of secondary complications.
- **Phase 4** occurs in patients who survive phase 3. It is marked by resolution of the hepatic damage. Normalization of liver function can take days to weeks, depending on the extent of hepatic necrosis.

Smaller ingestions (typically < 15 g) may not progress beyond phase 1 or phase 2. Fatalities occur during phase 3 and are caused by complications of fulminant hepatic failure.

Treatment

Management of patients with suspected acetaminophen overdose begins with the same supportive care used in any toxic ingestion. This treatment includes establishing IV access and performing ECG monitoring in unstable patients. If the suspected ingestion occurred within 2 hours of presentation, gastric decontamination with syrup of ipecac or gastric lavage should be performed, particularly if serum levels are not immediately available. However, syrup of ipecac may cause prolonged vomiting, which could hinder absorption of the antidote *N*-acetylcysteine (NAC). Activated charcoal effectively binds acetaminophen in the GI tract and decreases acetaminophen absorption, but controversy exists over its use because the charcoal also adsorbs the antidote NAC. In addition, charcoal may cause nausea and vomiting, further inhibiting NAC absorption. This issue continues to be studied and debated. It is essential to confirm or exclude coingestants because additional therapy may be required if other drugs are involved.

NAC is the antidote of choice for acetaminophen toxicity. It readily enters the hepatocytes and either is converted to active glutathione or inactivates NAPQI. The standard

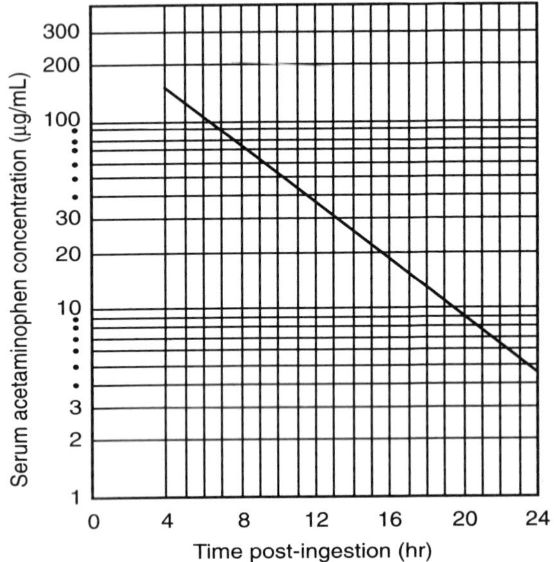

Figure 89–1. The Rumack-Matthew nomogram, used for predicting the risk of hepatotoxicity and the need for NAC administration in patients with acetaminophen poisoning. Patients with values shown above the diagonal line require *N*-acetylcysteine therapy. (Modified from Rumack BH, Matthew H. Acetaminophen poisoning and toxicity. *Pediatrics* 1975;55:871–876. Reproduced with permission of *Pediatrics*.)

method of estimating severity and deciding whether NAC treatment is indicated is based on determination of the serum acetaminophen level 4 hours after ingestion and application of the Rumack-Matthew nomogram (Figure 89–1). Serum assays obtained less than 4 hours after ingestion provide unreliable estimates of the peak acetaminophen level. Without treatment, nearly two-thirds of patients with a serum acetaminophen concentration greater than the treatment level indicated by the nomogram have significant liver damage (aspartate aminotransferase level > 1000 IU/L), and approximately 5% die. General indications for NAC administration are:

- Serum concentrations in the possibly toxic range, according to the Rumack-Matthew nomogram (Figure 89–1), e.g., > 150 μg/mL 4 hours after ingestion.
- Known or suspected ingestion of ≥ 7.5 g acetaminophen (in an adult) within 24 hours of presentation and inability to obtain serum acetaminophen assay results immediately.
- Presentation > 24 hours after ingestion, with measur-

able acetaminophen levels or biochemical evidence of hepatic injury (i.e., elevated liver enzyme levels).

The loading dose is 140 mg/kg as a 10% (1.4 mL/kg) or 20% (0.7 mL/kg) solution diluted to an approximately 5% final solution in fruit juice or soda. Seventeen maintenance doses of 70 mg/kg are given every 4 hours, in the same concentration and dilution. If NAC was initiated while the result of a serum acetaminophen level (obtained within 4–24 hours after ingestion) was pending, and the serum level is in the nontoxic range on the nomogram, maintenance doses can be discontinued.

Adverse effects of NAC include nausea, vomiting, diarrhea, and allergic reactions. Vomiting is a problematic side effect because it can interfere with absorption of the antidote. Parenteral (IV) acetylcysteine may be available through some poison control centers, but it has not been approved for general use in the United States. If vomiting occurs, metoclopramide 1 mg/kg IV or IM may be given 30 minutes before each dose of NAC. Prochlorperazine 10 mg IV and diphenhydramine 25–50 mg IV may be added to this regimen. Droperidol (1.25–2.5 mg IV, given 30–60 minutes before each dose, has also been used. Administration of NAC through a nasogastric or nasoduodenal tube may be helpful.

NAC should be given as soon as possible because its efficacy decreases progressively 8–16 hours after ingestion. The situation is complicated when the time and quantity of ingestion are not known. In some cases, the elicited information is incorrect. Several clinical studies suggest that NAC is ineffective if it is administered more than 24 hours after ingestion. However, newer information suggests that NAC may have therapeutic value, even in patients with established acetaminophen-induced hepatic failure. Postulated mechanisms include the free radical–scavenging properties of NAC and its positive effects on oxygen delivery.

Serum glucose levels should be monitored serially. If hypoglycemia is suspected, dextrose should be administered by rapid infusion (e.g., 25 g dextrose as a 50% solution given IV over 1–2 minutes) while serum glucose results are awaited. For patients who enter phases 2 and 3, other complications of evolving hepatic failure should be anticipated, and appropriate therapeutic measures initiated as needed.

Suggested Readings

Black M. Hepatotoxic and hepatoprotective potential of histamine (H_2)-receptor antagonists. *Am J Med* 1987;83(suppl 6A):68–75.

Reviews effects of H_2-receptor blocking agents on acetaminophen metabolism.

Keays R, Harrison PM, Wendon JA, et al. Intravenous acetylcysteine in paracetamol induced fulminant hepatic failure: A prospective controlled trial. *Br Med J* 1991;303:1026–1029.

Demonstrates efficacy of IV N-acetylcysteine in improving survival in group of patients with established acetaminophen-induced hepatic failure.

Lewis RK, Paloucek FP. Assessment and treatment of acetaminophen overdose. *Clin Pharmacol* 1991;10:765–774.

Review article covering hepatic and nonhepatic mechanisms of toxicity, clinical features and assessment of toxicity, and several supportive care controversies, including the issue of co-administration of activated charcoal and acetylcysteine, various route and dose regimens for acetylcysteine, and use of cimetadine (53 references).

Kumar S, Rex DK. Failure of physicians to recognize acetaminophen hepatotoxicity in chronic alcoholics. *Arch Intern Med* 1991;151:1189–1191.

Case series of hospitalized patients in whom acetaminophen-induced liver damage went unrecognized. Points out that this situation likely occurred because patients did not show obvious signs of overdose, as with suicide-associated ingestions; acetaminophen levels may be zero or within therapeutic range in these patients; and syndrome may be confused with alcoholic hepatitis, viral hepatitis, or hepatic necrosis caused by circulatory shock.

Rumack BH, Peterson RC, Koch CG, et al. Acetaminophen overdose: 662 cases with evaluation of oral acetylcysteine treatment. *Arch Intern Med* 1981;141:380–385.

Early study applying the Rumack-Matthew nomogram. Significantly greater efficacy was achieved when acetylcysteine was administered within 16 hours of ingestion compared with administration 16–24 hours postingestion.

Smilkstein MJ, Knapp GL, Kulig KW, et al. Efficacy of oral N-acetylcysteine in the treatment of acetaminophen overdose. Analysis of the National Multicenter Study (1976–1985). *N Engl J Med* 1988; 319:1557–1562.

Of 11,195 cases of suspected acetaminophen overdose in this study, 2540 patients were treated with a course of N-acetylcysteine. There were 11 deaths among patients receiving N-acetylcysteine, but no deaths among those receiving N-acetylcysteine within 16 hours of ingestion.

CHAPTER 90

Lithium Toxicity

(See Chapter 146)

James E. Cisek

Pharmacokinetics

Lithium crosses the cellular membrane slowly, accounting for the delay in therapeutic benefit. With lithium intoxication, there is a similar delay in redistribution out of the brain, accounting for the slow clinical improvement despite low serum levels. The therapeutic serum concentration ranges from 0.6–1.4 mmol/L. The volume of distribution of lithium is 0.6 L/kg. Elimination is through the kidney. Lithium is filtered in the glomerulus, and approximately 80% is reabsorbed in the proximal tubule. Excretion is decreased in sodium-depleted states and in patients with renal insufficiency. Thus, any underlying disease associated with sodium depletion or the concurrent use of thiazide diuretics will predispose to toxicity.

Signs and Symptoms

Fatigue, lethargy, weakness, intention tremor, disturbances in concentration and memory, cutaneous reactions, and certain other manifestations can occur, even at therapeutic serum levels. At toxic levels, a wide variety of signs and symptoms can occur, including:

- **CNS:** tremor, hyperreflexia, myoclonus, seizures, slurred speech, visual disturbances, ataxia, choreoathetosis, confusion, lethargy, coma, malignant neuroleptic syndrome.
- **Cardiovascular:** sinus node dysfunction, intraventricular conduction defects, U waves, T wave inversion, sinus bradycardia, ventricular dysrhythmias, hypotension.
- **GI:** anorexia, nausea, vomiting, diarrhea, excessive salivation, abdominal pain.
- **Renal:** nephrogenic diabetes insipidus, nephrotic syndrome, renal failure.
- **Metabolic:** hypothyroidism, hypercalcemia, hyperglycemia.
- **Teratogenesis:** potential tricuspid valve abnormalities, Ebstein's anomaly, neonatal hypothyroidism, hypotonia.

General Principles of Treatment

- Cardiac monitoring is used; and early intubation may be considered.
- Serum lithium level and routine laboratory assays are obtained, including serum electrolytes, glucose, urea nitrogen, and creatinine levels.
- Whole-gut lavage is initiated with polyethylene glycol solution (GoLytely®) 40 mL/kg/hr (1–2 L/hr for an adult of average size). Bowel sounds must be present. Lithium is not adsorbed by activated charcoal.
- Fluid and sodium deficits are replaced, and diuresis of 1–2 mL/kg/hr is promoted with IV saline.

Clinical improvement is usually slow because intracellular lithium must cross cell membranes and be eliminated by the kidney. Long-term toxicity generally responds more slowly than acute ingestion.

Hemodialysis

Hemodialysis effectively removes lithium from the blood. It is generally recommended in cases of moderate to severe intoxication. This category includes patients with a serum lithium level higher than 3.5–4 mmol/L, regardless of symptoms; patients with underlying renal insufficiency; and unstable patients. Peritoneal dialysis is only one-third as efficient as hemodialysis for clearing lithium. Dialysis may be necessary for serum levels of 2.0–4.0 mmol/L if renal elimination is impaired. This condition can be assessed by obtaining two or more serum lithium levels 3 hours apart and plotting the log of drug concentration versus time. Dialysis should be considered if linear extrapolation to a concentration of 0.6 mmol/L shows a corresponding elimination time of more than 36 hours. Once initiated, dialysis should be continued until the serum lithium level is less than 1 mmol/L. Serum concentrations may rebound 6–12 hours after dialysis is discontinued, and repeated dialysis may be necessary.

Suggested Readings

Amdisen A. Clinical features and management of lithium poisoning. *Med Toxicol Adverse Drug Exp* 1988;3:18–32.
(76 references).

Groleau G, Barish R, Tso E, et al. Lithium intoxication: Manifestations and management. *Am J Emerg Med* 1987;5:527–532.
Report of two cases showing role of predisposing factors and drug interactions, plus review of pathophysiology, manifestations, and approaches to treatment of lithium intoxication (39 references).

Kelleher SP, Raciti A, Arbeit LA. Reduced or absent serum anion gap as a marker of severe lithium carbonate intoxication. *Arch Intern Med* 1986;146:1839–1840.

Describes two patients with lithium intoxication who had decreased anion gap, and explains mechanisms of this potential diagnostic clue.

Simard M, Gumbiner B, Lee A, et al. Lithium carbonate intoxication: A case report and review of the literature. *Arch Intern Med* 1989;149:36–46.

Excellent comprehensive review (208 references).

CHAPTER 91

Cardiac Glycoside Toxicity

(See Chapter 146)

James E. Cisek

Digoxin is the most commonly prescribed cardiac glycoside in the United States. The clinical toxicity of all cardiac glycosides is similar. Ingestion of plants containing cardiac glycosides (e.g., foxglove, oleander, and lily of the valley) can also result in clinical toxicity. Although the minimal lethal dose in humans is not well established, the mortality rate is approximately 50% in patients with serum digoxin concentrations greater than 6 ng/mL.

Digoxin is 25% protein bound to alpha-1-glycoprotein, has a large volume of distribution (6 L/kg in adults), and has a half-life of approximately 36 hours. The kidney excretes approximately 70% of digoxin unchanged. On the other hand, digitoxin is metabolized by the liver and has a half-life of approximately 5 days.

Signs and Symptoms

- **Cardiac:** accelerated atrial rhythms, with second-degree atrioventricular block; accelerated junctional rhythm, with or without underlying atrial fibrillation; bradycardia; first-, second-, or third-degree heart block; premature ventricular contractions; bigeminy; ventricular tachycardia; ventricular fibrillation; asystole.
- **CNS:** fatigue, malaise, confusion, hallucinations, blurred vision, color perceptual changes, seeing haloes around sources of light.
- **GI:** anorexia, nausea, vomiting, diarrhea, abdominal pain.
- **Metabolic:** electrolyte disturbances, particularly hyperkalemia.

Dysrhythmias are the most common cardiac manifestation, and nearly any rhythm disturbance can occur.

Factors Predisposing to Toxicity

A number of diseases, metabolic disorders, and drugs increase the susceptibility to toxicity, including:

- **Underlying cardiovascular disease,** particularly infiltrative myocardial diseases such as amyloidosis.
- **Other diseases,** including chronic pulmonary disease, renal insufficiency, and hypothyroidism.
- **Acid–base disturbances,** if accompanied by either alkalemia or severe acidemia.
- **Electrolyte disturbances,** including hypokalemia, hypomagnesemia, and hypercalcemia.
- **Drugs:** antiarrhythmics (e.g., quinidine, amiodarone); calcium channel blocking agents; catecholamines; steroids and nonsteroidal anti-inflammatory drugs; diuretics (e.g., spironolactone, triamterene); antibiotics (e.g., erythromycin or tetracycline).

Plasma Concentrations of Cardiac Glycosides

Serum levels of digoxin cannot be interpreted fully until at least 4 hours after acute ingestion. Correlating clinical symptoms with serum levels is difficult because toxicity can occur with serum levels that are within the therapeutic range. However, most patients with toxic signs have levels greater than 2 ng/mL. A circulating digoxin-like immunoreactive substance can cause an artifactual increase in the serum digoxin level. This endogenous material is present in the blood of neonates, seriously ill older infants, pregnant women, and patients with a variety of underlying diseases, including hepatic and cardiac failure, but especially renal failure. Serum digoxin levels in these clinical circumstances may therefore be difficult to interpret. The clinical significance of this substance is unknown. Hyperbilirubinemia and spironolactone use may also spuriously elevate serum digoxin levels.

Treatment of Toxicity

General Principles

- Serum digoxin and potassium levels are obtained.
- Gastric lavage is performed after acute ingestion.
- Activated charcoal is administered at a dose of 1 g/kg.
- Fluid, electrolyte, and acid–base disturbances, particularly hypokalemia or hyperkalemia, are addressed.
- Continuous ECG monitoring is essential.

- Bradydysrhythmias are treated with atropine or temporary pacing by transvenous or transcutaneous methods; isoproterenol may precipitate dysrhythmias.
- Lidocaine or phenytoin is useful for treating ventricular dysrhythmias; magnesium sulfate may also be effective.
- Antiarrhythmics that prolong PR, QRS, and QT intervals should be avoided (e.g., procainamide, quinidine).
- Calcium channel and β-adrenergic blocking agents may have additive adverse effects on cardiac conduction.
- Calcium administration may worsen cardiac toxicity.

Because digitoxin undergoes enterohepatic recirculation, GI excretion of this cardiac glycoside is hastened by enteral administration of the binding agents cholestyramine and colestipol. Repeated doses of activated charcoal may have similar utility.

Hemodialysis is ineffective in enhancing elimination, but may be necessary if there is refractory hyperkalemia.

Cardiac Glycoside-Specific Antibodies (Digibind®). These Fab antibody fragments reverse toxicity by binding to digoxin in the extracellular fluid, causing a decrease in free extracellular drug concentration. This effect promotes the release of digoxin from receptor sites by mass action. Indications include severe intractable rhythm disturbances and hyperkalemia (serum potassium concentration > 5.5 mmol/L). Each vial of glycoside-specific antibody contains 40 mg Fab fragments, which will bind 0.6 mg digoxin or digitoxin. Each vial costs approximately $200 (US). Dose calculation is based on total body load of cardiac glycoside. Total body load can be determined with the following formula:

$$\text{Body load} = \frac{\text{Serum digoxin concentration} \times 5.6 \times \text{Body weight}}{1000}$$

where body load is expressed in milligrams, serum digoxin concentration is expressed in nanograms per milliliter, and body weight is expressed in kilograms. Alternatively, the total body load can be determined by the following formula:

$$\text{Body load} = \text{Number of tablets ingested} \times \text{Milligrams per tablet} \times 0.8$$

The coefficient 0.8 is deleted from the above equation if the ingestion involves digoxin elixer, a liquid capsule digoxin preparation (Lanoxicaps®), or digitoxin. The number of required vials may then be calculated as:

$$\text{Number of vials} = \frac{\text{Body load}}{0.6}$$

The drug is administered through a 0.22-μm/filter over 30 minutes or by bolus infusion, according to the clinical stability of the patient. Potential adverse effects include exacerbation of congestive heart failure, accelerated ventricular rate in patients with atrial fibrillation or flutter, hypokalemia, and allergic reactions. Before administration, a plan should be established for the management of accelerated ventricular rate if it occurs. Skin testing has been conventionally recommended before administration of antibody fragments, but is probably unnecessary in patients at low risk for an allergic reaction. The total serum glycoside level may increase dramatically after treatment, but it does not reflect the clinical state of intoxication. Therefore, serum levels are uninterpretable after administration of antibody fragments. In patients with renal failure, recurrent toxicity is possible 1 week or more after treatment because of degradation of the digoxin–Fab complexes.

Suggested Readings

Bismuth C, Gaultier M, Como F, et al. Hyperkalemia in acute digitalis poisoning: Prognostic significance and therapeutic implications. *Clin Toxicol* 1973;6:153–162.
Assessment of clinical importance of hyperkalemia in digitalis intoxication.

Morris RG, Frewin DB, Saccoia NC, et al. Interference from digoxin-like immunoreactive substances in commercial digoxin kit assay methods. *Eur J Clin Pharmacol* 1990;39:359–363.
Reviews aspects of digoxin-like immunoreactive substances.

Somberg JC. Digitalis: Neurally mediated arrhythmogenic and coronary vasoconstrictor properties. *Clin Pharmacol* 1985;25:529–539.
Basic science analysis of CNS effects of cardiac glycosides.

Stolshek BS, Osterhout SK, Dunham G. The role of digoxin-specific antibodies in the treatment of digitalis poisoning. *Med Toxicol Adverse Drug Exp* 1988;3:167–171.
Good review article on Fab therapy.

Wenger TL, Butler VP, Haber E, et al. Treatment of 63 severely digitalis-toxic patients with digoxin-specific antibody fragments. *J Am Coll Cardiol* 1985;5:118–123.
Elegant analysis of response to Fab therapy.

CHAPTER 92

Theophylline Intoxication

(See Chapters 109 and 146)

David S. Cooling

The upper therapeutic limit for serum theophylline is 20 mg/L. Theophylline intoxication is commonly seen in patients taking a one-time overdose with the intention of committing suicide. It is also commonly seen in patients taking theophylline preparations over a long period for obstructive lung disease; these patients may become intoxicated as a result of repeated overmedication.

Clinical Manifestations

- **GI:** nausea, vomiting, diarrhea, abdominal pain, hemorrhage.
- **Cardiovascular:** tachydysrhythmias, hypotension, cardiac arrest.
- **Neurologic:** irritability, tremor, headache, lethargy, seizures, coma.

The correlation between severity of symptoms and serum theophylline levels is different in acute (a single ingestion) and long-term intoxication. Life-threatening toxicity (e.g., seizures, hypotension, serious dysrhythmias, and cardiac arrest) usually does not occur until serum concentrations are significantly elevated (> 100 mg/L in acute toxicity; > 40 mg/L in chronic toxicity). Patients with underlying seizure disorders may have convulsions at lower levels of toxicity. In patients with acute toxicity, symptoms are more severe at higher serum levels. In contrast, there is little correlation between serum drug levels and symptoms in patients with chronic intoxication, and life-threatening manifestations may occur without warning. Ingestion of sustained-release preparations can cause delayed attainment of peak serum concentrations and delayed toxic manifestations.

Management of Acute Ingestions

Management of patients with severe theophylline intoxication includes:

- **Initial stabilization,** which may necessitate endotracheal intubation or cardiopulmonary resuscitation.
- **Close monitoring,** e.g., for unstable vital signs, cardiac dysrhythmias, seizures, respiratory arrest. ICU admission is necessary for patients who are symptomatic or who have serum levels that are more than mildly elevated. Supportive treatment should be provided.
- **IV administration** of concentrated dextrose, thiamine, naloxone, or flumazenil is routinely considered for patients with altered mental statuses.
- **Serum tests** are performed immediately, including theophylline level, glucose level, electrolyte levels, and other routine laboratory tests. Serum theophylline assays are repeated every 2–4 hours until the peak level is established.
- **Gastric evacuation** can be considered, particularly if the

patient is seen within a few hours of ingestion, if the ingestion involves sustained-release preparations, or if delayed gastric emptying is suspected.

- **Activated charcoal,** 0.5 g/kg, is administered PO or by nasogastric tube every 2–4 hours until the serum theophylline level is < 25 mg/L. Antiemetics may be necessary to suppress vomiting.
- **Cathartic** (e.g., 0.5–1 g/kg sorbitol solution) is given with the first dose of charcoal.
- **Charcoal hemoperfusion** should be considered in severe cases. Hemodialysis is less effective, but can be used if hemoperfusion is unavailable.

Conventional treatment should be initiated to treat seizures, hypotension, and cardiac dysrhythmias. Many patients with theophylline intoxication have underlying bronchospastic disease. Thus, β-adrenergic blocking agents are at least relatively contraindicated for the treatment of tachydysrhythmias. Hypotension also may be exacerbated by β-adrenergic antagonists. However, if other agents are unsuccessful or cannot be used, the ultra–short-acting β-adrenergic antagonist esmolol can be used because any deleterious effects can be reversed relatively rapidly by discontinuing the esmolol infusion.

Enterally administered activated charcoal adsorbs theophylline that remains in the GI tract. In addition, it effectively removes theophylline that has been absorbed systemically by establishing a concentration gradient across the intestinal mucosa, between the bowel lumen and the bloodstream, analogous to dialysis.

Charcoal hemoperfusion (or hemodialysis, if hemoperfusion is unavailable) is an alternative to enterally administered activated charcoal. Although hemoperfusion decreases serum theophylline levels rapidly, this therapy is usually not available immediately, it requires specialized equipment and personnel, and it is associated with potential complications, including:

- Difficulty obtaining central vascular access.
- Hypotension associated with extracorporeal circulation.
- Thrombocytopenia and leukopenia.
- Hemolysis and anemia.
- Hypocalcemia, hypophosphatemia, and hypoglycemia.

It may be considered in any of the following situations:

- Life-threatening theophylline intoxication.
- Patient whose condition is deteriorating despite conventional treatment.
- Patient who cannot tolerate enteral administration of activated charcoal (e.g., because of intractable vomiting or bowel obstruction).

- Serum theophylline concentration > 100 mg/L in acute intoxication.
- Serum theophylline concentration > 40–60 mg/L in chronic intoxication. The lower threshold is more applicable to patients with concomitant respiratory failure, congestive heart failure, or liver disease.

Suggested Readings

Corser BC, Youngs C, Baughman RP. Prolonged toxicity following massive ingestion of sustained-release theophylline preparation. *Chest* 1985;88:749–750.

Olson KR, Benowitz NL, Woo OF, et al. Theophylline overdose: Acute single ingestion versus chronic repeated overmedication. *Am J Emerg Med* 1985;3:386–394.

Of 15 patients with chronic theophylline intoxication (serum levels of 28–70 mg/L) 7 had seizures and 4 had serious dysrhythmias. In contrast, of 19 patients with acute single overdose (levels <100 mg/L) only 1 sustained seizures and 2 had serious dysrhythmias. However, of eight patients with single overdoses and levels greater than 100 mg/dL, 7 had seizures and 3 had serious dysrhythmias.

Parr MJ, Anaes FC, Day AC, et al. Theophylline poisoning: A review of 64 cases. *Intensive Care Med* 1990;16:394–398.

Demonstrates, as have other clinical studies, that leukocytosis, hyperglycemia, hypokalemia, and other electrolyte abnormalities are common in theophylline intoxication. Concludes that charcoal hemoperfusion may be safely reserved for patients in whom conservative measures are unsuccessful.

Seneff M, Scott J, Friedman B, et al. Acute theophylline toxicity and the use of esmolol to reverse cardiovascular instability. *Ann Emerg Med* 1990;19:671–673.

Case report describing use of esmolol in treatment of severe tachycardia caused by theophylline intoxication.

Sessler CN, Glauser FL, Cooper KR. Treatment of theophylline toxicity with oral activated charcoal. *Chest* 1985;87:325–329.

Report of 14 patients with serum theophylline levels ranging from 32 to 80 mg/L who were treated with oral activated charcoal. The 4 patients with the highest levels (average 77 mg/L) vomited all doses of oral charcoal, and 3 of these patients were treated with hemoperfusion.

Shannon M. Predictors of major toxicity after theophylline overdose. *Ann Intern Med* 1993;119:1161–1167.

Study of 249 patients referred after theophylline intoxication, showing that the major factors associated with toxicity are peak serum theophylline concentration (>100 mg/L) in acute intoxications and patient age (>60 years) in chronic overmedication.

CHAPTER 93

Alcohol Intoxication and Withdrawal

(See Chapter 62)

Mark A. Kaufman

Acute Ethanol Intoxication

Ethanol is the most common drug that causes acute intoxication in the United States. It is rapidly absorbed from the GI tract and metabolized in the liver to acetaldehyde and acetate following zero-order kinetics. Metabolism also occurs by the microsomal enzyme pathway, which is inducible by long-term use of ethanol and certain other drugs, such as barbiturates and benzodiazepines. Consumption of 4 ounces of 90 proof liquor or 48 ounces of beer results in a blood ethanol level of approximately 100 mg/dL in a 70-kg person.

Clinical Manifestations. Although ethanol is a CNS depressant, small amounts produce an initial period of exuberant behavior because of a loss of inhibition. Intoxication correlates better with the rate of ingestion than with the blood ethanol concentration because tolerance to the effects of ethanol differs among individuals. This tolerance is a CNS adaption, not a metabolic phenomenon. Nevertheless, rough correlates of blood levels with clinical findings are as follows:

- **50–150 mg/dL:** heightened verbal and motor activity, altered judgment, impaired concentration and judgment.
- **150–250 mg/dL:** ataxia of gait, dysarthria, poor visual pursuit, nystagmus, lethargy interrupted by brief periods of heightened activity.
- **250–400 mg/dL:** incoherent speech; stupor, intermittently interrupted by brief periods of hostile verbal and physical behavior.
- **> 400 mg/dL:** coma, respiratory arrest.

Other systemic signs of ethanol intoxication include the characteristic breath odor, flushed face, hypotension, tachycardia, and hypothermia. Paradoxical intoxication is psychotic behavior that occurs after the ingestion of ethanol. A period of delusions, hallucinations, and paranoia lasting for several minutes to hours is followed by sleep and amnesia for the episode.

Patients admitted to the hospital with ethanol intoxication often may have other acute medical conditions, sometimes clinically occult, including:

- Subdural hematoma.
- Infection, such as pneumonia or meningitis.
- Encephalopathy from hepatic or renal insufficiency.
- Hypoglycemia or fluid and electrolyte derangements.
- Other substance abuse, such as methanol poisoning or drug overdose.

Because of their attendant morbidity and mortality rates, these potentially concomitant disorders should be systematically considered in patients with acute ethanol intoxication.

Treatment. Therapy is aimed at isolating the patient in a calm environment and providing reassurance, close observation, and monitoring of vital signs. In severe intoxication, respiratory support with mechanical ventilation may be required. Concentrated glucose and thiamine should be administered parenterally in case there is associated hypoglycemia or thiamine deficiency that is responsible for the sensorial changes. A multivitamin preparation is also routinely administered. Sedative agents are avoided. Fluid and electrolyte imbalances are common, and should be corrected. Once ingestion of ethanol ceases, the blood level typically decreases at a rate of 10–25 mg/dL/hour. Dialysis has been used to accelerate the reduction of blood ethanol concentration in some cases of profound intoxication. However, this intervention is rarely necessary unless there is an additional indication for dialysis, such as concomitant renal failure or methanol poisoning.

Ethanol Withdrawal

The presence of sustained or severe symptoms after the cessation of long-term ethanol ingestion is known as the alcohol withdrawal syndrome. Generally, it occurs only after at least several days of drinking with abrupt cessation. However, it can also occur when there is a dramatic reduction from enormous amounts of daily ethanol ingestion to much smaller volumes.

The withdrawal syndrome classically develops in four phases. Although patients do not always experience each phase or follow the classic progression, the syndrome typically evolves in the following sequence:

- **Tremulousness** often occurs within 6–12 hours of abstaining. The tremors are coarse, and primarily involve the hands. A common expression for this phase is *the shakes.* In addition, there may be anxiety, insomnia, anorexia, and heightened responsiveness to stimuli. Mild withdrawal may not progress beyond this phase.
- **Hallucinosis:** The second phase is characterized by per-

ceptual disturbances and hallucinations, typically occurring approximately 24 hours after the last drink. These disturbances are usually visual or tactile rather than auditory. They may consist of vivid dreams, illusions or misperceptions, and hallucinations involving people, insects, or animals (hence, a common description of this phase is *seeing pink elephants*). A sensation of insects crawling on the body (formication) is also common.
- **Seizures:** The third phase is heralded by brief convulsions, commonly known as *rum fits*. These typically occur 6–48 hours after cessation of ethanol consumption, and consist of a single, generalized seizure or a cluster of brief seizures occurring over a few hours. Focal seizures and status epilepticus can occur, but are less common and should increase the suspicion of an alternative etiology.
- **Delirium tremens:** The fourth phase typically begins 2–5 days after cessation of drinking. The delirium often occurs as extreme agitation or a global confusional state. It may alternate with periods of relative lucidity. There is increased autonomic activity, with hypertension, tachycardia, tachypnea, flushing, diaphoresis, mydriasis, and sometimes fever.

Alcohol withdrawal that progresses to delirium tremens has an associated mortality rate of approximately 15%. Death can be caused by fluid and electrolyte imbalances, cardiac dysrhythmias, sepsis, aspiration pneumonitis with adult repiratory distress syndrome and respiratory failure, and other associated disorders, such as pancreatitis or GI hemorrhage.

Treatment. Routine laboratory studies, including renal and hepatic function tests, creatine phosphokinase levels (to exclude rhabdomyolysis), serum electrolyte levels (including calcium, magnesium, and phosphorus), complete blood count (with platelet count), and coagulation studies should be performed. In some cases, further specific diagnostic studies (e.g., computed brain tomography, lumbar puncture) may be necessary to exclude alternative causes of seizures or delirium.

Treatment common to all patients with alcohol withdrawal includes:

- Glucose administration to correct or prevent hypoglycemia.
- Parenteral administration of thiamine (e.g., 100 mg IV or IM) and multivitamins.
- Correction of electrolyte imbalances. Hypokalemia, hypomagnesemia, and hypophosphatemia are common.
- IV hydration. Many patients require vigorous hydration.
- A search for concomitant medical problems that are

commonly associated with this disorder (e.g., GI bleeding, infections, pancreatitis).
- Administration of a sedative drug, titrated to effect.

Numerous sedative agents have been succesfully used in the treatment of alcohol withdrawal, including:

- **Paraldehyde,** a traditional agent for treating alcohol withdrawal. Although it is effective, it has been used much less frequently since the advent of benzodiazepines. IV and IM administration is associated with potential adverse effects that preclude its use by these routes for treating alcohol withdrawal.
- **Chlordiazepoxide.** 25–100 mg PO every 4–8 hours.
- **Diazepam.** 5–10 mg IV, repeated every 5–10 minutes until the patient is calm but awake, then 5–20 mg every 2–6 hours.
- **Pentobarbital.** 200 mg PO, repeated hourly until the desired degree of sedation is attained. Then an appropriate maintenance dose is given at 6-hour intervals.

Many other benzodiazepines and other sedative agents, including parenterally administered ethanol, have been used therapeutically; however, the benzodiazepines are most often used today, and are generally recommended. The route and frequency of administration is determined by the clinical severity of withdrawal. The dose required to induce sedation is variable. Often as little as 25 mg chlordiazepoxide PO four times daily is sufficient, whereas in rare cases, more than 1 g/day parenterally may be necessary. IM adminstration of benzodiazepines is generally not recommended because absorption is erratic by this route. The goal of treatment is to reduce symptoms without producing excessive sedation. The patient should be maintained in a state of calm alertness or in a state of mild somnolence from which he or she can be easily awakened. The sedative regimen is gradually tapered as tolerated, usually over a period of several days.

Other drugs that have been advocated for treating alcohol withdrawal include:

- **Propranolol.** 0.1–1 mg IV or 5–10 mg PO every 4–8 hours to control the hyperadrenergic effects associated with delirium tremens. Other β-adrenergic blocking agents have also been used. It is important to be aware of contraindications.
- **Clonidine.** 0.1–0.2 mg PO every 6–12 hours, or a single oral loading dose followed by application of a transdermal clonidine patch. This agent is also useful in controlling the hyperautonomic effects of delirium tremens.
- **Magnesium sulfate.** Although hypomagnesemia, particularly if symptomatic, should be corrected, there is little

evidence that routine magnesium supplementation has a therapeutic effect on alcohol withdrawal.

Phenothiazines and other neuroleptic agents are not generally recommended because they can be epileptogenic. The treatment of alcohol withdrawal–associated seizures with conventional anticonvulsants is controversial. Many authorities recommend avoiding specific anticonvulsants (e.g., phenytoin) unless there is another reason, such as an underlying idiopathic seizure disorder, an acute head injury, or a severe metabolic factor that may have precipitated the seizure. Others routinely treat all patients with withdrawal seizures during the acute period, usually with phenytoin. When used for sedation, benzodiazepines or barbiturates exert at least some degree of anticonvulsant effect by themselves.

Wernicke-Korsakoff Syndrome

Chronic ethanol abuse can lead to several disorders of the CNS and peripheral nervous system, including peripheral neuropathy, chronic cerebellar ataxia, Marchiafava-Bignami syndrome, central pontine myelinolysis, and Wernicke-Korsakoff syndrome. Among these, Wernicke-Korsakoff syndrome is the most likely to necessitate treatment in the ICU. It is composed of two syndromes, Wernicke's encephalopathy and Korsakoff's dementia. Both are caused by thiamine deficiency. Wernicke's encephalopathy consists of:

- Altered mental status, ranging from poor concentration and disorientation to lethargy.
- Abnormalities of extraocular movements, such as multidirectional nystagmus, restricted abduction, or frank ophthalmoplegia.
- Ataxia, primarily truncal and often preventing ambulation.

Wernicke's encephalopathy is primarily a clinical diagnosis. Reduced blood transketolase level is a marker of thiamine deficiency, but is not usually necessary to establish the diagnosis. Korsakoff's dementia is a disorder of memory that may appear to evolve as part of the recovery from Wernicke's encephalopathy. It is characterized by the triad of memory loss, learning deficits, and confabulation. Some patients with acute alcohol intoxication or withdrawal may exhibit features of Wernicke-Korsakoff syndrome without actually having thiamine deficiency. The routine administration of thiamine in these settings is based on this difficulty in clinically excluding Wernicke-Korsakoff syndrome and the simplicity and safety of thiamine supplementation.

Treatment or prevention consists of IV or IM thiamine

administration (e.g., ≥ 50 mg/day). Patients at risk for this syndrome often have other vitamin deficiencies as well; therefore, a multivitamin preparation is also routinely administered.

Suggested Readings

Baumgartner GR, Rowen RC. Transdermal clonidine versus chlordiazepoxide in alcohol withdrawal: A randomized, controlled clinical trial. *South Med J* 1991;84:312–321.

Prospective, double-blind study showing effectiveness of transdermal clonidine for treatment of alcohol withdrawal.

Charnes ME, Simon RP, Greenberg DA. Ethanol and the nervous system. *N Engl J Med* 1989;321:442–454.

Concise review of neurologic consequences of ethanol (192 references).

Guthrie SK. The treatment of alcohol withdrawal. *Pharmacotherapy* 1989;9:131–143.

Reviews many classes of agents used to treat acute ethanol withdrawal syndrome.

Harper CG, Giles M, Finlay-Jones R. Clinical signs in the Wernicke-Korsakoff complex: A retrospective analysis of 131 cases diagnosed at necropsy. *J Neurol Neurosurg Psychiatry* 1986;49:341–345.

Emphasizes underdiagnosis of the condition, suggesting that rigid clinical criteria are needed.

Lechtenberg R, Worner TM. Seizure risk with recurrent alcohol detoxification. *Arch Neurol* 1990;47:535–538.

Large, retrospective series detailing experience with seizures associated with multiple episodes of alcohol withdrawal.

CHAPTER 94

Toxic Alcohol and Glycol Poisoning

(See Chapter 146)

James A. Kruse

Methanol Poisoning

Methanol, or wood alcohol, is widely available in commercial solvents and in paint and automotive products. The lethal dose is highly variable, ranging from less than 10 mL to more than 500 mL. Although the alcohol itself is relatively innocuous, it is metabolized to the toxic byproducts formaldehyde and formic acid, which are responsible for its ocular and CNS toxicity.

Clinical Manifestations. Poisoning can occur as a result of accidental or intentional ingestion. The latter frequently occurs in desperate or intoxicated alcoholics who use methanol-containing products as an alcohol substitute. Because of the relatively slow conversion of methanol to its toxic metabolites, there is frequently a delay between the time of ingestion and the development of toxic signs and symptoms. This delay typically ranges from 12–24 hours. Toxic signs and symptoms include:

- **Ocular:** blurred vision, scintillations, decreased visual acuity, scotomata, unreactive pupils, papilledema, partial or complete blindness. Blindness may be permanent in survivors.
- **CNS:** drunkenness, stupor, coma, seizures, meningeal signs, cerebral edema, basal ganglia infarction.
- **GI:** nausea, vomiting, epigastric pain, gastritis, GI hemorrhage, pancreatitis.
- **Respiratory:** faint odor of methanol or formaldehyde on breath, Kussmaul respirations, respiratory failure.

Severe degrees of poisoning may be associated with profound metabolic acidosis, circulatory shock, and death.

Laboratory findings include:

- **Metabolic acidosis,** recognized by analysis of serum CO_2 content and arterial blood gases. It is caused mainly by formic acid, but an element of lactic acidosis can also occur, especially if there is circulatory shock.
- **Increased anion gap** as a result of the accumulation of formate (and potentially lactate) anions.
- **Positive serum methanol assay,** which confirms the diagnosis. However, if results of this assay are not immediately available, initiation of therapy should not be delayed if a presumptive diagnosis can be made.
- **Increased serum osmole gap** calculated from simultaneously obtained measurements of serum osmolality (Osm_s), sodium (Na_s), glucose ($glucose_s$), urea nitrogen (UN_s), and ethanol ($ethanol_s$).

The osmole gap is calculated by:

$$\text{osmole gap} = Osm_s - (2 \times Na_s) + (Glucose_s/18) + (UN_s/2.8) + (Ethanol_s/4.6),$$

where Osm_s is measured in milliosmoles per kilogram water; sodium is expressed in millimoles per liter; and glucose, urea nitrogen, and ethanol are expressed in milligrams per deciliter. Normally, the osmole gap does not exceed 10–15 mOsm/kg H_2O. Higher values indicate an excessive concentration of osmotically active particles, such as methanol. Inclusion of ethanol in the above equation excludes the potential effect of this common coingestant on the osmole gap. In some cases, the patient is unable or unwilling to provide an accurate history of the toxic ingestion, and these simple laboratory findings are an important means of making an early presumptive diagnosis.

Treatment. After general supportive measures are instituted to ensure adequate ventilation, oxygenation, and circulation, and a presumptive or definitive diagnosis of methanol poisoning is made, the following therapy should be instituted:

- **$NaHCO_3$** is given to treat metabolic acidosis. Anecdotal reports suggest that this agent ameliorates toxic manifestations and may improve survival rates.
- **Ethanol** is administered to slow the conversion of methanol to its toxic metabolites by means of competitive inhibition of alcohol and aldehyde dehydrogenase. It is usually given IV (through a central vein) as a 10% solution; however, in mild cases of poisoning, it can be given PO (if the patient is sufficiently alert) or by nasogastric tube if it is sufficiently diluted (see Table 94–1).
- **Serial serum ethanol levels** (e.g., every 1–2 hours initially) should be obtained. The goal is to achieve and maintain a serum ethanol level of 100–150 mg/dL.
- **Folic acid** is given (e.g., 50–100 mg every 4 hours IV) to hasten the metabolic conversion of formic acid to CO_2. Folinic acid can also be used. These cofactors substantially decrease serum formate levels in animal models of methanol poisoning.
- **Hemodialysis,** to remove methanol and toxic metabolites from the body, should be instituted in all patients with ocular manifestations, in patients with renal impairment, in patients with peak serum methanol levels > 50 mg/dL, and in all patients with severe poisoning.

Gastric evacuation (by lavage) is likely of little value in most cases because methanol is rapidly absorbed. It can be used if the patient seeks treatment promptly after the ingestion. Syrup of ipecac should not be used because patients may have an impaired level of consciousness, which may increase the risk of aspiration. Attention to fluid balance is important because ethanol therapy necessitates large volumes of administered fluids.

Ethylene Glycol Poisoning

Ethylene glycol is a colorless, essentially odorless liquid with a sweet taste. It is widely available as the main constituent of most automotive antifreeze preparations. The lethal dose is variable, but generally ranges from 1–2 mg/kg. In common with methanol, ethylene glycol is nontoxic, but is metabolized to several byproducts (such as glycolic and glycoxylic acids) that are responsible for its toxicity.

TABLE 94–1

STANDARD THERAPEUTIC ETHANOL DOSING TO ACHIEVE SERUM ETHANOL CONCENTRATION OF 100 mg/dL*

Parameter	Nondrinker	Chronic Drinker
Loading dose		
Amount of absolute ethanol (mg/kg)†	600	600
Volume of 43% oral solution (mL/kg)‡	1.80	1.80
Volume of 90% oral solution (mL/kg)§	0.86	0.86
Volume of 10% parenteral solution (mL/kg)‖	7.6	7.6
Maintenance dose (not on dialysis)		
Amount of absolute ethanol (mg/kg/hr)†	66	154
Volume of 43% oral solution (mL/kg/hr)‡	0.20	0.46
Volume of 90% oral solution (mL/kg/hr)§	0.10	0.21
Volume of 10% parenteral solution (mL/kg/hr)‖	0.83	1.96
Maintenance dose (during dialysis)		
Amount of absolute ethanol (mg/kg/hr)†	169	257
Volume of 43% oral solution (mL/kg/hr)‡	0.50	0.77
Volume of 90% oral solution (mL/kg/hr)§	0.24	0.37
Volume of 10% parenteral solution (mL/kg/hr)‖	2.13	3.26

*Assumes typical volume of distribution and elimination kinetics; actual dosing should be titrated with frequent serum ethanol assays. Enterally administered solutions must be diluted to a final concentration of < 40% (preferably < 20%) ethanol.

†Specific gravity = 0.79.

‡Ethanol content = 34 g/dL (equivalent to 86 proof undiluted liquor).

§Ethanol content = 7.1 g/dL.

‖Ethanol content = 7.9 g/dL.

(Reprinted with permission from Kruse JA. Methanol poisoning. *Intensive Care Med* 1992;18:391–397, and based on data from McCoy HG, Cipolle RJ, Ehlers SM, et al. Severe methanol poisoning: Application of a pharmacokinetic model for ethanol therapy and hemodialysis. *Am J Med* 1979;67:804–807.)

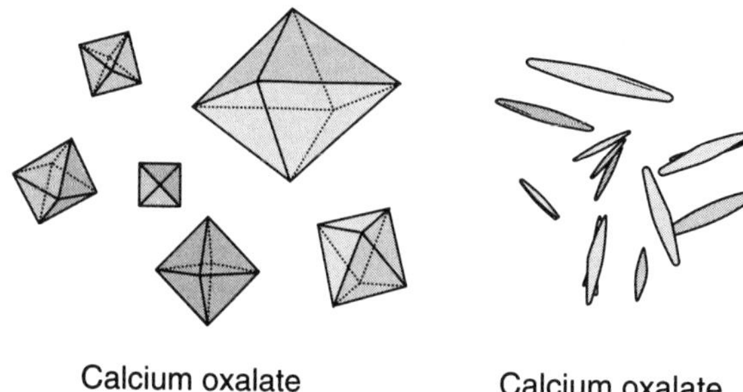

Figure 94–1. The two forms of urinary calcium oxalate crystals frequently observed in ethylene glycol poisoning. The dihydrate form assumes an octahedral configuration, which gives the appearance of an envelope under light microscopy. Other crystalline configurations have been described for the monohydrate form besides that shown. (From Kruse JA. Ethylene glycol intoxication. *J Intensive Care Med* 1992;7:234–243. Reprinted by permission of Blackwell Scientific Publications, Inc.)

Clinical manifestations include:

- **CNS effects,** which may occur within 30 minutes of ingestion. They include confusion, ataxia, lethargy, coma, and seizures.
- **Cardiopulmonary effects,** which typically occur 12–24 hours after ingestion. They include pulmonary edema, which can be severe enough to warrant mechanical ventilation, and circulatory shock.
- **Renal failure,** caused by acute tubular necrosis, classically occurs within 24–72 hours after ingestion. It may be severe enough to lead to uremia and require dialysis.

Laboratory findings include:

- **Metabolic acidosis,** which can be profoundly severe. It is chiefly caused by accumulation of the metabolite glycolic acid.
- **Increased anion gap,** caused by the accumulation of glycolate, the anion of glycolic acid.
- **Positive serum ethylene glycol assay,** which confirms the diagnosis. However, this assay is not immediately available at many centers. Initiation of therapy should not be delayed if a presumptive diagnosis can be made before this toxicologic assay result is available.
- **Crystalluria,** caused by precipitation of calcium oxalate in the renal tubules; oxalic acid is a terminal metabolite of ethylene glycol (Figure 94–1). Lack of crystalluria does not exclude the possibility of ethylene glycol intoxication.
- **Increased serum osmole gap,** as a result of high circulat-

ing concentrations of ethylene glycol and its metabolites.
- **Hypocalcemia,** which may occur because of the formation of calcium oxalate precipitates in urine and systemic tissues.

As with methanol intoxication, ethylene glycol intoxication is sometimes occult. The findings of high anion gap metabolic acidosis, increased osmole gap, and a compatible clinical setting are presumptive evidence of either form of poisoning.

Treatment is similar to that of methanol poisoning. It consists of:

- **Supportive measures** as the first priority. Adequate oxygenation, ventilation, and perfusion are ensured. Gastric evacuation may be used if the patient is treated soon after ingestion. Anticonvulsants, mechanical ventilation, and vasoactive drug therapy may be necessary.
- **$NaHCO_3$** to treat metabolic acidosis. Limited experimental evidence supports the idea that alkali therapy improves survival.
- **Ethanol,** administered in the same manner as for methanol poisoning (see earlier material in this chapter and Table 94–1).
- **Hemodialysis** to remove ethylene glycol and its metabolites from the body. All patients with toxic symptoms, patients with evidence of renal dysfunction, patients with peak serum ethylene glycol levels > 50 mg/dL, and patients with severe poisoning should undergo hemodialysis.
- **Calcium** has been recommended to intentionally precipitate oxalate in vivo. Because this effect may have deleterious effects, calcium administration is not recommended unless there is symptomatic hypocalcemia.
- **Pyridoxine** (vitamin B_6), which is given parenterally, based on experimental and indirect evidence that deficiency of this cofactor may result in impaired metabolism of glyoxylic acid.
- **Thiamine,** which may promote the breakdown of glyoxylic acid to less toxic intermediates.
- **Folic acid,** which may be given in doses of 50–100 mg every 4 hours IV to facilitate the metabolism of formate to CO_2. There is some evidence that at least small amounts of formic acid are generated during the metabolism of ethylene glycol.

Alkali, ethanol, and hemodialysis are the mainstays of specific treatment for both methanol and ethylene glycol poisoning. The efficacy of vitamin therapy for ethylene glycol poisoning is unproven, but the treatment is innocuous.

Isopropanol Poisoning

Isopropanol (isopropyl alcohol) is a colorless liquid with a distinctive odor and a burning taste. It is widely available as rubbing alcohol, but is also found in a variety of commercially available cleaning, automotive, and other products. Its only metabolite is acetone.

Clinical Manifestations. The characteristic odor of acetone or isopropanol may be present on the patient's breath. Other findings are:

- **GI effects** are common. They include nausea, vomiting, abdominal pain, hemorrhagic gastritis, and diarrhea.
- **CNS effects** include confusion, dizziness, headache, slurred speech, ataxia, miosis, lethargy, obtundation, and coma.
- **Hemodynamic effects** include hypotension, bradycardia, and frank circulatory shock.
- **Respiratory effects** include dyspnea, hypoxemia, pulmonary edema, and respiratory failure.
- **Miscellaneous effects** include flushing, myopathy, renal dysfunction, rhabdomyolysis, hemolysis, and hypothermia.

Laboratory findings include:

- **Elevated serum acetone** level as a result of the accumulation of this metabolite of isopropanol.
- **Increased serum osmole gap** because of high circulating concentrations of isopropanol and acetone.
- **Acid–base status** that is characteristically normal, i.e., there is no metabolic acidosis because neither isopropanol nor acetone is an acid. However, in some cases, there may be some degree of metabolic acidosis as a result of lactate accumulation. This accumulation may be caused by anaerobic generation of lactate if there is concomitant circulatory shock. It may also result from the accumulation of reduced nicotinamide-adenine dinucleotide during the conversion of isopropanol to acetone, leading to the formation of lactate from pyruvate.
- **Normal anion gap,** unless there is lactic acidosis. Neither isopropanol nor its metabolite acetone is an anion.
- **Positive serum isopropanol assay** result confirms the diagnosis.
- **Increased serum creatinine** level. This increase may be spurious because certain creatinine assays yield a falsely elevated result in the presence of high serum acetone concentrations.

Treatment

- **Gastric lavage** has been effective, even when there has been a significant delay between ingestion and treatment. Induced vomiting is contraindicated. Activated charcoal may be administered, but is probably not helpful.

- **Continuous nasogastric suctioning** is of speculative benefit based on the possibility that there is recirculation of absorbed isopropanol back into the GI tract through salivary or gastric secretion.
- **Respiratory support** with endotracheal intubation (and mechanical ventilation) is required in patients with a severely depressed sensorium, those undergoing gastric lavage, and those with impending or frank respiratory failure.
- **Treatment of shock** may include fluid therapy, inotropic agents, and vasopressor agents. Pulmonary artery catheterization may be helpful to guide these aspects of therapy.
- **Dialysis.** Both hemodialysis and peritoneal dialysis have been used, although the latter is less effective. Dialysis should be considered in patients with high serum isopropanol levels (e.g., $\geq$ 400 mg/dL), coma, or hypotension.

Suggested Readings

Gaudet MP, Fraser GL. Isopropanol ingestion: Case report with pharmacokinetic analysis. *Am J Emerg Med* 1989;7:297–299.

Kruse JA. Methanol poisoning. *Intensive Care Med* 1992;18:391–397.
Comprehensive review of toxicology, metabolism, clinical manifestations, laboratory findings, diagnosis, and treatment of methanol poisoning. The mechanism of action of folate therapy is explained (58 references).

Kruse JA, Cadnapaphornchai P. The serum osmole gap. *J Crit Care* 1994;9:185–197.
Detailed description of derivation, clinical utility, and limitations of serum osmole gap (114 references).

Winter ML, Ellis MD, Snodgrass WR. Urine fluorescence using a Wood's lamp to detect the antifreeze additive sodium fluorescein: A qualitative adjunctive test in suspected ethylene glycol ingestions. *Ann Emerg Med* 1990;19:663–667.
Describes novel method for identifying ethylene glycol poisoning by observing yellow-green fluorescence of patient's urine when it is exposed to ultraviolet light. Fluorescence is caused by presence of a dye added to many antifreeze preparations to aid in identification of automotive cooling system leaks. A variety of factors can lead to false-positive and false-negative results, however.

Miscellaneous Topics

CHAPTER 95

Preoperative Care

(See Chapter 137)

Richard D. Harvey and
Dennis J. Crnkovich

The central purpose of the preoperative evaluation is to minimize the risks of surgery. Risks are minimized by careful identification of medical conditions that increase operative risk and by application of appropriate perioperative management of these conditions. The preoperative evaluation consists primarily of a complete history and physical examination, along with subsequent testing as directed by the clinical findings to determine the severity of the known or suspected conditions that may affect surgical risk. Commonly recommended preoperative tests include chest radiography, ECG, complete blood count, serum chemistry profile (including electrolytes, blood urea nitrogen, and creatinine), urinalysis, and prothrombin time. More extensive testing may be indicated to evaluate an identified clinical problem.

Cardiovascular Disease

Studies have shown that the risk of perioperative myocardial infarction (MI) in an adult 30 years of age or older is less than 1%, but increases to approximately 7% in patients with a history of MI. However, if the patient has had an MI within 3 months before surgery, the risk of a postoperative MI approaches 40%. At 3–6 months after MI, the risk is approximately 16%. Goldman and associates developed a method of risk estimation based on signs and symptoms of cardiovascular disease (Table 95–1). This method is useful in identifying patients at risk for cardiac complications, but it underestimates the risk in those with symptomatic peripheral vascular disease and in those undergoing abdominal aortic surgery.

For patients identified as high risk (Goldman class III [13–25 points] or IV [> 26 points], unstable angina, or recent MI), surgery should be delayed when possible to permit further evaluation and treatment as indicated. Goldman class IV status carries a 39% mortality rate, a 12% risk of life-threatening complications, and a 78% risk of serious postoperative cardiac complications. By comparison, class III is associated with a 3% mortality rate, and class II, with a 1% mortality rate. In some settings, surgery

TABLE 95–1

THE GOLDMAN CARDIAC RISK INDEX

Risk Factor	Points
Signs of congestive heart failure (S_3 gallop, jugular venous distension)	11
Myocardial infarction within previous 6 months	10
Rhythm other than sinus or premature atrial contractions	7
> 5 premature ventricular contractions/min*	7
Age > 70 years	5
Emergency operation	4
Significant aortic stenosis	3
Intraperitoneal, intrathoracic, or aortic operation†	3
Poor general medical condition‡	3

*Premature ventricular contractions in the otherwise healthy patient with a normal heart are probably not associated with increased risk.

†Elective abdominal aortic surgery carries a higher risk than predicted by the original index. Also, symptomatic peripheral vascular disease in the patient with stable angina is associated with increased cardiac risk.

‡For example, respiratory failure (arterial oxygen tension [PaO_2] < 60 torr or arterial carbon dioxide tension [$PaCO_2$] > 50 torr); renal failure (serum urea nitrogen level > 50 mg/dL or creatinine level > 3 mg/dL); chronic liver disease; or bedridden from noncardiac cause.

(Adapted from information appearing in *The New England Journal of Medicine:* Goldman L, Caldera DL, Nussbaum SR, et al. Multifactorial index of cardiac risk in noncardiac surgical procedures. *N Engl J Med* 1977;297:845–850.)

cannot be delayed, and certain high-risk patients benefit from invasive hemodynamic monitoring preoperatively (see Table 137–6 in the main text).

Pulmonary Diseases

Atelectasis is the most common postsurgical pulmonary complication. Other complications include mucous plugging, bronchitis, pneumonia, bronchospasm, hypoxemia, pulmonary hypertension, and right-sided congestive heart failure, any of which, alone or in combination, may lead to postoperative respiratory failure. Important preoperative pulmonary risk factors include the patient's age, weight, and smoking status, and the type of operation to be performed. Lung resection and thoracic surgery without lung resection carry the highest risk, followed by upper and lower abdominal surgery.

Those at increased risk should be evaluated further with pulmonary function testing and arterial blood gas analysis. This group includes those with evident lung disease determined by history or physical examination, all smokers who are being considered for thoracic surgery, significantly obese patients, and patients older than 70 years. The following findings predict an increased risk of postoperative complications:

- Arterial carbon dioxide tension ($Pa{CO_2}$) > 45 torr.
- Forced expiratory volume in 1 second (FEV_1) < 2.0 L.
- Forced vital capacity < 50% predicted.
- Maximal voluntary ventilation < 50% predicted.
- Ratio of residual volume to total lung capacity > 50%.

Patients undergoing pulmonary resection are at particularly increased risk of postoperative morbidity and mortality. If results from arterial blood gas analysis and spirometry are borderline (e.g., FEV_1 < 2.0 L), split-lung perfusion scanning may be performed to better estimate the contribution of each lobe to total lung function. Predicted postoperative FEV_1 of greater than 0.8 L is generally acceptable. Other findings that are useful to predict significant mortality risk in this setting include exercise testing results that show increased pulmonary vascular resistance (> 190 dyne · sec · cm^{-5}) and reduced maximum oxygen consumption (< 1.0 L/min).

Hepatic Disease

Severe hepatic disease is a considerable risk for patients undergoing surgery, and it is difficult to predict the response of these patients to the stress of surgery. Therefore, all patients with clinical or laboratory evidence of hepatic disease should undergo further preoperative assessment. The preoperative goal in patients with significant liver disease is to improve general status, control ascites, correct any coagulopathy, control GI bleeding, improve nutritional status, and decrease ammonia absorption from the gut.

Perioperatively, it is important to prevent dehydration, hypokalemia, and alkalosis. For those with acute hepatitis, surgery should be delayed if possible until several weeks after the liver function test results have normalized. The Child-Turcotte Classification (Table 95–2) is useful for estimating surgical risk from the severity of hepatic cirrhosis.

Renal Disease

All forms of chronic renal disease (including chronic renal failure from any cause, renovascular hypertension, and polycystic kidney disease) increase the risk of perioperative fluid and electrolyte imbalances. In the setting of nonemergent acute renal failure or acute worsening of chronic renal failure, the management of the renal disease should take precedence over surgery. Careful preoperative optimization of volume status is critical because of the large fluid shifts associated with surgery. This step is espe-

TABLE 95-2

THE CHILD-TURCOTTE CLASSIFICATION SYSTEM

Factor	Class A	Class B	Class C
Serum albumin (g/dL)	> 3.5	3.0–3.5	< 3.0
Serum bilirubin (mg/dL)	< 2.0	2.0–3.0	> 3.0
Ascites	None	Mild	Severe
Encephalopathy	None	Mild	Severe
Nutritional status	Normal	Good	Poor
Surgical mortality rate (%)	10	30	> 70

cially important in abdominal surgery because of the potentially large volumes lost through the gut or sequestered in the abdomen. Invasive hemodynamic monitoring may be helpful in certain situations.

Electrolyte and acid–base status should be carefully evaluated preoperatively and followed closely postoperatively. Potassium and hydrogen ion and excretion are impaired as renal function declines. This situation can lead to serious problems. Acidosis may be treated preoperatively with bicarbonate administration or dialysis. A pH of 7.25 or greater is desirable preoperatively. Hyperkalemia can be treated with dietary restriction, diuretics, bicarbonate administration or, in those with marked renal dysfunction, dialysis. The preoperative potassium level should be less than 5.5 mmol/L.

Other important considerations in the patient with chronic renal disease are calcium balance, anemia, bleeding diatheses, and avoidance of potentially nephrotoxic agents.

Endocrine Disease

Patients with diabetes mellitus require close perioperative monitoring because of potential complications related to glycemic control, electrolyte imbalance, and comorbid conditions, especially atherosclerotic vascular disease. Patients undergoing elective surgery should maintain blood glucose levels of less than 250 mg/dL. Hyperglycemia may contribute to poor wound healing and infection.

Hypothyroidism and hyperthyroidism increase surgical risk. Thyroid replacement for hypothyroidism should be initiated preoperatively when possible. An exception is the nonmyxedematous patient undergoing coronary artery bypass, in whom replacement should begin postoperatively. Hyperthyroidism requires preoperative treatment because of the 10–32% risk of precipitating thyroid storm.

Preoperative treatment in the emergent setting consists of treatment with β-adrenergic blocking agents, propylthiouracil, and hydrocortisone.

Surgical stress and anesthesia cause a dramatic increase in corticosteroid requirements. Levels may return to baseline within 72 hours after uncomplicated surgery. Adrenal insufficiency must be considered preoperatively to avoid potentially life-threatening postoperative adrenal crisis. Adrenal suppression can occur in patients taking exogenous corticosteroids (> 2 weeks of adrenal-suppressing doses in the previous 6 months or current steroid use). It mandates perioperative steroid replacement. A recommended replacement schedule is 100 mg hydrocortisone given the evening before surgery, 1 hour preoperatively, intraoperatively, and every 6 hours postoperatively.

Patients with pheochromocytoma are at high risk of perioperative hypertensive crisis. They are often volume depleted because of high circulating levels of catecholamines, and they need volume replacement. Both α- and β-adrenergic blocking agents are needed to prevent hypertensive crisis. Invasive hemodynamic monitoring is an important tool in these patients to closely monitor volume status and blood pressure.

Hematologic Disease

Anemia is an operative concern because of the need for adequate oxygen delivery during the increased stress of surgery. Clinically stable patients with a stable hematocrit value of 20–30% generally tolerate major surgery well. In patients with chronic anemia and a hematocrit value less than 18%, or in those with less severe anemia but who are hemodynamically unstable because of blood loss, oxygen delivery is compromised and transfusion is needed. In elective surgery where significant blood loss is expected, autologous blood transfusion should be considered.

Thrombocytopenia presents an increased risk of surgical bleeding. Patients with platelet counts of less than 50,000 mm^{-3} should undergo evaluation and treatment preoperatively. Because of their antiplatelet effects, aspirin should be avoided for 1–2 weeks before surgery and other nonsteroidal anti-inflammatory drugs should be avoided for 1–2 days before surgery.

Deep vein thrombosis is the most common complication in the postoperative period; therefore, prevention is important. Preoperative anticoagulation is primarily employed in patients undergoing hip surgery, and it can be accomplished with either heparin or warfarin. Postoperatively, low-dose subcutaneous heparin (5,000 units every 8–12 hours) or pneumatic compression devices should be used until the patient is ambulatory.

Suggested Readings

Berlauk JF, Abrams JH, Gilmour IJ, et al. Preoperative optimization of cardiovascular hemodynamics improves outcome in peripheral vascular surgery: A prospective, randomized clinical trial. *Ann Surg* 1991;214:289–297.

Study of 89 patients randomized to preoperative invasive hemodynamic monitoring and optimization versus control group. Optimization interventions consisted of fluid loading, afterload reduction, or inotropic support. Mortality and morbidity rates were lower in optimized group compared with control group.

Deron SJ, Kotler MN. Noncardiac surgery in the cardiac patient. *Am Heart J* 1988;116:831–838.

Reviews effects of angina pectoris, prior myocardial infarction, revascularization, ventricular dysfunction, valvular disease, hypertension, and dysrhythmias on surgical risk.

Gass GD, Olsen GN. Preoperative pulmonary function testing to predict operative morbidity and mortality. *Chest* 1986;89:127–135.

Reviews literature on usefulness of preoperative pulmonary function testing (55 references).

Goldman L, Caldera DL, Nussbaum SR, et al. Multifactorial index of cardiac risk in noncardiac surgical procedures. *N Engl J Med* 1977;297:845–850.

Original description of Goldman surgical risk classification system. Instrument was developed from data on 1001 patients older than 40 years who underwent noncardiac surgery at Massachusetts General Hospital.

Merli GJ, Weitz HH. Preoperative consultation. *Med Clin North Am* 1987;71:353–590.

Issue consists of 17 articles on preoperative evaluation and management. Included are articles specific to patients with lung, heart, kidney, liver, endocrine, neurologic, oncologic, obstetric, and other diseases. There are also articles on antibiotic and thromboembolic prophylaxis and on nutritional management.

CHAPTER 96

Trauma

(See Chapter 138)

Toshio Nagamoto and
Dane J. Nichols

Traumatic injuries are the fourth leading cause of death in the United States. These injuries account for greater loss of life than any other major disease group. The timing of trauma-related death shows a trimodal distribution:

- **Immediate,** usually caused by disruption of major blood vessels or CNS injury.
- **Early,** related to intracranial hemorrhage, laceration of major organs, or massive blood loss from multiple injuries.

- **Late,** stemming from multiple organ failure, sepsis, or sequelae of closed head injury.

CNS Trauma

Closed Head Injury. Outcome from head injury correlates with the Glasgow Coma Score (see Chapter 6 in this book). Patients with scores greater than 8 have an associated mortality rate of 1–6%, whereas those with scores less than 8 may have a mortality rate of as high as 30%. Because of the poor prognosis in the latter group, intracranial pressure monitoring should be considered to optimize management. General measures include preserving cerebral perfusion pressure, controlling brain metabolism, and preventing or treating secondary injuries.

- **Initial management.** As many as half of head-injured patients with coma have other abnormalities, including anemia, hypotension, hypoxemia, or hypercarbia, that may contribute to cerebral injury. Stabilization of blood pressure with colloidal fluids and prompt endotracheal intubation and initiation of mechanical ventilation are the mainstays of therapy. Once the patient is resuscitated, volume replacement should be restricted to isotonic fluids, which may be given at 50–75% of maintenance levels (0.75–1 mL/kg/hr). Antipyretics are administered to patients with fever and may reduce brain metabolism.
- **Cerebral circulatory management.** Cerebral perfusion pressure (CPP) is the difference between mean arterial pressure (MAP) and intracranial pressure (ICP):

$$\text{CPP} = \text{MAP} - \text{ICP}.$$

  The minimum goal of therapy for CPP is 50 mm Hg; however, 70–80 mm Hg is preferred. After circulating volume is restored, control of ICP is given high priority.
- **ICP management.** Initial measures include correction of hypoxemia (i.e., maintaining arterial oxygen tension [Pa_{O_2}] $>$ 60 torr), therapeutic hyperventilation (arterial carbon dioxide tension [Pa_{CO_2}] 25–30 torr), and prevention of excessive motor activity. Increased intrathoracic pressure associated with coughing or positive end-expiratory pressure can be mitigated by the judicious use of nondepolarizing muscle relaxants. Mannitol in doses of 1 g/kg can be infused over 10–15 minutes and repeated every 4–6 hours as necessary to maintain ICP $<$ 20 mm Hg. Serum osmolality should be maintained $<$ 320 mOsm/kg H_2O. Barbiturates are not used prophylactically, but may have a role in patients with refractory elevations of ICP. Prevention or treatment of barbiturate-induced cardiovascular de-

pression through the use of volume expansion or inotropic support is essential.

- **Antihypertensive therapy.** If there are no contraindications, hypertension can be treated with β-adrenergic blocking agents (e.g., esmolol or labetalol). These agents may be preferable to nitroprusside, nitroglycerine, or hydralazine.
- **Seizure prophylaxis.** The risk of post-traumatic seizures is low; however, many clinicians administer phenytoin prophylactically during the acute phase. Patients at particular risk include those with intracranial hemorrhage or skull fracture.
- **Deep vein thrombosis (DVT) prophylaxis** is routinely implemented. In patients at risk for CNS bleeding, pneumatic compression devices are used instead of anticoagulants for this purpose. Prophylaxis against stress-related gastric bleeding should also be routinely used.

Spinal Cord Injury. Approximately 10,000 cases of spinal cord injury occur each year, 60% of which involve the cervical cord. The fifth and sixth cervical vertebrae are the most commonly dislocated or fractured bony elements in nonlethal injury to the spine. Lateral neck films miss approximately 15% of significant injuries; therefore, anterior–posterior and odontoid views should also be obtained routinely.

Limiting secondary injuries is of critical importance. Neck stabilization followed by kinetic bed therapy reduces the risk of complications. Hemodynamic monitoring with the use of inotropic or vasoactive drug therapy may be necessary if there is associated spinal shock. Systolic blood pressure should be maintained at greater than 100 mm Hg, if possible. Administration of methylprednisolone (30 mg/kg followed by 5.4 mg/kg/hr for 23 hours) is now considered standard practice for the immediate treatment of spinal cord injury. Delay beyond 6–12 hours after injury may significantly reduce the chance of benefit. Increased risk of sepsis, GI hemorrhage, and hyperglycemia occurs with corticosteroid therapy.

Thoracic Trauma

Evaluation of the extent of injury to the thorax is based on findings from the history, physical examination, chest radiograph, and other complimentary studies, such as computed tomography (CT), ECG, echocardiography, angiography, and bronchoscopy. Immediate life-threatening concerns include massive hemothorax, open or tension pneumothorax, airway obstruction or disruption, flail chest, and cardiac injuries, such as pericardial tamponade.

Bony Injuries. Rib fractures are the most frequently encountered chest injuries. The location of the fractures may point to more serious internal injuries involving abdominal organs, lung parenchyma, the heart, or major blood vessels. If segmental fractures occur in adjacent ribs, flail chest, with associated paradoxical ventilation, may develop. Management of thoracic cage injuries hinges on maintaining pulmonary toilet through the use of intercostal nerve blocks, epidural analgesia, and respiratory therapy. Operative stabilization of bony structures of the thorax is rarely indicated, with the exception of sternal fractures. Endotracheal intubation and mechanical ventilation may be necessary in patients with flail chest and in patients who cannot maintain adequate gas exchange.

Hemothorax and Pneumothorax. These conditions require placement of a large-bore (e.g., 40 Fr) chest tube in most instances. If more than 1,500 mL of blood is initially obtained, or if drainage exceeds 200 mL/hr, thoracotomy should be performed to identify the source of ongoing hemorrhage. Failure to adequately drain the pleural space or expand a collapsed lung may occur with improperly placed chest tubes, inadequate vacuum aspiration, or occlusion of tubes or airways by blood clots. CT scanning may be helpful in this setting for localizing the position of drainage tubes within the chest.

Parenchymal Lung Injuries. Pulmonary contusion follows blunt trauma in 30–40% of cases. If uncomplicated, resolution is usually complete in less than 2 weeks. The course may be complicated by pulmonary hematoma, laceration, post-traumatic cavitation, or adult respiratory distress syndrome.

Airway or Esophageal Injury. Persistent cough, hemoptysis, pneumomediastinum, or subcutaneous emphysema suggests the possibility of airway disruption. In addition, aspiration of tube feeding, inability to obtain an adequate endotracheal cuff seal, and distension of the stomach during mechanical ventilation can occur as a result of fistula formation between the trachea and esophagus. Diagnostic bronchoscopy followed by surgical repair should be performed when these conditions are recognized. Isolated esophageal injuries are rare, but are suggested by the presence of substernal pain, extraparenchymal air, and pleural effusions associated with signs of sepsis. The diagnosis is established by barium swallow, CT, and esophagoscopy.

Cardiac Trauma. Myocardial contusion can follow blunt trauma. It usually involves the right ventricle. It is associated with serum creatine phosphokinase level (MB fraction) elevation, ST segment changes, and regional wall motion abnormalities. Thus, differentiation from peritraumatic myocardial infarction may be difficult. Fortunately, overt cardiac failure is uncommon. Hemodynamic monitoring is generally not required, but may be helpful during the intraoperative period.

Abdominal Trauma

Significant, life-threatening abdominal injuries are frequently overlooked. In a large minority of patients, peritoneal signs are absent. Diagnostic peritoneal lavage (DPL) and CT are therefore essential during the early evaluation period, and often prove complimentary. The former result is considered positive if there are more than 100,000 red blood cells/mm^3, if there are more than 500 white blood cells/mm^3, if peritoneal fluid amylase or bilirubin concentration is out of proportion to serum levels, or if food particles are obtained. CT may be particularly helpful in evaluating for retroperitoneal and pelvic injuries.

Splenic Injury. Laceration of the spleen is the most common injury from blunt trauma that leads to operative intervention. DPL is the gold standard for diagnosis, although CT is proving valuable in predicting the likelihood of splenic preservation. Patients who remain hemodynamically stable, require fewer than two units of blood, and have minimal evidence of splenic trauma by CT can be safely observed. Vaccination against pneumococcus is routinely given before discharge.

Hepatic Injury. Because of its size and location, the liver is the second most commonly injured organ in the abdomen. Nonoperative management is feasible in the hemodynamically stable patient if the transfusion requirement is less than two units of blood and if CT evidence of hepatic injury is minor. However, a 72-hour period of observation in an ICU setting is mandatory for these patients. Complications of hepatic injury include the need for massive blood-product transfusions, bile leakage, and sepsis. Large-volume transfusion can result in hypothermia. Increasing ambient temperature, warming IV fluids, covering exposed body parts and, if necessary, providing warm-water irrigation of body cavities may be helpful in raising core temperature. Finally, massive transfusion requirements have been associated with hemorrhagic diatheses and an increased risk of late sepsis.

Genitourinary Injuries. Renal contusions usually manifest as gross hematuria. IV pyelography or contrast CT studies should be performed when urinalysis shows > 30 red blood cells per high-power field. Management involves bed rest and liberal fluid administration in the hemodynamically stable patient without evidence of major organ lacerations or pedicle injury. Vascular injuries should be repaired promptly because delay jeopardizes organ viability. Disruption of the collecting system should be suspected when the creatinine concentration of drainage fluids exceeds that of serum, or when azotemia develops in the face of normal creatinine clearance. Evaluation of the urethra and bladder by retrograde cystography should be performed if meatal blood, scrotal hematoma, or a high-riding prostate is found on physical examination.

Intestinal Injury. Penetrating trauma causes most intestinal injuries. Injuries caused by blunt trauma are less common and more difficult to recognize. The areas most often involved are the proximal jejunum, distal ileum, and sigmoid colon. DPL is helpful in the diagnosis, whereas CT generally is not. Patients who are at risk and continue to have abdominal pain and fever should undergo DPL or exploratory laparotomy. Patients with extensive perineal injuries or pelvic fractures should be evaluated for rectal injury with proctosigmoidoscopy.

Pancreatic injury is often difficult to diagnose secondary to its retroperitoneal location. CT is the diagnostic modality of choice. The cornerstone of therapy is ductal repair and debridement of devitalized tissue. Closed suction drainage may reduce the incidence of intra-abdominal abscess formation. Large drainage volumes and sustained elevations of amylase levels in the drainage fluid suggest ductal disruption.

Orthopedic and Extremity Injuries. Pelvic fractures are the most common orthopedic injury. Assessment of this type of injury begins with an anterior–posterior radiograph of the pelvis in addition to a rectal examination. DPL is superior to CT in establishing significant blood loss associated with pelvic fracture. Large transfusion requirements are usually seen in these cases. For continued hemodynamic instability, pneumatic antishock garments inflated to 30–40 mm Hg control bleeding in approximately two-thirds of patients. Angiography with therapeutic embolization is an alternative for those whose initial treatment is unsuccessful. Extremity fractures carry the risk of vascular injury, compartment syndrome, and fat embolism. Early stabilization is associated with a decreased morbidity rate. Operative intervention should proceed as soon as the patient's life-threatening injuries are controlled. Doppler blood flow studies are useful as a screening tool for vascular injuries; however, anteriography is the gold standard for diagnosis. Ischemic syndromes and crush injuries may lead to compartment syndrome. In conscious patients, pain that is out of proportion to the physical examination findings often heralds compartment syndrome. If intracompartmental pressure is evaluated directly, all compartments in the suspected extremity should be assessed. Decompression fasciotomy may be necessary for compartment pressure $>$ 30 mm Hg.

Other Considerations

Patients receiving more than 10 units of blood in 24 hours have an increased risk of transfusion-related complications and sepsis. However, factor depletion, thrombocytopenia, citrate toxicity, hypocalcemia, and hyperkalemia caused by massive transfusions are uncommon. In patients without previous hemostatic problems, continued bleeding most often reflects inadequate surgical hemostasis, associated hypothermia, or disseminated intravascular coagulation related to inadequate resuscitation. Prophylactic transfusion of plasma and platelets is discouraged.

Septic complications are reduced by early initiation of enteral alimentation. Therefore, enteral nutrition should be considered in all patients once they are resuscitated from circulatory shock. For patients receiving parenteral nutrition, a dedicated central IV access port for nutrient delivery should be established.

Suggested Readings

Borel C, Hanley D, Diringer MN, et al. Intensive care management of severe head injury. *Chest* 1990;98:180–189.

Describes current strategies for limiting secondary neuronal injury with emphasis on controlling intracranial pressure.

Clemmer TP, Fairfax WR. Critical care management of chest injury. *Crit Care Clin* 1986;2:759–773.

Practical guidelines for initial evaluation and management of patients with all types of chest injuries.

Collins JA. Recent developments in the area of massive transfusion. *World J Surg* 1987;11:75–81.

Excellent review detailing metabolic and hemostatic outcomes associated with massive transfusion.

Feliciano DV. Diagnostic modalities in abdominal trauma: Peritoneal lavage, ultrasonography, computed tomography scanning and arteriography. *Surg Clin North Am* 1991;71:241–256.

Compares various diagnostic techniques used to establish presence and extent of abdominal injury.

Heyland DK, Cook DJ, Guyatt GH. Enteral nutrition in the critically ill patient: A critical review of the evidence. *Intensive Care Med* 1993;19:435–442.

Reviews experimental and clinical evidence supporting role of enteral feeding in reducing hormonal and septic complications of critical illness.

CHAPTER 97

Obstetrics and Gynecology in the ICU

(See Chapter 139)

Meenakshy K. Aiyer
and Dane J. Nichols

Improvements in supportive care have led to a reduction in maternal deaths related to toxemia, sepsis, ectopic pregnancy, and peripartum hemorrhage. Despite these advances, embolic events continue to have high associated mortality rates. Complications in the critically ill obstetric and gynecologic population can be broadly divided into four categories: hemorrhagic shock, coagulopathies, septic conditions, and pregnancy-induced hypertension (PIH).

General Considerations

In patients with hemodynamic instability, obtaining secure vascular access is the first priority. Two large-bore IV catheters should be established for rapid volume infusion. Arterial catheterization allows continuous assessment of blood pressure as well as access for blood sampling for laboratory studies. The bladder should be catheterized to evaluate the adequacy of renal perfusion. Supplemental oxygen is routinely provided to ensure adequate saturation of circulating hemoglobin.

- **IV fluids.** There is no clear consensus regarding preference for crystalloids over colloids; however, the volume required for resuscitation is considerably less with the latter. In patients with PIH or cardiac disease, colloids may be advantageous because of the preservation of colloid oncotic pressure. The anticoagulant effects of dextran preclude its use in the obstetrical setting.
- **Blood products.** Packed red blood cells are the volume expander of choice in the hemorrhaging patient. Prophylactic administration of both fresh-frozen plasma and platelets in patients without previous difficulty with hemostasis is discouraged. Replacement therapy should be based on documented need.
- **Inotropes and vasopressors.** Except as a temporizing measure, vasopressors are contraindicated in pure hypovolemic or hemorrhagic shock. Vasopressor and inotropic agents may be necessary if there is evidence of

cardiogenic or septic shock, but should be reserved for situations in which maternal survival is in question. Experimental evidence suggests that there is a decrease in uterine blood flow at dopamine infusion rates > 10 μg/kg/min.

- **Cesarean section.** In maternal cardiac arrest, immediate cesarean section improves maternal and fetal outcome. Also, delivery leads to more effective cardiopulmonary resuscitation (CPR). Removal of the placenta at the time of surgery is encouraged.

Hemorrhagic Shock

The average blood volume expansion during pregnancy is approximately 1,500 mL. Typically, 500 mL is lost during normal vaginal delivery compared with 1000 mL during elective repeat cesarean section. However, hemorrhage can be easily underestimated. Relative bradycardia may occur with intraperitoneal bleeding. Specific etiologies that lead to life-threatening hemorrhage include:

- **Uterine atony,** which is the most common cause of postpartum hemorrhage, occurring in 5% of deliveries. Initial management includes exploration of the uterine cavity, fundal massage, and oxytocin administered IV or IM. Methylergonovine 0.2 mg IM can be used in patients without a history of antepartum hypertension. Prostaglandin analogues, given IV or IM, have been used in refractory cases, but may be associated with increased intrapulmonary shunting. Potential surgical interventions after unsuccessful medical therapy include hypogastric artery ligation or embolization and hysterectomy.
- **Placenta previa,** which is associated with high parity and previous cesarean section. The diagnosis is best established by prepartum ultrasonography. With antenatal transfusion, tocolytic therapy, and elective delivery, perinatal mortality rates are less than 13%. Management of profuse bleeding hinges on immediate cesarean section and arterial ligation or hysterectomy.
- **Abruptio placentae,** which occurs in 1 of every 120 deliveries and is associated with hypertension, parity, cocaine use, and previous abruptio placentae. Ultrasonography rarely identifies retroplacental or subchorionic clot. Management is dictated by fetal well-being and maternal coagulation status. Amniotomy may be helpful; cesarean section is indicated for severe hemorrhage or coagulopathy.
- **Ectopic pregnancy.** The classic triad is abdominal pain, amenorrhea, and irregular vaginal bleeding associated with inappropriately low human chorionic gonadotropin levels (HCG). Failure of the HCG level to increase

by at least two-thirds within 48 hours during the first 6 weeks should raise suspicion. Detection of the intrauterine sac by ultrasonography should be possible at β-subunit levels of 3,600 mIU with the transvaginal approach and at 6,500 mIU with the transabdominal window. The treatment of this condition is surgical.

- **Obstetric trauma.** Significant blood loss may occur secondary to obstetric laceration, occult hematomas in the vagina and retroperitoneum, uterine rupture (occurring in 1 of every 2,000 deliveries), and spontaneous hepatic rupture. Spontaneous hepatic rupture is associated with PIH and multiparity, and should be suspected in patients with right upper quadrant pain, decreasing hematocrit level, and altered liver function test results. Paracentesis, radionuclide liver–spleen scanning, or CT can be used to confirm the diagnosis.
- **Blunt trauma,** which carries a 28% risk of fetomaternal hemorrhage. There is increased risk of splenic rupture, which may be delayed. Evaluation includes assessment of Rh status in addition to fetal monitoring. Peritoneal lavage is considered safe and accurate in pregnancy.
- **Penetrating trauma.** Gunshot wounds are associated with nearly a 90% incidence of fetal injury. Laparotomy is therefore indicated whenever there is an abdominal gunshot wound to exclude visceral injury. Delivery is reserved for cases of extreme cardiovascular instability, an obstructed operating field, and fetal hemorrhage or distress.

Acquired Coagulopathy

- **Abruptio placentae.** In abruption associated with fetal demise, the incidence of hypofibrinogenemia approaches 40%. Treatment consists of prompt delivery, administration of clotting factors, and red blood cell replacement.
- **Amniotic fluid embolism** occurs in 1 of every 20,000–80,000 deliveries. It has an associated mortality rate of approximately 80%. Clinical features include chills, restlessness, dyspnea, cyanosis, altered mental status, and hemodynamic instability characterized by high pulmonary artery occlusion pressure and poor left ventricular performance. The finding of fetal squamous cells and mucin in the maternal circulation is suggestive, but not pathognomonic, of this condition. In patients who survive beyond the first hour, acquired coagulopathy, with subsequent hemorrhage, develops in approximately 40%. Therapy is largely supportive. The role of heparin is controversial.
- **Retained dead fetus.** Coagulopathy is rare before the fifth week after fetal demise. Treatment varies depending on whether the patient is in labor. Cryopreci-

priate can be given to correct hypofibrinogenemia. In the absence of labor, IV heparin can be given until fibrinogen levels are > 200–300 mg/dL and the platelet count is > 60,000 mm^{-3}. Labor is induced 6 hours after heparin is discontinued.

Pregnancy-Induced Hypertension

PIH complicates 25% of pregnancies in the United States. It is the second most common cause of late maternal death. The clinical expression is variable, and can involve virtually any organ system (for the differential diagnosis, see Table 139–11 in the main text). Criteria for diagnosis include: systolic blood pressure > 140 mm Hg, diastolic blood pressure > 90 mm Hg, or an increase from baseline value of > 30 mm Hg and 15 mm Hg, respectively; proteinuria of > 300 mg/day or urine protein concentration ≥ 1 g/L on two random urinalyses 6 hours apart; and generalized edema, with associated weight gain of more than 5 pounds in 1 week.

- **General management.** Many aspects of care are controversial, and concern timing of delivery, fluid therapy, and the role of invasive hemodynamic monitoring. However, there is general agreement that deteriorating maternal or fetal condition is an indication for prompt delivery.
- **Fluid therapy.** Usually only maintenance IV fluid is required (e.g., infusion rates of 75–125 mL/hr). In severe PIH, further fluid loading may be necessary, and may minimize the risk of hypotension during vasodilator therapy. Fluid loading often improves oxygen transport variables. Crystalloids have been recommended by some as the fluid of choice, unless colloid oncotic pressure is < 12 mm Hg.
- **Hemodynamic monitoring.** The indications for invasive monitoring are based on the severity of PIH and evidence of end-organ dysfunction. Pulmonary edema, continuing oliguria, refractory hypertension, New York Heart Association class III or class IV heart failure, suspicion of tissue-level ischemia, and septic shock are situations in which monitoring is generally helpful.
- **Antiseizure prophylaxis.** Magnesium sulfate is the standard therapy for eclampsia. Typical dosing regimens employ a 4–6-g IV loading dose followed by a 1–2-g/hr maintenance infusion. The higher ranges, however, are more predictable in achieving therapeutic serum levels (4–7 mEq/L). Caution should be used in patients with underlying renal insufficiency. Serial monitoring of serum magnesium levels and patellar reflexes is mandatory. For seizure activity that cannot be controlled by magnesium administration, thiopental or

sodium amobarbital may be given. Further seizure activity mandates CT.

- **Antihypertensive therapy** is generally recommended when systolic blood pressure is 160–170 mm Hg or diastolic blood pressure is > 110 mm Hg, although lower thresholds may be used in the peripartum period or if eclampsia supervenes. Hydralazine is the most commonly employed agent. It may be given as a continuous IV infusion or as 5–10-mg IV boluses repeated at 20-minute intervals to a total dose of up to 40 mg. The calcium channel blocking agents nifedipine and verapamil have been used successfully to treat PIH. The former is typically given as 10–20 mg at 3–6-hour intervals. Labetalol is also a useful agent because of its ability to increase uteroplacental perfusion and promote fetal lung maturation. It may be given IV in escalating bolus fashion every 10 minutes beginning at 10 mg, or as a continuous infusion at 1–2 mg/min. The total dose should not exceed 300 mg/day. Diuretics, angiotensin-converting enzyme inhibitors, and nitroprusside are not recommended in the management of PIH.
- **Hematologic complications.** Endothelial injury is believed to underlie many of the hematologic complications of PIH. Increased Factor VIII antigen activity occurs, along with decreased levels of antithrombin III. The constellation of intravascular hemolysis, hepatic dysfunction, coagulation defects, and thrombocytopenia defines the HELLP syndrome (*H*emolysis, *E*levated *L*iver function test results, *L*ow *P*latelet levels), which complicates 3–12% of preeclamptic pregnancies. Symptoms of malaise, nausea, vomiting, and epigastric or right upper quadrant pain increase the suspicion of its development. Delivery is the only definitive treatment known. Blood-product transfusion should be limited secondary to the increased risk of postpartum infection. General goals include maintaining platelet counts > 30,000 mm^{-3} and fibrinogen levels > 100 mg/dL.

Septic Complications

Septic shock is a rare complication in obstetrics, and may carry a lower mortality rate than in the general population. Genitourinary tract organisms account for most episodes. Combination antibiotics, including IV clindamycin (900 mg every 8 hours), ampicillin (2 g every 6 hours), and gentamicin (1.5 mg/kg every 8 hours), adjusted to renal function and serum levels, provide adequate initial empiric coverage in most instances. Urine, blood, amniotic fluid, and endometrial cultures aid in identifying the source and adjusting antibiotic therapy.

- **Septic abortion.** Sepsis occasionally occurs after abortion or chorionic villus sampling. Treatment includes broad-spectrum antibiotic therapy and evacuation of uterine contents. Lack of response (observed in approximately 5% of cases) should prompt exploratory laparotomy.
- **Chorioamnionitis.** Uterine infection occurs in approximately 1% of deliveries. The diagnosis is based on the finding of foul-smelling amniotic fluid, vaginal fluid leakage, and uterine tenderness, plus fever, leukocytosis, or tachycardia in mother or child. Treatment consists of IV antibiotics, hydration, and prompt delivery. The vaginal route is preferred if maternal and fetal conditions are stable.
- **Endometritis** is uncommon after vaginal delivery. Lack of response to broad-spectrum antibiotics occurs with intramyometrial abscess and septic pelvic vein thrombophlebitis.
- **Pyelonephritis.** Approximately 1–2% of pregnancies are complicated by this infection. *Escherichia coli* accounts for most infections. Fever that lasts more than 72 hours after the initiation of treatment should prompt a search for obstruction, renal abscess, or an alternative site of infection.
- **Toxic shock syndrome** is caused by the systemic absorption of *Staphylococcus aureus* exotoxin. Clinical features include fever > 102°F, diffuse erythrodermal rash followed by desquamation, hemodynamic instability, and multiple organ system dysfunction. Hemodynamic support and antistaphylococcal antibiotic therapy are the mainstays of therapy.
- **Septic pelvic thrombophlebitis** is rare in the antepartum period. The diagnosis is often difficult, with only 30% of patients having a tender, thrombosed vessel detectable on pelvic examination. CT and MRI have also shown diagnostic promise. There is a high (45%) incidence of associated pulmonary infarction, and this finding may aid in the diagnosis. Treatment includes broad-spectrum antibiotics in addition to a 10-day course of IV heparin. A patient whose condition does not improve or who has evidence of previous or intercurrent thromboembolism should undergo surgical intervention.

Suggested Readings

Barton JR, Sibai BM. Care of the pregnancy complicated by HELLP syndrome. *Gastroenterol Clin North Am* 1992;21:937–950.
Provides management guidelines for care of patients with this syndrome.

McCrae KR, Samuels P, Schreiber AD. Pregnancy-associated thrombocytopenia: Pathogenesis and management. *Blood* 1992;80:2697–2714.
Provides in-depth coverage of illnesses leading to thrombocytopenia in this population.

Nolan TE, Wakefield ML, Devoe LD. Invasive hemodynamic monitoring in obstetrics: A critical review of its indications, benefits, complications, and alternatives. *Chest* 1992;101:1429–1433.
Summarizes major studies evaluating use of invasive monitoring in obstetric population.
Sibai BM. Hypertension in pregnancy. *Obstet Gynecol Clin North Am* 1992;19:615–632.
Comprehensive review of management strategies for pregnancy-associated hypertension along with discussion of morbidity and mortality issues.

CHAPTER 98

Hypothermia

(See Chapter 142)

Beverly D. Bartley and Dennis J. Crnkovich

Primary (or accidental) hypothermia is caused by environmental exposure (see Table 142–1 in the main text). Secondary hypothermia is caused by hypothalamic thermoregulatory dysfunction secondary to underlying illness or the effects of drugs. Conditions that are sometimes associated with secondary hypothermia include sepsis, hypoglycemia, hypothyroidism, and certain forms of CNS injury and disease (see Table 142–4 in the main text). Numerous drugs and toxins have been reported in association with hypothermia, including:

- **Sedative drugs,** e.g., ethanol, barbiturates, glutethimide, methaqualone, morphine, heroin.
- **Neuroleptic and related agents,** e.g., phenothiazines, meprobamate, lithium, tricyclic antidepressants.
- **Anesthetic agents,** e.g., halothane, ether.
- **Endocrine-related drugs,** e.g., hypoglycemic agents, antithyroid medications.
- **Paralytic agents,** e.g., organophosphates, neuromuscular blocking agents.
- **Antihypertensives,** e.g., prazosin, reserpine.

Clinical Manifestations

The diagnosis is obvious in patients with a history of immersion or exposure to cold, but must also be considered in any patient with pale, cyanotic, or cold skin; altered mentation; or bradycardia, with or without characteristic

ECG changes. It is important to use thermometers that record low temperatures; some clinical mercury thermometers do not record temperatures less than 94°F (34.4°C). The severity of hypothermia can be classified as follows:

- **Mild,** i.e., core temperature of 93–98°F (34–36.5°C). The patient is conscious, but may exhibit shivering, mild confusion, memory impairment, tachypnea, tachycardia, ataxia, or polyuria. The patient may also be completely asymptomatic.
- **Moderate,** i.e., core temperature of 82–92°F (28–33.5°C). The patient is confused, weak, and dysarthric, and may display inappropriate behavior, such as paradoxical undressing. There may be severe bradycardia, hypotension, and slow, shallow respirations.
- **Severe,** i.e., core temperature < 82°F (28°C). Most patients are unresponsive, and may appear to be in rigor mortis. Areflexia, fixed and dilated pupils, nonpalpable pulses, and apnea may be present.

Osborn waves (or J waves) are characteristic ECG deflections involving the J point and early ST segment. They are usually observed when the core temperature is less than 32°C. The EEG reading may be flat at core temperatures less than 77°F (25°C). However, determination of death, either conventionally or according to brain death criteria, can be made only after the core body temperature is near normal and resuscitative measures have failed.

Management of Hypothermia

Initial field care consists of gently moving the patient to shelter, removing wet clothing, and insulating the patient from the environment. Glucose-containing drinks may be helpful if the patient is awake and alert. Once the patient is in an emergency facility, management consists mainly of performing external rewarming measures, infusing large amounts of warmed IV fluids (5% dextrose in normal saline without potassium), and continuously monitoring ECG and core temperature.

Resuscitation. Intubation and mechanical ventilation are often necessary in the obtunded or comatose patient, but orotracheal intubation may be difficult because of rigidity of the jaw muscles. After IV access is established, patients with altered mental status are given concentrated dextrose, thiamine, and naloxone. Hypovolemia is common and should be treated with fluid loading. Hypotension that does not respond to volume resuscitation should be treated with vasopressors. Hypothermic patients are at greatest risk for dysrhythmias during the rewarming process. Unnecessary movement of the patient should be avoided because it may precipitate dysrhythmias. Bretylium may have particular utility for treating ventricular tachydysrhythmias. Some have also recommended it to prevent ventricular fibrillation in severely hypothermic patients. Electrical defibrillation is unlikely to be successful until the core temperature is greater than 30°C.

Rewarming Techniques. Passive rewarming methods are used in all hypothermic patients. The choice of active rewarming method is based on the available resources, experience of the staff, and severity of the hypothermia. Use of active internal and external techniques is controversial because some methods may be associated with increased rates of morbidity and mortality.

Passive Rewarming. Wet clothing is removed, the patient is moved to a warm room, and blankets are applied. This method is the least invasive, but slowest rewarming method. It typically increases temperature at a rate of approximately 0.4°C/hr. Passive methods alone may suffice for patients with core temperatures greater than 30°F who are hemodynamically stable.

Active External Rewarming. These methods involve heating the skin, and may be associated with a phenomenon known as afterdrop. Afterdrop occurs as a result of warming-induced peripheral vasodilation, with central movement of peripheral blood causing the core temperature to decrease further. The underperfused peripheral areas may also be associated with more severe degrees of hyperkalemia and metabolic acidosis. Commonly used methods include application of heating blankets and the use of warming lights. Rewarming should be directed to the patient's trunk rather than limited to the extremities. Warm-water immersion has been used, but has not gained widespread acceptance because of the above risks and the potential difficulties inherent in managing a cardiac emergency while the patient is underwater.

Active Core Rewarming. Central body rewarming can be achieved by a variety of methods. One of the simplest is inhalation of heated, humidified gas through the mechanical ventilator circuit, delivered at a temperature of 40°C. The increase in core temperature is usually less than 1°C/hr. Infusion of warmed (e.g., 38–40°C) IV fluids is also relatively simple. Body cavity lavage with warmed saline or dialysate has also been advocated. Peritoneal, mediastinal, and pleural lavage and hemodialysis have been used. With peritoneal lavage, the increase in temperature is typically 4–6°C/hr. Less invasive methods, such as colonic or bladder irrigation, or lavage with intragastric or esophageal balloons, have been similarly applied. In extreme cases, cardiopulmonary bypass has been used at some centers to increase temperature rapidly (3–10°C/hr) as well as to support the patient hemodynamically.

Diagnostic Studies. Routine laboratory studies should include a 12-lead ECG; chest radiograph; complete blood count with differential and platelet count; assays for serum levels of electrolytes, glucose, urea nitrogen, creatinine, amylase, creatinine phosphokinase, lactate dehydrogenase, alkaline phosphatase, transaminases, and blood levels of lactate, fibrinogen, and fibrin split products; prothrombin time; partial thromboplastin time; blood cultures; and arterial blood gas studies. Arterial blood gas values are temperature dependent. However, because the normal ranges for arterial pH and gas tensions change in proportion to temperature, it is probably unnecessary to adjust measured values for body temperature. Thyroid and adrenal function tests may be appropriate in some cases, particularly if there is no history of clear-cut exposure. Toxicologic analyses, including ethanol, may also be indicated. The metabolism of drugs and toxins is significantly reduced in hypothermia. Because of the increased risk of provoking life-threatening dysrhythmias, pulmonary artery catheterization is avoided until rewarming is complete. Computed tomography of the head is indicated in patients whose neurologic condition does not improve once normal temperature is restored, and in patients with seizures or focal neurologic deficits.

Treatment of Underlying Disease. Any underlying cause should be adequately evaluated and treated. Documented or suspected hypoglycemia is treated with IV injection of 50% dextrose (25–50 g). Patients with altered mental status should also routinely receive thiamine and naloxone. Moderate hyperglycemia is not treated. Myxedema is treated with 300–500 μg thyroxine IV followed by 50–100 μg every 24 hours. Routine coadministration of corticosteroids is prudent to avoid precipitating adrenal insufficiency. Patients with hypothermia caused by sepsis require appropriate cultures and initiation of empiric antibiotic treatment. The management of frostbite and other local cold injuries is discussed in Chapter 142 in the main text.

Suggested Readings

Brunette DD, Biros M, Mlinek EJ, et al. Internal cardiac massage and mediastinal irrigation in hypothermic cardiac arrest. *Am J Emerg Med* 1992;10:32–34.

Describes two cases of hypothermia in which cardiac arrest developed during rewarming. Both patients were resuscitated with neurologic recovery after undergoing emergency thoracotomy, internal cardiac massage, and warming by mediastinal irrigation.

Danzl DF, Pozos RS, Auerbach PS, et al. Multicenter hypothermia survey. *Ann Emerg Med* 1987;16:1042–1055.

Findings of a survey from 13 institutions covering over 400 cases of hypothermia. Modifications to cardiopulmonary resuscitation standards and hypothermia survival index are proposed.

Jolly BT, Ghezzi KT. Accidental hypothermia. *Emerg Med Clin North Am* 1992;10:311–327.

Covers initial evaluation and management of patient with exposure hypothermia. Variety of rewarming techniques is reviewed (63 references).

Schaller M-D, Fischer AP, Perret CH. Hyperkalemia: A prognostic factor during acute severe hypothermia. *JAMA* 1990;264:1842–1845.
Retrospective study showing that patients with cardiac arrest caused by accidental hypothermia could not be resuscitated if admission serum potassium level was extremely elevated (6.8–24.5 mmol/L).
Weinberg AD. Hypothermia. *Ann Emerg Med* 1993;22:370–377.
Reviews clinical features and general principals of treatment, including moving the hypothermic patient, laboratory evaluations, and therapeutic interventions. Also addresses when to terminate resuscitative efforts.

CHAPTER 99

Heat Injury and Hyperthermic Syndromes

(See Chapters 61 and 141)

Angela Schupp, Dennis J. Crnkovich, and Mark A. Kaufman

Heat Injuries

(see pages 1626–1631 in the main text)

The three primary syndromes of systemic heat injury are heat cramps, heat exhaustion, and heat stroke. For all three, treatment consists of rapid cooling, rehydration, and supportive care. Heat stroke is a medical emergency with a high mortality rate. Prompt recognition and treatment are important in preventing a poor outcome. Burn injuries are discussed in detail in Chapter 140 of the main text.

Predisposing Factors. A variety of factors predispose to heat injury. These include:

- **Patient-related factors,** such as dehydration, fever or infection, obesity, fatigue, overdressing, extremes of age, nonacclimatization, strenuous exercise with high motivation (e.g., military recruits, athletes), sleep deprivation.
- **Weather-related factors,** such as high temperature, high humidity, no wind.
- **Medical conditions,** such as angina pectoris, cardiomyopathy, stroke, dementia, parkinsonism, alcoholism, autonomic dysfunction, cystic fibrosis, scleroderma, burn scars, diabetes mellitus, hyperthyroidism, hypoka-

lemia, malnutrition, obstructive lung disease, psychiatric disease, status epilepticus.
- **Drugs,** such as aspirin, alcohol, haloperidol, phenothiazines, lithium, antiparkinsonian medications, amphetamines, β-blocking agents, barbiturates, diuretics, thyroid replacement therapy.

Heat Cramps. These painful spasms of heavily exercised muscles may be accompanied by nausea, vomiting, and fatigue. Hemoconcentration is common; rhabdomyolysis can also occur. Treatment consists of rest in a cool environment, passive stretching, and oral fluid and electrolyte replacement.

Heat Exhaustion. Symptoms include headache, irritability, profuse sweating, cramps, nausea, and light-headedness. Core temperature is generally less than 39°C. Orthostatic hypotension, altered mental status, incoordination, hemoconcentration, and azotemia may be present. The treatment is rest, gradual surface cooling, and oral or IV rehydration.

Heatstroke. External heatstroke is caused by overproduction of heat from excessive exertion in hot, humid weather. Heatstroke typically occurs in patients with impaired thermoregulatory mechanisms as a result of age, debilitation, the use of drugs, CNS disorders, or other predisposing factors; however, it can occur in otherwise healthy subjects. Patients with severe heatstroke are highly susceptible to rhabdomyolysis, and are therefore at risk for acute renal failure.

Core temperature may exceed 41°C. There may be altered mental status, hypotension, tachycardia, tachypnea (panting), and little or no sweating. Late manifestations include seizures, coma, and hypovolemic shock. Irreversible or fatal brain injury can develop secondary to severe hyperthermia. Laboratory findings may include hypernatremia, hypokalemia (hyperkalemia in some cases of rhabdomyolysis or acute renal failure), hypocalcemia, hyperphosphatemia, elevated creatinine phosphokinase (CPK) levels, lactic acidosis, respiratory alkalosis, leukocytosis, hemoconcentration, thrombocytopenia, azotemia, and myoglobinuria.

Specific initial treatment can include:

- Moving the patient to a cool environment.
- Placing bags of ice over the great vessels of the neck, axillae, and groin; fanning; and covering the patient with cool, wet sheets.
- Rapid administration of isotonic IV fluids.

Antipyretics are often ineffective. Chlorpromazine can be administered to minimize shivering during surface cooling. Supportive care includes accurate monitoring of intake and output with a Foley catheter and, in severe cases, central venous pressure monitoring. Patients should be assessed for electrolyte disturbances, rhabdomyolysis, renal failure, disseminated intravascular coagulation (DIC), and hepatic necrosis (see Table 141–4 in the main text for routine diagnostic studies). Cooling measures are discontinued when body temperature is less than 39°C.

Hyperpyretic-Rigidity Syndrome

(see pages 698–706 in the main text)

Hyperpyretic-rigidity syndrome (HRS), also known as neuroleptic malignant syndrome, is caused by drugs that block postsynaptic dopamine receptors (i.e., neuroleptic drugs). These include major tranquilizers, such as phenothiazines and butyrophenones, and certain antiemetics. This syndrome occurs in fewer than 1% of patients receiving neuroleptics. It is unrelated to dosage or duration of use. It can occur at any time during the course of treatment, but it typically begins during the first 2 weeks of drug administration, and develops over a few days. Patients receiving lithium along with a neuroleptic agent appear to be at increased risk. Another cause is abrupt discontinuation of antiparkinsonian medication, particularly levodopa.

Clinical manifestations include:

- **Hyperthermia,** often significant, and potentially fatal.
- **Alterations in consciousness,** including lethargy, agitation, or coma.
- **Increased muscle tone,** often with tense muscular rigidity, and sometimes accompanied by slowness of movement (bradykinesia), sustained positioning of limbs and body (dystonia), or extrapyramidal-type involuntary movements.
- **Elevated serum CPK levels** and other evidence of rhabdomyolysis.
- **Autonomic nervous system dysfunction,** with fluctuations in blood pressure, heart rate, respiratory rate, and in some cases, diaphoresis, pallor, urinary retention, and incontinence.

The differential diagnosis includes CNS infection or sepsis, heatstroke, malignant hyperthermia, and lethal catatonia. Lethal catatonia is a syndrome of severe rigidity and hyperpyrexia that occurs after several days of worsening psychotic behavior. Sustained posturing is a classic finding. It occurs more often in mania than in schizophrenia, and is clinically difficult to distinguish from HRS.

Treatment begins with prompt discontinuation of the precipitating neuroleptic or reinstitution of antiparkinsonian drugs. Antipyretic drugs are administered, and a cooling blanket is used to reduce body temperature. Vital signs are closely monitored, and serum CPK levels are measured daily. Vigorous IV hydration is implemented to reduce the risk of myoglobinuric renal failure.

Bromocriptine, an ergot derivative that stimulates dopamine (DA_2) receptors, is the mainstay of therapy for HRS. Initial doses of 2.5–10 mg every 8 hours are increased by 5 mg/day until clinical improvement is seen. Total daily doses of as high as 100 mg/day may be necessary. The drug is continued for at least 10 days after the syndrome is controlled, and then it is slowly tapered. Depot neuroleptics, administered as IM doses every few weeks, can precipitate HRS and necessitate a prolonged course of bromocriptine treatment.

Dantrolene sodium, a direct skeletal muscle relaxant that increases calcium uptake into the sarcoplasmic reticulum, is used to relieve muscular rigidity and reduce muscle injury. Because it does not cross the blood–brain barrier, it has no CNS effects. The initial IV dose is 0.25 mg/kg every 6–12 hours, followed by maintenance doses of up to 3 mg/kg/day. The oral dose is 25–600 mg/day, in divided doses. This drug has been associated with hepatotoxicity, particularly when used at doses of more than 10 mg/kg/day for prolonged periods.

The antiparkinsonian drugs amantadine and levodopa and the anticholinergics all have dopaminergic properties. They have been used effectively to treat HRS. Neuromuscular blockade has been used as adjunctive therapy when bromocriptine and dantrolene do not control the syndrome, but this approach has the disadvantage of obscuring clinical assessment of the CNS.

Malignant Hyperthermia

(see pages 1631–1632 in the main text)

This rare disorder is precipitated by the use of volatile anesthetic agents (e.g., halothane) or succinyl choline in genetically susceptible patients (see Table 141–7 in the main text). There is usually dramatic onset of hyperpyrexia, accompanied by muscular rigidity and sometimes by hypoxia, hypercapnia, respiratory and metabolic acidosis, DIC, seizures, and severe rhabdomyolysis. Unlike HRS, this syndrome has no primary autonomic nervous system involvement, but tachydysrhythmias may occur.

Treatment consists of:

- Changing the anesthesia machine (including the tubing and soda lime).
- Hyperventilating the patient with 100% oxygen.
- Halting the surgical procedure, discontinuing anesthetics, and arranging for transfer to the ICU.
- Initiating external cooling measures, but avoiding induced hypothermia.

- Administering dantrolene at an initial dose of 1–3 mg/kg IV, followed by 1–2 mg/kg at 10-minute intervals, to a total dose of 10 mg/kg. Maintenance doses of 1–3 mg/kg IV are continued every 6–12 hours for at least several doses. IV or oral dosing may be continued for several days.
- Monitoring for and treating fluid and electrolyte derangements (particularly hyperkalemia), DIC, rhabdomyolysis (evaluated with serum CPK levels), and acute renal failure.

Droperidol and procainamide have also been advocated, the latter for its antiarrhythmic properties and both drugs for their ability to induce calcium reuptake into the sarcoplasmic reticulum. Vigorous hydration and the use of diuretics may decrease the risk of renal failure if significant rhabdomyolysis develops.

Suggested Readings

Baca L, Martinelli L. Neuroleptic malignant syndrome: A unique association with a tricyclic antidepressant. *Neurology* 1990;40:1797–1798.
Case report and review supporting contention that tricyclic antidepressant drugs, nonneuroleptic agents that do not alter central dopamine levels, can cause neuroleptic malignant syndrome.

Heiman-Patterson TD. Neuroleptic malignant syndrome and malignant hyperthermia. *Med Clin North Am* 1993;77:477–492.
Detailed review of both disorders (101 references).

Knochel JP. Heat stroke and related heat stress disorders. *Dis Month* 1989;35:313–377.
Lengthy review of subject, with special attention to pathophysiology. Includes extensive bibliography (298 references).

Strazis KP, Fox AW. Malignant hyperthermia: A review of published cases. *Anesth Analg* 1993;77:297–304.
Covers epidemiology, precipitating drugs, and mortality rate associated with malignant hyperthermia.

White JD, Kamath R, Nucci R, et al. Evaporative versus iced peritoneal lavage treatment of heatstroke: Comparative efficacy in a canine model. *Am J Emerg Med* 1993;11:1–3.
In animal model of heatstroke, simple, noninvasive evaporative cooling measures were as rapid and effective as iced peritoneal lavage.

CHAPTER 100

Electrical Injuries

(See Chapter 143)

James K. Adams and Dennis J. Crnkovich

Clinical Manifestations

Cutaneous and Musculoskeletal. Burns that involve large areas of the body surface are a striking feature of electrical injuries. The actual entry and exit sites of the current are sometimes shown by burned or charred skin. Typical entrance sites are the head and upper extremities, and exit sites often involve the lower extremities. Lightning injuries sometimes show a linear, fern-like pattern at contact sites. Even when cutaneous signs of injury are minimal, severe rhabdomyolysis may be present and can lead to compartment syndrome. Skeletal injuries, including fractures of the long bones or vertebral bodies, can occur as a result of electrically induced tetany. Also, because most (nonlightning) electrical injuries are occupational, secondary traumatic injuries, such as a fall from a power line, should be recognized.

Cardiac. Dysrhythmias are the most common cause of immediate death in patients with electrical injuries. Currents greater than 2 amperes can induce asystole, whereas a current of only 0.1 ampere may induce ventricular fibrillation. Other common dysrhythmias include atrial fibrillation, supraventricular tachydysrhythmias, and frequent premature ventricular contractions. Conduction disturbances and nonspecific ST segment and T wave changes also can be seen. Myocardial infarction (MI) is usually caused by a high-voltage injury. It differs from MI occurring in coronary artery disease in that electrically induced MI usually is not followed by serious dysrhythmias. Also, ECG changes may take as long as 4 days to appear, and serum enzyme patterns are altered secondary to trauma. Elevated serum creatinine phosphokinase (CPK) level, including elevated MB fraction, may result from electrical injury to skeletal muscle, even in the absence of myocardial injury.

Neurologic. Serious electrical injury can cause mental confusion, loss of consciousness, or seizures. Spinal cord injuries can occur as well, and may be immediately apparent or delayed in presentation. Injury to the peripheral nerves, particularly the median or ulnar nerves, is not uncommon. Reflex sympathetic dystrophy has also been described.

Vascular. Thrombus formation may be precipitated by electrically induced elevation in tissue temperature. The result may be ischemia and gangrene. Vascular injury can also lead to aneurysm formation.

Renal and Metabolic. Acute myoglobinuric renal failure may occur as a consequence of rhabdomyolysis. Rhabdomyolysis can lead to hyperkalemia, especially if there is concomitant renal failure. Lactic acidosis may result from local tissue ischemia or cardiogenic shock.

GI. Nausea, vomiting, and abdominal pain may occur. Stress ulceration, perforation of a hollow viscus, and paralytic ileus also may be seen.

Infection. Sepsis is the leading cause of death in electrical injuries once the patient has been initially resuscitated. Necrotic areas of injury are frequently the source of infection. Gram-positive cocci and *Pseudomonas* species are the most commonly encountered pathogens. Other possible septic complications include clostridial myositis, pneumonia, and osteomyelitis.

Prehospital Treatment

The patient must be removed from the source of electrical current as quickly and safely as possible. Next, cardiopulmonary status is quickly assessed and, if necessary, cardiopulmonary resuscitation (CPR) is promptly initiated. Most survivors recover to spontaneous respirations within 30 minutes, but complete recoveries have been documented even after prolonged cardiopulmonary arrest.

Hospital Management

- Airway patency and adequacy of ventilation are assured in patients with altered sensorium and those who have had a cardiac arrest. CPR is initiated if required.
- Fluid resuscitation is performed with isotonic fluids, such as lactated Ringer's solution or normal saline. Blood transfusion may be needed in patients with concomitant trauma and bleeding. For serious injuries, invasive hemodynamic monitoring may be helpful to ensure that fluid administration is adequate and to avoid overhydration.
- Arterial blood gas values, hemoglobin level, serum electrolyte levels, CPK level, and urine myoglobin level are monitored, and routine laboratory tests are performed.
- The requirement for continuous ECG monitoring is controversial. However, until a consensus is reached, this monitoring may be prudent during the initial 48 hours.

- Radiographs of the chest, abdomen, spine, or extremities are obtained if warranted by the history or physical examination findings.
- Rhabdomyolysis and myoglobinuria are treated by establishing brisk diuresis, avoiding hypovolemia, and attempting to alkalinize the urine with IV sodium bicarbonate.
- Peripheral pulses and neurologic function are assessed periodically for evidence of compartment syndrome. Changes in compartmental pressures or diminished pedal pulses may necessitate fasciotomy.
- Debridement of necrotic tissue is critical in avoiding infection. Patients with substantial tissue injury should receive tetanus toxoid and penicillin G (10–20 million units/day) for anticlostridial prophylaxis. Silver sulfadiazine or mafenide may be used for local treatment.
- Neurologic dysfunction is common in electrical injuries. However, in patients with severe impairment who do not show steady improvement in mental status, other etiologies, such as intracranial hemorrhage or anoxic encephalopathy, should be considered.

Suggested Readings

Browne BJ, Gaasch WR. Electrical injuries and lightning. *Emerg Med Clin North Am* 1992;10:211–229.

Good general review (105 references).

Fontanarosa PB. Elecrical shock and lightning strike. *Ann Emerg Med* 1993;22:378–387.

General review that surveys major issues and provides commentaries. Also describes various research initiatives (101 references).

Grube BJ, Heimback DM, Engrav LH, et al. Neurologic consequences of electrical burns. *J Trauma* 1990;30:254–258.

Clinical study concluding that immediate coma associated with electrical injury resolves unless associated with anoxic CNS damage.

Hammond JS, Ward CG. Myocardial damage and electrical injuries: Significance of early elevation of CPK-MB isoenzymes. *South Med J* 1986;79:414–419.

Clinical study suggesting that elevated serum creatinine phosphokinase MB levels may be a spurious indicator of myocardial damage in some cases of electrical injury.

Purdue GF, Hunt JL. Electrocardiographic monitoring after electrical injury: Necessity or luxury. *J Trauma* 1986;26:166–167.

Reviews cases of 48 patients who had high-voltage (>1000 volts) electrical injuries. No serious dysrhythmias occurred among those who had normal ECG reading on admission.

CHAPTER 101

Anaphylaxis

(See Chapter 144)

Marilyn T. Haupt and
Richard W. Carlson

Anaphylaxis is an acute, life-threatening, frequently explosive clinical response to environmental stimuli. A list of commonly implicated agents is given in Table 144–1 in the main text. In susceptible patients, anaphylaxis may lead to upper airway edema, bronchospasm, an increase in vascular permeability, acute respiratory failure, and circulatory shock from the acute release of inflammatory mediators. Prompt recognition and early treatment may be lifesaving. Therefore, it is essential for physicians to recognize anaphylaxis promptly and to distinguish it from acute conditions that resemble it. After the initial acute management is completed, the critical care specialist must be prepared to manage advanced manifestations with a rational therapeutic approach.

The classic anaphylactic response is a type I immune response involving antigen, immunoglobulin, and IgE immunoglobulin-specific effector cells (tissue-based mast cells and circulating basophils) and resulting in the release of inflammatory mediators. However, unlike other type I reactions (e.g., allergic rhinitis, allergic asthma), anaphylaxis is generalized rather than restricted to local sites. Agents that typically produce classic anaphylactic reactions include the penicillins, hymenoptera stings (bees, wasps, hornets, and fire ants), and egg albumin.

Anaphylactoid reactions are clinically identical to classic anaphylaxis. However, a nonimmune release of mediators derived from mast cells and basophils has been implicated in these reactions. Agents that produce anaphylactoid reactions include radiographic contrast dyes, opiates, salicylates, and other nonsteroidal anti-inflammatory agents.

Clinical Features

Although the clinical presentation of anaphylaxis is variable, most patients have severe, rapidly progressive symptoms after exposure to the antigen. The symptoms may be modified by the portal of entry for the antigen as well as by the rate of absorption and degree of hypersensitivity to the antigen. Accordingly, GI symptoms (nausea, vomiting, abdominal cramps, diarrhea) may precede more severe systemic symptoms after ingestion of an antigen. Inhalation of an antigen may produce nasal coryza, a sensation of tightness or a lump in the throat, hoarseness, stridor, wheezing, and dyspnea. Introduction of an antigen through the skin may produce local pruritus, urticaria, and swelling before the development of systemic symptoms. IV injection of an antigen may precipitate circulatory shock without preceding cutaneous or respiratory manifestations.

The most life-threatening reactions are usually explosive, often occurring within minutes of exposure to the antigen. Patients with these reactions may describe a feeling of impending doom before more defined symptoms develop. Generalized cutaneous abnormalities may be observed. They include erythema, urticaria, and flushing. Swelling of the periorbital and perioral areas is characteristic. Upper and lower airway abnormalities are frequently observed and pose a major threat to life. Swelling of the posterior pharynx, uvula, tonsils, and vocal cords may develop rapidly. Auscultation may show generalized wheezing and prolongation of expiration. Signs of pulmonary edema, usually of the permeability type, may be present, and are often severe. Forced exhalation through a swollen glottis may lead to acute pneumothoraces and acute pulmonary emphysema. Signs of circulatory shock, including progressive hypotension, oliguria, and lactic acidosis, are seen as plasma continues to escape the circulation. Adverse cardiac effects, including myocardial ischemia, infarction, and dysrhythmias, are occasionally observed, and may occur after epinephrine administration. The clinical features of anaphylaxis may respond quickly to treatment or, in severe cases, may last for several hours to several days. An initial favorable response to treatment may be followed by a late-phase reaction, which is a recurrence of symptoms approximately 6–12 hours after the initial reaction.

Initial Management

Initial assessment of the patient with suspected anaphylaxis should be brief because immediate therapeutic interventions are required. Appropriate evaluations should be performed quickly to exclude the variety of conditions that can simulate anaphylaxis. Examples include vasovagal episodes, acute pulmonary events (e.g., asthmatic attacks, pulmonary edema, pulmonary embolus, spontaneous pneumothorax, foreign body aspiration), acute cardiac events (e.g., supraventricular and ventricular tachycardias, acute myocardial infarction), drug overdoses, and insulin shock.

When a diagnosis of anaphylaxis is reasonably certain, treatment should proceed rapidly, using a team approach. Treatment includes:

- Provision of a patent airway.
- Removal of the toxin at the site of introduction (e.g., removal of the insect stinger, thorough washing of the skin at the exposure site).
- Delay of the systemic absorption of the toxin (a proximal constricting band is applied if the site is an extremity, but arterial blood flow must not be occluded).
- Administration of epinephrine (0.3–0.5 mL of 1:1000 solution) subcutaneously at the exposure site to retard systemic absorption of venom.
- Establishment of IV access for fluid therapy.

Mild cases may only require the above measures. Severe cases warrant additional consideration as described below. These patients are susceptible to late-phase reactions, and severe symptoms may occur as long as 12 hours after the initial attack. Serious cases necessitate further emergency treatment, admission to an ICU, and use of the following measures:

- **Endotracheal intubation** may be necessary if stridor caused by laryngeal or upper respiratory tract edema develops. Frequent assessment for hoarseness, stridor, tachypnea, and signs of upper airway obstruction is required. Supplemental oxygen is given as necessary.
- **Frequent monitoring** of blood pressure, heart rate, urine output, and other indicators of impending circulatory compromise.
- **Chest radiograph** should be obtained immediately and closely scrutinized for pneumothoraces and acute pulmonary emphysema.
- **Continuous ECG monitoring** is performed during the initial period to detect serious dysrhythmias and signs of cardiac ischemia.
- **Mechanical ventilation** is instituted in patients who require endotracheal intubation, particularly if spontaneous ventilation is uncertain or impaired. Positive end-expiratory pressure is provided as needed.
- **Hemodynamic monitoring** may be necessary for patients who have circulatory shock and impaired pulmonary gas exchange. Fluid therapy and inotropic vasopressor drug therapy require titration to achieve optimal organ perfusion and systemic oxygen delivery.

The mainstay of pharmacologic therapy for anaphylaxis is epinephrine. The α- and β-adrenergic properties of epinephrine are of proven efficacy in reversing bronchoconstriction and hypotension associated with anaphylaxis. Two dilutions of epinephrine are commonly available: 1:1000 and 1:10,000. Most authors recommend that, for mild cases, 0.3–0.5 mL 1:1000 solution (0.3–0.5 mg) be given subcutaneously. This dose may be repeated at 5–10-minute intervals if symptoms do not improve. The dose of epinephrine for IV administration in severe anaphylaxis is controversial. Most authors recommend an initial dose of 0.3–0.5 mg (1:10,000 dilution). However, to avoid myocardial ischemia or infarction, some recommend a starting dose of 0.1 mg infused over 5–10 minutes at 1:100,000 dilution (0.1 mL 1:1000 dilution mixed in 10 mL normal saline, or 1 mL 1:10,000 dilution mixed in 10 mL normal saline). This cautious starting dose may need to be repeated at frequent intervals if symptoms do not improve. The cardiac rhythm should be monitored in all patients who receive IV epinephrine.

Fluid therapy effectively reverses the intravascular volume deficits that are characteristic of anaphylaxis. Colloidal fluids, such as 5% human serum albumin or 6% hydroxyethyl starch, are rational choices because they mimic the oncotic properties and electrolyte concentrations of plasma. Crystalloidal fluids may also be used, although considerably more crystalloid than colloid is required to achieve comparable intravascular volume repletion. Reversal of hemoconcentration is a reasonable resuscitative goal for stable patients. However, in unstable patients with wide fluctuations in vital signs and worsening pulmonary function, fluid therapy should be administered according to hemodynamic and pulmonary assessments.

If hypotension and other signs of circulatory shock persist after the initial administration of epinephrine and fluids, further vasoactive and inotropic support is necessary. Continuous IV infusions of epinephrine, norepinephrine, or dopamine may be required.

Additional Therapeutic Options

- **Antihistamines** are frequently given to patients with anaphylaxis because of their safety and theoretical, although unproven, efficacy. Diphenhydramine, a histamine H_1-receptor antagonist, may be given IV at 4–6-hour intervals in doses of 25–50 mg. The H_2-blocking agent cimetidine may be given IV (300 mg in 50 mL normal saline over 5 minutes) and repeated at 6–8-hour intervals.
- **Aminophylline** is effective in alleviating bronchospasm. In severe cases, a loading dose of 4–6 mg/kg aminophylline is infused over 20 minutes, followed by a continuous infusion of 0.2–0.9 mg/kg/hr. Mild bronchospasm may be treated with anhydrous theophylline 200–400 mg PO twice daily.
- **Corticosteroids** should be administered in severe cases because they increase tissue responsiveness to β-agonists, inhibit histamine synthesis, and attenuate late-phase reactions. Hydrocortisone 100–200 mg may be given IV and repeated at 4–6-hour intervals for 24 hours, and rapidly tapered.

- **Nebulized epinephrine** (0.5 mL of a 2.25% solution of racemic epinephrine diluted in 3.5 mL distilled water) may be administered for mild laryngeal edema. Severe laryngeal edema associated with respiratory distress or stridor should be treated with intubation of the trachea.
- **Inhalational β-agonist drugs** (e.g., 0.2–0.3 mL of a 5% solution of metaproterenol in 2.5 mL saline, every 2–4 hours by nebulization) may be useful in the treatment of persistent bronchospasm.

Suggested Readings

Lasser EC, Berry CC, Talner LB, et al. Pretreatment with corticosteroids to alleviate reactions to intravenous contrast material. *N Engl J Med* 1987;317:845–849.

Documents effectiveness of measures to prevent anaphylactic reactions to contrast medicine.

Serafin WE, Austin KF. Mediators of immediate hypersensitivity reactions. *N Engl J Med* 1987;317:30–34.

Summarizes biochemical and inflammatory mediators that are typical of anaphylactic reactions.

Valentine MD. Anaphylaxis and stinging insect hypersensitivity. *JAMA* 1992;268:2830–2834.

Discusses insect venom anaphylaxis and appropriate treatment and immunotherapy.

Weiss ME, Adkinson NF. Immediate hypersensitivity reactions to penicillin and related antibiotics. *Clin Allergy* 1988;18:515–540.

Discusses mechanism and approach to treatment of penicillin anaphylaxis and to other β-lactam antibiotics (97 references).

Wong S, Dykewicz MS, Patterson R. Idiopathic anaphylaxis: A clinical summary of 175 patients. *Arch Intern Med* 1990;150:1323–1328.

Describes clinical features of idiopathic anaphylaxis and response to acute and prophylactic treatment.

INDEX

Pages in *italics* indicate illustrations; those followed by t refer to tables.